Recent Results in Cancer Research

Volume 194

For further volumes:
http://www.springer.com/series/392

Richard P. Baum · Frank Rösch
Editors

Theranostics, Gallium-68, and Other Radionuclides

A Pathway to Personalized Diagnosis and Treatment

Springer

Editors
Prof. Dr. Richard P. Baum
ENETS Center of Excellence
THERANOSTICS Center for Molecular Radiotherapy and Molecular Imaging
Bad Berka
Germany

Prof. Frank Rösch
Institut für Kernchemie
Universität Mainz
Mainz
Germany

ISSN 0080-0015
ISBN 978-3-642-27993-5 ISBN 978-3-642-27994-2 (eBook)
DOI 10.1007/978-3-642-27994-2
Springer Heidelberg New York Dordrecht London

Library of Congress Control Number: 2012940457

Printed on acid-free paper

Springer is part of Springer Science+Business Media (www.springer.com)

Contents

Part I
Generators

$^{68}Ge/^{68}Ga$ Generators: Past, Present, and Future

F. Rösch

Abstract

In 1964, first $^{68}Ge/^{68}Ga$ radionuclide generators were described. Although the generator design was by far not adequate to our today's level of chemical, radiopharmaceutical and medical expectations, it perfectly met the needs of molecular imaging of this period. ^{68}Ga-EDTA as directly eluted from the generators entered the field of functional diagnosis, in particular for brain imaging. A new type of generators became commercially available in the first years of the 21st century. Generator eluates based on hydrochloric acid provided "cationic" ^{68}Ga instead of "inert" ^{68}Ga-complexes and opened new pathways of Me^{III} based radiopharmaceutical chemistry. The impressive success of utilizing ^{68}Ga- DOTA-octreotides and PET/CT instead of e.g., ^{111}In-DTPA-octreoscan and SPECT paved the way not only towards clinical acceptance of this particular tracer for imaging neuroendocrine tracers, but to the realisation of the great potential of the $^{68}Ge/^{68}Ga$ generator for modern nuclear medicine in general. The last decade has seen a ^{68}Ga rush. Increasing applications of generator based ^{68}Ga radiopharmaceuticals (for diagnosis alone, but increasingly for treatment planning thanks to the inherent option as expressed by THERANOSTICS), now ask for further developments – towards the optimization of $^{68}Ge/^{68}Ga$ generators both from chemical and regulatory points of view. Dedicated chelators may be required to broaden the feasibility of ^{68}Ga labeling of more sensitive targeting vectors and generator chemistry may be adopted to those chelators – or vice versa. This review describes the development and the current status of $^{68}Ge/^{68}Ga$ radionuclide generators.

F. Rösch (✉)
Institute of Nuclear Chemistry, Johannes Gutenberg-University,
55128 Mainz, Germany
e-mail: froesch@uni-mainz.de

R. P. Baum and F. Rösch (eds.), *Theranostics, Gallium-68, and Other Radionuclides*,
Recent Results in Cancer Research 194, DOI: 10.1007/978-3-642-27994-2_1,

Contents

1 Introduction

Today, gallium-68 is seeing a renaissance in terms of new ^{68}Ge/^{68}Ga radionuclide generators, sophisticated ^{68}Ga radiopharmaceuticals, and state-of-the-art clinical diagnoses via positron emission tomography (PET)/computed tomography (CT) (Roesch and Riss 2010). Why this "renaissance"?

^{68}Ga represents one of the very early radionuclides applied to PET imaging at a time when even the term PET itself was not established, long before the usage of, e.g., fluorine-18. Moreover, due to the availability of this positron emitter via the first ^{68}Ge/^{68}Ga generators (Gleason 1960; Greene and Tucker 1961; Yano and Anger 1964), Hal Anger could create the first positron scintillation camera at the start of the 1960s.

Driven thus by the combination of old-fashioned radiochemistry and first-generation ^{68}Ge/^{68}Ga radionuclide generators available in the early 1960s, in particular those providing ^{68}Ga-ethylene diamine tetraacetic acid (EDTA) eluates, and dramatic improvements of tomographic detection systems, several ^{68}Ga tracers for imaging of various diseases were investigated, mainly for imaging the human brain. Hundreds of patients were almost immediately investigated in the USA with ^{68}Ga-ethylene diamine tetraacetic acid (EDTA), and others from 1963 onwards.

Although several publications described "improved" ^{68}Ge/^{68}Ga radionuclide generators, the impact of ^{68}Ga imaging faded away in the late 1970s, mainly for two reasons: the generator design itself appeared inadequate for the various requirements of ^{68}Ga radiopharmaceutical synthesis, and those available through existing technology had minor clinical relevance, in particular in view of the parallel and rapid developments of the new classes of ^{99m}Tc- and ^{18}F-labeled diagnostics. Nevertheless, numerous papers in the 1970s and 1980s described the use of inorganic matrixes as well as organic resins, selectively adsorbing ^{68}Ge and providing ^{68}Ga desorption within hydrochloric acid solutions at weak (0.1–1.0 N) or strong (>1 N) concentrations, respectively.

Thanks to the pioneering achievement of radiochemists in Obninsk, Russia, a new type of ^{68}Ge/^{68}Ga generator became commercially available in the early years of the 21st century (Razbash et al. 2005). Generator eluates based on hydrochloric acid provided "cationic" ^{68}Ga instead of "inert" ^{68}Ga complexes, opening new pathways of Me^{III}-based radiopharmaceutical chemistry. Again conicidentally, the ^{68}Ga cation was introduced immediately into existing designs of magnetic resonance imaging (MRI) and single-photon emission computed tomography (SPECT) imaging probes, namely diethylene triamine pentaacetic acid (DTPA)- or dodecane-N,N',N",N"'-tetraacetic acid (DOTA)-based derivatives. The impressive success of utilizing ^{68}Ga-DOTA-octreotides and PET/CT instead of, e.g., ^{111}In-DTPA-octreoscan paved the way not only to the clinical acceptance of this particular tracer for neuroendocrine imaging, but to the realization of the great potential of the $^{68}Ge/^{68}Ga$ generator for modern nuclear medicine in general.

Consequently, the last decade (from 2000 on) has seen a ^{68}Ga rush. Increasing applications of generator-based ^{68}Ga radiopharmaceuticals (for diagnosis alone, but increasingly for treatment planning thanks to the inherent option as expressed by theranostics) (Roesch and Baum 2011), have driven progressive developments towards the optimization of $^{68}Ge/^{68}Ga$ generators from both the chemical and regulatory points of view. Dedicated chelators may be required to broaden the possibilities of ^{68}Ga labeling of more sensitive targeting vectors. Last but not least, the concept of ^{68}Ga radiopharmaceutical chemistry should be applied to an increasing number of targeting vectors, addressing the clinically most relevant diseases.

It maybe a vision, or maybe a dream, but within a decade from now, $^{68}Ge/^{68}Ga$ generator-based ^{68}Ga diagnostics may approach rank 3 or 4 of clinical impact molecular imaging, following ^{99m}Tc-, ^{18}F-, and radioiodine-based tracers.

2 The Early Years (1960–1970): The Dawn of ^{68}Ga

The first $^{68}Ge/^{68}Ga$ radionuclide generator was described in 1960 (Gleason 1960) as "a positron cow." The title immediately delivers the message of applying the concept of a radionuclide generator to a positron-emitting radionuclide. The latter was itself a new entry into radiopharmaceutical chemistry and nuclear medicine molecular imaging in vivo. The generator chemistry was liquid–liquid extraction, and the whole processing was by far not revealing the real features of today's radionuclide generator systems. Here are some key sentences from Gleason's paper:

> The Germanium-68 comes to us from the cyclotron in a solution buffered to pH 6.4. … the accumulated gallium can be milked off every three to four hours. …A 35 per cent solution of fresh acetyl-acetone in cyclohexane is mixed vigorously for two minutes with the germanium solution and yields on numerous tests a 70–80 per cent recovery of available gallium in the solvent. The gallium is collected by mixing for two minutes with a solution of 0.1 N HCl. … (1 milligram of $GaCl_3$ is added to the germanium solution every three to four separations to insure adequate carrier for the very small amounts of radioactive gallium present) … The gallium chloride is neutralized with normal sodium hydroxide, yielding a solution containing one milligram or less of gallium chloride, containing 2–3 millicuries of Gallium-68. … No Germanium-68 is carried over under these circumstances.

Nevertheless, a variety of ^{68}Ga compounds were synthesized, cf. Shealy et al. 1964:

> *Gallium versenate*: 10 milligrams of sodium versenate ... added to the extraction product and the mixture heated for two minutes. This is injected intravenously and scanning begun about twenty minutes later. ... We have not yet had sufficient quantity to start scans at one hour which would be desirable.
>
> *Gallium protoporphyrin*: The neutralized gallium is added to one milligram protoporphyrin ... and heated for five minutes. The solution is injected intravenously and scanning begun 45–60 minutes later.
>
> *Gallium phthalocyanate*: The neutralized gallium chloride, $GaCl_3$, is added to 30 milligrams sodium phthalocyanate ..., and after heating for one minute this is injected intravenously.
>
> "*Ionic*" *gallium*: The neutralized solution is injected intravenously... scanning is begun 30 to 60 minutes later.
>
> *Sodium gallate*: 1 N Sodium hydroxide is added to the neutral gallium to bring the solution to pH 9. This is injected intravenously, and scanning begins 30 to 60 minutes later.
>
> *Sodium galloarsenate*: Neutralized gallium chloride is added to 1 milligram sodium arsenate in a strongly basic solution and autoclaved for fifteen minutes.
>
> In all these compounds an excess of chelating agent or of solution is present. Purer preparations might be more useful but have not been made yet.

2.1 Further Generator Developments: Al_2O_3-Based EDTA-Eluted Generators

Because of these inherent drawbacks of the first generator, soon after, two improved generator concepts were described. The liquid–liquid extraction chemistry introduced by Gleason was substituted by a solid-phase-based ion exchange system (Greene and Tucker 1961; Yano and Anger 1964). [Nevertheless, an improved liquid–liquid extraction version was described in 1978 (Erhardt and Welch 1978), cf. Fig. 1].

The concept of the solid-phase-based generator is illustrated in Fig. 2; the original sketch is taken from the original publication by Yano and Anger (1964), cf. Fig. 3.

These solid-phase chromatographic generators offered excellent radiochemical characteristics. Using an alumina column and EDTA as eluent (10 mL 0.005 M EDTA), ^{68}Ga was easily and repeatedly eluted in 95% yield without the need to introduce stable Ga^{III} as carrier.

> Gallium 68, the daughter of 270-day germanium 68 ..., is obtained by passing edetate solution through an alumina column upon which ^{68}Ge is placed. The edetate becomes labeled with the short half-life ^{68}Ga, while the ^{68}Ge remains on the column to be "milked" again. ... Sterility is insured by using a suitable eluting solution and sterilizing the eluent with a Millipore filter (Yano and Anger 1964).

The eluate fraction contained as little as $<1.4 \times 10^{-5}$% of the parent ^{68}Ge. Before injection, 0.5 mL 18% NaCl solution was added to the eluate. This system served as a convenient and economical source of ^{68}Ga-EDTA. Indeed, nuclear medicine physicians such as Gottschalk and others made extensive use of this tracer.

Gleason 1960	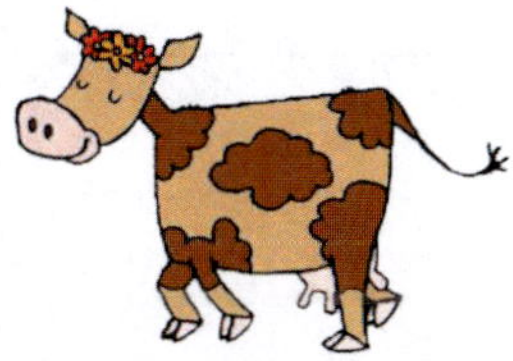	A positron cow
Greene and Tucker 1964	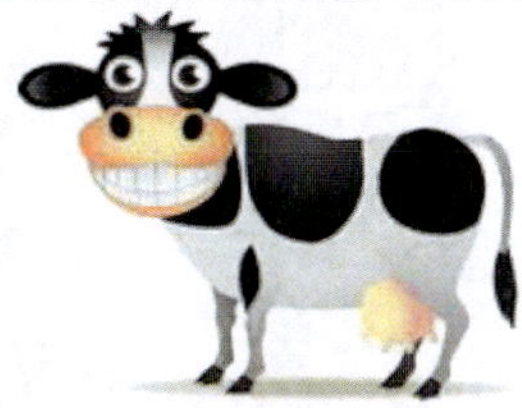	An improved gallium-68 cow
Yano and Anger 1964	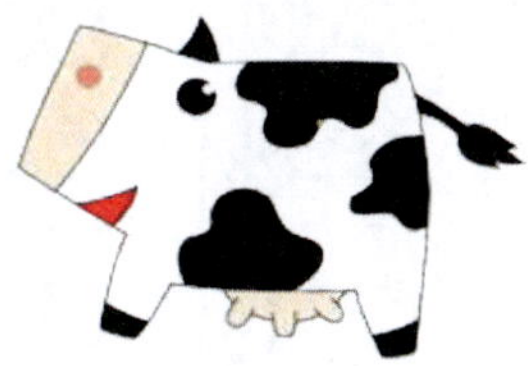	A gallium-68 positron cow for medical use.

Fig. 1 Progress in $^{68}Ge/^{68}Ga$ radionuclide generators I: design of cows towards medicine

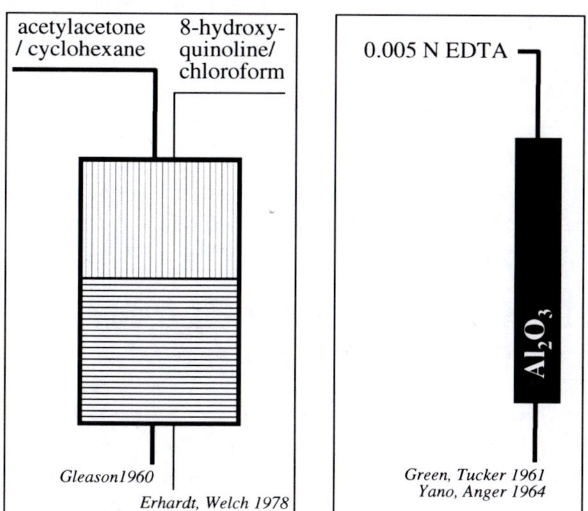

Fig. 2 Progress in $^{68}Ge/^{68}Ga$ radionuclide generators II: from liquid–liquid extraction to solid-phase-based elution

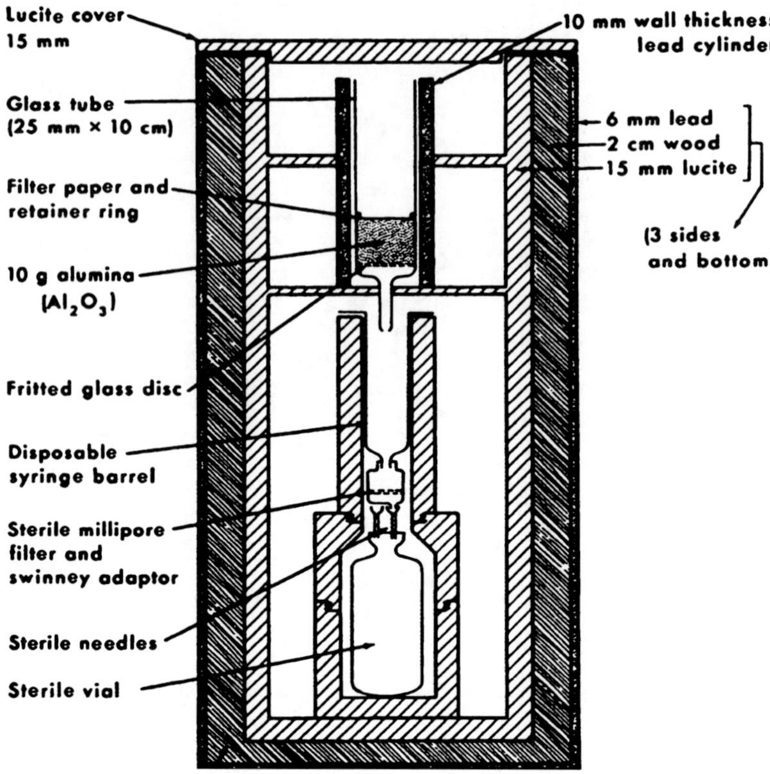

Fig. 3 Solid-phase-based (alumina) elution (by EDTA solution), taken from the original publication by Yano and Anger (1964)

In a way, this radionuclide generator was basically a synthesis unit of a relevant radiopharmaceutical, ^{68}Ga-EDTA (named "veronate" at that time).

2.2 ^{68}Ga-EDTA: The PET Pharmaceutical, Development of Positron Scintillation Cameras

Around 1960, radioisotopic brain scanning using a number of agents was being evaluated. Among the most satisfactory were the positron emitters arsenic-74 (as arsenate), copper-64 (as versenate), and mercury-203 (as neohydrin).

In this context, Shealy et al. (1964) concluded the following:

> Unfortunately these preparations present some technical difficulties and have not achieved widespread use. In searching for another positron-emitter, it is necessary to find one which for use with present equipment has a half-life of at least one hour, but has a biological half-life of not more than a few days. Further, it should be readily obtainable and incorporable

> into a chemical form of high specific uptake and of low toxicity. Such an element is Gallium-68 with a half-life of 66 minutes. It is particularly useful because it emits 85 per cent positrons with few non-annihilation gammas. It is a natural decay product of Germanium-68, which has a half-life of 250 days. Such a continuous and relatively inexpensive supply of isotope is desirable if the scanning test is to become widely used. A short-lived isotope such as Ga88 is of particular interest for use with camera-type detection systems. ...These show promise of reducing scanning time from the present hours to minutes.

^{68}Ga-EDTA and in a few cases more ^{68}Ga tracers have been adapted for human applications quite quickly by various groups in the USA. (EDTA itself and its relation to Ca^{II} were established well known to be nontoxic.) For early applications, see, e.g., Gottschalk and Anger (1964a, b) and Schaer et al. (1965). Systematic application for brain imaging was reported, with medical impact seriously depending on the type of imaging applied. Conventional imaging appeared to by relatively difficult, and relatively high activities of ^{68}Ga-EDTA were needed for valuable medical information. A typical sac of these years is illustrated in Fig. 4.

Hal Anger thus started to develop the basics of positron imaging tomography (see, e.g., Anger and Gottschalk 1963; Gottschalk 1996, 2004), arguing as follows (Gottschalk and Anger 1964a, b) (Fig. 5):

> ... We seriously question whether satisfactory results can be obtained with the conventional positron scanner. Recent phantom studies indicate that the positron scintillation camera using G68 EDTA will detect lesions ½ the volume that can be detected by the conventional positron scanner using As74. The increase in sensitivity is obtained even though the phantom was set up to simulate our clinical condition where brain pictures are obtained in 4–10 minutes with a dose of 350–750 microcuries of Ga68-EDTA. Shealy et al., however, found that 2–3 millicuries of Ga68-EDTA was sometimes an inadequate dose with their positron scanner.

Despite these new features and the great success of ^{68}Ga-EDTA molecular imaging, there was an obvious limitation of the generator application, as it was in practice limited exclusively to synthesis of ^{68}Ga-EDTA. Transfer of ^{68}Ga out of the thermodynamically very stable ($\log K = 21.7$) eluate species ^{68}Ga-EDTA was not straightforward. Yano and Anger (1964) reported, that "attempts are being made… to freed ^{68}Ga… from the EDTA complex." The procedure, however, was far from user friendly. The time required was given as 30 min, and the transfer yield at 10 mg Ga carrier was 60% (Yano and Anger 1964). The protocol was as follows:

> (1) The cow is milked with 10 mL of 0.005 M EDTA solution, and the ^{68}Ga is collected in a 40 mL centrifuge tube. (2) 10–20 mg of carrier $GaCl_3$ in HCl solution is added. (3) The 0.5 mL of saturated ammonium acetate solution is added. (4) Concentrated NH_4OH is added drop wise (about 1 mL) to precipitate $Ga(OH)_3$ at pH 6.0. (5) The solution is heated in a boiling water bath for 10 min to coagulate the $Ga(OH)_3$. (6) The solution is centrifuged, and the supernatant solution is discarded. (7) The $Ga(OH)_3$ is dissolved with a minimum volume of hot 20% NaOH. (8) The solution is acidified with about 1 mL of concentrated HCl.

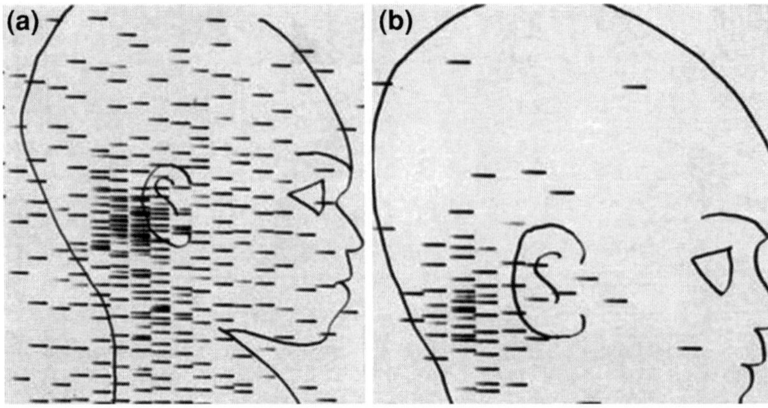

Fig. 4 "Cisternal blockade in an infant with posterior spread of a glioma of the optic chiasm. Five hundred μc of ^{68}Ga were given via the lumbar route. In the first scan (Scan **a**) an early rise to the cerebellar cisterns is found. Later scans, including Scan **b**, showed that the isotope remained in the posterior fossa and did not pass upward" (McQueen and Abbassioun 1968)

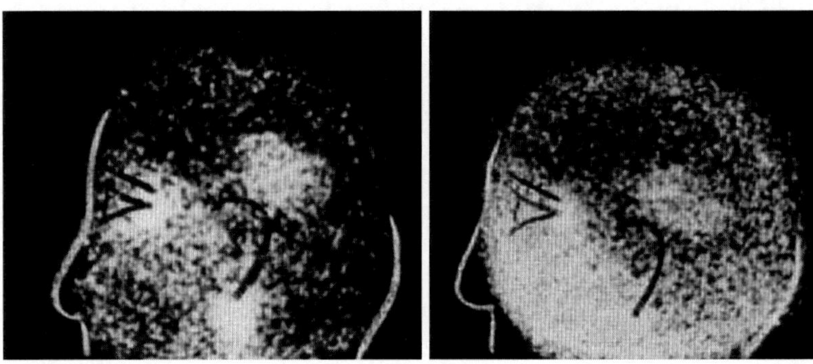

Fig. 5 ^{68}Ga-EDTA brain scan acquired with the Anger positron camera circa 1962, showing the tomographic capability. The brain tumor is in best focus in the left image, taken at about the level of the temporal horn (Anger and Gottschalk 1963, 1964a, b)

3 Hibernating ^{68}Ga Medical Applications, but New Chemistry Ahead

The impact of ^{68}Ga imaging started to fade away in the late 1970s, mainly because of two reasons: the generator design itself appeared inadequate for the various requirements of ^{68}Ga radiopharmaceutical synthesis, and those available through existing technology had minor clinical relevance, in particular in view of the parallel and rapid developments of the new classes of ^{99m}Tc- and ^{18}F-labeled diagnostics.

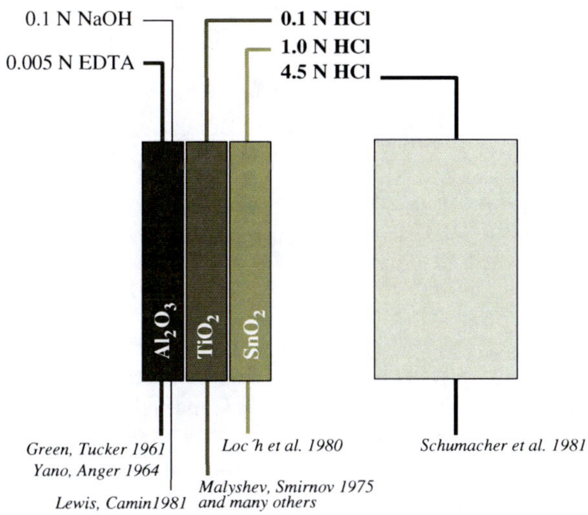

Fig. 6 $^{68}Ge/^{68}Ga$ radionuclide generator concepts developed in the 1970s and 1980s towards "cationic" generators

At the same time, however, numerous basic radiochemical papers in the 1970s and 1980s described the use of inorganic matrixes as well as organic resins, selectively adsorbing ^{68}Ge and providing ^{68}Ga desorption within hydrochloric acid solutions of weak (0.1–1.0 N) or strong (>1 N) concentrations, respectively.

In fact, the challenge was to design radiochemical separation systems to provide cationic ^{68}Ga eluate species available for versatile radiolabeling chemistry. Ga(III) exists as cationic species [either pure water-hydrated aquo-complexes such as the hexa-aqua cation $Ga(H_2O)_6^{3+}$, or similar monochloro or monohydroxo species]. This speciation is easily achieved in solutions of hydrochloric acid with pH ranging between approximately 0 and 2 (i.e., 0.01–1.0 N HCl). For this purpose, $Me^{IV}O_2$-type matrixes (Me = Sn, Ti, Zr, Ce, etc.) appeared to be adequate, effectively adsorbing $^{68}Ge^{IV}$ (e.g., Kopecky et al. 1973, 1974; Malyshev et al. 1975; Loc'h et al. 1980; Ambe 1988). Alternatively, organic resins have been developed, eluting ^{68}Ga in even stronger HCl (e.g., Arino et al. 1978; Neirinckx et al. 1980; Schumacher and Maier-Borst 1981) (Fig. 6).

4 Commercial "Ionic" Generators

Thanks to the pioneering achievement of radiochemists in Obninsk, Russia, a new type of $^{68}Ge/^{68}Ga$ generator became commercially available in the first years of the 21st century (Razbash et al. 2005). Generator eluates based on hydrochloric acid provided "cationic" ^{68}Ga instead of "inert" ^{68}Ga complexes, opening new pathways of Me^{III}-based radiopharmaceutical chemistry (Fig. 7).

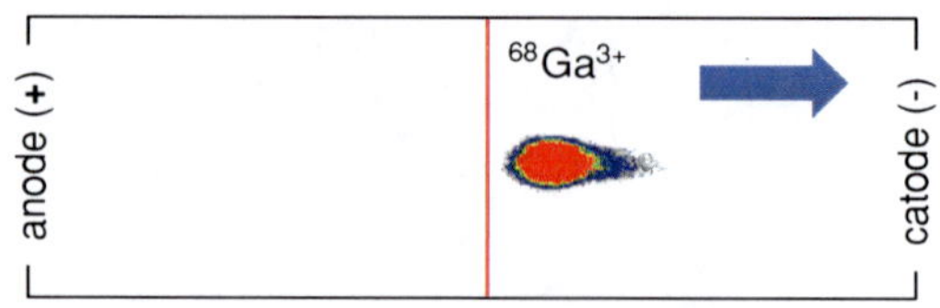

Fig. 7 Electrophoresis of a 0.1 N HCl ^{68}Ga generator eluate (EZAG Obninsk generator) demonstrating the presence of "cationic" ^{68}Ga. (parameters: 0.1 HCl, Whatman paper strip, $l = 19$ cm, $t = 5$ min, 191 V, 210 mA, 40 W)

Again conicidentally, the ^{68}Ga cation was introduced immediately into existing designs of MRI and SPECT imaging probes, namely DTPA- or DOTA-based derivatives. The impressive success of utilizing ^{68}Ga-DOTA-octreotides and PET/CT instead of, e.g., ^{111}In-DTPA-octreoscan paved the way not only to the clinical acceptance of this particular tracer for neuroendocrine imaging, but to the realization of the great potential of the ^{68}Ge/^{68}Ga generator for modern nuclear medicine in general.

While commercial "ionic" generators thus entered clinical environments, questions on adequate use concerning radiation safety, legal requirements, and labeling of medical tracers became increasingly relevant.

Problem 1 The long physical half-life of the parent in principle should allow usage of at least 1 year. However, the shelf-life of the generators did not necessarily parallel this long physical half-life, partly due to decreasing quality of the generator itself in terms of ^{68}Ga elution yield but mainly due to increasing breakthrough of ^{68}Ge. ^{68}Ge breakthrough reduction and/or removal of ^{68}Ge from the eluate is thus an important radiochemical challenge.

Problem 2 ^{68}Ga generator eluates are neither chemically nor radionuclidically pure. Nonradioactive metals such as $^{68}Zn^{II}$ (as generated in the generator as a decay product of ^{68}Ga), Fe^{III} as a general chemical impurity, and breakthrough $^{68}Ge^{IV}$ may represent metals competing with $^{68}Ga^{III}$ for coordinative labeling of radiopharmaceutical precursors. Again, removal of ^{68}Ge from the eluate is thus another important radiochemical challenge (Zhernosekov et al. 2007).

Problem 3 The new generation of ^{68}Ge/^{68}Ga radionuclide generators utilizes hydrochloric acid solutions for ^{68}Ga elution. The relatively high concentration of H^+ may protonate functional groups of ligands and bifunctional ligands needed for the labeling of ^{68}Ga. Finally, minimizing pH and volume of ^{68}Ga eluted prior to labeling should facilitate synthetic yield.

In this context, three approaches have been developed to address one or more of these problems. Two processes include chemical separation strategies and may be termed "post-processing," while a third technology is simple fractionation of the

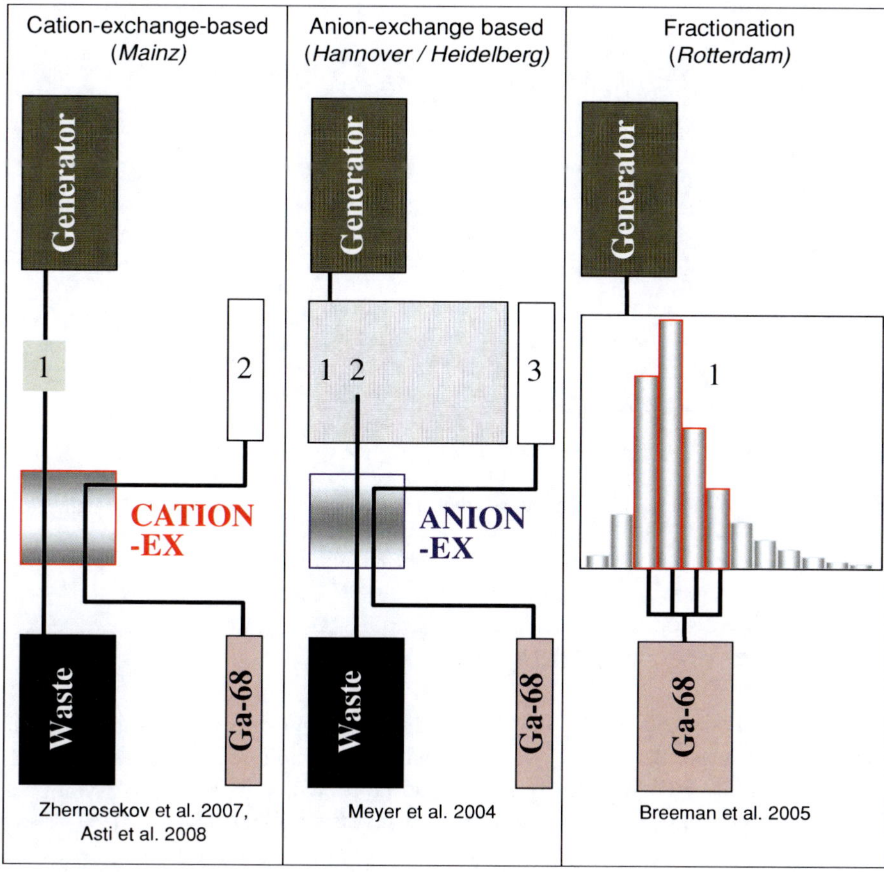

Fig. 8 Overview on post-processing technologies for commercial $^{68}Ge/^{68}Ga$ radionuclide generators

eluate, i.e., isolating eluate fractions with the highest ^{68}Ga concentration. The three methods are illustrated schematically in Fig. 8.

In most cases, these generators are being used in direct connection with one of the three post-eluate processing technologies mentioned. In particular, cation-exchange-based post-processing guarantees almost complete removal of metallic impurities, in particular ^{68}Ge. It thus avoids transfer of critical ^{68}Ge levels into the radiopharmaceutical preparation and guarantees safe use of the systems, which is of upmost relevance from the legal point of view, i.e., addressing safety criteria for routine clinical use (see Fig. 9).

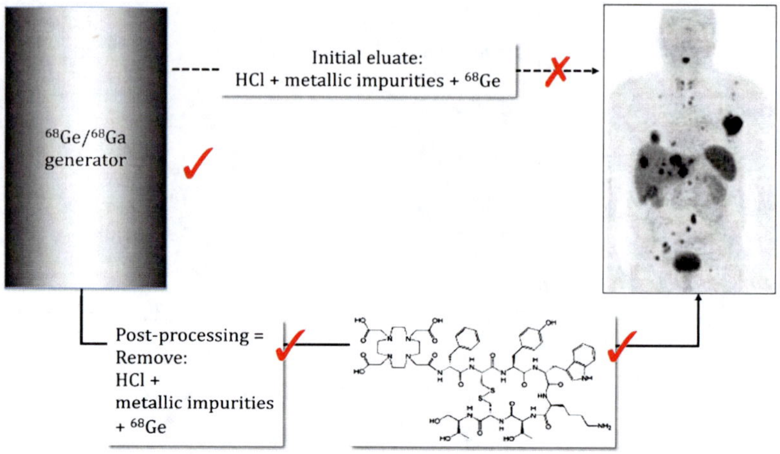

Fig. 9 $^{68}Ge/^{68}Ga$ radionuclide generators with integrated post-processing providing chemically pure and safe (^{68}Ge isolated) ^{68}Ga fractions ready for ^{68}Ga labeling

5 Current State/Outlook

Generators: Today, several $^{68}Ge/^{68}Ga$ radionuclide generators are commercially available, either TiO_2- or SnO_2-based or using an organic resin. ^{68}Ga eluate yields range from about 70% to 80% for fresh generators, with a more or less pronounced decrease over time. ^{68}Ge breakthrough is at levels of about 0.01–0.001% or even better for fresh generators, with increasing percentages over longer periods of generator usage. In combination with post-processing technologies, ^{68}Ga radiopharmaceuticals are being synthesized routinely and safely. Thus, times have been a-changin′, as predicted in 1964 (Zimmermann 1964) at the same time as the Yano and Anger paper (1964), since the early $^{68}Ge/^{68}Ga$ radionuclide generator systems developed about half a century ago.

Nuclear data: Interestingly, times have been a-changin′ for nuclear decay data of both generator parent and daughter. Figure 10 schematically compares "old" and current values for half-life and positron branching (Burrows 2002; Schönfeld 1999). The most recent values are $t_{1/2}$ of 270.95 days and 67.71 min for ^{68}Ge and ^{68}Ga, respectively, with 89.14% positron branching of ^{68}Ga.

Future developments: Figure 10 illustrates some future directions.

Concerning solid-phase-based ion exchange chromatographic $^{68}Ge/^{68}Ga$ radionuclide generators, some improvements may be made within the resin material itself, helping to decrease ^{68}Ge release over time of generator usage. Recent publications hint at the potential of sophisticated nanoparticles. In parallel, good manufacturing practice (GMP)-certified and licensed commercial generators are needed to satisfy the increasing requirements by legal authorities.

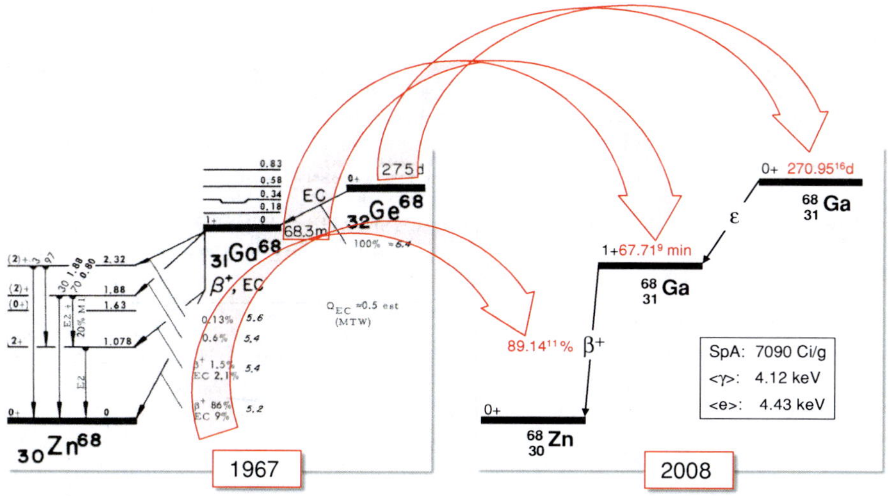

Fig. 10 Sketch of some future directions in $^{68}Ge/^{68}Ga$ radionuclide generators and related research and technology

Elution by generators may further be integrated into improved online, fast, efficient post-processing procedures managed by automated modules. Optionally, these post-processing technologies should allow for versatile labeling protocols, including, e.g., transfer from aqueous to nonaqueous solutions (addressing potential lipophilic ^{68}Ga tracers) (Zoller et al. 2010) or on-resin, solid-phase-supported labeling reactions.

$^{68}Ge/^{68}Ga$ radionuclide generator performance may be facilitated by developing new ligands and bifunctional ligands for coordinating ^{68}Ga specifically, i.e., ideally discriminating Fe^{III} and Zn^{II}, or by allowing complex formation under a broader range of pH.

With the existing state-of-the-art $^{68}Ge/^{68}Ga$ radionuclide generators and post-processing technologies, and thanks to the exciting ^{68}Ga radiopharmaceuticals available and under development, in another decade from now, $^{68}Ge/^{68}Ga$ generator-based ^{68}Ga diagnostics may approach rank 3 or 4 of clinical impact molecular imaging, following ^{99m}Tc-, ^{18}F-, and radioiodine-based tracers. A particular impact will be in the field of oncology, in view of the concept of theranostics and personalized patient treatment strategies, as none of the other major imaging radionuclides is able to bridge quantitative diagnoses by PET/CT with subsequent endoradionuclidic therapies as can be done with ^{68}Ga, the β-emitters ^{90}Y and ^{177}Lu, or α-emitters such as ^{213}Bi and possibly ^{225}Ac.

References

Ambe S (1988) Germanium-68-gallium-68 generator with alpha-ferric oxide support. Appl Radiat Isot 39:49

Anger HO, Gottschalk A (1963) Localzation of brain tumors with the positron scintillation camera. JNM 4:326

Arino H, Skraba WJ, Kramer HH (1978) A new $^{68}Ge/^{68}Ga$ radioisotope generator system. Int J Appl Radiat Isot 29:117
Asti M, De Pietri G, Fraternali A, Grassi E, Sghedoni R, Fioroni F, Roesch F, Versari A, Salvo D (2008) Validation of $^{68}Ge/^{68}Ga$ generator processing by chemical purification for routine clinical application of ^{68}Ga-DOTATOC. Nucl Med Biol 35:721
Burrows TW (2002) Nuclear data sheets for A = 6.8. Nucl Data Sheets 97:1–127
Breeman WAP, de Jong M, de Blois E, Bernard BF, Konijnenberg M, Krenning EP (2005) Radiolabelling DOTA-peptides with ^{68}Ga. Eur J Nucl Med 32:478
Erhardt GJ, Welch MK (1978) A new germanium-68/gallium-68 generator. J Nucl Med 19: 925–929
Gleason GI (1960) A positron cow. Int J Appl Radiat Isot 8:90
Greene WT, Tucker WD (1961) An improved gallium-68 cow. Int J Appl Radiat Isot 12:62
Gottschalk A, Anger HO (1964a) The sensivity of the positron scintillation camera for detecting simulated brain tumors with Gallium-68 EDTA. Am J Roentgen 92:174
Gottschalk A, Anger HO (1964b) Letter to the editor. J Nucl Med 5(3):569
Gottschalk A (1996) The early years with Hal Anger. Sem Nucl Med 26(3):171
Gottschalk A (2004) Hal Anger: Nuclear medicine's quiet genius. J Nucl Med 45(23): 13 N, 26 N
Kopecky P, Mudrová B, Svoboda K (1973) The study of conditions for the preparation and utilization of ^{68}Ge-^{68}Ga generator. Int J Appl Radiat Isot 24:73
Kopecky P, Mudrová B (1974) ^{68}Ge-^{68}Ga generator for the production of ^{68}Ga in an ionic form. Int J Appl Radiat Isot 25:263
Lewis RE, Camin LL (1981) Germanium-68/Gallium-68 generator for the one step elution of ionic gallium-68. J Lab Compds Radiopharm 18, 16
Loc'h C, Maziere B, Comar D (1980) A new generator for ionic gallium-68. J Nucl Med 21:171
Malyshev KV, Smirnov VV (1975) Gallium-68 yield from hydrated zirconium oxide-based generators. Sov Radiochim 17:137
McQueen JD, Abbassioun K (1968) Cisternal brain scanning with positron emitting isotopes. J Neurosurg 29(6):597
Meyer G-J, Mäcke HR, Schuhmacher J, Knapp WH, Hofmann M (2004) ^{68}Ga-labelled DOTA-derivatised peptide ligands. Eur J Nucl Med 31:1097
Neirinckx RD, Davis MA (1980) Potential column chromatography for ionic Ga-68 II: Organic ion exchangers as chromatographic supports. J Nucl Med 21:81
Razbash AA, Sevastianov YuG, Krasnov NN, Leonov AI, Pavlekin VE (2005) Germanium-68 row of products. Proceedings of the 5th International Conference on Isotopes, 5ICI, Brussels 25–29 April Medimond, Bologna, pp 147–151
Roesch F, Baum RP (2011) Generator-based PET radiopharmaceuticals for molecular imaging of tumours: On the way to THERANOSTICS. Dalton Trans 40(23):6104–6111
Roesch F, Riss PJ (2010) The Renaissance of the $^{68}Ge/^{68}Ga$ radionuclide generator initiates new developments in ^{68}Ga radiopharmaceutical chemistry. Curr Top Med Chem 10(16):1633–1668
Schaer LR, Anger HO, Gottschalk A (1965) Gallium Edetate ^{68}Ga experiences in brain-lesion detection with the positron camera. AMAM 198:139
Schumacher J, Maier-Borst W (1981) A new $^{68}Ge/^{68}Ga$ radioisotope generator system for production of ^{68}Ga in dilute HCl. Int J Appl Radiat Isot 32:31
Schönfeld E(1999) ^{68}Ge-^{68}Ga. Comments on evaluation—CEA ISBN 27272 02111 3
Shealy CN, Aronow S, Brownell GL (1964) Gallium-68 as a scanning agent for intracranial lesions. J Nucl Med 5:161
Yano Y, Anger HO (1964) A gallium-68 positron cow for medical use. J Nucl Med 5:484
Zhernosekov KP, Filosofov DV, Baum RP, Aschoff P, Bihl H, Razbash AA, Jahn M, Jennewein M, Rösch F (2007) Processing of generator-produced ^{68}Ga for medical application. J Nucl Med 48:1741
Zimmerman RA (1964) The Times They Are a-Changin'. Columbia Records
Zoller F, Riss PJ, Montforts F-P, Rösch F (2010) Efficient post-processing of aqueous generator eluates facilitates ^{68}Ga-labelling under anhydrous conditions. Radiochim Acta 98(3):157–160

Overview and Perspectives on Automation Strategies in ^{68}Ga Radiopharmaceutical Preparations

Stefano Boschi, Claudio Malizia and Filippo Lodi

Abstract

The renaissance of ^{68}Ga radiopharmacy has led to great advances in automation technology. The availability of a highly efficient, reliable, long-lived $^{68}Ge/^{68}Ga$ generator system along with a well-established coordination chemistry based on bifunctional chelating agents have been the bases of this development in ^{68}Ga radiopharmacy. Syntheses of ^{68}Ga peptides were originally performed by manual or semiautomated systems, but increasing clinical demand, radioprotection, and regulatory issues have driven extensive automation of their production process. Several automated systems, based on different post-processing of the ^{68}Ga generator eluate, on different engineering, and on fixed tubing or disposable cassette approaches, have been developed and are discussed in this chapter. Since automatic systems for preparation of radiopharmaceuticals should comply with qualification and validation protocols established by regulations current Good Manufacturing Practices (cGMP) and local regulations, some regulatory issues and the more relevant qualification protocols are also discussed.

S. Boschi (✉) · C. Malizia · F. Lodi
PET Radiopharmacy, Nuclear Medicine Department,
S.Orsola-Malpighi University Hospital, Bologna, Italy
e-mail: stefano.boschi@aosp.bo.it

S. Boschi
Radiofarmacia PET, U.O. Medicina Nucleare,
Pad.30 Polo Tecnologico, Azienda Ospedaliero Universitaria S.Orsola-Malpighi,
Via Massarenti 9, 40138 Bologna, Italy

R. P. Baum and F. Rösch (eds.), *Theranostics, Gallium-68, and Other Radionuclides*,
Recent Results in Cancer Research 194, DOI: 10.1007/978-3-642-27994-2_2,

Contents

1 Introduction

Positron emission tomography (PET) is an imaging modality which provides quantitative images of biological processes in vivo at molecular level. It provides clinically important information for tumor diagnosis and staging as well as for neurological applications.

Most of the PET radiopharmaceuticals are labeled with radionuclides (^{18}F, ^{11}C, ^{15}O, ^{13}N) which are produced by medical cyclotrons, thus limiting the availability of these short-lived tracers. Generator-produced radionuclides such as ^{68}Ga represent an important and interesting alternative to cyclotron-produced radionuclides because of some important advantages.

^{68}Ga decays 89% by positron emission, with E_{max} of 1.92 MeV, and 11% via electron capture. Its physical half-life of 67.71 min is compatible with the pharmacokinetics of most radiopharmaceuticals of low molecular weight.

In the early 1990s, Deutsch (1993) proposed the use of ^{68}Ga for PET, even if ^{68}Ga had been used since the early 1960s in nuclear medicine (Shealy et al. 1964; Hayes et al. 1965). Many reasons, however, underlie the enormous development of ^{68}Ga in the last seven years.

First of all, PET has become a routine clinical imaging modality in the last decade. Second, ^{68}Ge/^{68}Ga generators approached a reliable level of robustness, adequate for modern requirements of radiometal labeling chemistry in a clinical environment. Third, more favorable chemistry was developed, substituting open-chain complexing agents by macrocyclic 1,4,7,10,-tetraazacyclododecane-1,4,7,10 tetraacetic acid (DOTA)- and 1,4,7-triazacyclononane-N,N',N''-triacetic acid (NOTA)- derived conjugates.

These complexing agents provide outstanding characteristics to the radiopharmaceuticals, by shielding the Ga core effectively under physiological conditions, thus avoiding ligand exchange with the blood serum protein transferrin, which has very high affinity for Ga^{3+} ($K_{ST} = 20.3$) (Harris and Pecoraro 1983).

Optimization of these chelating structures in terms of thermodynamic stability and kinetic inertness as well as in terms of labeling efficiency and options for bifunctionality opens brilliant research and clinical perspectives.

One of the most important drivers for development of ^{68}Ga radiopharmacy has been the development of small tumor-affine peptides, most notably those targeting somatostatin receptors (Maecke et al. 2005). ^{68}Ga-DOTA-octreotide derivatives were the breakthrough vector molecules and fundamental to the development of present-day ^{68}Ga radiopharmacy and $^{68}Ge/^{68}Ga$ generators.

PET with ^{68}Ga-DOTA-conjugated peptides has brought about dramatic improvements in spatial resolution and is increasingly being used in many specialized centers. In particular, PET clearly offers higher resolution and improved pharmacokinetics as compared with somatostatin (SST) receptor scintigraphy, with promising results for detection of SST receptor-expressing tumors (Kowalski et al. 2003; Buchman et al. 2007), as well as providing prognostic information (Campana et al. 2010).

Syntheses of ^{68}Ga peptides were originally performed by manual or semiautomated systems. Radioprotection considerations and increasing regulatory demands may hamper wider clinical application of such systems. Extensive automation of the process is therefore needed to fulfill radioprotection as well as increasing regulatory requirements for hospital-based preparation of PET radiopharmaceuticals.

2 Approach to Automation: Considerations on ^{68}Ga Radiolabeling Process

The availability of a highly efficient, reliable, long-lived $^{68}Ge/^{68}Ga$ generator system has been the basis of the development in ^{68}Ga radiopharmacy. A very comprehensive review on $^{68}Ge/^{68}Ga$ generators and coordination chemistry is available in the literature (Roesch and Riss 2010). Different types of $^{68}Ge/^{68}Ga$ generator are described, with absorption of the parent radionuclide ^{68}Ge ($t_{1/2} = 270.8$ days) onto different solid column materials, such as organic pyrogallol–formaldehyde resins and metal oxides (mainly SnO_2 or TiO_2). Most of them are commercially available, and considerable efforts towards sterile, pharmaceutical-grade, cGMP-compliant generators are underway.

However, there are still some drawbacks to direct use of ^{68}Ga eluate for radiolabeling of peptides in clinical PET.

The most relevant issues are measurable activities of the long-lived parent radionuclide ^{68}Ge (i.e., ^{68}Ge breakthrough), the high eluate volume, and the high HCl concentration (0.1–1 M). In addition, metallic impurities such as Zn^{2+}, generated from the decay of ^{68}Ga, Ti^{4+} or other potential impurities from the column material, as well as Fe^{3+} could be present in the eluate. All these metallic impurities may adversely affect the ^{68}Ga yield as well as the specific activity of the labeled product.

It is important to underline that the concept of specific activity in this context is more related to the coformation of metal complex with the same ligand than to the presence of stable gallium isotopes.

Several approaches for processing generator-derived ^{68}Ga eluates have recently been described, each with a markedly different impact on the development of automatic systems for ^{68}Ga radiolabeling.

Processing of ^{68}Ga eluates by using strong anion exchange resins was introduced first (Meyer et al. 2004; Velikyan et al. 2004). ^{68}Ga is retained in 5.5 N HCl by forming an anionic tetrachloro complex $[^{68}GaCl_4]^-$ to remove cationic impurities and concentrate the generator eluate. This strategy separates ^{68}Ge, but does not allow direct loading of ^{68}Ga onto the anion exchange resin from 0.1 N HCl eluate.

Another approach to overcome these problems is to fractionate the initial generator eluate (Breeman et al. 2005). The rationale resides in the fact that about two-thirds of the total ^{68}Ga activity elutes within a $\sim$1–2 mL activity peak. However, ^{68}Ge and metallic impurities are only minimized, because of the lower eluate volume, rather than being chemically removed.

Zhernosekov et al. (2007) reported an efficient and simplified method for preparation of ^{68}Ga-labeled radiopharmaceuticals based on the different affinities of ^{68}Ga and other metals toward cation exchange resin in acetone/HCl solutions. This method combines volume reduction with almost complete removal of metallic contaminants as well as ^{68}Ge, thus providing concentrated ^{68}Ga in a useful form for direct radiolabeling.

Gallium posseses a well-established coordination chemistry. DOTA and NOTA bifunctional derivatives are easy to label with ^{68}Ga in a reproducible manner and with high yield in water or, most frequently, in buffers such as acetate or 4-(2-hydroxyethyl)-1-piperazineethanesulfonic acid (HEPES).

NOTA derivatives have the advantage of room-temperature labeling, while DOTA requires elevated temperatures and longer reaction times. Differences in the chelator system may also influence the pharmacokinetics, the affinity, and the tumor uptake of some new somatostatin antagonists (Fani et al. 2011).

Microwave heating was found to be efficient to accelerate and improve the complexation reaction of ^{68}Ga with bifunctional chelators, DOTA and NOTA, conjugated to peptides and oligonucleotides and to increase specific radioactivity (Velikyan et al. 2004).

The final part of the radiolabeling process is purification of the ^{68}Ga-DOTA-conjugated peptides. This is generally accomplished by solid-phase extraction (SPE). This step increases the radiochemical purity by removing free ^{68}Ga ions and acetate complex as well as colloidal ^{68}Ga, which is formed especially at higher pH.

The increasing clinical demand for such tracers has motivated automation of the radiolabeling process to facilitate the transition from manual or semiautomated systems to full automation. Drivers for this transition can be summarized as follows:

- **Radioprotection.** A fully automated synthesis process, including post-processing of the eluate, without user intervention leads to much lower hand doses to the operator.
- **Higher reproducibility and robustness.** A prevalidated process increases standardization robustness and synthesis reproducibility.

- **Better cGMP compliance.** Traceability of the complete process, including documentation of all process parameters and functions, is mandatory for fulfilling the requirements for patient application in clinical settings.
- **Better control on sterility.** A fully automated and validated cleaning routine after each process or use of the sterile disposable cassette approach can guarantee better control of sterility and apyrogenicity of the radiopharmaceutical.
- **Dissemination.** Standardized and fully validated technologies are easy to transfer to new institutions, thus increasing the number of patients studied.

3 Modules for ^{68}Ga Radiopharmaceuticals

A renaissance in ^{68}Ga radiopharmacy has resulted from the huge demand for ^{68}Ga-DOTA somatostatin analogs. Manual systems have been described (Meyer et al. 2004; Zhernosekov et al. 2007) and have definitely boosted the diffusion of such radiopharmaceuticals in clinical centers. Many of them are still in use, especially in countries with lower regulatory impact.

An example (Zhernosekov et al. 2007) is shown in Fig. 1. This manual system has been used for years in our laboratory, with some modification to improve operator radioprotection (Di Pierro et al. 2008), with excellent results in terms of radiochemical yield and robustness.

A manual, easy-to-use, self-shielded system including an organic-based ^{68}Ge/^{68}Ga generator is available on the market from ITG (ITG Isotope Technologies Garching GmbH, Garching, Germany). The system is equipped with a sterile single-use kit, no post-processing of ^{68}Ga eluate is needed, and it has a built-in filter integrity test device (Fig. 2).

Supply of automatic systems has considerably increased in the last few years. Several automated systems are commercially available, combining generator elution, post-processing, ^{68}Ga labeling reactions, and purification of ^{68}Ga-labeled peptide with pharmaceutical characteristics.

3.1 Classification and Characteristics of Automated Systems

A tentative classification of the available automated systems could be based on:

- **Post-processing approach:** anionic, fractionation, cationic
- **System engineering:** fully equipped compact system, modular system
- **Fluid path:** fixed tubing system, disposable sterile cassette.

All the post-processing approaches mentioned in Sect. 2 have been adopted in developing and engineering automatic systems. The choice of post-processing approach is based on scientific considerations which fall outside the scope of this chapter.

There are, however, commercial reasons often based on collaborations and spin-offs between academia and companies which have actually led to preferential implementation of one of the post-processing approaches.

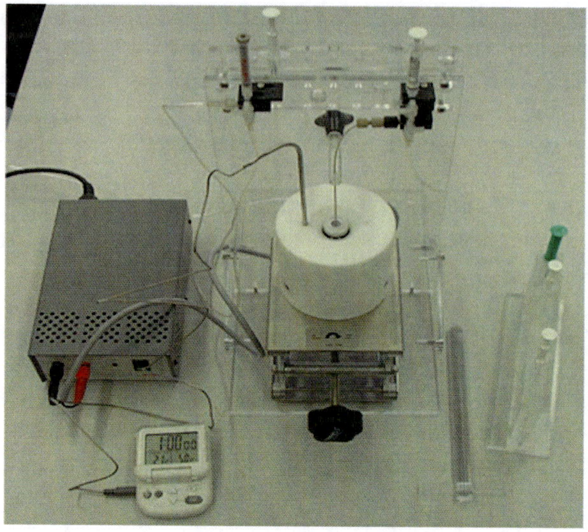

Fig. 1 Manual system for ^{68}Ga radiolabeling (Zhernosekov et al. 2007)

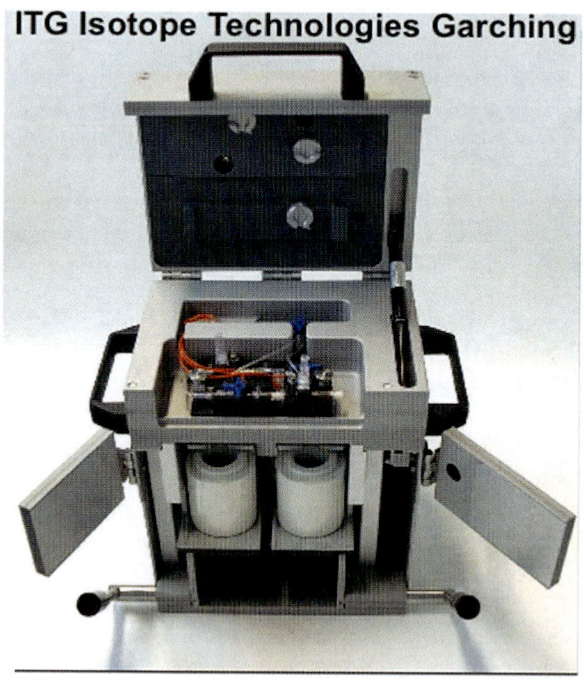

Fig. 2 Manual self-shielded system

Moreover, fractionation was widely used, at least in the early years, because it is intrinsically easy to use and cost effective, and it shorten synthesis time.

Some companies still offer a choice of systems adopting different post-processing approaches.

Data from the literature evidence differences in the radiochemical yield of the whole ^{68}Ga-DOTA-peptide labeling process among different post-processing approaches.

The 60% decay corrected (d.c.) radiochemical yield was reported using a fully automated system with a fractionation protocol (Decristoforo et al. 2007) and 30 μg DOTA-D-Phe^{1}-Tyr^{3}-octreotide (DOTATOC) in acetate buffer. Different amount of peptide used, strong influence of the type of buffer (Bauwens et al. 2010), and incubation parameters make comparison among automatic systems using different post-processing approaches extremely difficult.

A radiochemical yield of 95% was reported by cation exchange-based post-processing because of the high purity of the ^{68}Ga eluted from AG50 X8 resin (Zhernosekov et al. 2007). Since this method requires manual interference in the labeling procedure, this protocol was completely automated by using a miniaturized multi-use column with a cation exchange resin (AG 50 W-X4) similar to that described by Zhernosekov and, successively, using a commercial, disposable cation exchange cartridge (Ocak et al. 2010).

Replacement of a multiple-use resin by a single-use cartridge has led to better cGMP compliance and simplification of the process, as cleaning and reconditioning of the column for multiple uses is avoided. Better microbiological safety with respect to sterility and pyrogens should also be considered. Inactive metal impurities, except Zn, are less reduced than with a permanent cation exchanger but without problems for synthesis.

Comparative decay/non-decay corrected yields of ^{68}Ga-DOTATOC, with using different post-processing approach synthesis methods were reported by the same author (Ocak et al. 2010). These values ranged from 67% d.c. for the fractionation method to 77–84% d.c. using different cationic post-processing and different buffer. The longer overall synthesis time with fully automated prepurification as compared with a fractionated system (Decristoforo et al. 2007) was compensated by the advantage of using all available activity of ^{68}Ga by concentration on the cation exchanger, thus balancing the radiochemical yield.

Commercial automatic systems based on fractionation, anionic, and cationic post-processing are shown in Figs. 3, 4, 5.

Fully equipped, ready-to-use, compact systems are available from companies such as Iason, Veenstra, Comecer, and Raytest (Figs. 3, 4, 5). These systems represent turnkey solutions, suitable for cGMP pharmaceutical environments, but, at least in principle, with limited flexibility.

Increasing flexibility can be achieved by "modular" systems or systems based on expandable platforms (Eckert and Ziegler, Scintomics). Automation of a broad spectrum of procedures for radiolabeling, isotope purification, routine tracer production, and other radiopharmaceutical processes is possible with such systems.

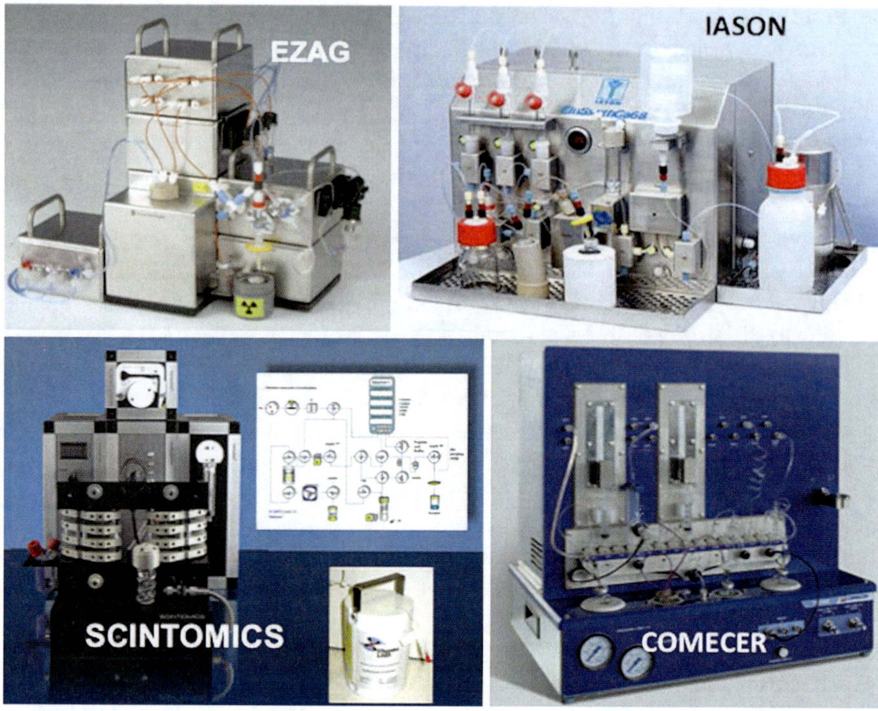

Fig. 3 Fractionation-based automatic systems

System integrated components, such as handling parts, sensors, pumps, valves, regulators, heaters, high-performance liquid chromatography (HPLC) equipment, etc., allow for a high level of flexibility in the construction of customized modules.

It is important to underline that the need for flexibility and regulatory requirements are often conflicting, since regulations pose some hurdles to the production of radiopharmaceuticals for clinical use. The different chemistry approaches used, the many types of PET tracer required for research and clinical studies, and the limited resources in production facilities call for flexible systems. On the other hand, regulations for small-scale hospital radiopharmaceutical preparation are based on risk analysis-based validation plans, extensive qualification/validation protocols, and full documentation and traceability, thus reducing the possibility of implementing flexible processes.

Since regulations (cGMP or local, national pharmacopoeia regulations) are becoming mandatory for radiopharmaceutical preparations, a current trend in engineering of automatic systems is to move from fixed tubing to cassette systems.

Single-use sterile cassettes avoid time-consuming cleaning validation procedures as well as intense cleaning and sanitation routines. By changing the cassette, multiple syntheses can be easily performed even for various tracers and with different radionuclides.

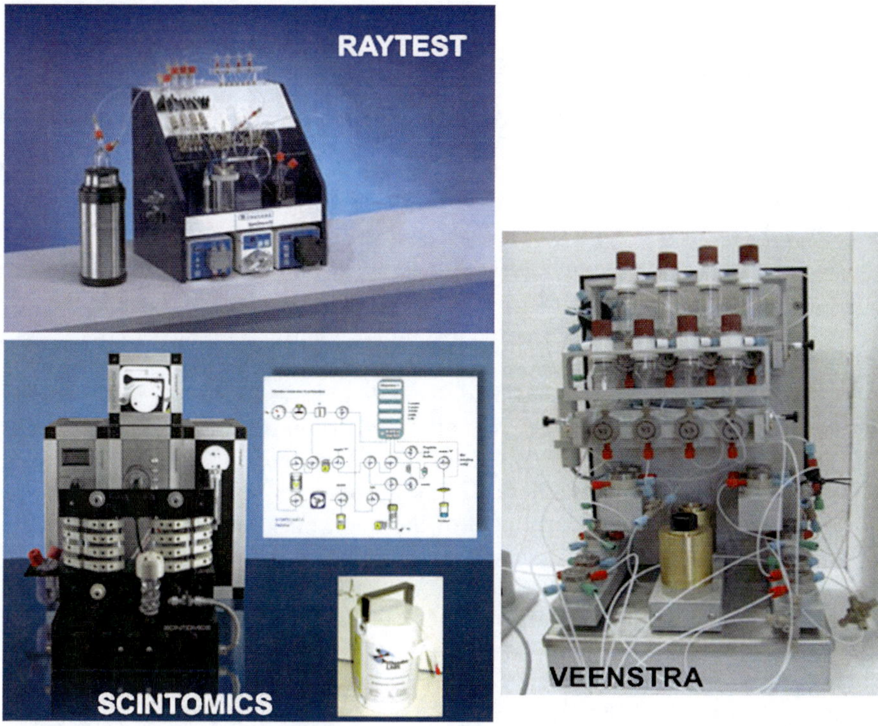

Fig. 4 Anionic exchange-based automatic systems

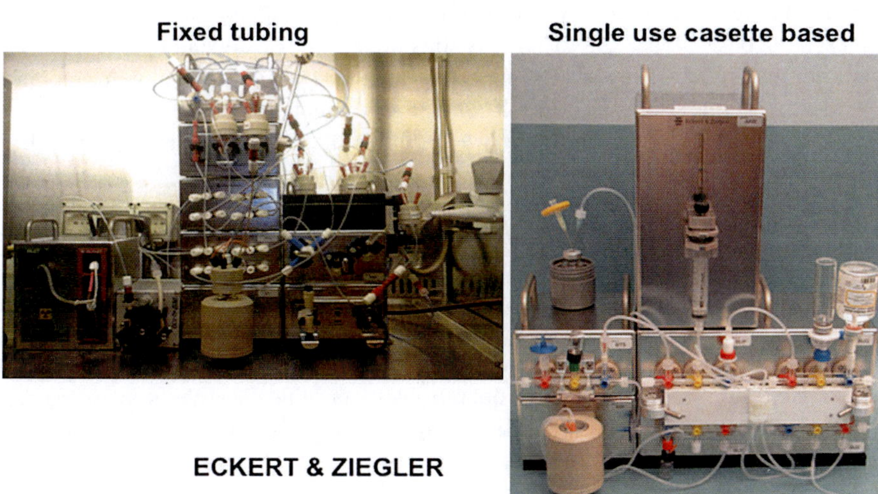

Fig. 5 Cationic exchange-based automatic systems

This is particularly attractive for management of neuroendocrine tumors, since radiolabeling of DOTA-somatostatin analogs with ^{68}Ga for tumor staging and labeling of the same compound with a radionuclide such as ^{177}Lu or ^{90}Y for therapy become feasible. By simply changing the cassette, it is possible to avoid the delicate cleaning validation process to guarantee complete removal of ^{90}Y or ^{177}Lu.

^{68}Ga/^{177}Lu/^{90}Y/^{111}In-DOTA peptides have been synthesized with high purity, high radiochemical yield (>80% d.c. for ^{68}Ga-DOTA peptides and 90% d.c. for ^{177}Lu/^{90}Y/^{111}In-DOTA peptides), and acceptable synthesis time (Petrik et al. 2011). Sterile, single-use, disposable cassettes assembled under cGMP-compliant clean-room conditions guarantee better control of sterility and apyrogenicity of the radiopharmaceutical preparation, even if complete control of these parameters relies only on a fully validated process.

Eckert and Ziegler engineered a self-shielded cassette-based solution for routine production, becoming an integral part of the synthesis system. Only single-use cassettes are located inside the shielded area, allowing weight reduction to one-tenth of that of a conventional hot cell. The system can be placed in virtually any laboratory, without any reinforcement of the floor, thus facilitating dissemination of the methodology.

Many companies are moving toward single-use disposable kits or a cassette approach. GE Healthcare has drawn up the Gallea project for development of a cassette system for ^{68}Ga radiopharmaceutical preparations based on the Fastlab platform.

Cassette systems have also some drawbacks if compared with fixed tubing systems: first, the high cassette cost and the reliance on the cassette manufacturer; second, reduced flexibility. Optimized and fully validated cassettes for each radiopharmaceutical are needed, and the development of new cassette systems strongly relies only on marketing considerations. Third, the fluid path of the cassette is often engineered by commercially available disposable medical devices (tubes, stopcock valves, kits for intravenous injection). Leaks and bubbles are then possible, and special care should be taken to assess all components and connections to avoid malfunctioning resulting in low radiochemical yield.

A comprehensive comparison between tubing and cassette systems is presented in Table 1.

Since the majority of these systems have been developed and/or upgraded in the second part of the 2000s, the various software packages are generally characterized by intuitive user interfaces that comply with cGMP and good laboratory practices (GLP) requirements. Some software complies also with GAMP5 guidelines, or with more extensive requirements such as FDA 21CFR part 11.

The software controls all aspects of the synthesis, many of them being easy to program by simple drag-and-drop operations of graphical symbols, and provides complete traceability of the process through audit trails and extensive documentation of the radiopharmaceutical preparation.

Table 1 Comparison between cassette and tubing systems

	Cassette	Tubing
Synthesis pathways	Fractionated, precleaning with disposable cation exchange cartridge	Fractionated, precleaning with one-way, permanent cation exchange cartridge
Handling	Very easy	Easy
Cleaning	None	Fully automatic cleaning procedure, validation of cleaning procedure needed
Sterility	All parts in contact with media are sterile	System needs cleaning and disinfection to maintain sterility
Costs	Costs for cassette, reliance on manufacturer	Tubing replacement (min. yearly), personnel cost because of time for cleaning and handling
Flexibility	Only limited	Full
Cross-contamination	None, various tracers and nuclides such as ^{90}Y, ^{111}In, and ^{177}Lu on the same system with different cassettes	Cannot be excluded, use of various nuclides not tolerated by authorities
GMP	Fully compliant	

3.2 Automation and Regulatory Aspects

As with any other medicinal products, it is mandatory to ensure that quality and safety of ^{68}Ga radiopharmaceuticals are adequate for their intended use.

Substantial differences between US and EU regulation for preparation of radiopharmaceuticals are still evident, in spite of efforts towards worldwide harmonized regulation in the field of medicinal products for human use. Furthermore, different interpretation of European regulations among EU countries as well as local, specific GMP-like regulations generates differences in the requirements demanded by national regulatory authorities.

In recent years, the trend has been for implementation of cGMP regulation for PET radiopharmaceutical preparations, even if the cost and difficulty of cGMP enforcement in academic and hospital environments could hamper the development of clinical and research applications of these medicinal products. Besides cGMP, there are several guidelines such as GAMP® 5 which provide guidance to achieve compliant GxP computerized systems using a flexible risk-based approach.

To achieve the quality objective, however, a comprehensively designed and correctly implemented quality assurance system is of utmost importance. Accordingly, all equipment, instruments, and technologies which may affect the quality of the product should undergo proper qualification protocols. Written and approved protocols specifying critical steps, acceptance criteria, and how qualification will be conducted should be established.

Automatic systems for synthesis of radiopharmaceuticals which will be installed in radiopharmacies should therefore comply with qualification and validation protocols which are established by regulations (cGMP, GMP-like, or local regulations).

Annex 15 of the EU Guide to Good Manufacturing Practice (cGMP) provides important definitions of the qualification protocols that should be implemented. They are derived from the validation master plan, which includes all the strategies and protocols for the entire validation plan and can be listed as follows:

Design qualification (DQ): documented verification that the proposed design of the facilities, systems, and equipment is suitable for the intended purpose.

Installation qualification (IQ): documented verification that the system is installed according to the specifications and complies with approved design and manufacturer's recommendations.

Operational qualification (OQ): documented verification that the system performs as intended throughout the established operating ranges.

Performance qualification (PQ): documented verification that the system performs according to the process specifications, assuring reproducibility, robustness, and product quality.

Successful OQ should allow the finalization of calibration, operating, and cleaning procedures, operator training, and preventative maintenance requirements. It should permit formal "release" of the system.

The qualification protocols described above should be derived from well-established specification protocols implemented by the manufacturer, starting from the user requirement, through functional and design specifications. The protocols and the documents derived from them are the prerequisite for complete and successful IQ, OQ, and PQ.

Continuous interaction between users and manufacturers could be extremely helpful to better define the requirements and, consequently, specifications. Manufacturers should definitely provide documental and technical support for qualification plans to be implemented at sites.

A risk-based approach to a compliant system is shown in Fig. 6.

4 Perspectives

The renaissance of ^{68}Ga radiopharmacy has led to great advances in automation technology in the last five years. Different automation strategies are now available, which can also be tailored to different needs. Also, sites with no experience can receive a turnkey system and adequate training.

Automation technologies have implemented different prepurification approaches leading to increased chemical and radionuclidic purity (minimizing ^{68}Ge breakthrough) as well as high specific radioactivity of the final preparation.

The fundamental advantages of using automated systems reside in their improved reproducibility, higher throughput, easier handling, improved response to clinical demand, and cGMP-compliant production.

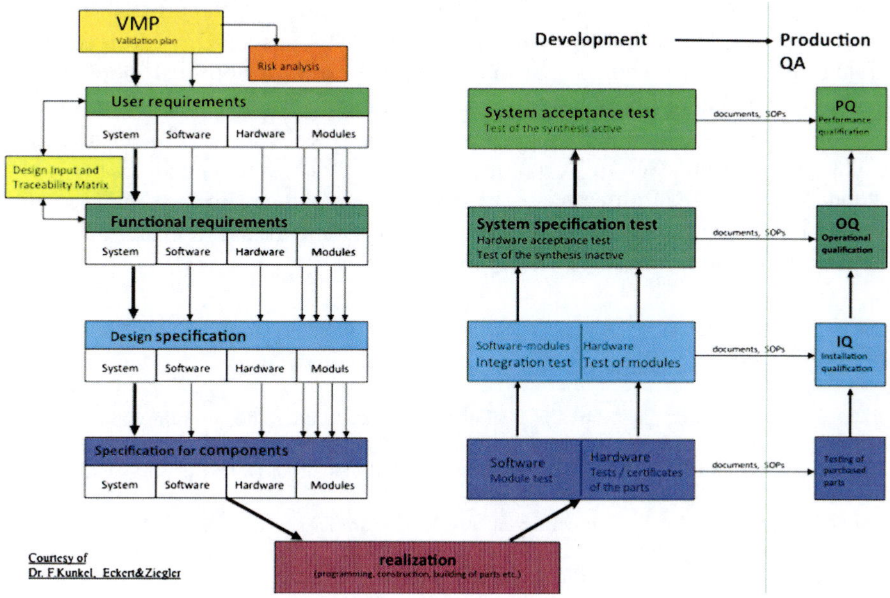

Fig. 6 A risk-based approach to a compliant system

Available systems are well established, and many centers have already performed hundreds of syntheses in a reproducible and robust manner.

Preloaded cassette-based modules, manufactured under cGMP standards, could represent a further improvement in terms of safety and compliance with regulations, but huge investments are needed, and the clinical demand is not as great as for ^{18}F-fluorodeoxyglucose (FDG).

Further development toward miniaturization is possible. Microfluidic approaches could open interesting perspectives, at least for ^{68}Ga labeling. Major concerns are, however, radiolysis due to the high concentration of radionuclide and surface effects.

Development of ^{68}Ga radiopharmaceuticals as freeze-dried kits, similar to ^{99}Mo/^{99m}Tc-generator-based ^{99m}Tc radiopharmaceuticals, may indeed be an alternative to cyclotron-based radiopharmaceuticals. Use of bifunctional chelating agents based on NOTA scaffold might allow for simple kit-based radiopharmaceuticals (Velikyan et al. 2008).

Detailed discussion on kit development issues lies beyond the scope of this chapter. Anyway, moving towards kit-based preparations will require simplified post-processing technology. Remaining differences between generators and eluates should be overcome by new generator concepts which avoid metal-base matrixes and utilize HCl at less than 0.1 M to achieve optimum conditions for high yield and quick, room-temperature labeling. More effort is needed on generators themselves than on automation technology.

The availability of a commercial $^{68}Ge/^{68}Ga$ generator with potential for routine application and a favorable chemistry using DOTA- and NOTA-derived bifunctional chelators has opened a brilliant future for almost unlimited application of ^{68}Ga in all fields of noninvasive molecular imaging with radioactive probes.

Automation technology has grown together with the huge clinical demand for ^{68}Ga-DOTA somatostatin receptor agonists, which have become the golden standard for PET/CT imaging of neuroendocrine tumors, to become one of the most important tools for bridging the development and application of new ^{68}Ga-radiolabeled molecules into clinical practice.

References

Bauwens M, Chekol R, Vanbilloen H et al (2010) Optimal buffer choice of the radiosynthesis of ^{68}Ga-Dotatoc for clinical application. Nucl Med Biol 31(8):753–758

Breeman WAP, de Jong M, de Blois E et al (2005) Radiolabelling DOTA-peptide with ^{68}Ga. Eur J Nucl Med 32:478–485

Buchmann I, Henze M, Engelbrecht S et al (2007) Comparison of ^{68}Ga-DOTATOC PET and ^{111}In-DTPAOC (octreoscan) SPECT in patients with neuroendocrine tumours. Eur J Nucl Med Mol Imaging 34(10):1617–1626

Campana D, Ambrosini V, Pezzilli R et al (2010) Standardized uptake values of ^{68}Ga-DOTANOC PET: a promising prognostic tool in neuroendocrine tumors. J Nucl Med 51(3):353–359

Deutsch E (1993) Clinical PET: its time has come? J Nucl Med 34:1132–1133

Decristoforo C, Knopp R, Von Guggenberg E et al (2007) A fully automated synthesis for the preparation of ^{68}Ga-labelled peptides. Nucl Med Commun 28(11):870–875

Di Pierro D, Rizzello A, Cicoria G et al (2008) Radiolabelling, quality control and radiochemical purity assessment of the octreotide analogue ^{68}Ga DOTA NOC. Appl Radiat Isot 66:1091–1096

Fani M, Del Pozzo L, Abiraj K et al (2011) PET of somatostatin receptor-positive tumors using ^{64}Cu and ^{68}Ga somatostatin antagonists: the chelate makes the difference. J Nucl Med 52(7):1110–1118

GAMP® 5: A risk-based approach to compliant GxP computerized systems. ISPE 2008

Hayes RL, Carlton JE, Byrd BL (1965) Bone scaning with gallium-68: a carrier effect. J Nucl Med 6:605–610

Harris WR, Pecoraro V (1983) Thermodynamic binding constants for gallium transferrin. Biochemistry 22:292–299

Kowalski J, Henze M, Schuhmacher J et al (2003) Evaluation of positron emission tomography imaging using [^{68}Ga]-DOTA-D-Phe1-Tyr3-octreotide in comparison to [111In]-DTPAOC SPECT. First results in patients with neuroendocrine tumors. Mol Imaging Biol 5:42–48

Maecke HR, Hofmann M, Haberkorn U (2005) ^{68}Ga peptides in tumor imaging. J Nucl Med 46:172S–176S

Meyer GJ, Maecke H, Schuhmacher J et al (2004) ^{68}Ga- labelled DOTA-derivatised peptide ligands. Eur J Nucl Med Mol Imaging 31:1097–1104

Ocak M, Antretter M, Knopp R et al (2010) Full automation of 68 Ga labelling of DOTA-peptides including cation exchange prepurification. Appl Radiat Isot 68:297–302

Petrik M, Knetsch PA, Knopp R et al (2011) Radiolabelling of peptides for PET, SPECT and therapeutic applications using a fully automated disposable cassette system. Nucl Med Commun 32(10):887–895

Roesch F, Riss PJ (2010) The reinassance of the $^{68}Ge/^{68}Ga$ radionuclide generator initiates new developments in ^{68}Ga radiopharmaceutical chemistry. Curr Top Med Chem 10:1633–1668

Shealey CN, Aronow S, Brownell GL (1964) Gallium-68 as a scanning agents for intracranial lesions. J Nucl Med 5:161–167
Velikyan I, Beyer GJ, Langstrom B (2004) Microwave-supported preparation of ^{68}Ga bioconjugates with high specific radioactivity. Bioconjugate Chem 15(3):554–560
Velikyan I, Maecke H, Langstrom B (2008) Convenient preparation of ^{68}Ga-based PET radiopharmaceuticals at room temperature. Bioconjugate Chem 19:569–573
Zhernosekov KP, Filosofov DV, Baum RP et al (2007) Processing of generator-produced Ga-68 for medical application. J Nucl Med 48(10):1741–1748

Post-Processing via Cation Exchange Cartridges: Versatile Options

F. Rösch

Abstract

New ^{68}Ge/^{68}Ga radionuclide generators provide the positron emitter ^{68}Ga ($T_{1/2}$ = 67.7 min) as an easily available and relatively inexpensive source of a PET nuclide for labeling of interesting targeting vectors. However, currently available "ionic" ^{68}Ge/^{68}Ga radionuclide generators are not necessarily optimized for the routine synthesis of ^{68}Ga-labeled radiopharmaceuticals in a clinical environment. Post-processing of ^{68}Ge/^{68}Ga generators using cation exchange resins provides chemically and radiochemically pure ^{68}Ga with 97±2% within less than 4 min, with ^{68}Ge almost completely removed, and ready for online labeling. This simple, fast, and efficient technology can be extended for new applications. The options are (a) to transfer ^{68}Ga from the cation exchange resin onto an anion exchange resin, to remove acetone, and to further purify the ^{68}Ga, (b) to obtain ^{68}Ga in pure non-aqueous solution via $^{68}Ga(acac)_3$ as a synthon for syntheses in organic solvents, and (c) to create an option toward instantaneous determination of ^{68}Ge breakthrough, what may be required prior to the release of ^{68}Ga radiopharmaceutical preparations.

Abbreviations

TODGA N,N,N',N'-tetra-n-octyldiglycolamide

F. Rösch (✉)
Institute of Nuclear Chemistry,
Johannes Gutenberg-University,
55128 Mainz, Germany
e-mail: froesch@uni-mainz.de

R. P. Baum and F. Rösch (eds.), *Theranostics, Gallium-68, and Other Radionuclides*,
Recent Results in Cancer Research 194, DOI: 10.1007/978-3-642-27994-2_3,

Contents

1 Introduction

New ^{68}Ge/^{68}Ga radionuclide generators provide the positron emitter ^{68}Ga ($t_{1/2}$ = 67.7 min) as an easily available and relatively inexpensive PET nuclide for labeling interesting targeting vectors. The ^{68}Ge/^{68}Ga radionuclide generator provides an excellent source of positron-emitting ^{68}Ga for application of ^{68}Ga-labeled compounds using PET. However, currently available "ionic" ^{68}Ge/^{68}Ga radionuclide generators are not necessarily optimized for routine synthesis of ^{68}Ga-labeled radiopharmaceuticals in a clinical environment. The eluates have rather large volume (up to 5–10 mL for a complete generator elution), high acidity (0.1–1.0 N, depending on the generator type), initial ^{68}Ge breakthrough in the range 10^{-3}–10^{-2}%, increasing with time or usage frequency, and metallic impurities such as stable Zn^{II} (generated by on-generator decay of ^{68}Ga), Ti^{IV}, Sn^{IV}, or other metals as a consequence of use of metal oxide-based generator matrixes.

We have developed an effective post-processing method for ^{68}Ge/^{68}Ga generators to provide high ^{68}Ga recovery, removal of ^{68}Ge, removal of metallic impurities, and minimized volumes for labeling. This is easily achieved by online passage of the generator eluate through a small cation exchange resin (CEX). Subsequently, ^{68}Ga is eluted in 400 μL of a second mixture of acetone and HCl (N2) from the cation exchanger. The ^{68}Ga recovery is as high as 97% within 3 min, the additional removal of ^{68}Ge reaches four orders of magnitude, and the removal of metallic impurities including the inherent stable Zn^{II} is almost quantitative. Finally, the volume for subsequent labeling is just 400 μL at low acid concentration, resulting in excellent yields of ^{68}Ga synthesis reactions. The chemical procedure has in part been adopted by commercial modules combining generator elution, post-processing, and radiopharmaceutical syntheses.

In extending this concept, the temporarily absorption of highly purified ^{68}Ga on the small cation exchange cartridge appears to be an ideal starting point for various further options. The present chapter introduces various directions:

1. The purified, solid-phase-adsorbed ^{68}Ga was subsequently subject to anion exchange-based processing to achieve ^{68}Ga fractions free of any organic component such as acetone (Loktionova et al. 2011).

2. The other approach investigated was to use it for versatile synthesis of ^{68}Ga tracers under nonhydrous conditions. A convenient method was investigated for ^{68}Ga-labeling using solid phase (cation exchange resin)-derived ^{68}Ga-acetyl-acetonate, ^{68}Ga(acac)$_3$. The initial aqueous generator eluate was transferred online to a cationic exchange resin to quantitatively absorb ^{68}Ga as described before as usual. From this resin, ^{68}Ga was eluted with different acetone–based, nonaqueous solvent systems, providing n.c.a. ^{68}Ga(acac)$_3$ as labeling agent. More than 95% of the initially eluted ^{68}Ga was eluted from the cationic exchange resin with 600 μL of 98% acetone/2% acetylacetone mixture.
   ^{68}Ga-labeled water-insoluble porphyrin derivatives were chosen as model compounds for a proof of principle for labeling of lipophilic compounds. Labeling of these model compounds was performed in chloroform (Zoller et al. 2010).
3. Finally, the extreme potential of the cation exchange resin introduced by us (Zhernosekov et al. 2007) to almost quantitatively discriminate chemically between ^{68}Ga^{III} and ^{68}Ge^{IV} may be extended to analyze the breakthrough of a ^{68}Ge/^{68}Ga radionuclide generator. The concept lies in separating ^{68}Ga online quantitatively from ^{68}Ge, which passes completely the cation exchange resin into the waste vial. If ^{68}Ga-free, the count rate measured in that vial will represent the increasing generation of ^{68}Ga from that ^{68}Ge. This facilitates instant measurement of ^{68}Ge levels even within about 1 h post elution.

2 The Initial Cation Exchange-Based Post-Purification Concept

The generator eluate, e.g., 10 mL 0.1 M HCl (but maybe also 20 mL from two successive generators), and maybe any volume of HCl eluates of different concentration (e.g., ranging from about 0.01 N to about 0.6 N), is transferred directly and online to a cation exchange resin, ideally AG 400 Wx8, minus 400 mesh (but maybe also similar resins after adopting to the specific requirements).

^{68}Ga is thereby adsorbed quantitatively online. Chemical impurities such as Fe^{III}, Zn^{II}, Ti^{IV}, but also a significant part of the breakthrough ^{68}Ge are almost completely eluted from the cation exchange column into waste (Fig. 1a).

In an additional washing step using 1 mL of HCl/acetone mixture (solution N1), remaining impurities are removed from the cation exchange cartridge, while ^{68}Ga efficiently stays in the resin (Fig. 1b).

Finally, the transfer of purified ^{68}Ga from the resin into a (labeling) vial is almost quantitative. Applying 400 μL of 0.05 N HCl/98% acetone (solution N2), overall, 97 ± 2% of the ^{68}Ga initially obtained from the generator is isolated by even 3 min after the elution procedure (Fig. 1c).

This ^{68}Ga is chemically pure. The ^{68}Ge content/breakthrough is decreased from $>10^{-3}$ initially to $<10^{-7}$% finally. The final volume of the purified ^{68}Ga fraction is low, as is the pH (400 μL 0.05 N HCl/acetone). As the purified ^{68}Ga is eluted directly into a labeling vial containing amounts of precursor, the removal of

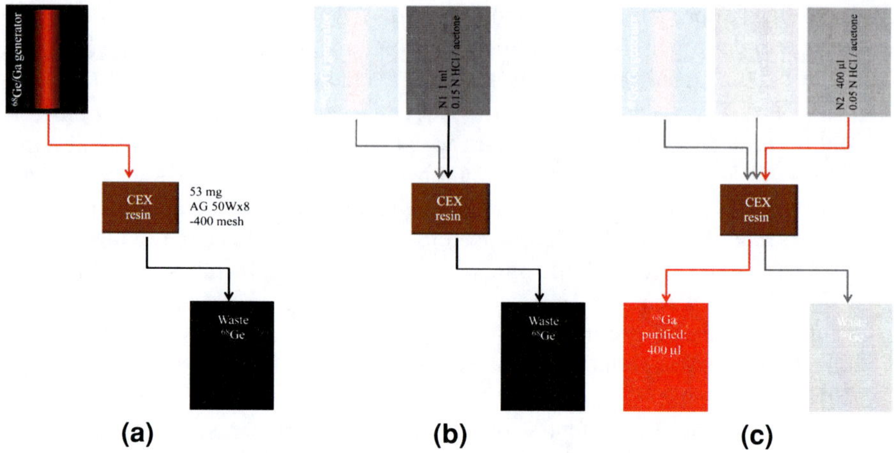

Fig. 1 Successive steps of post-processing of $^{68}Ge/^{68}Ga$ radionuclide generator eluates via cation exchangers (Zhernosekov et al. 2007; Asti et al. 2008). **a** ^{68}Ga is adsorbed online by passing the $^{68}Ge/^{68}Ga$ radionuclide generator eluate through a 53 mg cation exchange (CEX) AG 50 Wx8 cartridge. Chemical impurities such as Fe^{III}, Zn^{II}, Ti^{IV}, but also a significant part of the breakthrough ^{68}Ge are eluted almost completely from the cation exchange column into waste. **b** In an additional washing step using 1 mL of 0.15 N HCl/acetone mixture (solution N1), remaining Fe^{III}, Zn^{II}, Ti^{IV}, and ^{68}Ge are removed from the cation exchange cartridge, while ^{68}Ga efficiently stays in the resin. **c** Transfer of purified ^{68}Ga from the CEX resin into a (labeling) vial by applying 400 μL of 0.05 N HCl/98% acetone (solution N2). Overall, 97 ± 2% of the ^{68}Ga initially obtained from the generator is isolated even by 3 min after the elution procedure

metallic impurities results in high labeling yields and ^{68}Ga radiopharmaceuticals of high specific activities. For, e.g., DOTATOC, labeling is achieved in pure water (adding 5 mL ultrapure water to the precursor creates a final pH of 2.3 after adding the ^{68}Ga fraction of 400 μL 0.05 N HCl/acetone), thus avoiding any addition of buffers. About >95% labeling at 10 min of >450 MBq/nmol DOTATOC is obtained. Overall, ca. 65% product yields are achieved (not corrected for decay) with respect to the initially eluted ^{68}Ga.

3 Combined Cation and Anion Exchange-Based Post-Processing

The radionuclide ^{68}Ga is desorbed from the resin quantitatively with 0.4 mL of 0.05 N HCl/98% acetone solution (N2). Contents of the acetone in the reaction mixture are low and nontoxic (Zhernosekov et al. 2007; Roesch 2010). They are easily reduced to nondetectable levels within labeling procedures at elevated temperature. They might be, however, avoided for direct in vivo applications or for radiolabeling reactions performed under high temperature or for chemical reactions requiring pure aqueous media exclusively.

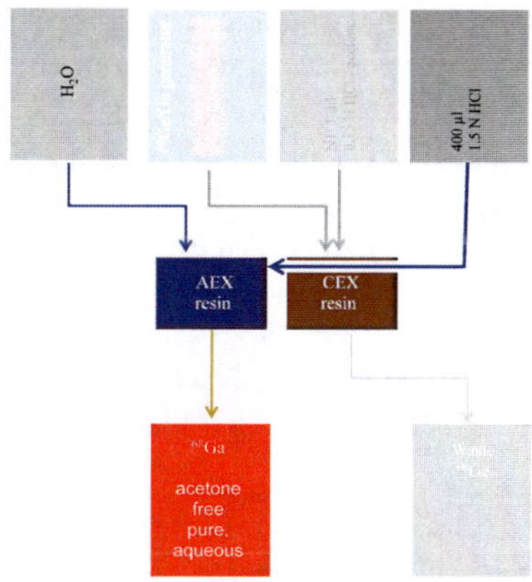

Fig. 2 Essentials of the combined cation (CEX) and anion exchanger (AEX)-based post-processing (Loktionova et al. 2011). The purified, solid-phase-adsorbed ^{68}Ga is effectively transfered to subsequent anion exchange-based processing and eluted from it using, e.g., water

The aim of present work is to develop an improved column-based chemical strategy combining anion exchange (AEX) processing. Direct preconcentration of ^{68}Ga from the original eluate and its purification are supposed to be performed on the cation exchanger according to Zhernosekov et al. (2007). This ^{68}Ga can be eluted with hydrochloric acid solutions of >2 N concentration. For effective transfer of the purified ^{68}Ga into the aqueous phase of low acidity and small volume a secondary microcolumn, now AEX based, is introduced into the process, which allows direct readsorption of gallium eluted form the cation exchanger. From the AEX, ^{68}Ga can be finally striped with a small volume of pure water. For this purpose a typical anion exchanger and a novel extraction chromatographic resin based on N,N,N',N'-tetra-n-octyldiglycolamide (TODGA) is applied (Loktionova et al. 2011).

A conceptual flow sheet of the system, including the combination of cation exchange and anion exchange, e.g., AG 1 × 8 or TODGA, columns is presented in Fig. 2. The columns are connected consecutively via three-way valves. In the first step, 7 mL 0.1 N HCl passes through the generator and the cation exchange resin into the waste. Step 2 involves eluting the cation exchanger with 1 mL of hydrochloric acid/acetone solution N1 into the waste. The third step is the nearly quantitative transfer of ^{68}Ga from the cation exchange column onto the anion exchanger resins with 3 mL of 5 or 4 M HCl. [This represents a significant improvement compared with other anion exchange-based procedures, as high concentrations of HCl and large volumes are avoided (Schumacher and Maier-Borst 1981; Meyer et al. 2004)]. While ^{68}Ga is quantitatively adsorbed on both resins, the 3 mL of HCl continues to the waste vial, thereby removing the acetone introduced at the CEX step via solution N1. (Use of acetone may even be completely avoided by removing the high-performance purification of ^{68}Ga from metallic impurities via solution N1. However, in view of the idea of almost completely removing ^{68}Zn, as much Fe as possible, and in particular ^{68}Ge, this special feature of the process should be retained.)

From the supplementary anion exchange, e.g., AG or TODGA columns, ^{68}Ga is eluted using 0.3 or 1.0 mL water, respectively, into the product vial. With 98% effectivity for the cation exchange part, 92 and 98% yields were obtained for desorbing ^{68}Ga from the anion exchange and chromatographic TODGA columns, respectively. The overall yield in the final 0.3–1.0 mL water fraction is 87 ± 5% (for AG 400 1-X8) and 96% (for TODGA resin) with respect to the initial generator eluate.

4 Post-Processing Towards Nonaqueous Systems for Labeling Lipophilic Compounds

While almost all currently used ^{68}Ga radiopharmaceuticals, particularly labeling precursors, are compounds that are easily soluble in aqueous solutions, some promising ^{68}Ga tracers requiring nonaqueous synthesis conditions may be developed (Roesch and Riss 2010; Riss et al. 2010). The other direction for continuing development of the cation exchange post-processing thus proposes a convenient method for ^{68}Ga-labeling under anhydrous conditions using solid-phase-derived gallium acetylacetonate, [^{68}Ga]Ga(acac)$_3$. Again, the initial aqueous generator eluate is first transferred online to a cation exchange resin (SCX in the present case) and ^{68}Ga is absorbed quantitatively. From this resin, ^{68}Ga is eluted with different acetone-based, nonaqueous solvent systems (Zoller et al. 2010). The resin is washed with solution N1 (0.15 N, 20% in acetone, 1 mL). The resin is dried in a stream of argon for 2 min, followed by elution of the trapped radioactivity as a [^{68}Ga]Ga(acac)$_3$ complex using 2% acetylacetone in acetone in volumes ranging from 200 to 1,600 μL. For comparison, the cation exchange resin was also eluted with 97.6% acetone/0.05 M HCl or 100% acetone in the same manner (Fig. 3). More than 95% of the generator-eluted ^{68}Ga was obtained from the cation exchange resin with 600 μL of 98% acetone/2% acetylacetone mixture, providing n.c.a. [^{68}Ga]Ga(acac)$_3$ as labeling agent. The identity and purity of the labeling agent were verified via radio-thin-layer chromatography (TLC) using 1 μL sample aliquots on reverse-phase TLC sheets. Radio-TLC was developed in ethyl acetate:ethanol 1:1 (v/v) with [^{68}Ga]Ga(acac)$_3$ $R_f = 0.85$ and ^{68}Ga^{3+} $R_f = 0.0$.

Water-insoluble macrocyclic polypyrrole derivatives were chosen as model compounds for a proof of principle of labeling of lipophilic compounds with ^{68}Ga (Zoller et al. 2010). Labeling of two different porphyrin derivatives, *meso*-tetraphenyl-porphyrin (Tpp) and 3-(1-hydroxyheptyl) deuteroporphyrin dimethyl-ester (HHDPD), was performed in chloroform in a focused microwave synthesis system in yields of up to 90% within 5 min using phenol as co-ligand. Moreover, new co-ligands were investigated to be more effective and significantly less toxic than phenol. Among the phenol alternatives, gentisic acid (2,5-dihydroxybenzoic acid, DHB, 5 mg) emerged as the most useful, nontoxic phenol substitute. It facilitates reduction of the load of co-ligand by 95% while providing increased labeling yield of 97%. ^{68}Ga-labeled porphyrins may facilitate medical applications for molecular imaging via positron emission tomography (Zoller et al. 2010). Purification of the labeled ^{68}Ga porphyrin derivatives was performed via solid-phase extraction,

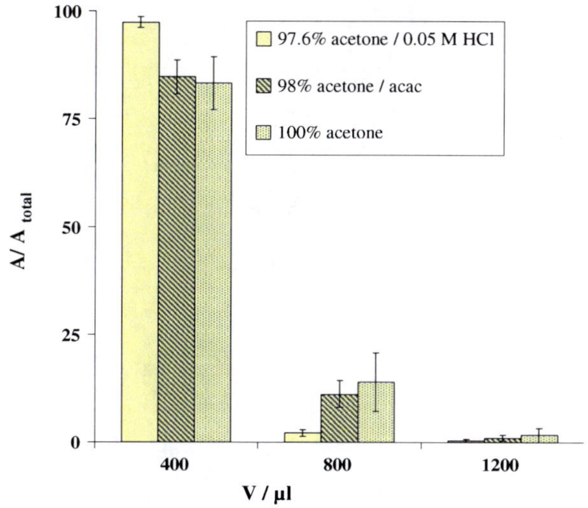

Fig. 3 Elution profile of gallium-68 from the cation exchange SCX resin using different acetone systems ($n = 4$). The SCX column was loaded with 150 µL of these solutions first, and the resin-bound ^{68}Ga was allowed to equilibrate with the eluent for 2 min

resulting in radiochemical purity (RCP) of 98 ± 1% for ^{68}Ga-Tpp and 95 ± 2% for ^{68}Ga-HHDPD. RCP was verified via radio-TLC and radio-HPLC. Overall radiochemical yields of 73 ± 6% for [^{68}Ga]Tpp and 50 ± 9% for [^{68}Ga]HHDPD were achieved. Total time of synthesis, consisting of generator elution, post-processing, labeling, and purification, was 17 min for both compounds.

In conclusion, n.c.a. [^{68}Ga]Ga(acac)$_3$ as labeling synthon for synthesis in nonaqueous media was obtained in high yield by adopting cation exchange-based post-processing of ^{68}Ge/^{68}Ga radionuclide generator. Based on these results, the novel procedure providing n.c.a. [^{68}Ga]Ga(acac)$_3$ offers a wide scope of applications for this labeling agent.

5 Instant Quantification of Generator ^{68}Ge Breakthrough

Finally, the extreme potential of the cation exchange resin (Zhernosekov et al. 2007) to almost quantitatively discriminate chemically between $^{68}Ga^{III}$ and $^{68}Ge^{IV}$ was applied to analyze the breakthrough of a ^{68}Ge/^{68}Ga radionuclide generator. The concept lies in separating ^{68}Ga online quantitatively from ^{68}Ge, which passes completely the cation exchange resin into the waste vial. If ^{68}Ga-free, the (relative) count rate or (absolute) activity measured in that vial will represent the increasing generation of ^{68}Ga from that ^{68}Ge. This facilitates instant measurement of ^{68}Ge levels even within about 1 h post elution. The scheme of the procedure is illustrated in Fig. 4.

A 2-year-old ^{68}Ge/^{68}Ga generator (EZAG, Obninsk) was used with yield of ^{68}Ga of about 100 MBq and breakthrough of ^{68}Ge of about 85 kBq. The generator was eluted with 5 mL 0.1 M HCl. For separation, cation exchange AG 50 W-X8 and

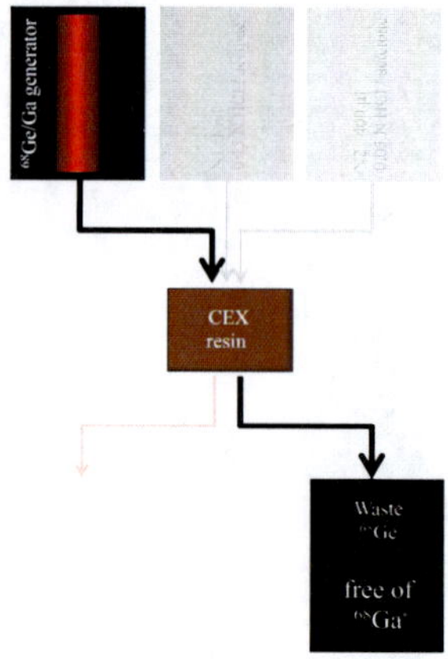

Fig. 4 Principle of online isolation of ^{68}Ga on the cation exchange resin to provide ^{68}Ge solutions completely free of ^{68}Ga

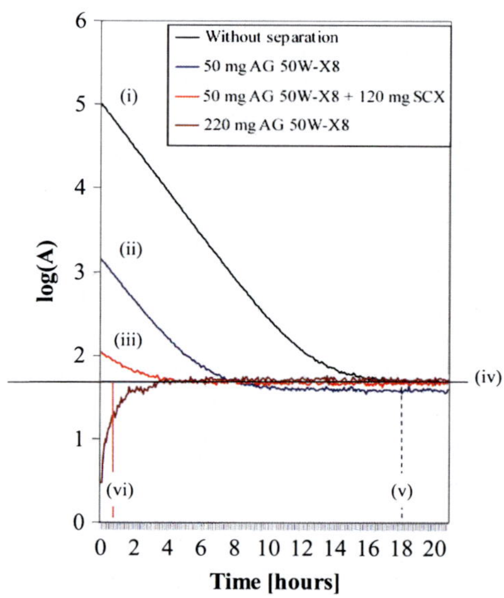

Fig. 5 Effects of removing ^{68}Ga from ^{68}Ge breakthrough for selected cation exchange resins. ^{68}Ga activities measured in kBq: *1* for initial, nonprocessed ^{68}Ge/^{68}Ga radionuclide generator eluate over time; *2 3*, and *4* for ^{68}Ge waste solutions after application of 50 mg AG50 Wx8, 50 mg AG50 Wx8 + 120 mg SCX, and 220 mg AG50 Wx8, respectively; *4* in equilibrium, reflecting the level of ^{68}Ge activity achieved at different time-points after elution; *5* after about 18 h without purification; *6* half of the ^{68}Ga equilibrium activity measured at 67.7 min post elution, representing 50% of the ^{68}Ge activity present

SCX resins were used separately and in various combinations, such as 50 mg AG 50 W-X, 50 mg AG 50 W-X8 + 30 mg SCX, 50 mg AG 50 W-X8 + 120 mg SCX, 220 mg AG 50 W-X8, and 220 mg AG 50 W-X8 + 120 mg SCX. In the case of using two resins, the generator was eluted first through the AG 50 W-X8 and then through the SCX column. Results are indicated in Fig. 5.

Measurements of absolute ^{68}Ga activity were performed by Curie-meter every 5 min (automated mode) during at least 20 h. For control, a sample without separation was also measured.

^{68}Ge was quantitatively separated from ^{68}Ga using cation exchange columns AG 50 W-X8 and SCX, either separately in the case of 220 mg AG 50 W-X8 or in combination. ^{68}Ge can thus be quantified directly after the initial elution, by just letting the ^{68}Ga increase for one (or ½) half-life of 67.7 min.

6 Conclusions

Post-processing of ^{68}Ge/^{68}Ga radionuclide generators using cation exchange resin provides chemically and radiochemically pure (97 ± 2%) ^{68}Ga within 4 min, with ^{68}Ge almost completely removed, and ready for online labeling (Zhernosekov et al. 2007). This simple, fast, and efficient technology can easily be extended for new applications. The concept is to:

1. Retain online cation exchange purification.
2. Guarantee removal of chemical impurities and ^{68}Ge breakthrough.
3. Achieve high ^{68}Ga transfer from cation exchange resin.

- Subsequently, by use of 1.5 N HCl to transfer ^{68}Ga from cation exchange resin to anion exchange resin, acetone is removed and the ^{68}Ga is further purified. ^{68}Ga quantitatively free of ^{68}Ge breakthrough is observed in acetone-free, pure aqueous solution of highest chemical purity at ca. 80% with respect to the initial generator eluate ^{68}Ga activity.
- In a second option, ^{68}Ga is obtained in pure nonaqueous solution via $^{68}Ga(acac)_3$ as a synthon for syntheses in organic solvents at ca. 70% with respect to the initial generator eluate.
- Moreover, just an increase in the quantity of cation exchanger used provides an elegant option towards instantaneous ^{68}Ge analytics, which may be required prior to release of ^{68}Ga radiopharmaceutical preparations.
- In the future, another option may be investigated, namely to synthesize ^{68}Ga radiopharmaceuticals "on-resin" by carefully adopting adequate solvents containing the labeling precursor, the resin material, residence time, temperature, etc.

References

Asti M, De Pietri G, Fraternali A, Grassi E, Sghedoni R, Fioroni F, Roesch F, Versari A, Salvo D (2008) Validation of ^{68}Ge/^{68}Ga generator processing by chemical purification for routine clinical application of ^{68}Ga-DOTATOC. Nucl Med Biol 35(6):721–724

Loktionova NS, Belozub AN, Filosofov DV, Zhernosekov KP, Wagner T, Türler A, Rösch F (2011) Improved column-based radiochemical processing of the generator produced ^{68}Ga. Appl Radiat Isot 69:942–946

Meyer G-J, Mäcke HR, Schuhmacher J, Knapp WH, Hofmann M (2004) ^{68}Ga-labelled DOTA-derivatised peptide ligands. Eur J Nucl Med 31:1097

Roesch F (2010) Impurity in ^{68}Ga-peptide preparation using processed generator eluate. J Nucl Med 51:496

Roesch F, Riss PJ (2010) The Renaissance of the ^{68}Ge/^{68}Ga radionuclide generator initiates new developments in ^{68}Ga radiopharmaceutical chemistry. Curr Top Med Chem 10(16): 1633–1668

Riss P, Hanik N, Rösch F (2010) Studies towards the development of lipophilic bifunctional N_3S_3 chelators for ^{68}Ga. Radiochim Acta 98/8:519–523

Schumacher J, Maier-Borst W (1981) A new ^{68}Ge/^{68}Ga radioisotope generator system for production of ^{68}Ga in dilute HCl. Int J Appl Radiat Isot 32:31

Zhernosekov KP, Filosofov DV, Baum RP, Aschoff P, Bihl H, Razbash AA, Jahn M, Jennewein M, Rösch F (2007) Processing of generator-produced ^{68}Ga for medical application. J Nucl Med 48:1741

Zoller F, Riss PJ, Montforts F-P, Rösch F (2010) Efficient post-processing of aqueous generator eluates facilitates ^{68}Ga-labelling under anhydrous conditions. Radiochim Acta 98(3):157–160

^{68}Ga Generator Integrated System: Elution–Purification–Concentration Integration

Van So Le

Abstract

A ^{68}Ge/^{68}Ga generator combined with an automated ^{68}Ga eluate purification–concentration unit [*radioisotope generator integrated system* (RADIGIS)], specially designed for ^{68}Ga processing (RADIGIS-^{68}Ga), was developed. The high-stability sorbents of a nanocrystalline structure Zr-Ti ceramic matrix were used for immobilizing the ^{68}Ge, and the ^{68}Ga was eluted from the sorbent column with 3.5 mL 0.05–0.1 M HCl solution following an optimized ^{68}Ga-elution schedule. The ^{68}Ge breakthrough $<10^{-3}$% and no ^{68}Ge zone spreading/drift found in PET imaging of the ^{68}Ga generator column prove the excellent performance of the sorbents. ^{68}Ga eluate was purified on a small column of salt-form ion exchange resin using an aqueous alcohol solution mixture of hydrochloric and ascorbic acids, and halide salts. An alkali solution was used for stripping ^{68}Ga from the ion exchange resin column to obtain a purified ^{68}Ga solution, which is conditioned with acidic solution to obtain a final ^{68}Ga product in either 0.75 mL 0.5 M NaCl solution of pH 3–4 or 0.5 M sodium acetate or citrate solution of pH 5. The ^{68}Ge content in purified ^{68}Ga solution was $<10^{-6}$%. An insignificant metallic contamination including ^{68}Zn found in the ^{68}Ga solution and its alkalinity–acidity were evaluated with respect to ^{68}Ga radiolabeling efficacy for DOTATATE and DOTATOC ligands. Quality control protocols were also developed to evaluate the quality of ^{68}Ga solution.

V. S. Le (✉)
ANSTO LifeSciences, Australian Nuclear Science and Technology Organisation,
MEDISOTEC—Medical Isotope Techniques 14(1) Dwyer Street,
Gymea, NSW 2227, Australia
e-mail: Vansole01@gmail.com

R. P. Baum and F. Rösch (eds.), *Theranostics, Gallium-68, and Other Radionuclides*,
Recent Results in Cancer Research 194, DOI: 10.1007/978-3-642-27994-2_4,

Contents

1 Introduction

The short-lived radioactive isotopes produced from radionuclide generators are effectively used in diagnostic nuclear medicine and in biomedical research. The ^{99m}Tc generator is a well-known example and most widely used in single-photon emission computed tomography (SPECT) for diagnostic imaging. Today, with the fast expansion of advanced superior techniques for tomographic reconstruction in positron emission tomography (PET) imaging, the supply of positron-emitting radionuclides becomes crucial. The use of short-lived radioisotopes ^{18}F, ^{11}C, and ^{15}O in PET imaging is well established. Unfortunately, all of these short-lived (half-life less than 2 h) positron-emitting radionuclides are only available from onsite, expensive cyclotrons operating in a handful of major hospitals. Expansion of the use of positron-emitting radionuclides produced from radionuclide generators is always desirable, subsequently benefiting the superiority of the PET-based molecular imaging technique.

It has been known that, among the possible generator-produced positron-emitting nuclides, the ^{68}Ga isotope, with its desirable half-life of 68 min and generated from the long-lived parent ^{68}Ge with 287-day half-life, has the greatest potential for wide and cost-effective application in daily clinical PET practice.

Biomedically, current nuclear medicine applications of ^{68}Ga isotope and ongoing research activities are based on its favorable properties as follows: Gallium element is itself known as a second chemotherapy agent, after platinum, due to its high and specific affinity toward tumor tissues. Well-known coordination chemistry of gallium is advantageous for radiolabeling of radiopharmaceuticals. The readiness of the ^{68}Ga radioactive isotope to couple to small biomolecules makes it potentially an alternative to ^{18}F- and ^{11}C-based PET radiopharmacy. Several chelate compounds developed for radiolabeling of peptides and/or protein entities with metallic radionuclides are well suited to ^{68}Ga labeling. Today, ^{68}Ga finds significant applications in conventional nuclear medicine practice, including ^{68}Ga-EDTA (EDTA = Ethylenediaminetetraacetic acid) for detection of blood–brain barrier integrity and ^{68}Ga-PLED (PLED = *N, N'*-bis(pyridoxyl)ethylenediamine-*N, N'*-diacetic acid) or ^{68}Ga-EDTA for renal function investigation. ^{68}Ga-based targeting PET radiopharmaceuticals under phase III clinical trial are ^{68}Ga-DOTA-NOC (DOTA = 1, 4, 7, 10-tetraazacyclododecane-1, 4, 7, 10-tetraacetic acid, NOC= 1-Nal^3-octreotide), ^{68}Ga-DOTA-TATE (DOTA = 1, 4, 7, 10-tetraazacyclododecane-1, 4, 7, 10-tetraacetic acid, TATE = [tyr^3, thr^8]-octreotide), ^{68}Ga-DOTA-lanreotide, and ^{68}Ga-DOTA-TOC (DOTA = 1, 4, 7, 10-tetraazacyclododecane-1, 4, 7, 10-tetraacetic acid, TOC = D-phe^1-tyr^3-octreotide), which are used for PET imaging of several subtypes of somatostatin receptors for imaging of neuroendocrine tumors; ^{68}Ga-DOTA-bombesin for PET imaging of gastrointestinal stromal, colon, and prostate cancer; and ^{68}Ga-AMBA (AMBA = DO3A-CH(2)CO-G-[4-aminobenzoyl]-QWAVGHLM-NH(2)) for study on NMB (non-peptide neuromedin B) and GRP-R (gastrin releasing peptide receptors) bombesin receptors on medullary thyroid cancer.

In terms of nuclear physics, ^{68}Ga is considered as a second important β^+ emitter (after ^{18}F) efficiently used in PET imaging with the following favorable characteristics: High positron abundance and good PET imaging resolution are the most important features of ^{68}Ga when used for biomedical imaging. Decay via β^+ particles (with the 511-keV annihilation gamma-ray of 178.2% intensity) occurs in 89.14% of atoms. The 836.02-keV positron radiation gives a PET imaging resolution of about 2.3 mm (bone) to 11.5 mm (lung) for living tissues (compared with 0.65–2.7 mm in the case of ^{18}F). These values are well within the system resolution of modern PET cameras (4–5 mm) and even high-resolution PET systems (3 mm). A further advantage is that there is no associated gamma impact on PET images. The insignificant amounts of associated gamma emissions (0.03407%) falling into the commonly used PET energy window of 350–700 keV have almost no impact on PET images. From the radiation point of view, ^{68}Ga conforms well with conventional radiation safety. The $\Gamma_{20\mathrm{keV}}$ exposure rate constant of 0.179 μSv.m^2/MBq.h (compared with 0.188 μSv.m^2/MBq.h for ^{18}F) makes use of ^{18}FDG [(^{18}F)fluorodeoxyglucose] standard radiation safety automatic infusion systems feasible. In terms of economy and convenience of use, ^{68}Ga offers the advantages of cost-effectiveness and on-demand availability: The long-lived parent nuclide ^{68}Ge can deliver cost-effective PET imaging due to the generator shelf-life of approximately 2 years. The ^{68}Ge/^{68}Ga generator also renders ^{68}Ga-based PET radiopharmacy independent of an onsite cyclotron. This means that this generator is ideally suited to on-demand availability of β^+ emitters for biomedical experiments and clinical targeting imaging, both in remote PET centers without a cyclotron and even in cyclotron-operating PET centers. The ability to formulate kits and the simplicity/elegance of its use are further good reasons to use ^{68}Ga in daily clinical practice. It is predicted by experts that ^{68}Ga will become the ^{99m}Tc for PET/CT (X-ray computed tomography, also Computed tomography). The potential for provision of kit-formulated precursors along with a ^{68}Ga generator, similar to ^{99m}Tc in vivo kits, will make this generator become the mainstay for nuclear medicine molecular imaging in the very near future.

To date, various $^{68}Ge/^{68}Ga$ generator systems have been developed using two different techniques. First, solvent extraction techniques using acetyl acetone-carbon tetrachloride/dilute HCl solution and 8-hydroxyquinoline/chloroform have been applied by different research groups (Erhardt and Wetch 1978).

Column technique-based $^{68}Ge/^{68}Ga$ generators were developed using different sorbents as generator column packing materials and either alkaline or acidic solutions or aqueous solutions containing complexing agents as eluents to separate ^{68}Ga by elution from its parent nuclide ^{68}Ge, which was immobilized on the column.

Among the column techniques applied, the following are worth mentioning: An organic ion exchanger resin (Bio-Rad AG1-X8) column-based ^{68}Ga generator with elution of dilute HF solution as well as synthetic chelate resin (condensation of pyrogallol and formaldehyde) column-based ^{68}Ga generators have been studied (Neirinckx and Davis 1980; Neirinckx et al. 1982; Neirinckx and Davis 1981a, b; Schuhmacher and Maier-Borst 1981). Recently, solid-phase extraction resins have been studied for ^{68}Ga generator production. Dipentyl pentylphosphonate (UTEVA) resin was used for selectively retaining ^{68}Ga in 4 M HCl solution while ^{68}Ge remained unadsorbed, followed by eluting the ^{68}Ga from the column with 0.1 M HCl solution (McAlister and Horwitz 2009). Diaion CRB 02 resin (*N*-methyl-D-glucamine) was studied for selective immobilization of ^{68}Ge, with elution of ^{68}Ga performed with a citrate solution (Hsin-Li 2009). Unfortunately, the radiation degradation sensitivity of the organic matrix of both ion exchange resins and solid-phase extraction resin was unfavorable over the expected lifetime of the ^{68}Ga generator (around 2 years).

Alumina column combined with elution with 0.005 M EDTA solution (Greene and Tucker 1961; Kopecky et al. 1973) or high-temperature-treated alumina column combined with elution with 0.1–0.2 M HCl solution (Egamediev et al. 2000; Kopecky and Mudrova 1974) has also been applied for $^{68}Ge/^{68}Ga$ generator development. Alumina column-based ^{68}Ga generators with alkaline solution elution have also been patented (Lewis and Milford 1982). The high content of Al^{3+} ion in the ^{68}Ga eluate, the use of complexing agent EDTA-containing solution for elution, and ^{68}Ga eluate of low specific volume are the major disadvantages for labeling PET radiopharmaceuticals.

Silica gel was among the earliest sorbents studied for ^{68}Ga generator preparation (Caletka and Kotas 1974; Lievens and Hoste 1974; Neirinckx and Davis 1979). Recently, an improved technology using silica gel as a nonmetallic sorbent for ^{68}Ga generator production has been developed. As a result of this development, ITG company is commercializing a silica gel-based ^{68}Ga generator today.

A tin dioxide column-based ^{68}Ga generator using elution with 0.6–1.0 M HCl solutions has been developed and is among the currently used generator systems (Aardaneh and Van der Walt 2006; Loc'h et al. 1980; Waters et al. 1983; McElvany et al. 1984). Tin dioxide column-based generators with 0.6 M HCl solution elution are now commercialized by IDB Holland BV. However, the high content of metallic ion impurities in the ^{68}Ga eluate, the use of stronger acidic solution for the elution, and the ^{68}Ga eluate of low specific volume are undesirable factors for processing of coordination chemistry labeling of PET radiopharmaceuticals.

Titanium dioxide, silicon dioxide, glass microsphere sorbent, and cerium dioxide column-based ^{68}Ga generators with 0.1 M HCl solution elution have been reported in literature (Kozlova et al. 1994; Neirinckx and Davis 1979; Bao and Song 1996; Erhardt and Wetch 1992). Besides the low specific volume of ^{68}Ga eluate obtained, the problem of metallic impurities from dissolution of the column packing materials remains to be solved. Presently, commercial ^{68}Ge/^{68}Ga generators are available. These generators are based on a modified titanium dioxide column with 0.1 M HCl solution elution, commercialized by Eckert and Ziegler Eurotope GmbH-Berlin and Cyclotron Co. Ltd., Obninsk.

Hydrous zirconium oxide column-based ^{68}Ga generators with 0.1–0.5 M HCl or HNO_3 solution elution have been studied (Pao et al. 1981; Neirinckx and Davis 1979). Undesirable large volumes of eluents were necessary to elute ^{68}Ga from the zirconium dioxide column, and low ^{68}Ga elution yield was reported. An improved technology using nanozirconia sorbent to immobilize ^{68}Ge followed by ^{68}Ga elution with 0.01 M HCl solution has recently been developed (Chakravarty et al. 2011). Despite leaching of Zr^{4+} ions from the sorbent substrate, which may require more peptide DOTA-TATE to achieve high-yield labeling, the encouraging results are under evaluation.

A tetravalent lanthanide oxide CeO_2 was studied for immobilizing ^{68}Ge for ^{68}Ga generator preparation (Bao and Song 1996). However, the adsorption/elution performance of this sorbent remains far from practical application in useful ^{68}Ga generator production.

Polyantimonic acid column-based ^{68}Ga generators developed using elution with sodium oxalate solution are unsuitable for radiolabeling targeted radiopharmaceuticals due to stable complex formation of ^{68}Ga ions with oxalate ions (Arino et al. 1978).

The development of a valuable ^{68}Ga generator, capable of providing a ^{68}Ga eluate suitable for biomedical application, requires different specific technical solutions. These include a sorbent for immobilizing the parent nuclide ^{68}Ge, a suitable eluent used for elution of the daughter nuclide ^{68}Ga, and the component parts and materials used for the setup of the generator. Presently, commercial ^{68}Ge/^{68}Ga generators using tin dioxide, titanium oxide, or silica gel sorbent for ^{68}Ge immobilization are available. However, the 5 mL dilute HCl solution required for ^{68}Ga elution and the unavoidably high metallic ion contamination makes these generators' utilization for labeling radiopharmaceuticals impossible. Moreover, the critical level of ^{68}Ge breakthrough and acidity of the ^{68}Ga eluate produced from the above-mentioned generator systems also present a disadvantage, and so further development of alternative sorbents is required for generator performance improvement.

Regarding the sorbents used in radionuclide generator technology, in addition to the high chemical separation specificity requirement, both high radiation resistance and chemical stability are equally needed. The sorbent used in a ^{68}Ga generator should be highly resistant to the high radiation dose delivered from the positron and gamma radiation emitted from the ^{68}Ge/^{68}Ga pair for the entire life of the generator, which is long due to the long half-life of the parent ^{68}Ge. For this reason, organic sorbents including ion exchange resins are likely not suitable for ^{68}Ga generator columns. Inorganic sorbents developed to date have hydrated amorphous structure, which has disadvantageous properties regarding chemical and physical stability. The low physical stability causes the sorbent particles to break easily, blocking the flow of fluid in the sorbent bed of the chromatographic column. The low chemical stability causes leaching of metal ions from the sorbent material into the separated solute product. Consequently, the product is contaminated with sorbent metal ions. To avoid these disadvantageous properties of amorphous inorganic sorbents, crystalline metal oxide-based sorbents should be developed to improve the performance of inorganic sorbents.

Components for generator setup should be nonmetallic to avoid metallic ion contamination of ^{68}Ga eluate and also be highly resistant to high radiation dose for the long lifetime relevant to the advantageously long-lived parent nuclide ^{68}Ge. The chromatographic column of the generator, including fritted disks located at the ends, should be made from either quartz or plastic material such as polyetheretherketone (PEEK). Components made of borosilicate glass should not be used, to avoid leaching of metallic ions into the ^{68}Ga solution during processing. Suprapure water and chemicals should be used for preparation and elution of the generator.

To be successfully applied for formulating ^{68}Ga-labeled targeted radiopharmaceuticals (molecular probes/tracers) currently used in clinical PET imaging, the ^{68}Ga eluate should be evaluated based on three utmost important parameters: The first, for radiation safety reasons, is that the ^{68}Ga solution produced from a ^{68}Ge/^{68}Ga generator should be of very high radionuclidic purity, or in other words, the ^{68}Ge parent nuclide contamination in the ^{68}Ga solution should be very low ($<10^{-3}$%) due to the long half-life of the ^{68}Ge radionuclide. Besides, the chemical impurities, particularly the metallic ion content in the ^{68}Ga solution, should be kept as low as possible to eliminate any concurrent coordination chemistry reactions which may reduce the ^{68}Ga labeling yield. Moreover, ^{68}Ga solution of high radioactive concentration is also an important factor affecting the capability for ^{68}Ga labeling of the nanomole quantities of biomedical tracers/molecular probes currently used in routine molecular imaging and in targeted radiopharmaceutical development. Additional parameters are that the ^{68}Ga eluate should be free from either complexing agents or organic solvent which may be harmful to both biomolecules and complexation of Ga^{3+} ions.

To be used in biomedical applications, especially for labeling of targeting radiopharmaceuticals useful in PET imaging as mentioned above, the ^{68}Ga eluate from the generator (generator column) should typically be purified to remove the trace amount of ^{68}Ge breakthrough and metallic ion impurities, then concentrated to increase the radioactive concentration. Although the solvent extraction technique for concentration–purification of ^{68}Ga eluate using the extractant methyl ethyl ketone has recently been studied (Bokhari et al. 2009), processes for purification and concentration of ^{68}Ga eluate are still preferably applied using a single column of either cationic or anionic ion exchange resins. A strong anionic exchanger resin column-based process and automated system were recently patented and published. ^{68}Ga eluate in 4 M HCl solution was passed through a strong anionic ion exchange resin column. ^{68}Ga retained on this column was then eluted with a small volume of distilled water (Mourtada et al. 2009; Velikyan et al. 2004b). This method is not capable of removing some important metallic ion impurities, such as Fe^{3+} or Zn^{2+}. The above-mentioned patent presents a complex and sophisticated apparatus, unfriendly to nonprofessional users. A strong cationic ion exchange resin-based method has also been reported and is currently in use. This technique is based on retaining $^{68}Ga^{3+}$ ions from the ^{68}Ga eluate onto a strong cationic ion exchange resin column; then, the co-adsorbed impurity metal ions are removed by washing the column with 0.15 M HCl solution containing 80% acetone. Finally, ^{68}Ga ions are eluted from the resin column with a small volume (around 0.5 mL) of 0.015 M HCl solution containing 98% acetone (Rösch et al. 2008; Zhernosekov et al. 2007). This method successfully removes the majority of impure metallic ions, including Fe^{3+} and Zn^{2+}; however, the acetone solvent can react with the HCl solution to form a polymer product. Consequently, the purification process will fail if the history of the acetone/HCl solution is unknown. It is also worth mentioning that polymeric residue in the $^{68}GaCl_3$ preparation after evaporation of acetone will affect the radiolabeling of radiopharmaceuticals, which are usually biomedical substances. In a similar manner, 98% acetone/2% acetylacetone mixture has also been used to elute ^{68}Ga from the cation exchange resin column for ^{68}Ga-labeling under anhydrous conditions (Zoller et al. 2010). All steps of these purification processes were performed manually.

Dual-column methods for ^{68}Ga purification–concentration were recently reported. Compared with the single-column method mentioned above, two columns of different resins connected in series with separate outlets and inlets for eluents were used. In the first option, a strong cationic resin column (column 1) followed by a strong anionic resin (column 2) (Pawlak et al. 2011) and in the second a strong cationic resin (column 1) and TODGA (N, N, N', N'-tetraoctyldiglycolamide) extraction resin (column 2) (Loktionova et al. 2011) were used. The dual-column technique, although resulting in ^{68}Ga solution of very high purity, is not practical due to its complicated tubing connection and thus elution processing. Therefore, there is a need in the art for a new method and fully automated apparatus that purifies and concentrates generator-produced ^{68}Ga eluate. The required apparatus should be easily adaptable for use with ^{68}Ga eluate produced from different ^{68}Ge/^{68}Ga generators which are commercially available and expecting further development.

A comprehensive project for ^{68}Ga generator development has been implemented in ANSTO, starting with synthesis of inorganic sorbents which offer suitable sorption/elution performance for useful ^{68}Ga generator system (high ^{68}Ga elution yield, low breakthrough of ^{68}Ge parent nuclide, and high chemical and radiation stability), followed by generator design and setup. A newly developed purification–concentration process using mild aqueous solutions was also developed to provide effective and safe ^{68}Ga production. As a result of our project, a radioisotope generator coupled/integrated with post-elution purification concentration (PC) processing apparatus [radioisotope generator integrated system (RADIGIS)], specially designed for ^{68}Ga solution processing (RADIGIS-^{68}Ga), has been developed. This system is a benchtop ^{68}Ga generator coupled with a programmable and automated purification–concentration processing unit. The first version of RADIGIS-^{68}Ga system (Model GAG-1-Plus), operated with the single PC column process and manual neutralization of purified ^{68}Ga solution, was developed in ANSTO. The second version (MEDI-Ga-2) with additional improved functions, including automatic neutralizing/conditioning process and alternative dual-PC column purification–concentration operation, is recently developed by MEDISOTEC. An automatic elution process ensures a low radiation dose exposure and reliable long-time operation for safe and cost-effective production of reproducible high-quality ^{68}Ga solution product. This system makes the ^{68}Ga production process safer and friendly to moderately skilled operators available in a daily hospital environment.

2 Nuclear Characteristics and Radioactive Transformation Equilibrium

The nuclear characteristics and principal decay scheme of ^{68}Ge and ^{68}Ga are shown in Fig. 1. The radioactive transformation equilibrium of the radionuclide pair ^{68}Ge/^{68}Ga is presented in Fig. 2. The half-life of the parent nuclide ^{68}Ge is much longer than that of the daughter ^{68}Ga, so this equilibrium is considered as a transient/secular process for which the maximum ^{68}Ga build-up time $t_{100\%\ \text{Build-up}}$ is calculated using the equation $t_{100\%\ \text{Build-up}} = [\ln(\lambda_{\text{Ga-68}}/\lambda_{\text{Ge-68}})]/(\lambda_{\text{Ga-68}} - \lambda_{\text{Ge-68}})$, and the approximate time required to reach 50% of the maximum ^{68}Ga build-up is $t_{50\%\ \text{Build-up}} = [\ln(2 \cdot \lambda_{\text{Ga-68}}/(\lambda_{\text{Ga-68}} + \lambda_{\text{Ge-68}}))]/(\lambda_{\text{Ga-68}} - \lambda_{\text{Ge-68}})$.

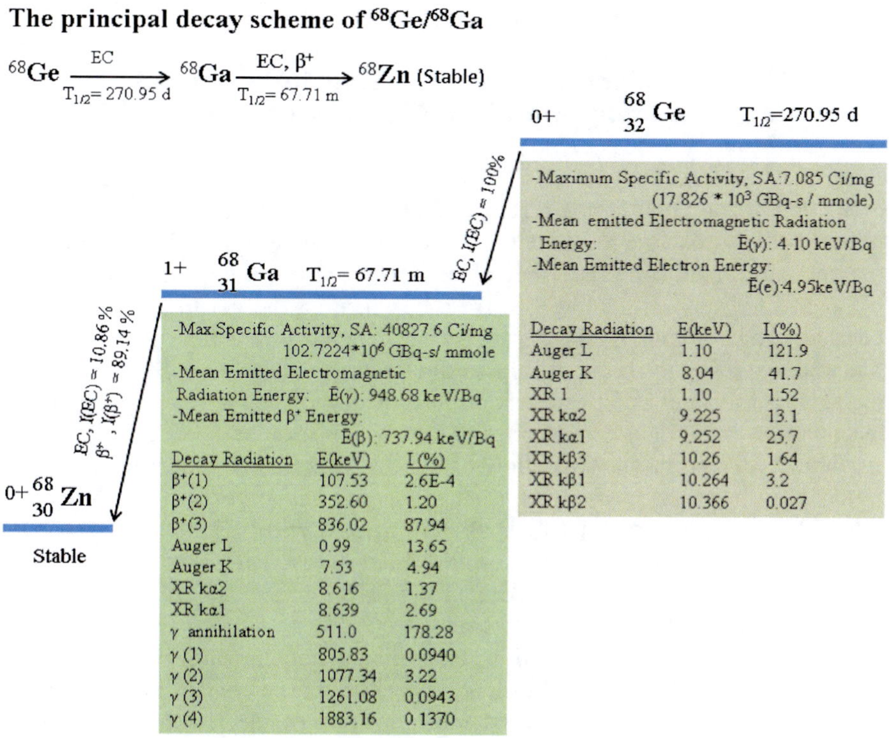

Fig. 1 Nuclear characteristics and principal decay scheme of ^{68}Ge and ^{68}Ga (Eckerman and Endo 2011; Browne and Firestone 1986)

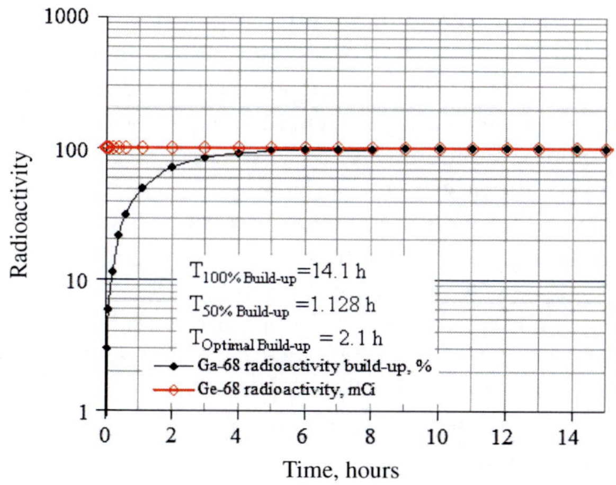

Fig. 2 Transient/secular equilibrium and radionuclide generator kinetics for the system ^{68}Ge/^{68}Ga

3 $^{68}Ge/^{68}Ga$ Separation and ^{68}Ga Generator

3.1 Nanocrystalline Ceramic Structure Sorbent Used for Chromatographic $^{68}Ge/^{68}Ga$ Separation

Sorbent synthesis: The synthesis methods were detailed in our previous work (Le et al. 2007, 2009a, b; Le 2011a, b). Briefly, the sorbent comprises a porous nanocrystalline powder of a metal oxide or mixed metal oxide. A process for making the sorbent comprises several steps: reacting a metal halide or a mixture of metal halides and an alcohol to form a gel, heating the gel to activate the condensation and/or polymerization reaction for the formation of a particulate material, exposing the particulate material to an oxidant to completely convert the metals to tetravalent state, and heating the powder to a temperature sufficient to at least partially melt or sinter particles of the powder so as to form the sorbent. In an example of the reaction, the following reactant mixtures, with different reactant ratios, have been used to prepare a range of different sorbents:

0.5 mol $ZrCl_4$ + 0.5 mol $TiCl_4$ + iPrOH for the sorbent ZT-11
0.75 mol $ZrCl_4$ + 0.25 mol $TiCl_4$ + iPrOH for the sorbent ZT-31
1.0 mol $ZrCl_4$ + iPrOH for the sorbent ZiSORB
1.0 mol $TiCl_4$ + iPrOH for the sorbent TiSORB

An exothermal chemical reaction starts immediately, raising the temperature of the reaction mixture at the end of reactant addition. The condensation reaction of the reactants is allowed to proceed under heating of the reaction mixture with thermostat control. The solid polymer gel material in powder form with particle sizes from 0.10 to 0.01 mm is then left to cool at room temperature overnight before starting further chemical treatment.

The solid polymer gel powder is treated in an alkali solution which contains oxidizing agent NaOCl: about 10 mL 0.5 M NaOH solution containing 1% by weight NaOCl is used per gram of solid polymer gel powder. The solid powder/oxidant solution mixture is gently shaken using a mechanical shaker for at least 4 h so as to convert the gel structure solid powder into a macroporous solid powder and to convert any lower-valence metallic ions to their original 4+ valence. The volume of solution required per gram of solid gel powder is determined so that the pH of solution at the process end is between 2 and 5. The solid matter is then separated by filtering through a sintered glass filter, washed several times with double-distilled water to remove all dissolved sodium and chloride ions, and dried at 80°C for 3 h to dryness to obtain a white solid powder. The resulting white solid powder is heated at a temperature in the range from about 500°C to about 900°C (the actual temperature depending on the particular sorbent being prepared). This may be conveniently performed in a furnace. A suitable heating time is about 3 h. The heating allows the nanoparticles of the powder to recrystallize and melt, and partially fuse so as to produce a solid powder of crystalline structure. The partial fusion and surface coordinative connection are thought to cross-link the particles to create a hard porous matrix of solid material. The initially formed solid is commonly in the form of white solid powder particles composed of different clusters of greater than about 100 nm in size. The clusters are aggregates of amorphous and semicrystalline nanoparticles (less than about 5 nm). The clusters appear to be held together by weak hydrogen bonds and van der Waals bonds. Consequently, the aggregate particles are macroporous and soft. During high-temperature heating (sintering) the amorphous and semicrystalline nanoparticles (less than about 5 nm) crystallize to form crystalline nanoparticles inside clusters. Simultaneously, these crystalline nanoparticles partially melt and combine with other nanoparticles inside the same cluster with interfacial coordinatively-bond/ordered structure to form larger porous crystalline particles. Because there is longer distance between the clusters than between nanoparticles within a single cluster, the nanoparticles belonging to different clusters do not combine with each other to form a single mass. Adjacent nanoparticles on the surface of clusters fuse to a limited area of the cluster surface to form a bridge to crosslink the clusters (at this stage, the clusters have already become larger crystalline particles) to form sorbent particles. In this way, meso/macroporosity formed between the former clusters can be maintained.

The high chemical and mechanical stability of the product is thought to result at least in part from the formation of stable crystalline monophase in the solid material. The crystalline structure of the product is stable when exposed to high radiation doses from radioactive materials. Doping by different amounts of metal ions (for example, Ti, Sn, or Ge) added to the zirconium chloride solution in the synthesis is thought to be responsible for a stabilized crystalline phase which makes the product chemically and mechanically stable. The doping of smaller ions, Ge^{4+}(radius 0.53 Å), Ti^{4+} (radius 0.605 Å) and Sn^{4+}(radius 0.69 Å), onto the matrix of larger ions Zr^{4+}(radius 0.8 Å) facilitates isomorphism-based adsorption of $^{68}Ge^{4+}$ ions from its acidic solution. The powders obtained using the above process have high stability and high porosity and may be used as a state-of-the-art sorbent for different chemical separation processes, for example, for separation of highly radioactive materials.

At the end of this heating process, the resulting powder is sieved. In particular, the fraction of particle size between about 50 and about 100 μm may be collected to be used as a sorbent for chromatographic column packing applied to chemical separation processes.

Structure and adsorption characteristics: The sorbents of a Ti-Zr ceramic structure (Le et al. 2011a, b) were used as a generator column packing material. Scanning electron microscopy (SEM) images showing the micro- and mesoporosity of the sorbent materials synthesized above are shown in Fig. 3. A tetragonal nanocrystalline Ti-Zr ceramic structure is present. A typical X-ray diffraction pattern of these sorbents is shown in Fig. 4.

The adsorption capacity for Ge^{4+} ions is approximately 120 mg Ge per gram sorbent in 0.1 M HCl solution. The distribution coefficient K_d >10,000 mL/g for carrier-free $^{68}Ge^{4+}$ ions and 2 mL/g for $^{68}Ga^{3+}$, when evaluated in 0.1 M HCl solution.

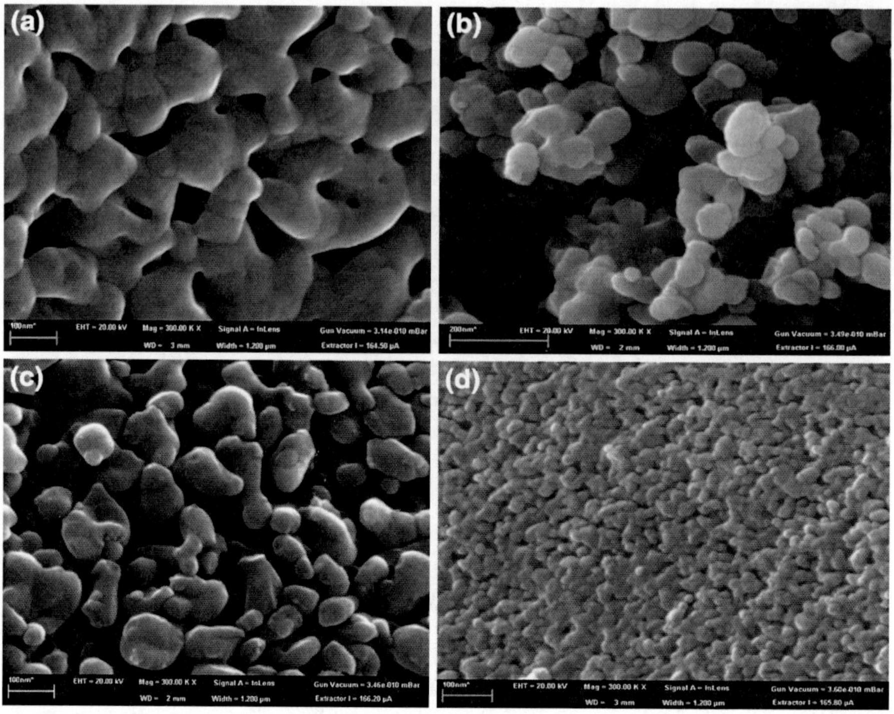

Fig. 3 SEM image of the Ti-Zr ceramic sorbent used for loading $^{68}Ge/^{68}Ga$ generator column. Sorbents: **a** ZT-11, **b** ZT-31, **c** ZiSORB, and **d** TiSORB

Strong adsorption of $^{68}Ge^{4+}$ ions is supposed to result from chemically coordinative bonds formed between germanium and oxygen atoms in the solid matrix of the sorbent material. The similar ionic radius of Ge^{4+} and Ti^{4+} ions (0.53 and 0.605 Å, respectively) facilitates isomorphism-based adsorption (doping) of $^{68}GeO_4$ groups onto the $(ZrTiO_4)_n$ matrix of the sorbent. The larger radius of the main component Zr^{4+} ions (0.8 Å), playing the role of the backbone of the solid matrix in the sorbent, reduces the bonding power of TiO_4 groups doped into the $(ZrTiO_4)_n$ matrix, and hence the rate of isomorphic doping/sorption of $^{68}GeO_4$ groups will be enhanced. So, the strong adsorption of $^{68}Ge^{4+}$ ions onto the Zr-Ti matrix-based ceramic sorbents is supported by an isomorphic incorporation mechanism. In contrast, the weak adsorption of Ga^{3+} ions is attributed to an amorphism process. The strong adsorption of Ge^{4+} ions supposed above is valued for other sorbents of similar structure, $(ZrSnO_4)_n$ and $(ZrGeO_4)_n$, which are recently investigated in our laboratories (Le 2011a, b).

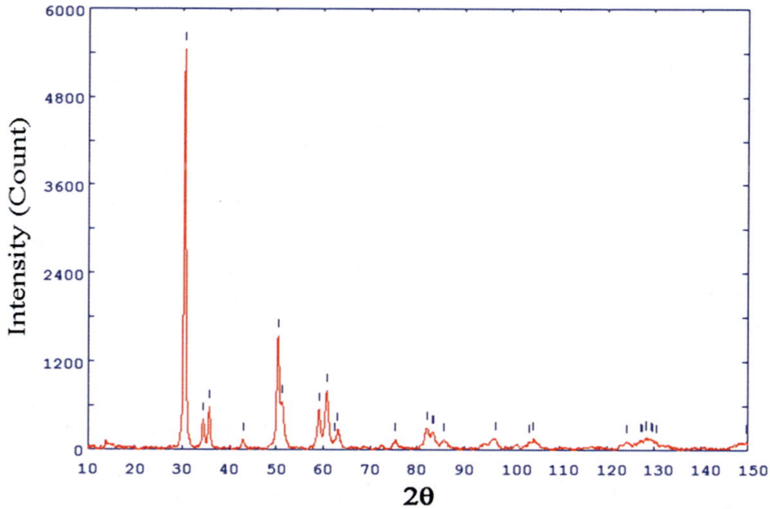

Fig. 4 Tetragonal structure X-ray diffraction pattern of nanocrystalline ceramic sorbent ZT-31

3.2 ^{68}Ga Generator Setup

Generator design: As discussed above, the sorbents synthesized above may be used to produce a ^{68}Ga generator (Figs. 13 and 14a). A chromatographic column is packed with the sorbent. A stock acidic ^{68}Ge solution is applied to the column to immobilize the ^{68}Ge parent nuclide on the sorbent. As the ^{68}Ge decays to generate the daughter nuclide ^{68}Ga, $^{68}Ga^{3+}$ ions are formed and weakly adsorbed on the column. Eluting the column with a dilute acidic solution will therefore generate a ^{68}Ga-containing eluate. Because the sorbent has much higher adsorption affinity for ^{68}Ge than for ^{68}Ga, the acidic eluate contains mainly $^{68}Ga^{3+}$ ions and a significantly lower amount of ^{68}Ge (^{68}Ge breakthrough). An apparatus or generator for separating ^{68}Ga from ^{68}Ge ions may therefore comprise: a column made from radiation-resistant material such as quartz glass and thermoplastic and having a column inlet and outlet, provided with filter fritted diskettes on both ends and closed by a plastic septum together with silicon rubber gaskets and being capped by aluminum clamping lids; a radiation protection shielding lead housing surrounding the column, provided with two ports for tubing to the column outlet and inlet; an acidic eluent supply system coupled to the sorbent column inlet; a pump to pass eluent or other liquid through the column as required, located downstream of the column and operating by suction; an outlet valve coupled to the column outlet, to stop the eluent or direct it to a product container; and an electronic controller for generator operation, designed to make the process reproducible and radiation safe.

To avoid any possible contamination by metallic ions of the ^{68}Ga solution produced by the ^{68}Ga generator, all components of the generator, including the chromatographic column and tubing lines, should be made of nonmetallic materials.

Due to the long half-life of the parent nuclide ^{68}Ge, the radiation stability of the nonmetallic materials used in the ^{68}Ge/^{68}Ga generator design should be evaluated to ensure an advantageously long operating lifetime of the ^{68}Ga generator. The radiation exposure dose of the materials used for the generator column and its fritted diskettes were therefore estimated for the generator design. The PEEK material intended to be used in the design of the generator column can withstand any radiation doses likely to be sustained during service. PEEK 450G can withstand over 1,000 Mrads (10 MGy) without any loss of mechanical properties. Radiation exposure from a single loading of 100 mCi of ^{68}Ge into the column is less than this 1,000 Mrads value (as shown below), and therefore radiation exposure is not a problem for the PEEK column. Using MicroShield software, the initial dose rate from the unshielded 100 mCi ^{68}Ge source is calculated to be 25 mGy/h at contact. It is assumed that the dose from the isotope is negligible after 10 half-lives (i.e., 68,880 h) and then the total dose can be calculated as follows: $D = \int_0^{68,880} 25e^{-0.0001t}dt = 249.7\,\text{Gy}$. The exposure limits of 2,600 Gy and 3,321 Gy for the 2-mm column segments of the PEEK column and its quartz frits, respectively, show that these generator parts are capable of withstanding the dose from the ^{68}Ge/^{68}Ga radioisotopes for the entire life of the isotope (10 half-lives). This is based on the conservative assumption that the entire dose is absorbed by the column for a single-use package.

^{68}Ge loading: The stock acidic ^{68}Ge solution is commonly a ^{68}Ge solution in 0.05–0.5 M HCl. A suitable ^{68}Ge concentration is from about 10 to 50 mCi ^{68}Ge/mL. The ^{68}Ge solution volume applied for each sorbent column is commonly about 2.0 to 5.0 mL. During application or loading of the stock acidic ^{68}Ge solution to the column, the ^{68}Ge solution flows through the column under gravity or by means of a peristaltic pump. The preferred flow rate of the solution is from 0.05 to 0.2 mL/min, depending on the size of the column. Following the loading of the stock acidic ^{68}Ge solution onto a sorbent column, the column is washed with 10 to 20 mL 0.1 M HCl solution. Then, the column is ready for regular elution (separation) of ^{68}Ga daughter radioisotope solution for regular use.

3.3 Generator Operation and Specification

^{68}Ga elution performance: A 1.0 g weight sorbent column was used for immobilizing the parent nuclide ^{68}Ge, and ^{68}Ga was eluted from the column with 3.5 mL 0.05–0.1 M HCl solution by dry elution or 5.0 mL by wet elution. The ^{68}Ga elution profile of the >18 mCi activity ^{68}Ga generator is shown in Fig. 5.

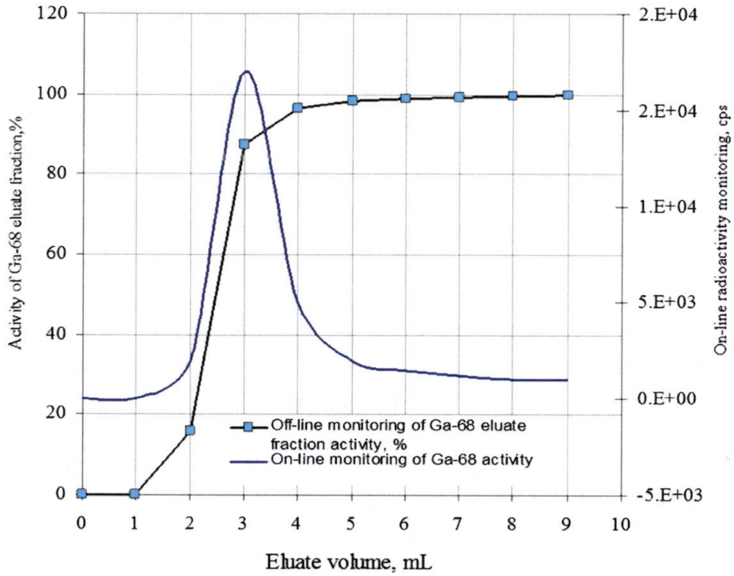

Fig. 5 ^{68}Ga elution profile of the ^{68}Ga generator (column: 5.0 mm i.d × 30.0 mm length; sorbent: 1.0 g sorbent ZT-31; ^{68}Ge radioactivity loaded on the generator column: 18 mCi; eluent: 0.1 M HCl)

As shown, more than 95% of the ^{68}Ga radioactivity was eluted in 3.5 mL 0.1 M HCl solution. A series of generators with ^{68}Ge activities from 5 to >18 mCi have been studied at ANSTO, and ^{68}Ga elution performed for 2 years. During this operation time, more than 300 elution cycles were performed, and the ^{68}Ga elution yield varied from 97.0% (at the first elution) to 71.0% (at the 301st elution). More detailed results are presented in Table 1.

^{68}Ge breakthrough and its evaluation: As described in (Sect. 5), the ^{68}Ge breakthrough in ^{68}Ga eluate from the generator was determined based on the counts of the 511-keV photopeak of ^{68}Ga activity, which is in radioactive equilibrium with the impure ^{68}Ge activity. Because the majority of the activity in the eluate is ^{68}Ga activity, which is not in equilibrium with the ^{68}Ge activity, for a certain measurement of impure ^{68}Ge activity of the ^{68}Ga-eluate sample, this sample should be left for a given time so that the majority of the ^{68}Ga activity has decayed to a reasonable degree to reduce the interference from nonequilibrium ^{68}Ga activity of the ^{68}Ga eluate sample. A relationship between the measurement certainty R, decay time t, and required ^{68}Ge breakthrough (impurity) limit L has been established and is shown in Fig. 6. As shown, a 25 h decay time is required for the ^{68}Ga eluate sample to be left to decay before starting a reliable gamma-ray spectrometric ^{68}Ge activity measurement (certainty degree $R = 98\%$). This calculation result complies with the required ^{68}Ge breakthrough (impurity) limit

Table 1 ^{68}Ga production performance of ^{68}Ga generator and RADIGIS-^{68}Ga system

Quality parameter	^{68}Ga generator: ^{68}Ga elution without post-elution purification			RADIGIS-^{68}Ga system: ^{68}Ga elution followed by post-elution purification–concentration		
^{68}Ga build-up time of the generator, h	2	24	96	2	24	96
Overall processing time, min	1	1	1	10	10	10
^{68}Ga solution volume, mL, and (acidity) of final product	5.0 (0.1 M HCl)	5.0 (0.1 M HCl)	5.0 (0.1 M HCl)	0.75 (0.5 M KOH)	0.75 (0.5 M KOH)	0.75 (0.5 M KOH)
^{68}Ga-elution yield, %	86.5 ± 0.8	85.6 ± 0.7	83.2 ± 0.5	–	–	–
Overall ^{68}Ga production yield, %	–	–	–	81.5 ± 0.8	80.6 ± 0.7	78.2 ± 0.5
^{68}Ge breakthrough, %	$<10^{-4}$	$\sim 10^{-4}$	$<10^{-3}$	$<10^{-6}$	$<10^{-6}$	$<10^{-6}$
^{68}Ga-DOTATATE labeling yield (HPLC method), %	~100	~100	~100	~100	~100	~100
^{68}Ga-DOTATOC labeling yield (HPLC method), %	~100	~100	~100	~100	~100	~100
Bacterial endotoxin, EU/mL	<2.50	<2.50	<2.50	<2.50	<2.50	<2.50
Metallic ion contamination, ppm or μg/mL						
Ca(II)	1.180	0.638	0.648	0.105	0.105	0.160
Sr(II)	0.008	0.005	0.079	<0.001	<0.001	<0.001
Ba(II)	0.130	0.212	<0.001	<0.001	<0.001	<0.001
Ni(II)	0.010	0.018	0.011	0.020	0.025	0.030
Co(II)	0.012	0.006	0.008	0.006	0.005	0.004
Cu(II)	0.014	0.024	0.027	0.021	0.021	0.025
Zn(II)	0.487	0.302	0.355	0.134	0.134	0.192
Cd(II)	0.001	0.002	0.002	0.001	0.001	0.001
Pb(II)	0.022	0.012	0.006	0.177	0.178	0.179
Al(III)	0.522	0.468	0.510	0.220	0.245	0.250
Y(III)	0.001	0.054	0.004	<0.001	<0.001	<0.001
Fe(III)	0.188	0.149	0.513	0.125	0.129	0.153
Lu(III)	<0.001	0.001	<0.001	<0.001	<0.001	<0.001
Yb(III)	<0.001	<0.001	<0.001	<0.001	<0.001	<0.001

(continued)

Table 1 (continued)

Quality parameter	^{68}Ga generator: ^{68}Ga elution without post-elution purification			RADIGIS-^{68}Ga system: ^{68}Ga elution followed by post-elution purification–concentration		
Ti(III)	3.084	3.582	3.416	0.083	0.063	0.059
Zr(III)	<0.001	<0.001	0.003	0.001	0.001	<0.001
Total metal contamination, μg/mL	5.659	5.473	6.182	0.893	0.907	1.514

$L = 10^{-3}\%$ of the activity of the ^{68}Ga eluate as stated in literature (EANM-Monograph-2464 2011).

The minimum activity $A_{0,P}$ of the ^{68}Ga eluate sample at time $t = 0$ needed for later measurement of the ^{68}Ge breakthrough activity after decaying for time t is calculated using the equation $A_{0,P} = 100 \times L_D \times e^{\lambda_i \times (\lambda - \lambda_i)^{-1} \times \ln(100 \times R/((100-R) \times L))}/L$, where the detection limit L_D is a spectrometric parameter of the available gamma-ray spectrometer used for the ^{68}Ga radioactivity measurement. λ_i and λ are decay constants of ^{68}Ge and ^{68}Ga, respectively (Le et al. 2012). The $A_{0,P}$ calculation above ensures insignificant interference in the ^{68}Ge breakthrough (impurity) activity measurement of the ^{68}Ga eluate sample with respect to a justified certainty degree R and a ^{68}Ge breakthrough (impurity) limit L required by regulatory compliance.

Based on this assessment method, breakthrough activity measurement of ^{68}Ga eluate sample of >117.55 μCi activity was justified after a delay of $t = 25.2$ h. The measurement was performed using a gamma-ray spectrometer with a 2.035 Bq detection limit (L_D) and counting time >30 min. The ^{68}Ge breakthrough activity in the ^{68}Ga eluate from our generators was $<10^{-3}\%$ for generators of 5–18 mCi ^{68}Ge activity. This result has also been confirmed by a visual observation technique using PET imaging. The PET image of the ^{68}Ga generator column after 300 elution cycles (Fig. 7) showed no significant spreading or drift of the ^{68}Ge zone along the column.

Optimization of ^{68}Ga elution: The maximum ^{68}Ga build-up time ($t_{100\%\ \mathrm{build\text{-}up}}$) for the ^{68}Ge/^{68}Ga generator system is 14.1 h. Despite the optimal ^{68}Ga build-up time ($t_{\mathrm{optimal\ build\text{-}up}}$) for the ^{68}Ge/^{68}Ga generator system of 2.0 h (Fig. 2) as evaluated at the 70% ^{68}Ga build-up in our optimization assessment, more effective utilization of hot ^{68}Ga atoms is found if only partial (commonly about 50% of the maximum) build-up of the gallium on the sorbent is allowed to occur before milking the gallium from the sorbent, repeating this several times. This can result in a more satisfactory ^{68}Ga/^{68}Zn ratio and higher overall ^{68}Ga radioactivity. ^{68}Ga radioactivity build-ups for consecutive elutions performed at 50% radioactivity build-up of ^{68}Ga are shown in Fig. 8.

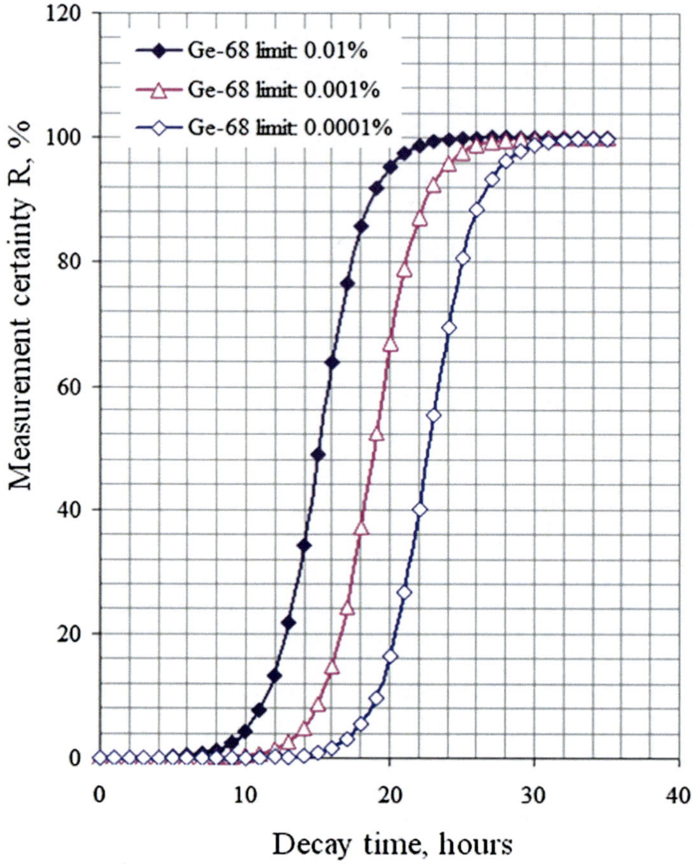

Fig. 6 Certainty parameter R versus decay time t of ^{68}Ga eluate at different required ^{68}Ge contamination limits L for detection of ^{68}Ge breakthrough. (R(%) $= 100 \times$ (Activity of ^{68}Ge) / (Activity of ^{68}Ge + Activity of ^{68}Ga); Poisson distribution 95% confidence interval, $C \pm 1.96\sqrt{C}$, with error <8.77%, >500 counts)

As the time required to reach 50% of the maximum amount of ^{68}Ga ($t_{50\%\ \mathrm{build\text{-}up}}$) is about 1.128 h, this is also the waiting period between subsequent elutions of the generator. One advantage of consecutive elution performed at 50% ^{68}Ga build-up is the improvement in the quality of ^{68}Ga solution in terms of reduction of Zn content in the eluate. An amount of 6.97×10^{-3} nmol Zn-68 was evaluated at the 50% ^{68}Ga build-up compared with the value of 0.2 nanomoles at the maximum ^{68}Ga build-up time ($t_{100\%\ \mathrm{build\text{-}up}} = 14.1$ h) for the ^{68}Ge/^{68}Ga generator system (Fig. 9). Using this elution plan, a ^{68}Ga/^{68}Zn molar ratio of approximately 3.0 in the eluate is achievable compared with the value of 0.1 at the time $t_{100\%\ \mathrm{build\text{-}up}}$ (Fig. 10).

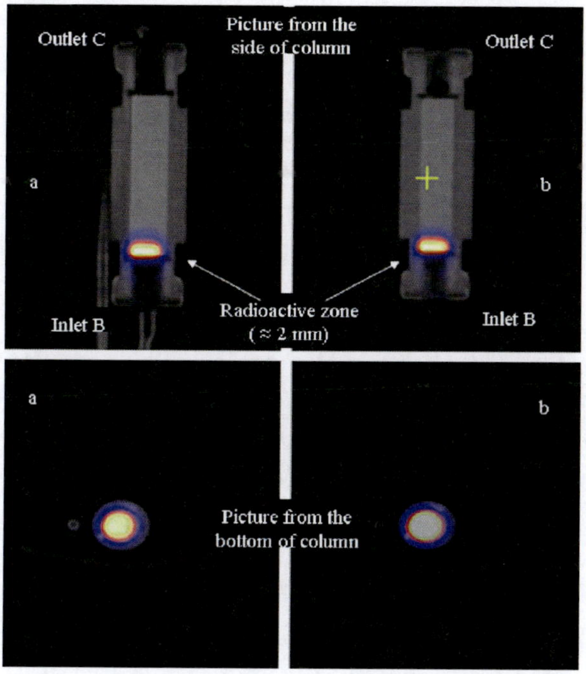

Fig. 7 PET imaging of the $^{68}Ge/^{68}Ga$ generator column after 300 ^{68}Ga elution cycles

This elution plan offers cost-effective utilization of this generator system. The total useful ^{68}Ga radioactivity gathered in 12 consecutive elutions (overall time period around 14 h) is six times higher than that eluted once at time $t_{100\%\ \text{build-up}} = 14.1$ h (calculated based on the same period of ^{68}Ga build-up time for the generator). Moreover, this 1.128 h-elution plan (with 50% ^{68}Ga build-up) conforms with the time required for labeling peptide radiopharmaceutical plus consequently performing PET imaging (around 1.0 h in total) before starting a subsequent ^{68}Ga generator elution. This statement is based on a unique dose of ^{68}Ga peptide injection prepared from the elution of 18 mCi activity ^{68}Ga generator as a whole.

3.4 $^{68}Zn^{2+}$ Formation and Its Influence on Coordination Chemistry of ^{68}Ga-Radiolabeling

As shown in the $^{68}Ge/^{68}Ga$ radioactive decay equilibrium in Fig. 1, ^{68}Ga generated from ^{68}Ge decays relatively rapidly to zinc. There is a defined amount of $^{68}Zn^{2+}$ ions that can accumulate on the sorbent and then possibly be eluted into the ^{68}Ga eluate during the generator elution operation. This quantity of ^{68}Zn is evaluated as

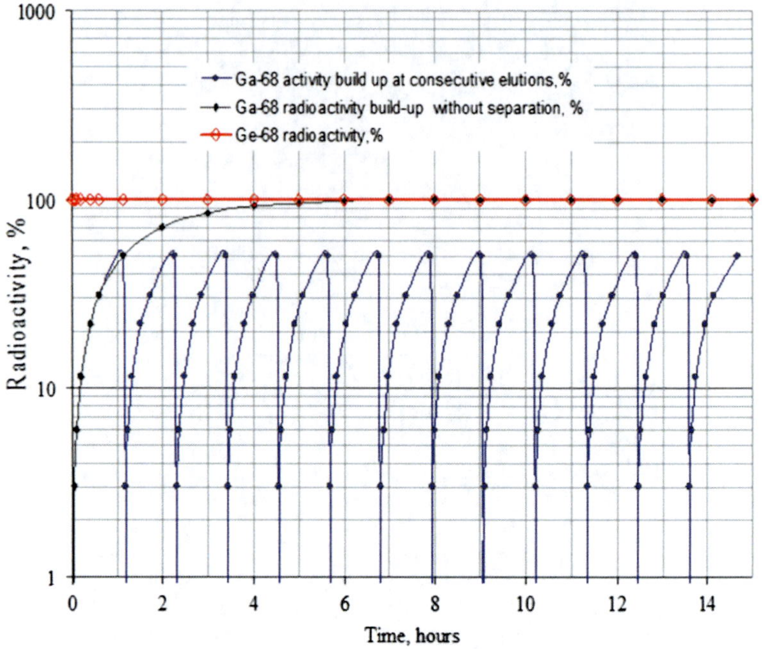

Fig. 8 ^{68}Ga radioactivity build-ups for consecutive elutions performed at 50% radioactivity build-up of ^{68}Ga

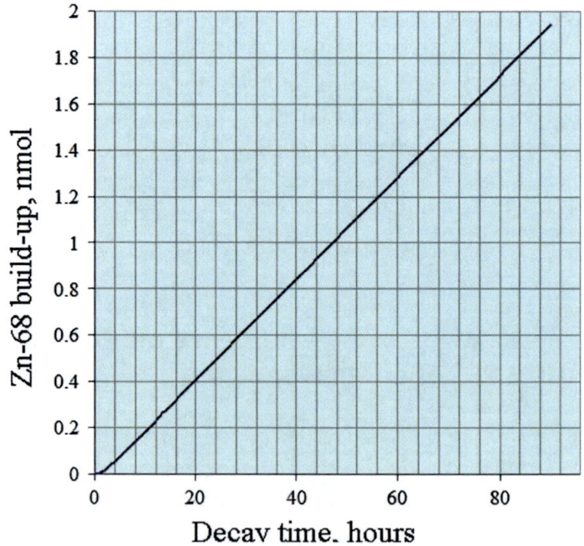

Fig. 9 ^{68}Zn build-up in the 100 mCi ^{68}Ga (0.207 μmol ^{68}Ge) generator

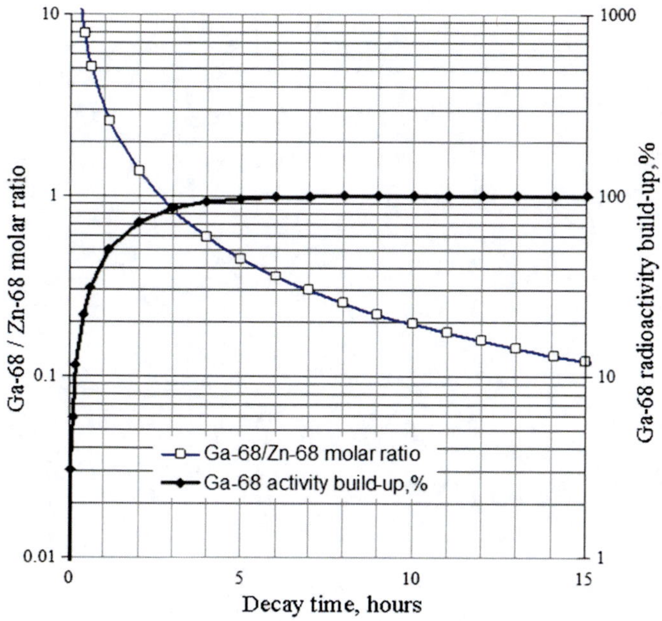

Fig. 10 ^{68}Zn formation rate versus ^{68}Ga build-up in the system ^{68}Ge/^{68}Ga

shown in Fig. 9. Because of the high capability for coordination competition of $^{68}Zn^{2+}$ ions to form complexes with common bifunctional ligands used for ^{68}Ga-radiolabeling target agents such as DOTATATE and DOTATOC (pK = 21.33 for Ga-DOTATATE and pK = 21.10 for Zn-DOTATATE), investigation of the effect of additional Zn^{2+} content on ^{68}Ga labeling of DOTATATE and DOTATOC ligands was performed. Different given amounts of Zn^{2+} were added to ^{68}Ga solution eluted from the generator at the 2 h equilibration time and purified using a cationic ion exchange resin column as described in Sect. 4. This elution–purification process ensures a minimal metallic contamination and a molar ratio ^{68}Ga/^{68}Zn < 1.0 in the ^{68}Ga eluate, as shown in Fig. 10. Labeling of DOTATATE and DOTATOC ligands with ^{68}Ga using these solutions was carried out, and the labeling yield was evaluated as described in Sect. 5. The investigation results obtained show that reaction mixture containing 5 nmols ligand and >4 nmols Zn^{2+} gave ^{68}Ga labeling yield less than 90% compared with a yield value of 100% for the reaction mixture containing <3 nmols Zn^{2+}. Comparing with the ^{68}Zn build-up values shown in Fig. 9, it can be stated that the ^{68}Zn build-up from 5 days of decay of ^{68}Ga eluate from the 100 mCi ^{68}Ga-generator may affect labeling of DOTATATE and DOTATOC ligands if the ligand quantity used for labeling is less than 5 nmols. Labeling <2 nmols ligands with ^{68}Ga eluate, which is eluted daily directly from the generator, should be avoided due to lack of reproducibility.

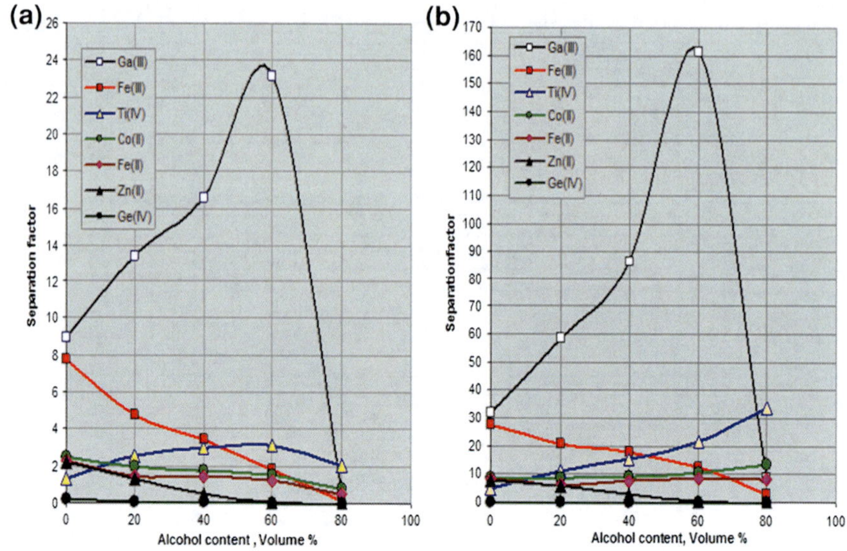

Fig. 11 Separation factor of metallic ions compared with K^+/Li^+ ions in acidic alcohol aqueous solution using salt-form cationic exchange resin AG50 W-X4: **a** K^+ form in 0.5 M HCl + 0.05 M KCl + 0.5% ascorbic acid + ethanol (or methanol) mixture, and **b** Li^+ form in 0.5 M HCl + 0.15 M LiCl + 0.5% ascorbic acid + ethanol (or methanol) mixture

4 Post-Elution Purification–Concentration of ^{68}Ga Eluate

4.1 Salt-Form Cationic Exchange Resin-Based Purification–Concentration Method

The process of purification–concentration of ^{68}Ga is based on the much higher adsorption selectivity or separation factor of Ga^{3+} ions compared with other metallic ions in the acidic alcohol aqueous solution/salt-form strong cationic exchange resin system. As shown in Fig. 11, an acidic solution containing more than 30% alcohol can be used for effective elimination of several metallic contaminants from ^{68}Ga eluate for purification–concentration purpose.

Based on the results obtained, the process of ^{68}Ga purification–concentration was set up as shown in Fig. 12. ^{68}Ga eluate of around 5–10 mL volume in 0.1 M HCl solution was purified on a small cationic exchanger column with aqueous alcohol solution mixture of hydrochloric and ascorbic acids, and halide salts. An alkali solution was used for elution of ^{68}Ga from the ion exchange resin column to obtain purified ^{68}Ga solution, which is neutralized with acidic solution to obtain a final ^{68}Ga product of pH 3–4 in 0.75 mL 0.5 M NaCl or 0.5 M sodium acetate solution. Metallic contamination of <3 nmol per mL was found in this product solution. The organic-solvent-free ^{68}Ga solution product, with acidity suitable for

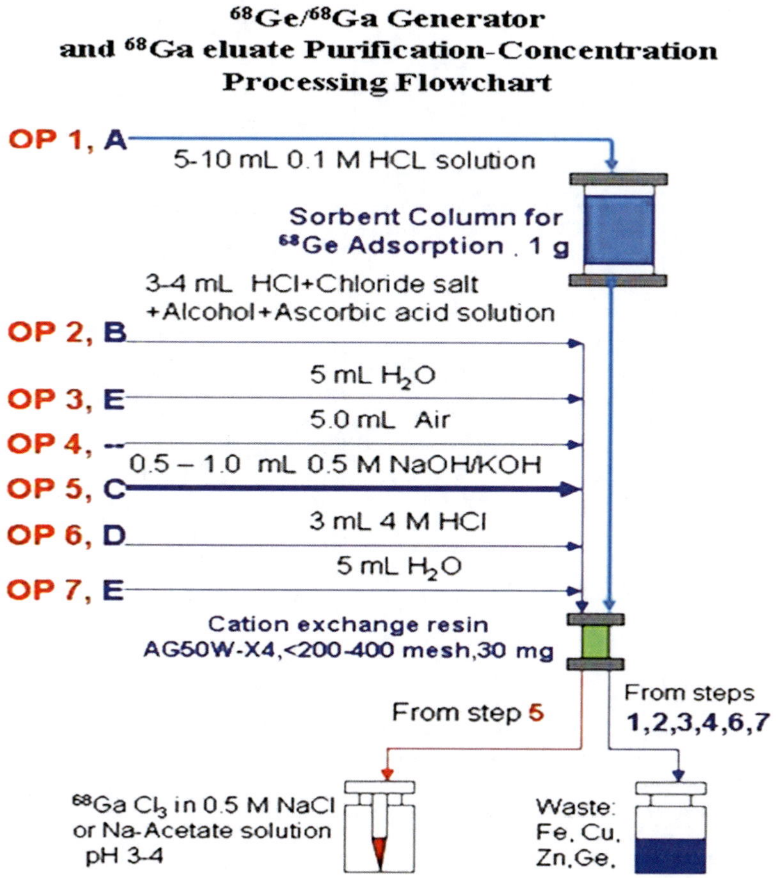

Fig. 12 Processing flowchart for elution and purification–concentration of ^{68}Ga from ^{68}Ga generator

coordination chemistry-based labeling of peptide ligands, was successfully used for preparation of DOTATATE and DOTATOC PET radiopharmaceuticals.

4.2 Automation Process and Setup of ^{68}Ga Radioisotope Generator Integrated System (RADIGIS-^{68}Ga)

The process of ^{68}Ga elution from the generator followed by ^{68}Ga eluate purification was performed using a low-cost automated benchtop radioisotope generator integrated system (RADIGIS) specially designed for elution–purification–concentration of ^{68}Ga radioisotope (RADIGIS-^{68}Ga) (Le 2011a, b). RADIGIS is a radioisotope separation integrated system developed for separation, purification, and concentration of different radionuclide solutions produced from different

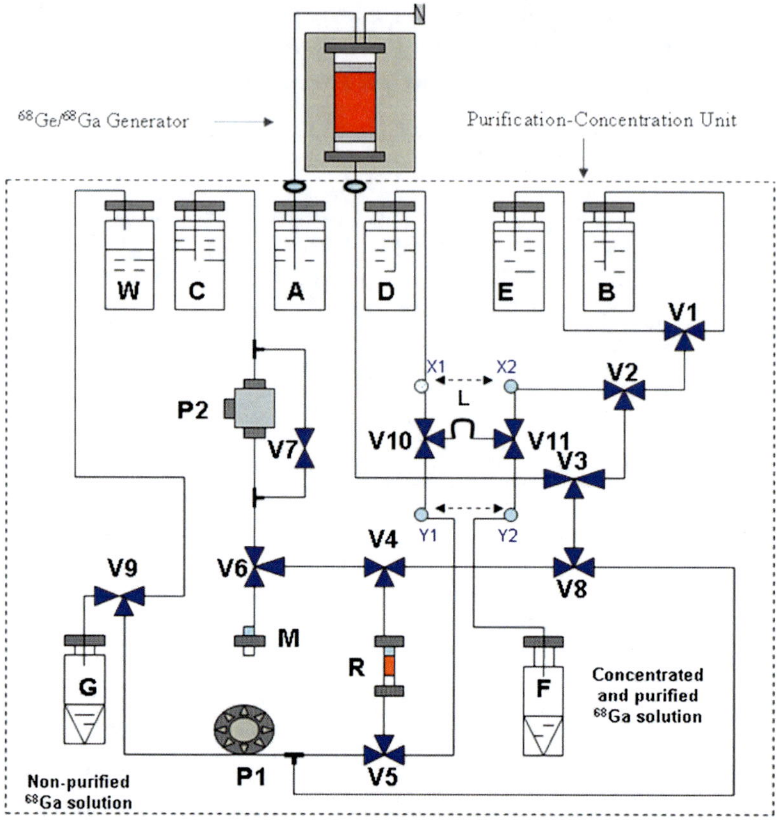

Fig. 13 Fluid flow diagram and setup of the RADIGIS-^{68}Ga system. P1, peristaltic pump; P2, microdisplacement pump; V, solenoid valve; A-E, solutions; W, waste; L, loop for neutralization; R, cationic ion exchange resin microcolumn; G, nonpurified ^{68}Ga eluate; F, purified ^{68}Ga solution

processes (Le et al. 2009a, Le 1990, 2003). This system was designed and manufactured (Fig. 14) based on the timing sequence of seven processing steps without feedback control. The chemical engineering steps of purification–concentration of ^{68}Ga eluted from the ^{68}Ga generator are described in Fig. 13. The variable flow rate of eluents used for elution/purification in this system also ensure the optimization of operating times with respect to different adsorption/desorption kinetics of ^{68}Ga ion species, which is controlled by the sorbent and ion exchange resin used in the generator and purification columns. This generator system also incorporates an automated neutralizer to adjust basic purified ^{68}Ga eluate from the cationic ion exchange resin column to the required pH using HCl and/or acetic acid. This operation mode offers alternative options to achieve three finished ^{68}Ga solution products: basic ^{68}Ga gallate solution, acidic ^{68}Ga chloride solution, and ^{68}Ga gallium complex solution (gallium acetate or citrate).

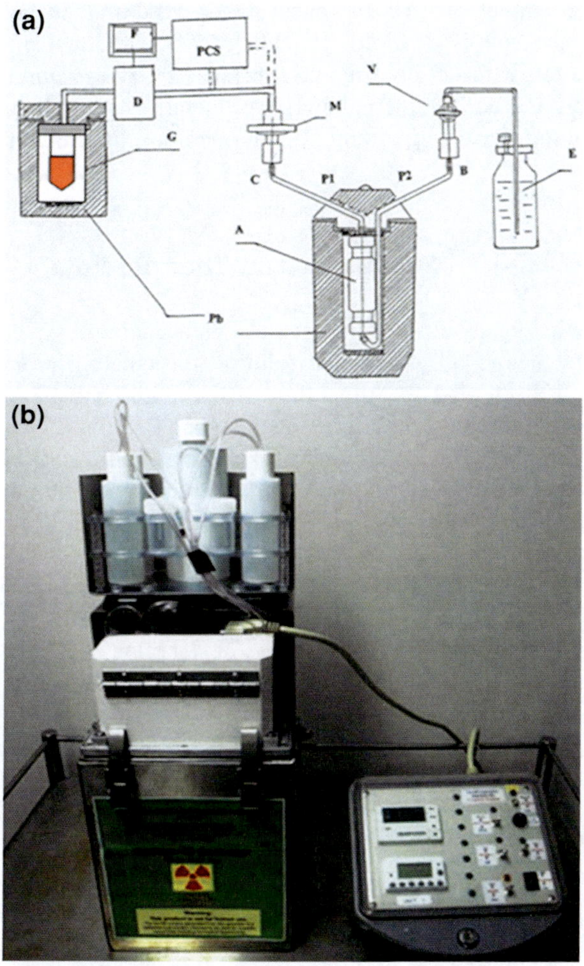

Fig. 14 RADIGIS-^{68}Ga: a ^{68}Ga radioisotope generator integrated system recently developed at ANSTO. **a** Outline of design (*A*, sorbent column; PCS, purification–concentration system; *D*, pump; *F*, controller; *G*, ^{68}Ga product; *E*, eluent; *M*, Millipore filter). **b** Photo of the real generator system

The ^{68}Ga radioisotope generator integrated system RADIGIS-^{68}Ga shown in Fig. 14 comprises a ^{68}Ga generator (housed in the lead container in the lower part of the system) and processing unit with the eluents for ^{68}Ga eluate purification (in the upper part) together with a control unit at the bottom right. This system offers the unique function of programmable elution with better product quality without radiation dose burden for operators as well as increased cost-effective utilization through an elution schedule conforming to daily clinical practice. Advantages of this integrated system are nonvariable elution performance (consistent ^{68}Ge breakthrough and ^{68}Ga elution yield), utilization of mild aqueous solutions for chemical processing (ensuring no risk of leakage, corrosion, and organic substance polymerization), providing a ^{68}Ga product of high purity and high concentration without any organic substance residues (avoiding the negative impact on labeling procedures), and no risk of metallic contaminant build-up in the purification column (ensuring a long system operating lifetime without significant maintenance).

4.3 Basic/Acidic ^{68}Ga Eluates and Their Radiolabeling

As mentioned in Sect. 4.2, our integrated ^{68}Ga generator system is capable of providing either acidic or basic ^{68}Ga solution for labeling radioligands. Therefore, it is worth discussing the capability of the acidic and basic ^{68}Ga solutions for coordination labeling of bifunctional ligands. Several experiments were performed to label DOTATATE and DOTATOC with acidic and basic ^{68}Ga solutions. It was found that both acidic and basic ^{68}Ga solutions gave identical labeling performance (radiolabeling yield and reproducibility) when the same labeling reaction conditions and manipulations were applied (except for the DOTATATE and DOTATOC ligand solution preparation). While ligands dissolved in H_2O are preferably labeled using acidic ^{68}Ga solution, we found that basic ^{68}Ga solution was more effective for labeling ligands in 0.1 M HCl solution. Details of the labeling process using basic ^{68}Ga solution are given in Sect. 5.1.

4.4 Performance of ^{68}Ga Generator and ^{68}Ga Radioisotope Generator Integrated System

The performance of ^{68}Ga generator systems was evaluated for years as described in Sect. 5.

The quality evaluation results are given in Table 1. It can be stated that the quality of our ^{68}Ga generator systems (^{68}Ga generator and RADIGIS-^{68}Ga system) was quite suitable for several biomedical studies and comparable to, if not better than, other ^{68}Ga generator systems currently used in nuclear medicine applications (Asti et al. 2008).

Effect of metallic contamination on ^{68}Ga labeling: To confirm the above statement, an additional conservative test was performed as follows. Three 1.0 mL 0.1 M HCl solutions, each containing 16 metals (listed in Table 1) with concentrations of 1.0, 0.8, and 0.3 ppm for each metal, were prepared. These solutions were added to nonpurified ^{68}Ga eluates from the ^{68}Ga generator used for the study given in Table 1. Then, the mixed solutions were used for ^{68}Ga-labeling of DOTATATE and DOTATOC ligands. Radiolabeling and yield determination were performed in the usual manner as described in Sect. 5. The results obtained showed that the mixed ^{68}Ga solutions containing <0.8 ppm of each metal (equivalent to total metal amount of 12.8 μg/mL) did not cause any reduction in radiolabeling yield. This result suggests that the metal contamination of the original nonpurified ^{68}Ga eluates given in Table 1 (whole content of 16 metals <6.18 μg/mL) is still far below the critical value (12.8 μg/mL) which may affect the radiolabeling capability of the ^{68}Ga eluates.

5 Quality Evaluation Experiments: Quality Control Protocols and Radiolabeling Efficacy Evaluation

The performance of the ^{68}Ga generators will be evaluated based on two investigations: quality evaluation and operation performance assessment for both the ^{68}Ga generator (without ^{68}Ga-eluate purification) and the ^{68}Ga generator integrated system (with purification–concentration of ^{68}Ga eluate). The procedures described below are selected from literature (Asti et al. 2008; Velikyan et al. 2004a; Zhernosekov et al. 2007; EANM-Monograph-2464 2011; Blois et al. 2011).

The radiolabeling procedures described in Sect. 5.1.2 were developed and optimized in our laboratory. The major feature of this procedure is the use of lower content of DOTATATE or DOTATOC ligands (5 nmols) for radiolabeling with the entire ^{68}Ga eluate (1.0 mL) eluted from the generators. The reduction in the ^{68}Ga eluate volume and in the mass of ligands used for labeling compared with the amounts described in literature (15 nmols ligand and 5 mL ^{68}Ga eluate) was planned to minimize the effect of metal contamination and increase the sensitivity of the evaluation investigation.

5.1 Quality Evaluation of ^{68}Ga Solution

- *Specifications required for evaluation*
  - ^{68}Ga radioactivity and ^{68}Ga separation yield
  - Radionuclidic purity
  - Radiochemical purity
  - Radiolabeling capability: labeling yield and quality of ^{68}Ga-labeled ligands
  - pH of ^{68}Ga solution
  - Metallic ion contamination of ^{68}Ga solution
  - Bacterial endotoxin of ^{68}Ga solution
- *Material and equipment requirements*
  - Coaxial HPGe detector coupled to 4,096-channel gamma-ray spectrometer
  - Radiation dose calibrator: a calibrated Capintec (USA) ionization chamber
  - Radioactive thin-layer chromatography (TLC) scanner such as the AR 2,000 imaging scanner (BioScan, USA)
  - Inductively coupled plasma mass spectrometry (ICP-MS) such as the 7,500 Ce ICP-MS analyzer (Agilent Santa Clara, USA) and/or inductively coupled plasma optical emission spectrometry (ICP-OES)

– pH-meter with microprobe
– Micropipettes
– TLC chromatography tank
– Radiolabeling microheater/reactor and water bath
– Sep-Pack light C-18 cartridge (Waters)
– TLC plates ITLC-SG (Pall Corporation, East Hill, NY, USA)
– TLC plates RP-18F (Merck, Whitehouse Station, NJ, USA)
– Milli-Q purity water (18.2 M′Ω cm, Millipore Corp.)
– Millipore 0.24-μm filter, disposable syringe, and glassware
– All chemicals used to be of analytical grade

5.1.1 Quality Control Procedures

- *Procedure for radioactivity measurement and ^{68}Ga separation yield determination*
  Radioactivity of ^{68}Ga solution is measured using a calibrated Capintec ionization chamber. The ^{68}Ga separation yield is calculated based on the calibrated radioactivity of produced ^{68}Ga solution and the actual activity of ^{68}Ge decay (or build-up of ^{68}Ga activity for a given time). An EXCEL calculation worksheet is preset for this calculation with the collected measurement data set.
- *Procedure for radionuclidic purity determination*
  – Radionuclidic purity of the ^{68}Ga solution is determined by measurement of ^{68}Ge activity (^{68}Ge breakthrough) in the ^{68}Ga solution sample.
  – Gamma-ray spectrometry is applied for radionuclidic purity determination. The measurement is made using a calibrated HPGe detector coupled to a multichannel gamma-ray spectrometry analyzer such as the Canberra series 85.
  – ^{68}Ga solution of activity 100–200 μCi ^{68}Ga is taken from the product and placed into a calibrated measurement vial together with 1.0 mL rinsing water (standard measurement vial of 1.0 mL solution is normally used).
  – The ^{68}Ga activity is measured first as described in preceding paragraph of this section. The result and time point of measurement are recorded. Then, the ^{68}Ge level (or ^{68}Ge breakthrough) in the ^{68}Ga solution is quantified after 25 h of decay of this sample.
  – The ^{68}Ge activity of the sample is determined by quantification of the 511-keV photopeak and calibrated at the time point of ^{68}Ga activity measurement. Samples of constant geometry (standard measurement vial of 1.0 mL solution is normally used) are counted with low (5%) dead time.
  – ^{68}Ge breakthrough level (%) = 100 × (^{68}Ge activity in the sample/^{68}Ga activity in the sample)
  – Radionuclidic purity of ^{68}Ga solution (%) = 100 − ^{68}Ge breakthrough level (%).
- *Procedure of radiochemical purity determination*
  Thin-layer chromatography (TLC) is applied for radiochemical purity determination.

The following system is used for determination of free $^{68}Ga^{3+}$ ions in the solution: TLC plate RP-18F (Merck, USA), mobile phase 0.1 M sodium citrate solution (pH = 5).

R_f value for free $^{68}Ga^{3+}$ ions is $R_f = 0.9$. R_f value for other ^{68}Ga species is $R_f \leq 0.5$.

- The above-mentioned TLC plate is cut into 2 × 20 cm strips, marked at 2 and 12 cm from the origin, placed into a 100°C oven to dry for approximately 0.5 h (strip activation), and allowed to cool at room temperature for 5 min.
- The activated strips are spotted with 5 μL of ^{68}Ga solution 2 cm from origin.
- They are placed immediately in a thin-layer chromatography tank containing the mobile phase, ensuring that the sample spot is above the solvent level.
- The chromatogram (TLC strip) is allowed to develop to 12 cm from the origin.
- The strips are dried in a 100°C oven for about 15 min.
- The strips are covered with tape on both front and back surfaces.
- The strips are placed on a TLC scanner for scanning of the radiochromatogram.
- After scanning is complete, the areas of all peaks found are integrated to determine the radiochemical purity using the following equation:
- Radiochemical purity (%) = 100 × (area of the peak with R_f of free Ga^{3+}/ area sum of all peaks)

- *pH measurement of ^{68}Ga solution*
  The pH value of any aqueous solution is measured by a calibrated pH-meter.
- *Procedure for metallic ion impurity determination using ICP-MS or ICP-OES*
  This process will be performed based on an analysis service contract. The contractor is qualified based on certification from a well-recognized institution. For the analysis sample submission, ^{68}Ga solution samples of 0.5 mL volume and decay time of longer than 24 h are required.
- *Bacterial endotoxin of ^{68}Ga solution*
  Bacterial endotoxin test is performed as described in US or EU pharmacopoeias.

5.1.2 Radiolabeling Efficacy Evaluation Based on Radiolabeling Ligands DOTATOC and DOTATATE with ^{68}Ga Solution

Radiolabeling is evaluated based on the labeling yield of commonly used ligand DOTATOC or DOTATATE.

Process of radiolabeling ligands with basic ^{68}Ga solution: 0.75 mL basic purified ^{68}Ga solution of given radioactivity received from a ^{68}Ga radioisotope generator integrated system RADIGIS-^{68}Ga is transferred directly into a reaction vial containing 5 nmols DOTATOC or DOTATATE ligand dissolved in 5 μL 0.1 M HCl (1.0 mM ligand solution). HEPES (4-(2-hydroxyethyl)piperazine-1-ethanesulfonic acid) buffer solution (375 μL, 1.0 M) is added to the reaction vial, and pH is adjusted to 4.0 using about 30 μL 4 M HCl solution. The mixture is heated to 95°C in an aluminum block-mantled microheater for 10 min, then transferred to quality control for radiolabeling yield determination by either SPE sorbent cartridge or HPLC method.

Radiolabeling yield determination with SPE sorbent cartridge: The reaction mixture labeled above is passed through a Sep-Pack light C-18 cartridge (Waters). Unreacted ^{68}Ga is then removed by washing the cartridge with 4 mL water. The ^{68}Ga-DOTATOC or ^{68}Ga-DOTATATE is eluted with 0.45 mL ethanol into the final vial, containing 5 mL saline, and activity is then measured using a Capintec radiation dose calibrator. Radiolabeling yield (%) = 100 × (activity of ^{68}Ga-ligand calibrated at the time point of activity measurement of the ^{68}Ga solution/^{68}Ga solution activity).

Radiolabeling yield determination with HPLC (high performance liquid chromatography): HPLC system from Waters consisting of a pump, gradient former, UV and high-sensitivity radiation detectors, and Rheodyne sample injector (PEEK, 100 μL) are coupled in series. A Phenomenex Synergi 4 μm Hydro-RP 80A HPLC column with dimensions of 250 × 4.6 mm packed with C18 with Polar Encapping (high hydrophobicity) of 4 μm particle size is used. The eluent system and gradient elution program are as follows:

Elution time, min	Flow rate, mL/min	% A (acetonitrile)	% B (water)	% C (1% TFA (trifluoroacetic acid) in water)
0	1	5	85	10
1	1	5	85	10
9	1	90	0	10
10	1	5	85	10
17	1	5	85	10

^{68}Ga-DOTATATE and/or ^{68}Ga-DOTATOC peak appears at 11–12 min, and $^{68}Ga^{3+}$ ions and hydrolyzed products are retained at 2–3 min.

Radiochemical purity control of ^{68}Ga-labeled ligand: Thin-layer chromatography is applied for radiochemical purity determination of ^{68}Ga-labeled DOTATOC and/or DOTATATE. Two thin-layer chromatography (TLC) systems are used for determination of free $^{68}Ga^{3+}$ ions and hydrolyzed ^{68}Ga in the solution.

TLC system 1: TLC plate RP-18F (Merck, Whitehouse Station, NJ, USA), mobile phase 0.1 M sodium citrate solution (pH 5).

R_f value for ^{68}Ga-DOTATOC or ^{68}Ga-DOTATATE is $R_f = 0.0$. R_f value for free $^{68}Ga^{3+}$ ions is $R_f = 0.9$

TLC system 2: TLC plates ITLC-SG (Pall Corporation, East Hill, NY, USA), mobile phase 1 M ammonium acetate/methanol (1:1) mixture.

R_f value for ^{68}Ga-DOTATOC or ^{68}Ga-DOTATATE is $R_f = 0.9$. R_f value for hydrolyzed ^{68}Ga is $R_f = 0.1$. TLC process:

- The above-mentioned TLC plate is cut into 2 × 20 cm strips and marked at 2 and 12 cm from the origin.

- The strips are placed in a 100°C oven and allowed to dry for approximately 0.5 h (strip activation), then allowed to cool at room temperature for 5 min.
- The activated strips are spotted with 10 μL of ^{68}Ga-DOTATOC or ^{68}Ga-DOTATATE solution 2 cm from the origin.
- They are placed immediately in a thin-layer chromatography tank containing the mobile phase, ensuring that the sample spot is above the solvent level.
- The chromatogram (TLC strip) is allowed to develop to 12 cm from the origin.
- The strips are dried in a 100°C oven for about 15 min.
- The strips are covered with tape on both front and back surfaces.
- The strips are placed on a TLC scanner for scanning of the radiochromatogram.
- After scanning is complete, the areas of all peaks found are integrated to determine the radiochemical purity using the following equation:
- Radiochemical purity (%) = 100 × (area of the peak with R_f of ^{68}Ga-DOTA-TOC or ^{68}Ga-DOTATATE/area sum of all peaks)

5.2 Operation Performance Assessment of Ga-68 Generator Systems

^{68}Ge/^{68}Ga generator column: Evaluation of the physical integrity and leakage of the column is required; Elution–purification–concentration system and programming: Evaluation on the robustness (regarding normal operation, failure, and any incident occurring) of the elution–purification–concentration module is required; Radiation protection: Evaluation on radiation safety is required.

Acknowledgments The author would like to thank the Australian Nuclear Science and Technology Organisation (ANSTO) for financial support for the Radionuclide Development Project (RRI-0168, including the Ga-68 generator). The author also acknowledges Michael Izard for his electronic installation, Hien Do for her valuable review, Paula Berghofer for English polishing, and Elisabeth Oehlke and Jackson Tim for generator elution and ^{68}Ga-radiolabeling evaluation. Pellegrini Paul and Myint Zaw are acknowledged for test elution of the first generator prototype. David Joel and Theresa Cao are acknowledged for SEM and ICP-OES analysis. William Townsend and Gerard Breen are acknowledged for generator packaging approval and engineering service.

References

Aardaneh K, Van der Walt TN (2006) Ga_2O for target, solvent extraction for radiochemical separation and SnO_2 for the preparation of a ^{68}Ge/^{68}Ga generator. J Radioanal Nucl Chem 268:25–32

Arino H, Skraba WJ, Kramer HH (1978) A new ^{68}Ge/^{68}Ga radioisotope generator system. Int J Appl Radiat Isot 29:117–120

Asti M, Pietri GD, Fraternali A et al (2008) Validation of ^{68}Ge/^{68}Ga generator processing by chemical purification for routine clinical application of ^{68}Ga-DOTATOC. Nucl Med Biol 35:721–724

Bao B, Song M (1996) A new ^{68}Ge/^{68}Ga generator based on CeO_2. J Radioanal Nucl Chem Lett 213:233–238

Blois E, Chan HS, Naidoo C et al (2011) Characteristics of Sn_2O-based $^{68}Ge/^{68}Ga$ generator and aspects of radiolabelling DOTA-peptides. Appl Radiat Isot 69:308–315
Bokhari TH, Mushtaq A, Khan IU (2009) Concentration of ^{68}Ga via solvent extraction. Appl Radiat Isot 67:100–102
Browne E, Firestone RB (1986) Ge-68 and Ga-68. In: Shirley VS (ed) Table of radioactive nuclides. Wiley, New York
Caletka R, Kotas P (1974) Separation of germanium from some elements by adsorption of silica gel. J Radioanal Chem 21:349–353
Chakravarty R, Shukla R, Ram R (2011) Development of a nano-zirconia based $^{68}Ge/^{68}Ga$ generator for biomedical applications. Nucl Med Biol 38:575–583
Eckerman KF, Endo A (2011) MIRD: radionuclide data and decay schemes, 2nd edn. The Society of Nuclear Medicine, Reston
Egamediev SKh, Khujaev S, Mamatkazina AKh (2000) Influence of preliminary treatment of aluminium oxide on the separation of ^{68}Ge-^{68}Ga radionuclide chain. J Radioanal Nucl Chem 246:593–596
Erhardt GJ, Wetch MJ (1978) A new Germanium-68/Gallium-68 generator. J Nucl Med 19:925–929
Erhardt GJ, Wetch MJ (1992) United States Patent no. 5,154,897
European Association of Nuclar Medicine EANM-Monograph 2464 (2011) Galliumchloride(68 Ga) solution for radiolabelling. Pharmeuropa 23:507–509
Greene MW, Tucker WD (1961) An improved Gallium-68 cow. Int J Appl Radiat Isot 12:62–63
Hsin-Li (2009) A new Ge-68/Ga-68 generator system using a higher sorption capacity resin as adsorbent for Ge-68. J Nucl Med 50:2137
Kopecky P, Mudrova B (1974) ^{68}Ge-^{68}Ga generator for the production of ^{68}Ga in an ionic form. Int J Appl Radiat Isot 25:263–268
Kopecky P, Mudrova B, Svoboda K (1973) The study of conditions for the preparation and utilization of ^{68}Ge-^{68}Ga generator. Int J Appl Radiat Isot 24:73–80
Kozlova MD, Malinin AB, Kodina GE (1994) Development of $^{68}Ge/^{68}Ga$ generator in institute of biophysics. J Lab Comp Radiopharm 35:282
Le VS (1990) Preparation of gel-type chromatographic ^{99m}Tc generators using titaniummolybdate and zirconium-molybdate columns containing (n,gamma) ^{99}Mo. IAEA Research Co-ordination Meeting, BRIT-Bombay, India
Le VS (2003) ^{99m}Tc generator preparation using (n,gamma) ^{99}Mo produced ex-natural molybdenum. Proceeding of the 2001 Workshop on the utilization of research reactors, November 2001 Beijing China. JAERIConf- 2003-004, 216–223 http://jolissrch-inter.tokai-sc.jaea.go.jp/pdfdata/JAERIConf-2003-004.pdf
Le VS (2011a) Sorbent material. WIPO (World Intellectual Property Organization), WO 2011/106847 A1
Le VS (2011b) ^{68}Gallium purification. WIPO (World Intellectual Property Organization), WO 2011/106846 A1
Le VS, Nguyen C D, Bui V C et al. (2007) Synthesis, characterization and application of PTC and PZC sorbents for preparation of chromatographic ^{99m}Tc and ^{188}Re generators. In: ANSTO publications online, http://apo.ansto.gov.au/dspace/handle/10238/3715
Le VS, Nguyen CD, Pellegrini P et al (2009a) Polymeric titanium oxychloride sorbent for $^{188}W/^{188}Re$ nuclide pair separation. Sep Sci Tech 44:1074–1098
Le VS, Nguyen CD, Bui VC et al (2009b) Preparation of inorganic polymer sorbents and their application in radionuclide generator technology. In: IAEA (ed) Therapeutic radionuclide generators: $^{90}Sr/^{90}Y$ and $^{188}W/^{188}Re$ generators, technical report series no. 470, IAEA, Vienna
Le VS, Izard M, Pellegrini P et al (2011a) Development of ^{68}Ga generator at ANSTO. In: ANSTO publications online, http://apo.ansto.gov.au/dspace/handle/10238/3701
Le VS, Morcos N, Oehlke E et al (2012) Methods of protocol development for radionuclidic purity test of radioisotope products used in nuclear medicine. J Radioanal Nucl Chem (submission)
Le VS, Izard M, Pellegrini P et al (2011b) Development of ^{68}Ga generator at ANSTO. Abstracts of poster presentations (chemistry). World J Nucl Med 10:86

Lewis RE, Milford N H (1982) Method and system for generating and collecting Gallium-68 using alkaline eluant. United States Patent 4,330,507

Lievens P, Hoste J (1974) Selective removal of germanium by retention on silica gel. Anal Chim Acta 70:462–464

Loc'h C, Maziere B, Comar D (1980) A new generator for ionic Gallium-68. J Nucl Med 21:171–173

Loktionova NS, Belozub AN, Filosofov DV, Zhernosekov KP, Wagner T, Turler A, Rösch F (2011) Improved column-based radiochemical processing of the generator produced ^{68}Ga. Appl Radiat Isot 69:942–946

McAlister DR, Horwitz EP (2009) Automated two column generator systems for medical radionuclides. Appl Radiat Isot 67:1985–1991

McElvany KD, Hopkins KT, Welch MJ (1984) Comparison of ^{68}Ge/^{68}Ga generator systems for radiopharmaceutical production. Int J Appl Radiat Isot 35:521–524

Mourtada F, Azhdarinia A, Yang D (2009) Automated system for formulating radiopharmaceuticals. United States Patent US 2008/0035542 A1

Neirinckx RD, Davis MA (1979) Potential column chromatography generators for ionic Ga-68 I. Inorganic substrate. J Nucl Med 20:1075–1079

Neirinckx RD, Davis MA (1980) Potential column chromatography generators for ionic Ga-68 II. Organic ion exchangers as chromatographic supports. J Nucl Med 21:81–83

Neirinckx RD, Davis MA (1981a) Generator for Gallium-68 and compositions obtained therefrom. United State Patent 4,264,468

Neirinckx RD, Davis MA (1981b) Generator for ionic Gallium-68 based on column chromatography. United State Patent 4,288,424

Neirinckx RD, Layne WW, Sawan SP et al (1982) Development of an ionic ^{68}Ge/^{68}Ga generator 3. Chelate resins as chromatographic substrates for germanium. Int J Appl Radiat Isot 33:259–266

Pao PJ, Silvester DJ, Waters SL (1981) A new method for the preparation of ^{68}Ga generators following proton bombardment of Gallium oxide targets. J Radioanal Chem 64:267–272

Pawlak D, Wojdowska W, Mikolajeczak R (2011) Method for post-elution concentration and acidity reduction of eluate obtained from SnO_2 based ^{68}Ge/^{68}Ga generator. Abstracts of poster presentations (chemistry). World J Nucl Med 10:78

Rösch F, Filosofov DV, Zhernosekov KP et al (2008) Method and device for isolating a chemically and radiochemically cleaned ^{68}Ga-radionuclide and for marking a marking precursor with the ^{68}Ga radionuclide. United States Patent Application Publication US2008/0277350 A1

Schuhmacher J, Maier-Borst W (1981) A new ^{68}Ge/^{68}Ga radioisotope generator system for production of ^{68}Ga in dilute HCl. Int J Appl Radiat Isot 32:31–36

Velikyan I, Beyer GJ, Langström B (2004a) Microwave-supported preparation of ^{68}Ga bioconjugates with high specific radioactivity. Bioconjugate Chem 15:554–560

Velikyan I, Langström B, Beyer GJ (2004b) Method of obtaining gallium-68 and use thereof and device for carrying out said method, WIPO (World Intellectual Property Organization), WO 2004/089517

Waters SL, Horlock PL, Kensett MJ (1983) The application of hydrous Tin(IV)Oxide in radiochemical separations and, in particular, for the ^{68}Ge/^{68}Ga and ^{82}Sr/^{82}Rb generator systems. Int J Appl Radiat Isot 34:1023

Zhernosekov KP, Filosofov DV, Baum RP et al (2007) Processing of generator-produced ^{68}Ga for medical application. J Nucl Med 48:1741–1748

Zoller F, Riss PJ, Montforts FP, Rösch F (2010) Efficient post-processing of aqueous generator eluates facilitates ^{68}Ga-labelling under anhydrous conditions. Radiochim Acta 98:157–160

Purification and Labeling Strategies for ^{68}Ga from ^{68}Ge/^{68}Ga Generator Eluate

Dirk Mueller, Ingo Klette and Richard P. Baum

Abstract

For successful labeling, ^{68}Ge/^{68}Ga generator eluate has to be concentrated (from 10 mL or more to less than 1 mL) and to be purified of metallic impurities, especially Fe(III), and ^{68}Ge breakthrough. Anionic, cationic and fractional elution methods are well known. We describe two new methods: (1) a combined cationic–anionic purification and (2) an easy-to-use and reliable cationic purification with NaCl solution. Using the first method, ^{68}Ga from 10 mL generator eluate was collected on a SCX cartridge, then eluted with 1.0 mL 5.5 M HCl directly on an anion exchanger (30 mg AG1X8). After drying with a stream of helium, ^{68}Ga was eluted with 0.4 mL water into the reaction vial. We provide as an example labeling of BPAMD. Using the second method, ^{68}Ga from 10 mL generator eluate was collected on a SCX cartridge, then eluted with a hydrochloric solution of sodium chloride (0.5 mL 5 M NaCl, 12.5 μL 5.5 M HCl) into the reaction vial, containing 40 μg DOTATOC and 0.5 mL 1 M ammonium acetate buffer pH 4.5. After heating for 7 min at 90°C, the reaction was finished. Radiochemical purity was higher than 95% without further purification. No ^{68}Ge breakthrough was found in the final product.

D. Mueller (✉) · I. Klette · R. P. Baum
Department of Nuclear Medicine, Centre for PETCT,
Zentralklinik Bad Berka, 99437 Bad Berka, Germany
e-mail: d.mueller.pet@zentralklinik-bad-berka.de

I. Klette
e-mail: ingo.klette@zentralklinik.de

R. P. Baum
e-mail: info@rpbaum.de

R. P. Baum and F. Rösch (eds.), *Theranostics, Gallium-68, and Other Radionuclides*,
Recent Results in Cancer Research 194, DOI: 10.1007/978-3-642-27994-2_5,

Contents

1 Introduction

1.1 History

The first ^{68}Ga radiopharmaceuticals and ^{68}Ge/^{68}Ga radionuclide generators were developed at the beginning of the 1960s, in parallel with the creation of the first positron scintillation cameras, long before imaging with ^{18}F (Rösch 2011). The first ^{68}Ge/^{68}Ga generators were self-made by radiochemical laboratories, mostly being based on EDTA elution (Hnatowich 1975). ^{68}Ge breakthrough was relatively high, as well as other metallic impurities. For a number of years now, a new type of ^{68}Ge/^{68}Ga generator has been commercially available (Obninsk, Russia), followed by diverse improvements from other manufacturers as well.

1.2 Current State

Molecular imaging of tumors by PET/CT using peptides radiolabeled for receptors is on the rise (Prasad and Baum 2010; Baum et al. 2010; Sainz-Esteban et al. 2010). The popularity of ^{68}Ga-labeled radiopharmaceuticals is rising due to their utility for molecular imaging, as well as the potential for on-demand production of ^{68}Ga for radiolabeling in the absence of cyclotron facilities. As generator technologies have matured to more consistently deliver high-purity ^{68}Ga over many months, the availability of highly adaptable postprocessing radiochemistry modules has also increased.

These developments suggest a rich future for generator-produced ^{68}Ga as an attractive candidate for radiolabeling of not only peptides but also other molecular targeting vectors such as carbohydrates, proteins, and oligonucleotides (Tolmachev et al. 2011; Fellner et al. 2010). Numerous methods for ^{68}Ga generator elution, purification, and radiolabeling of peptide radiopharmaceuticals have been advanced, being primarily based on three thematic ^{68}Ga eluate purification procedures found in the literature.

1.3 Basic Methods

1.3.1 Anionic Purification

In the first of these basic methods, Meyer et al. described ^{68}Ga labeling using an anionic purification step. In this procedure, ^{68}Ga chloride in the ^{68}Ge/^{68}Ga generator eluate is converted to the ^{68}Ga gallate anion by addition of concentrated HCl and then trapped on an anionic exchanger cartridge. After drying the cartridge with a stream of inert gas or air, the ^{68}Ga is eluted with water into the reaction vessel with chelator-modified peptide (Meyer et al. 2004). Although the obtained ^{68}Ga eluate has high chemical purity, an alternative to the intermediate conversion step using concentrated HCl may have advantages.

1.3.2 Cationic Purification

In a second approach, a labeling procedure based on a purification step of the ^{68}Ga eluate using a cation exchange resin was described by Zhernosekov et al. (2007). In this method, ^{68}Ga eluted from the generator is trapped by a cation exchange resin and then washed and eluted with two different hydrochloric acid/acetone solutions. The majority of the acetone is removed during the radiolabeling step, which is carried out at 100°C. This method has formed the basis for numerous effective strategies for purification of ^{68}Ga generator eluates and radiolabeling of peptides. To ensure that the final product is of sufficient radiochemical purity (>95%), a variation on this basic approach to ^{68}Ga purification and radiolabeling applies the same principles (Meyer et al. 2004) but includes also a final product purification using a C-18 cartridge, from which the final product is extracted with ethanol. The use of acetone/HCl may lead to detectable presence of mesityl oxide (4-methyl-3-penten-2-on) in the final product, although this can be avoided by using fresh preparations of the acetone/HCl eluent.

1.3.3 Fractional Elution

The third fundamental approach to ^{68}Ga labeling procedures uses the generator eluate directly based on fractional elution of the ^{68}Ge/^{68}Ga generator. In this method, early and late fractions of the 0.1 M HCl eluent containing ^{68}Ga are discarded, and an intermediate volume of eluted ^{68}Ga is collected and buffered to an appropriate pH for radiolabeling (e.g., with HEPES). Theoretically, a significant fraction of impurities are removed in early fractions of eluent (Breeman et al. 2005), and the fraction of eluent containing the highest concentration of pure ^{68}Ga is used for preparation of the radiopharmaceutical. Following the radiolabeling step, impurities such as free ^{68}Ga are removed by use of a C-18 cartridge and extraction with ethanol (as described above). The potential disadvantages of this method lie in that the procedure uses only a fraction of the elutable ^{68}Ga activity, which may reduce the achievable specific activity of the final radiopharmaceutical product, as well as the need for gas chromatographic analysis to establish the concentration of ethanol as an excipient in the final product.

2 Combined Cationic–Anionic Purification of $^{68}Ge/^{68}Ga$ Generator Eluate for Labeling of Fragile Peptides and Proteins

2.1 Aim

The combination of cationic and anionic purification of ^{68}Ga eluate should reduce the amount of concentrated HCl as well as the eluate volume. On the other hand, in the case of larger and fragile peptides or proteins such as DOTA-conjugated Affibody, the cationic concentration with the help of acetonic HCl followed by labeling with ^{68}Ga (Zhernosekov et al. 2007) requires high temperature to evaporate the acetone. The basic idea for this procedure is trapping of ^{68}Ga using a cation exchanger in a first step followed by elution of the precleaned ^{68}Ga with a minimal amount of 5.5 M HCl. The resulting ^{68}Ga tetrachlorogallate can then be collected using an anion exchanger in a second purification step (Mueller et al. 2009). This purification procedure for the $^{68}Ge/^{68}Ga$ eluate also eliminates acetone or other organic solvents.

2.2 Description

The $^{68}Ge/^{68}Ga$ generator was eluted with a total of 10 mL 0.1 M HCl, and the ^{68}Ga was collected on a SCX cartridge (Varian, Bond Elut-SCX, 100 mg, 1 mL). The activity was then eluted with 1.0 mL 5.5 M HCl and directly collected again on an anion exchanger cartridge (AG1X8, 30 mg, preconditioned with 1 mL 5.5 M HCl). After drying of the cartridge with a stream of helium (or air) for 1 min, 60% of the ^{68}Ga was eluted with 0.4–1.0 mL water into the reaction vial with 0.4 mL 1.5 M HEPES buffer and 100 μg DOTA-Affibody (DOTA-$Z_{Her2:342\text{-}pep2}$). The reaction mixture was heated to 80°C for 5 min.

For the anionic purification step, the authors developed a combined cartridge. For this purpose a 100 mg SAX cartridge (Alltech SAX Extract Clean SAX, 100 mg, 1.5 mL) was covered with 70 mg AG1X8 (BIO-RAD, 200–400 Mesh). If this cartridge is used, up to 80% of ^{68}Ga is elutable.

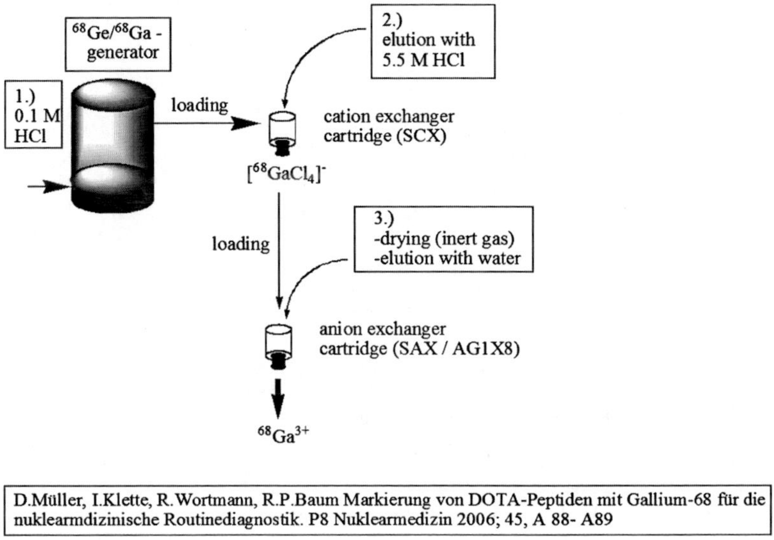

Fig. 1 Purification procedure, schematic drawing

2.3 Advantages

This procedure leads to a final product with radiochemical purity greater than 95% without further purification steps. The described purification delivers ^{68}Ga in high chemical and radiochemical purity. Use of acetone or ethanol during the labeling procedure is not necessary, so that GC investigation is not essential for release. This method allows labeling of fragile peptides with molecular mass higher than DOTA-D-Phe1-Tyr3-octreotide (DOTATOC) such as DOTA-Affibody (DOTA-$Z_{Her2:342\text{-}pep2}$) or proteins (Mueller et al. 2006, 2009) (Figs. 1, 2, 3).

2.4 Example: Synthesis of ^{68}Ga-BPAMD

2.4.1 Introduction

For the ^{68}Ga-labeled bisphosphonate monoamide derivative of DOTA (BPAMD) for patient studies, the combined cationic/anionic ^{68}Ga eluent purification was successfully used in our department. The widely used cationic labeling procedure (Zhernosekov et al. 2007) leads to a nonphysiologic final product with pH lower than 2. Neutralization of the final product with sodium hydrogencarbonate (8.4%) is not possible, because of the decomposition of ^{68}Ga-BPAMD. Furthermore, the final product contains nonreacted and free ^{68}Ga^{3+} in different concentrations, so that a purification step is necessary. The combined purification method avoids these problems.

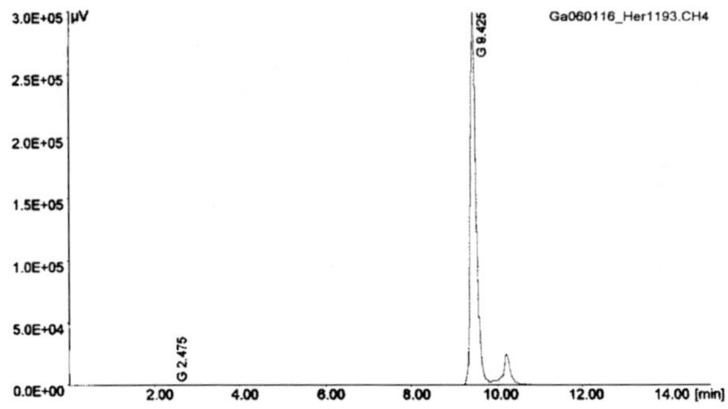

#	Name	RT	Height[µV]	Area[µV.Sec]	%Area
1	Ga68-Chlorid	2.475	153	1342.000	0.04
2	Ga68-Her2	9.425	300552	3119761.500	99.96

Total Area of Peak = 3121103.500 [µV.Sec]

Fig. 2 HPLC of the final product. Column: RP-18, LiChroCART 250-4, LiChrospher 100, RP-18e (5 µm); solvent A: acetonitrile solution in water (5%), 0.1% TFA; solvent B: 95% acetonitrile solution in water, 0.1% TFA; flow rate: 1.2 mL/min; gradient: from 0–2 min 100% A, 3–15 min to 100% B. $^{68}GaCl_3$: (R_t = 2.5 min) 0.04%, ^{68}Ga-Affibody: (R_t = 9.4 min) 99.96%

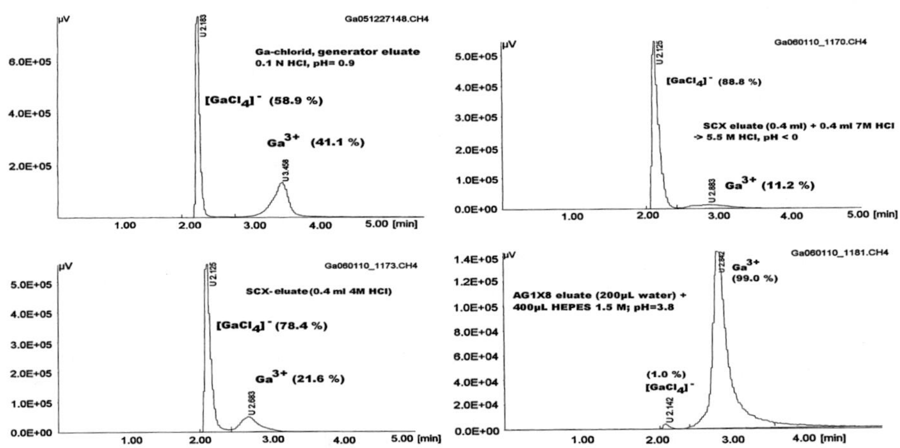

Fig. 3 HPLC of $^{68}GaCl_3$ samples at different HCl concentrations. Column RP-18, LiChroCART 250-4, LiChrospher 100, RP-18e (5 µm); solvent A: acetonitrile solution in water (5%), 0.1% TFA; solvent B: 95% acetonitrile solution in water, 0.1% TFA; flow rate: 1.2 mL/min; gradient: from 0–2 min 100% A, 3–5 min to 30% B

2.4.2 Labeling Procedure

The ^{68}Ga generator was eluted with a total of 10 mL 0.1 M HCl, and the ^{68}Ga was collected on a SCX cartridge (Varian, Bond Elut-SCX, 100 mg, 1 mL). This cartridge was then eluted with 5.5 M HCl directly through an anion exchanger cartridge.

For this anionic purification step we used a combined SAX cartridge (Alltech SAX Extract Clean SAX, 100 mg/1.5 mL), covered with 70 mg AG1X8 (BIO-RAD,

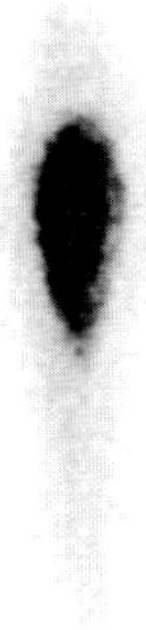

Fig. 4 TLC of sterile filtered reaction solution synthesized by the combined cationic–anionic purification method (ITLC-SG; solvent: 0.1 M citric acid)

200–400 Mesh, hydroxide form), preconditioned with 1 mL 5.5 M HCl. The cartridge was dried with a stream of inert gas or air for 1 min, and ^{68}Ga was then eluted with 1 mL water followed by elution with 0.5 mL aqueous 1.5 M ammonium acetate solution into the reaction vial with 1 mL water, 0.5 mL aqueous 1.5 M ammonium acetate solution, and 20 μg BPAMD. Then, the reaction mixture was heated to 100°C for 12 min.

2.4.3 Results

The $^{68}Ga^{3+}$ was completely bonded, and after sterile filtration the radiochemical yield was about 55% (n.d.c.). This procedure leads to a final product with radiochemical purity greater than 95% without further purification steps. The pH of the final solution is about 4. Determination of other impurities by gas chromatography is not necessary. No organic solvents were added. The use of our developed combined SAX/AG1X8 cartridge increased the yield significantly. The instant thin layer chromatography (ITLC) quality control (Fig. 4) determines free $^{68}Ga^{3+}$ as well as potentially formed ^{68}Ga hydroxide.

We thereby developed a reproducible and applicable labeling procedure for synthesis of ^{68}Ga-BPAMD. The reaction delivers the product with radiochemical purity higher than 95%. Subsequent purification is not necessary, and the pH of the reaction solution is about 4.

3 A New Highly Efficient NaCl-Based Cationic $^{68}Ge/^{68}Ga$ Generator Eluate Purification: The Basis for Effective ^{68}Ga Labeling

3.1 Aim

The aim is to develop efficient ^{68}Ga labeling procedures for routine application in clinical practice. The purification procedure for the $^{68}Ge/^{68}Ga$ eluate should reduce handling with concentrated HCl, and should form the labeled final product in high

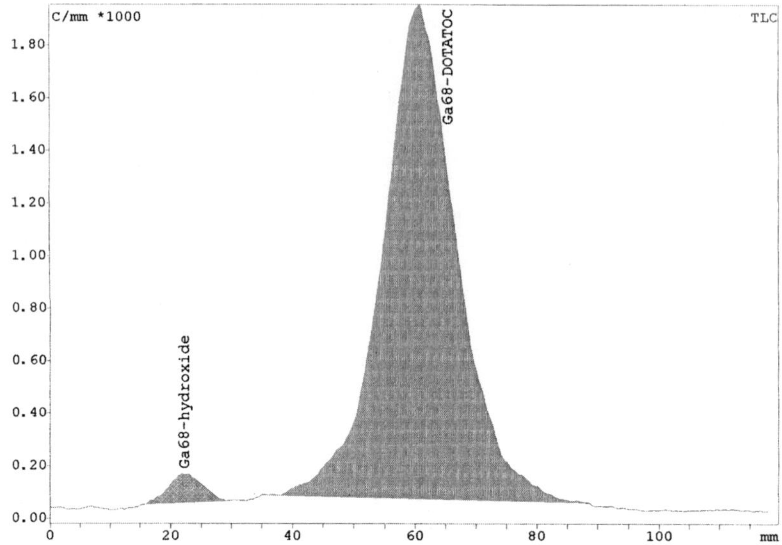

Fig. 5 ITLC-SG of the final reaction mixture; eluent: acetonitrile/water 1:1; ^{68}Ga-hydroxide/-chloride ($R_f = 0$): 2.4% ^{68}Ga-DOTATOC ($R_f = 0.5$): 97.6%

yield with high purity. Use of acetone or other organic solvents or compounds such as HEPES should be avoided. Handling should be reduced to a minimum of simple steps and should allow transfer to an automated system.

3.2 Labeling Strategy

Our strategy was influenced in part by the methods mentioned above, with the finer points of the new approach inspired by a reported procedure in which a rinse step for an OASIS WAX cartridge with 5 M NaCl solution was used to remove the 5.5 M HCl (de Blois et al. 2011). The use of only one ion exchange cartridge, but without use of organic solvents and high purification ability, were part of this method, combined with a search for a suitable buffer system. For DOTA-conjugated peptides, we exemplarily used DOTATOC.

3.3 Description of the Method

All reagents were purchased from commercial sources and used as received. The mentioned cartridges are commercially available. For all experiments a ^{68}Ga generator from Obninsk (Eckert and Ziegler Europe) and IGG100 ^{68}Ga generator (Eckert and Ziegler Europe) were used. The generator was eluted with 10 mL 0.1 M HCl (Merck, Germany). The ^{68}Ga of the generator eluate was collected on a SCX cartridge (VARIAN, Bond Elut-SCX, 100 mg, 1 mL; preconditioned with

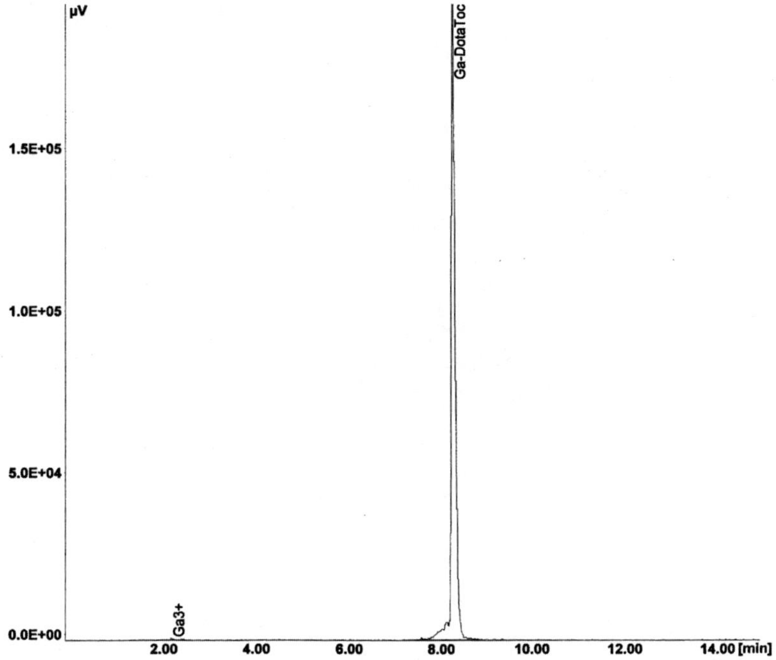

Fig. 6 HPLC of the final product. Column: RP-18, LiChroCART 250-4, LiChrospher 100, RP-18e (5 µm); solvent A: 5% acetonitrile in water, 0.1% TFA; solvent B: 95% acetonitrile in water, 0.1% TFA; flow rate: 1.2 mL/min; gradient: from 0–2 min 100% A, 3–15 min to 100% B. $^{68}Ga^{3+}$ ($R_t = 2.3$ min) 0.6%, ^{68}Ga-DOTATOC ($R_t = 8.4$ min): 99.4%

1 mL 5.5 M HCl, 10 mL water) and then eluted with hydrochloric solution of sodium chloride (0.5 mL 5.0 M NaCl, 12.5 µL 5.5 M HCl) into the reaction vial with 40 µg DOTATOC, 3 mL water, and 250 µL 1 M ammonium acetate buffer (3.9 g NH_4Ac, 50 mL water, 1 mL HCl conc., adjusted with acetic acid to pH 4.5). After heating the solution for 7 min at 90°C, the reaction was finished.

This method works very reliably on an automated synthesis module. The concentration of unbound ^{68}Ga is lower than 5%. The radiochemical purity of the labeled DOTATOC is higher than 95%. The reaction mixture contains no toxic substances or substances of concern, so subsequent purification is not required. After sterile filtration, the radiochemical yield is about 82% (n.d.c.).

3.4 Results

We developed a new, easy-to-handle, highly effective NaCl-based cationic method for ^{68}Ge/^{68}Ga generator eluate purification. With this procedure, the radiochemical yield for labeling of DOTATOC with ^{68}Ga is about 82%. A subsequent purification

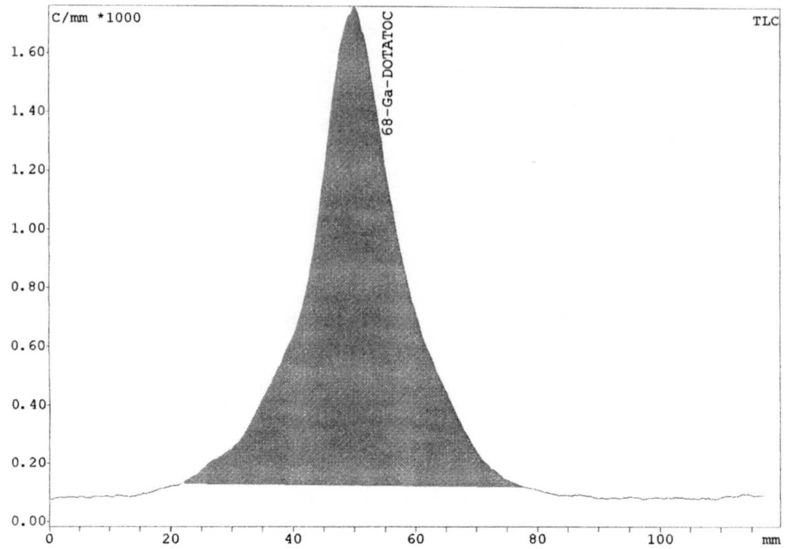

Fig. 7 ITLC-SG of the final product after sterile filtration; eluent: acetonitrile/water 1:1

step is not necessary. The final solution contains no organic solvents, and a GC investigation is not essential for release (Figs. 5, 6, 7).

References

Baum RP, Prasad V, Müller D, Schuchardt C, Orlova A, Wennborg A, Tolmachev V, Feldwisch J (2010) Molecular imaging of HER2-expressing malignant tumors in breast cancer patients using synthetic 111In- or 68 Ga-labeled affibody molecules. J Nucl Med 51:892–897

Breeman WA, de Jong M, de Blois E, Bernard BF, Konijnenberg M, Krenning EP (2005) Radiolabeling DOTA-peptides with 68 Ga. Eur J Nucl Med Mol Imaging 32:478–485

de Blois E, Sze Chan H, Naidoo C, Prince D, Krenning EP, Breeman WA (2011) Characteristics of SnO_2 based $^{68}Ge/^{68}Ga$ generator and aspects of radiolabeling DOTA-peptides. Appl Radiat Isot 69:308–315

Fellner M, Baum RP, Kubcek V, Hermann P, Lukes I, Prasad VFR (2010) PET/CT imaging of osteoblastic bone metastases with 68 Ga-bisphosphonates: first human study. Eur J Nucl Med Mol Imaging 37:834

Hnatowich DJ (1975) A method for the preparation and quality control of ^{68}Ga radiopharmaceuticals. J Nucl Med 16:764

Meyer GJ, Mäcke H, Schuhmacher J, Knapp WH, Hofmann M (2004) 68 Ga-labelled DOTA- derivatised peptide ligands. Eur J Nucl Med Mol Imaging 31:1097–1104

Mueller D, Klette I, Wortmann R, Baum RP (2006) Markierung von DOTA-peptiden mit gallium- 68 für die nuklearmedizinische Routinediagnostik. Nuklearmedizin 45:A88–A89

Mueller D, Klette I, Gottschaldt M, Baum RP (2009) Radiolabeling of fragile macroligands with ^{68}Ga. J Labelled Compd Radiopharm 52:477

Prasad V, Baum RP (2010) Biodistribution of the Ga-68 labeled somatostatin analogue DOTA- NOC in patients with neuroendocrine tumors: characterization of uptake in normal organs and tumor lesions. Q J Nucl Med Mol Imaging 54:61–67

Rösch F (2011) $^{68}Ge/^{68}Ga$- generators – past, present and future. World J Nucl Med 10:26

Sainz-Esteban A, Prasad V, Baum RP (2010) Interesting image. Pancreatic neuroendocrine tumor with involvement of the inferior mesenteric vein diagnosed by Ga-68 DOTA-TATE PET/CT. Clin Nucl Med 35:40–41

Tolmachev V, Altai M, Sandström M, Perols A, Eriksson Karlström AH, Boschetti F, Orlova A (2011) Evaluation of a maleimido derivative of NOTA for site-specific labeling of affibody molecules. Bioconjug Chem 22:894–902

Zhernosekov KP, Filosofov DV, Baum RP, Aschoff P, Bihl H, Razbash AA, Jahn M, Jennewein M, Rösch F (2007) Processing of generator produced 68 Ga for medical application. J Nucl Med 48:1741–1748

^{67}Ga and ^{68}Ga Purification Studies: Preliminary Results

R. F. Costa, M. F. Barboza and J. A. Osso Jr

Abstract

The positron emission tomography technique is very useful for diagnosis of several diseases. ^{68}Ga is a positron emitter with half-life of 67.7 min. As it is available from ^{68}Ge/^{68}Ga generator systems, it is not necessary to have a nearby cyclotron. However, the eluate from commercial generators contains high levels of metallic impurities, which compete with ^{68}Ga in biomolecular labeling. Thus, a subsequent purification step is needed after generator elution. Here we present the results of two different methods developed for handmade purification of ^{68}Ga and ^{67}Ga for subsequent radiolabeling of biomolecules. Two purification methods were employed. The first one uses a cation exchange resin, and ^{68}Ga is eluted with a solution of acetone/acid. The second method of purification is performed by column chromatography solvent extraction, with ^{68}Ga recovery in deionized water. The best result was achieved with cationic resin AG50W-X8 (>400 mesh). However, the resin is not commercially available. The extraction chromatography column based on absorption of diisopropyl ether in XAD-16 is the most promising purification method. Although the levels of ^{68}Ga recovery and purification were smaller with the cationic resin method, its advantage is the ^{68}Ga recovery in deionized water.

R. F. Costa (✉) · M. F. Barboza · J. A. Osso Jr
Diretoria de Radiofarmácia, Instituto de Pesquisas Energéticas e Nucleares (IPEN/CNEN-SP), Cidade Universitária, Av. Prof. Lineu Prestes, 2242, São Paulo, SP CEP 05508-000, Brazil
e-mail: renatafcosta@usp.br

R. P. Baum and F. Rösch (eds.), *Theranostics, Gallium-68, and Other Radionuclides*, Recent Results in Cancer Research 194, DOI: 10.1007/978-3-642-27994-2_6,

Contents

1 Introduction

For more than 50 years, long-lived $^{68}Ge/^{68}Ga$ generators have been in development. The advantage of obtaining ^{68}Ga through a generator system is that it is not necessary to have an in-house cyclotron, which is a considerable convenience for PET centers with no nearby cyclotron (Roesch and Riss 2010). ^{68}Ga disintegrates 89% by positron emission with low photon emission (1,077 keV, 3.22%) and has physical half-life of 67.7 min, compatible with the pharmacokinetics of low-weight biomolecules such as peptides and antibody fragments. Moreover, its established metallic chemistry allows it to be stably bound to the carrier peptide sequence via a suitable bifunctional chelator such as 1,4,7,10-tetraazacyclododecane-1,4,7,10-tetraacetic acid (DOTA), which is most widely used in labeling processes (Velikyan 2005). All these reasons, combined with the development of PET/CT technology, have improved the field of clinical practice of molecular imaging, such as in neuroendocrine diagnosis.

However, the eluate from one such commercial generator (Cyclotron Co. Ltd., Russian Federation) still contains high levels of long-lived ^{68}Ge, besides other metallic impurities such as Fe^{3+} and Zn^{2+}, which compete with ^{68}Ga, resulting in consequent reduction of the labeling yield of biomolecules (Zhernosekov et al. 2007). Furthermore, successful clinical application of these peptides demands high specific radioactivity, considering the limited amount of receptors, the high binding affinity to receptors, and the possibility of pharmacological side-effects (Velikyan et al. 2008). Thus, the lower the amount of impurities in the eluate, the smaller the competition between the radiolabeled and unlabeled peptide at the receptor, and the better the imaging quality. To reduce impurities, a subsequent purification step is needed after generator elution. The aim of this work is to present the results of two different methods developed for handmade purification of ^{67}Ga and ^{68}Ga for subsequent radiolabeling of biomolecules.

2 Materials and Methods

2.1 $^{68}Ge/^{68}Ga$ Generator and ^{67}Ga

A commercial $^{68}Ge/^{68}Ga$ generator based on a TiO_2 phase adsorbing ^{68}Ge was obtained from Cyclotron Co. (Obninsk, Russian Federation), with activity of 1,110 MBq (30 mCi). ^{68}Ga was manually eluted with 5 mL 0.1 mol L^{-1} HCl during 2 min. The $^{68}Ge/^{68}Ga$ generator was evaluated for 6 months. ^{67}Ga, obtained from MDS Nordion®, was used as surrogate for ^{68}Ga. Radioactivity was measured by Capintec®. The amount of chemical impurities present in ^{67}Ga and ^{68}Ga was evaluated by ICP-OES (Varian, EUA) before and after purification. The metals analyzed were Cu, Fe, Ge, Ni, Ti, and Zn.

2.2 Materials

Cation exchange resin AG50W-X8 (H+, 200–400 mesh) and Chelex 100® (Na^+, 100–200 mesh) were purchased from BioRad (USA). Cation exchange resin AG50W-X8 (H+, >400 mesh) was a donation. The adsorbent resin, XAD-16 (20–60 mesh) was obtained from Sigma-Aldrich (USA). Acetone, diisopropyl ether, hydrochloric acid (30%, Suprapure), titanium chloride, and sodium iodide were purchased from Merck (Germany). No metal material was used. Plastic materials were preferable; however, in some experiments, glass material had to be used.

2.3 Water Purification

Chelex 100® was used to purify deionized water, in all experiments. The deionized water was stirred with resin for at least 2 h and filtered. The efficiency of the process was analyzed by ICP-OES.

2.4 ^{68}Ga Purification on Cation Exchange Resin

The cation exchange purification method used AG50W-X8 (H+, 200–400 mesh and >400 mesh) previously conditioning with 0.1 mol L^{-1} HCl, based on Zhernosekov et al. (2007). A solution of ^{68}Ga in 0.1 mol L^{-1} HCl was loaded onto the column, and ^{68}Ga was further eluted with a solution of acetone/12 mol L^{-1} HCl (97:0.4)%. Two column geometries were tested, containing 0.5 and 0.05 mL resin, as shown in Fig. 1.

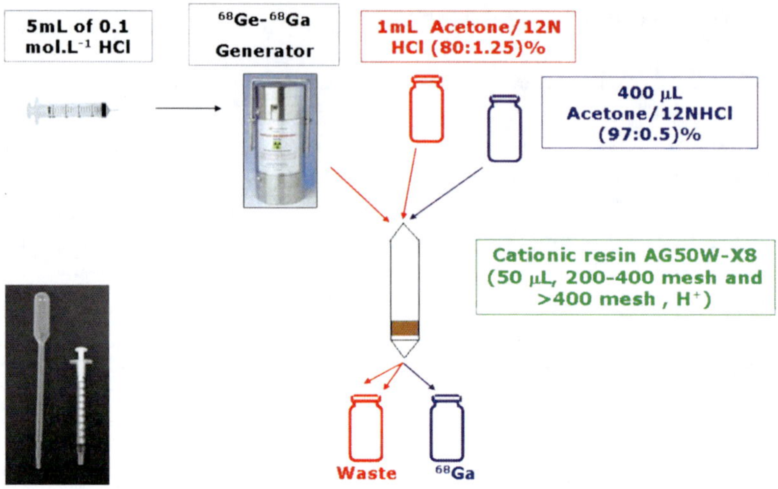

Fig. 1 Homemade ^{68}Ga purification with cationic resin

2.5 ^{67}Ga/^{68}Ga Purification: Isopropyl Ether Extraction System

2.5.1 Liquid–Liquid Solvent Extraction

The second method of purification was conventional solvent extraction using diisopropyl ether (Nachtrieb and Fryxell 1949; Brown 1971). ^{67}Ga was diluted in 3.5 mL 7 mol L^{-1} HCl and extracted three times with 3.5 mL diisopropyl ether. The resulting solution, 10.5 mL diisopropyl ether containing ^{67}Ga, was equilibrated three times with 10.0 mL deionized water, where ^{67}Ga was back-extracted to the aqueous phase. To reduce the final volume containing radioactive gallium, the volume of extraction was reduced to 4.0 mL.

2.5.2 Column Chromatography Solvent Extraction

The purification studies shifted towards preparation of an extraction chromatography column based on absorption of diisopropyl ether in XAD-16. The resin was washed with ethanol and water once. The dried resin (1 g) was kept in contact with 1.4 mL diisopropyl ether during 24 h at 4°C.

The first column was a 10 mm glass column and the second column was a micropipette, as shown in Fig. 2. Furthermore, addition of $TiCl_3$ and 1% NaI to reduce Fe(III) present in the solution to Fe(II) was also studied. $TiCl_3$ can reduce Fe(III), however it is a contaminant for ^{68}Ga labeling. Iodide can also reduce Fe(III), albeit less effectively than $TiCl_3$. Fe(III) and Ga(III) have chemical similarity, which makes Fe(III) a competitor with Ga(III) in labeling procedures.

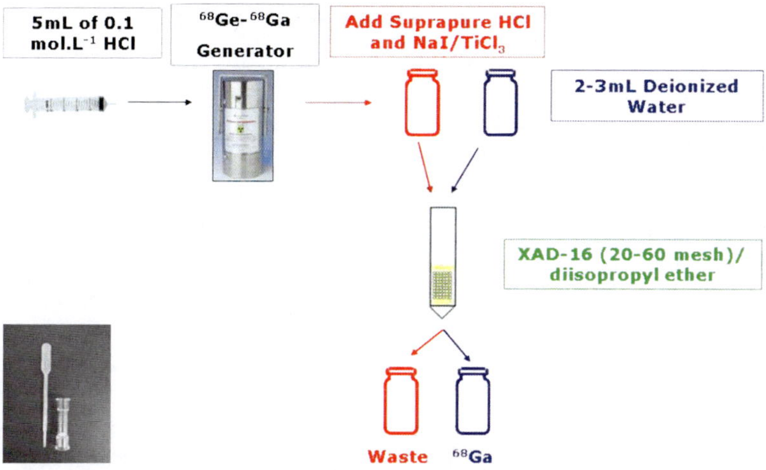

Fig. 2 Homemade ^{67}Ga/^{68}Ga purification with extraction chromatography column

3 Results and Discussion

3.1 ^{68}Ge/^{68}Ga Generator Performance

Figure 3 shows the ^{68}Ge/^{68}Ga generator efficiency, averaging (71.2 ± 4.0)%. The ^{68}Ge/^{68}Ga generator was relatively new, having been calibrated in January 2011. It is essential to obtain good results for elution of the ^{68}Ge/^{68}Ga generator, mainly in case of manual elution, in terms of elution yield and time for the process.

In addition, Fig. 4 shows the importance of often eluting the ^{68}Ge/^{68}Ga generator. Elution was performed every day, and the levels of impurities were reduced.

3.2 Water Purification

The results of analyses showed that the main contaminants, Fe and Zn, were reduced after Chelex 100® purification, by (82 ± 5)% and (91 ± 10)% ($n = 3$), respectively. Other analyzed metals, such as Cu, Ge, Ti, and Ni, were not significantly present in deionized water.

3.3 ^{67}Ga/^{68}Ga Purification on Cation Exchange Resin

The first purification method was applied in a syringe used as chromatography column with volume of 0.5 mL of AG50W-X8 (200–400 mesh). Although the results for reduction of metals (87.0 ± 3.6, $n = 3$) and ^{68}Ga yield (70.9 ± 2.8, $n = 3$) were good, the processing time was 15 min and the final volume containing

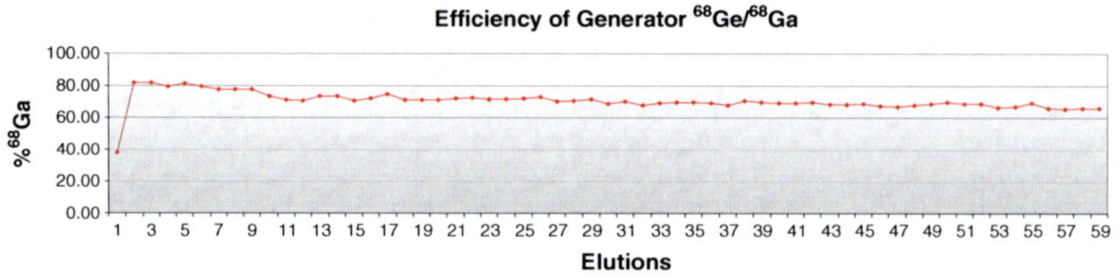

Fig. 3 $^{68}Ge/^{68}Ga$ generator efficiency measured during 6 months

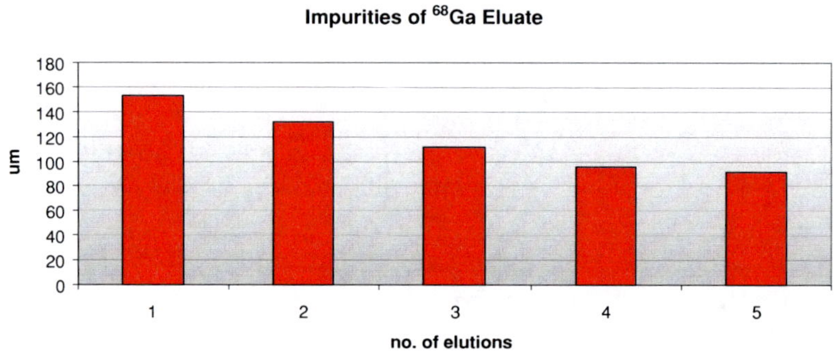

Fig. 4 Level of impurities measured in the eluate, performed five times consecutively

^{68}Ga was 1 mL acetone/12 mol L^{-1} HCl (97:0.4)%, which are both high considering the short half-life of ^{68}Ga radioisotope and the importance of reducing the final volume in order to minimize contaminants and the mass of acetone and hydrochloric acid.

The chromatography column was changed for a smaller one; consequently, the resin volume was reduced to 0.05 mL. With this effort, processing time was reduced to 5 min and the purified ^{68}Ga was recovered in 0.4 mL acetone/12 mol L^{-1} HCl (97:0.4)%. The reduction of metals was (97.0 $\pm$ 2.7)% ($n = 3$), however the ^{68}Ga yield was decreased to (60.3 $\pm$ 5.7)% ($n = 3$).

Using the same type of chromatography column, the cation exchange resin was changed. AG50W-X8 (>400 mesh) showed the best result of (77.5 $\pm$ 6.0)% ^{68}Ga yield ($n = 3$) with (98.0 $\pm$ 1.0)% reduction of total metals ($n = 3$).

3.4 $^{67}Ga/^{68}Ga$ Purification Using Isopropyl Ether Extraction System

3.4.1 Liquid–Liquid Solvent Extraction

The first experiments used ^{67}Ga in 7 mol L^{-1} HCl–diisopropyl ether. ^{67}Ga recovery was (72.5 $\pm$ 0.1)% ($n = 3$). Although the ^{67}Ga extraction was good, the final volume was 30 mL, inappropriate for labeling of small peptide quantities.

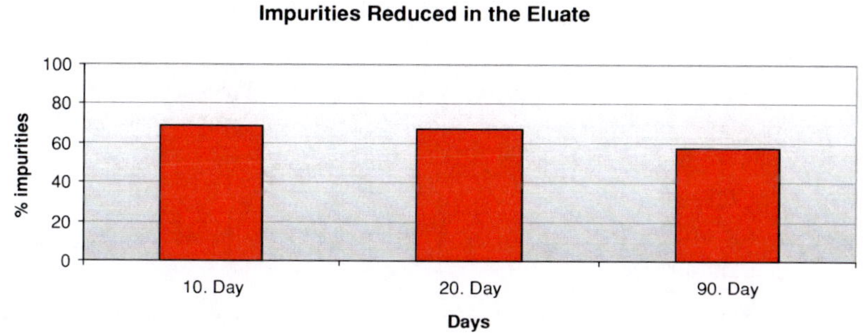

Fig. 5 Reduction of impurities present in the ^{68}Ga eluate with elution interval

Therefore, the volume was reduced to 4.0 mL, with ^{68}Ga recovery of (97.7 ± 1.3)% ($n = 3$). However, the presence of metals, considered contaminants, increased in both cases, and the process time was too long. Furthermore, the process required care during manipulation of volatile diisopropyl ether with radioactive isotope.

3.4.2 Column Chromatography Solvent Extraction

The recovery yield for solvent extraction in a 10 mm column with XAD-16 was 83.3% in 3 mL deionized water; the levels of contaminants decreased to 69% compared with the first procedure. The level was decreased to 67% (1 day after the first purification) and 57% (9 days after the first purification) in subsequent experiments, as shown in Fig. 5. ^{68}Ga recovery was decreased to 81 and 79% as well. The total processing time was reduced to 10 min with this methodology.

The column was changed for a smaller one. The process time was reduced to 5 min, and the final volume of ^{68}Ga was 1 mL in all experiments. Although ^{68}Ga recovery was decreased to 52% compared with the 10 mm glass column, the impurities were reduced to 82%. Two other purification procedures were realized. The level of impurities was reduced to 78 and 70%, respectively. However, the yield of ^{68}Ga recovery increased to 56% in both experiments.

Solution of $TiCl_3$ was added to the initial solution before passing through the microchromatography column. The ^{68}Ga recovery was 72%, and the impurities were reduced to 77%, Fe(III) was 56% lower, and the amount of Ti in the sample was 110 μg, much higher when compared with the other methods, where the amounts of Ti were less than 1 μg.

The experiments with addition of 1% NaI resulted in 58% recovery of ^{68}Ga, and total impurities were reduced to 74%; Fe(III) was 72% lower. Without adding a reducing agent to the ^{68}Ga initial solution, the level of Fe(III) was decreased to 70%, slightly less than the result with addition of 1% NaI.

Table 1 summarizes the most relevant data about all the purification methods of $^{67}Ga/^{68}Ga$.

Table 1 Data for the different ^{68}Ga purification methodologies

Purification method	Resin	$^{67}Ga/^{68}Ga$ recovery (%)	Impurities (%)	Final volume (mL)	Elution
Standard 1 mL syringe	AG50WX8 (200–400 mesh)	70.9 ± 2.8	87.0 ± 3.6	1.0	Acetone/12 mol L^{-1} HCl (97:0.4)%
Micropipette	AG50WX8 (200–400 mesh)	60.3 ± 5.74	97.0 ± 2.65	0.4	Acetone/12 mol L^{-1} HCl (97:0.4)%
Micropipette	AG50WX8 (>400 mesh)	77.5 ± 6.0	98.0 ± 1.0	0.4	Acetone/12 mol L^{-1} HCl (97:0.4)%
Extraction solvent	–	72.5 ± 0.1	–	30.0	Deionized water
Extraction solvent	–	97.7 ± 1.3	–	4.0	Deionized water
Glass column-10 mm	XAD-16	83.3	69.0	3.0	Deionized water
Micropipette	XAD-16	52.0	81.6	1.0	Deionized water
Micropipette	XAD-16 with 1% NaI	58.0	74.0	1.0	Deionized water
Micropipette	XAD-16 with $TiCl_3$	72.0	77.0	1.0	Deionized water

4 Conclusion

The best result was achieved with AG50W-X8 (>400 mesh), for which ^{68}Ga recovery and purification were better compared with other methods. However, the resin is not commercially available, and ^{68}Ga was eluted with a mixture of acetone/strong acid. The extraction chromatography column based on absorption of diisopropyl ether in XAD-16 was the most promising purification method. Although the levels of ^{68}Ga recovery and purification were lower than for the cationic resin method, the advantage is the ^{68}Ga recovery in deionized water. Nevertheless, it is necessary to measure the mass of diisopropyl ether to perform subsequent labeling of biomolecules which does not require heating of the solution.

References

Brown LC (1971) Chemical processing of cyclotron produced ^{67}Ga. Int J Appl Radiat Isot 22:710–713

Nachtrieb NH, Fryxell RE (1949) The extraction of gallium chloride by isopropyl ether. J Am Chem Soc 71:4035–4039

Roesch F, Riss PJ (2010) The renaissance of the ^{68}Ge/^{68}Ga radionuclide generator initiates new developments in 68Ga radiopharmaceutical chemistry. Curr Top Med Chem 10:1633–1668

Velikyan I (2005) Synthesis, characterization and application of ^{68}Ga-labelled macromolecules. Dissertation-Uppsala University, Sweden

Velikyan I, Beyer GJ, Bergstrom-Pettermann E et al (2008) The importance of high specific radioactivity in the performance of ^{68}Ga-labeled peptide. Nucl Med Biol 35:529–536

Zhernosekov KP, Filosofov DV, Baum RP et al (2007) Processing of generator-produced ^{68}Ga for medical application. J Nucl Med 48:1741–1748

Part II
Radiochemistry and Radiopharmacy

The Diversity of ^{68}Ga-Based Imaging Agents

Irina Velikyan

Abstract

Development of new radiopharmaceuticals and their availability are crucial factors influencing the expansion of clinical nuclear medicine. The number of new ^{68}Ga-based imaging agents for positron emission tomography (PET) is increasing greatly. ^{68}Ga has been used for labeling of a broad range of molecules (small organic molecules, peptides, proteins, and oligonucleotides) as well as particles, thus demonstrating its potential to become a PET analog of the legendary generator-produced gamma-emitting ^{99m}Tc but with added value of higher sensitivity and resolution as well as quantitation and dynamic scanning. Further, the availability of technology for GMP-compliant automated tracer production can facilitate the introduction of new radiopharmaceuticals and enable standardized, harmonized multicenter studies to be conducted for regulatory approval. This chapter presents some examples of tracers for targeted, pretargeted, and nontargeted imaging with emphasis on the potential of ^{68}Ga to facilitate clinically practical PET development and to promote the PET technique worldwide for earlier and better diagnostics, and personalized medicine with the ultimate objective of improved therapeutic outcome.

Keywords

Positron emission tomography · ^{68}Ga · Radiochemistry

I. Velikyan (✉)
Department of Radiology, Oncology, and Radiation Science,
Uppsala University, SE-75285 Uppsala, Sweden
e-mail: irina.velikyan@bms.uu.se

I. Velikyan
PET-Centre, Centre for Medical Imaging,
Uppsala University Hospital, Uppsala, Sweden

R. P. Baum and F. Rösch (eds.), *Theranostics, Gallium-68, and Other Radionuclides*, Recent Results in Cancer Research 194, DOI: 10.1007/978-3-642-27994-2_7,

Contents

1 Introduction

Preparation of ^{68}Ga-based imaging agents is amenable to automation as well as kit-type production. Combined with the availability of ^{68}Ga ($t_{1/2} = 68$ min) from a ^{68}Ge/^{68}Ga generator, this makes PET clinical examinations possible at clinical centers remote from accelerators and distribution sites and also enriches the radiopharmaceutical arsenal at centers equipped with accelerators.

There are several types of commercial generator available on the market nowadays. All of them have the common advantage of providing ^{68}Ga in ionic form, thus allowing straightforward use for labeling chemistry. The molarity of the hydrochloric acid eluent used varies from 0.05 M to 1 M. Their common disadvantage is the relatively high volume of the eluate (5–7 mL), breakthrough of the long-lived parent ^{68}Ge ($t_{1/2} = 270.8$ days) as well as metal cation impurities. Simple solutions have been suggested to overcome some of these disadvantages. Thus, reduction of the generator eluate volume and consequent enhancement of the ^{68}Ga concentration was achieved by collection of the peak fraction of the generator eluate (Fig. 1) (Velikyan et al. 2004; Zhernosekov et al. 2007; Meyer et al. 2004; Asti et al. 2008). The void volume and elution profile may vary amongst generators, but commonly the peak fraction (1–2 mL) contains 60–90% of the total available radioactivity. Reduction of the concentration of contaminant metal ions including Zn as a product of ^{68}Ga decay in the generator eluate can be achieved by regular elution of the generator (Velikyan et al. 2004). In addition, elution 3–4 h prior to radiosynthesis is recommended, since the interfering metal ion concentration can thus be kept at its lower value while allowing accumulation of over 95% of the maximum possible radioactivity (Fig. 2) (Velikyan et al. 2004). Utilization of ion exchange chromatography allowed further ^{68}Ga concentration enhancement and purification of the generator eluate from some of the competing metal cations as well as ^{68}Ge (Velikyan et al. 2004; Zhernosekov et al. 2007; Meyer et al. 2004; Asti et al. 2008). Anion exchange chromatography allows for 30-fold decrease of

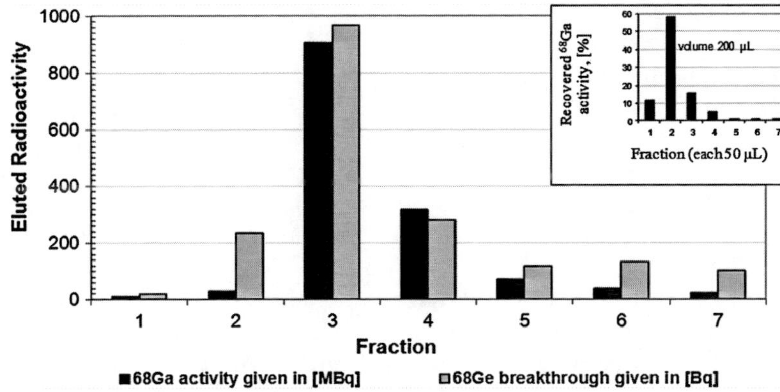

Fig. 1 Elution profile of a ^{68}Ge/^{68}Ga generator where one fraction was 1 mL (fraction 1 = 0.3 mL, fraction 7 = 0.7 mL) for total eluted volume of 6 mL. The profiles for ^{68}Ga elution and ^{68}Ge breakthrough are similar. Fraction 3 (1 mL) contains over 60% of the available ^{68}Ga activity. *Inset*: elution profile of ^{68}Ga eluted from the small SAX SPE Chromafix cartridge with small volumes of deionized water. More than 90% of the initial ^{68}Ga activity was obtained in 200 μL solution. Reproduced from Velikyan et al. (2004)

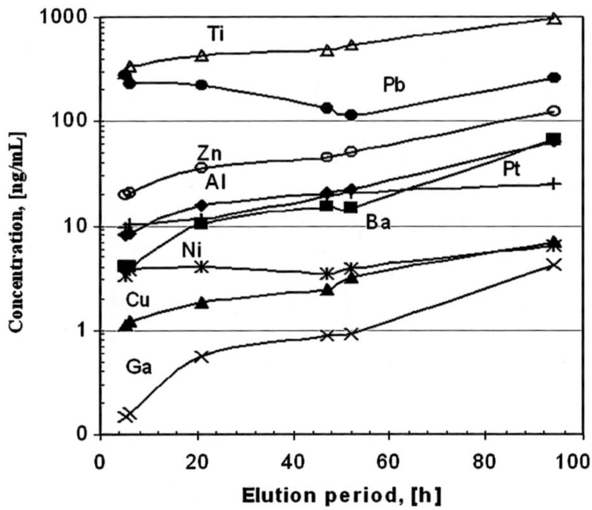

Fig. 2 Metal ion content in 6 mL generator eluate as a function of elution time period. Reproduced from Velikyan et al. (2004)

the volume and purification from long-lived ^{68}Ge as well as Al, In, and Ti (Velikyan et al. 2004). The initially available radioactivity and generator shelf-life are also enhanced, since eluates from several generators can be preconcentrated in one procedure, resulting in the same final volume of 200–300 μL HCl(aq) (Fig. 1, inset). Preconcentration and purification of generator eluate performed using cation exchange resins results in 400 μL solution of acetone/HCl mixture (Zhernosekov et al. 2007). The content of $^{68}Ge(IV)$, Zn(II), Ti(IV), and Fe(III) in the eluate is decreased, respectively, by factors of 10^4, 10^5, 10^2, and 10. These methods (Velikyan et al. 2004; Zhernosekov et al. 2007) were tested (Gebhardt et al. 2010) with the objective of automating the ^{68}Ga preconcentration procedure, and it was found that the content of radioactivity when using the cation exchange method (Zhernosekov et al. 2007) was too low for the desired applications, while the anion exchange method (Velikyan et al. 2004) demonstrated high reproducibility and high radioactivity content and concentration. It should be mentioned that these methods do not purify ^{68}Ga from its strongest competitor, Fe(III), completely.

Buffers with weak complexing strength are used in labeling synthesis to keep ^{68}Ga in solution, prevent precipitation and colloid formation, and provide pH required for formation of the desired complex. Use of 4-(2-hydroxyethyl)piperazine-1-ethanesulfonic acid (HEPES) buffer resulted in preparation of tracers with higher specific radioactivity as compared with sodium acetate (Velikyan et al. 2004). Such buffers as succinate, formate, tris, glutamate, lactate, oxalate, and tartrate lead to poor radiochemical yields (Bauwens et al. 2010).

Labeling with high specific radioactivity (SRA) provides a wide range of SRA values that can be adjusted by addition of the cold vector molecule. This provides the possibility for optimization of the SRA for each application, considering the tracer affinity as well as the target expression level in both diseased and normal tissue. In targeted and pretargeted imaging, the requirement for sufficiently high SRA is dictated by biological factors such as the limited amount of binding sites, tracer affinity, and possible pharmacological side-effects. It might also be of interest to explore the influence of SRA on the quantification precision and the possibility for refined evaluation of receptor binding parameters, especially to determine in vivo the total receptor number in, e.g., tumors.

The radioactivity incorporation and thus the specific radioactivity of tracers can be enhanced using microwave heating and preconcentrated ^{68}Ga (Velikyan et al. 2004; Velikyan 2005; Bergstrom et al. 2005; Blom et al. 2009; Lavén et al. 2004, 2005; Lendvai et al. 2005, 2008, 2009; Roivainen et al. 2004; Velikyan et al. 2004, 2008; Långström et al. 2008; Velikyan and Långström 2004; Velikyan et al. 2004, 2005; Tolmachev et al. 2010). Moreover, DOTA may have higher selectivity for Ga as compared with In and Fe under microwave heating conditions (Velikyan et al. 2008). The NOTA chelating moiety can be labeled at room temperature (Velikyan et al. 2008), providing mild reaction conditions for bioconjugates comprising temperature-sensitive, fragile macromolecules (Velikyan et al. 2008; Velikyan and Långström 2006; Riss et al. 2008).

Advancement in generator development and eluate quality enhancement methodologies in combination with macrocyclic chelators and most importantly the advent of receptor-targeted peptides, with the success story of SST, has accelerated applications involving ^{68}Ga. Radiotracers for targeted imaging of specific protein expression products (receptors, enzymes, and antigens), pretargeted imaging using small effector or hapten molecules, as well as nontargeted imaging of pulmonary and myocardial perfusion and ventilation are being developed. Imaging agents to monitor inflammation and infection as well as general downstream biologic properties such as proliferation, hypoxia, glycolysis, and angiogenesis have also been investigated (Velikyan 2011). The variety of potential applications is analogous to that of ^{99m}Tc. In addition, ^{68}Ga PET provides such benefits as higher sensitivity, resolution, quantitation, and dynamic scanning. Moreover, the similarity of the coordination chemistry of ^{68}Ga to that of therapeutic radionuclides such as ^{90}Y and ^{177}Lu might allow for theranostics. The contribution of imaging diagnostics to cancer therapy in terms of early disease detection, staging, therapy selection, and follow-up is leading to personalized medicine.

The core of clinical nuclear medicine advancement is the development of new radiopharmaceuticals and their availability. The examples below demonstrate the diversity and range of potential ^{68}Ga applications exemplified by targeted, pretargeted, and nontargeted imaging.

2 Targeted Imaging

Peptides labeled with a positron-emitting radionuclide can be used to make an accurate tumor diagnosis, determine staging, and quantify the radiation dose to tumors and critical organs, thus allowing dose planning and dose monitoring for successful radiotherapy, and to follow tumor response to chemo- and radiotherapy, thus providing personalized patient management (Lundqvist and Tolmachev 2002; Mutic et al. 2003; Kowalski et al. 2003; Baum et al. 2008; Reubi et al. 2005; Heppeler et al. 2000; Eisenwiener et al. 2002; Liu and Edwards 1999; Thakur 1995; Behr et al. 1999; Otte et al. 1997; de Jong et al. 1997; Schmitt et al. 2004; Pless et al. 2004; Meier et al. 2004; Tolmachev 1800; Maecke et al. 2005; Barone et al. 2005; Gambhir 2002; Carlsson et al. 2002; Tofilon et al. 2003; Carlsson et al. 2003; Forssell-Aronsson et al. 2002). The compatibility of ^{68}Ga with peptides for targeted imaging of such receptors as somatostatin, bombesin, human epidermal growth factor, integrin, vascular endothelial growth factor, cholecystokinin-2, gastrin-releasing peptide, melanocyte stimulation hormone, glucagon-like peptide 1, gonadotropin-releasing hormone, folate, neurotensin, and neuropeptide Y receptors has been demonstrated (Tolmachev 1800; Maschauer et al. 2010; Mathias et al. 2003; Fani et al. 2011; Schottelius et al. 2008; Demmer et al. 2008; Brom et al. 2010; Wild et al. 2010; Froidevaux et al. 2004; Cantorias et al. 2009; Wei et al. 2007; Zhang et al. 2007; Schuhmacher et al. 2005; Dimitrakopoulou-Strauss et al. 2007; Hofmann et al. 2004; Baum et al. 2007; Cagnolini et al. 2010; Mansi et al. 2011; Reubi and Maecke 2008). The corresponding ligands commonly have satisfactory pharmacokinetics with fast blood clearance, relatively low hepatobiliary excretion, and mostly renal elimination as well as excellent tissue penetration, minimal side-effects, and no or low antigenicity.

2.1 Imaging Somatostatin Receptors

Somatostatin receptor (SSTR) ligand analogs are the most well-developed and extensively investigated group of small regulatory peptides. Somatostatin receptors are expressed in neuroendocrine tumors, renal cell carcinoma, small cell lung cancer, breast cancer, prostate cancer, and malignant lymphoma (Reubi 2001). The receptor binding affinity, internalization, and biodistribution of different SST ligands have been shown to be dependent on the peptide constitution, chelator type (1,4,7,10-Tetraazacyclododecane-1,4,7,10-tetraacetic acid (DOTA), 1,4,7-triaza-cyclononane-1,4,7-triacetic acid (NOTA), desferrioxamine (DFO), diethylenetri-aminepentaacetic acid (DTPA), and their derivatives), metal cations (In, Y, Ga, Tc, Lu), linkers, and pharmacokinetic modifiers (Kowalski et al. 2003; Eisenwiener et al. 2002; Maecke 2005; Rivier et al. 2005; Wild et al. 2003; 2005; Ginj et al. 2005; Hofland et al. 1999; De Jong et al. 1998; Reubi et al. 2000; Froidevaux and Eberle 2002; Forrer et al. 2004; Schmitt et al. 2005; Smith-Jones et al. 1994; Froidevaux et al. 2002; Heppeler et al. 1999; Henze et al. 2001; Deshmukh et al. 2005; Hofmann et al. 2001; Pettinato et al. 2008; Antunes et al. 2007; Erchegyi et al. 2008; Grace et al. 2008a, b; Cescato et al. 2008; Fani et al. 2010).

Quantification is one of the prominent advantages of the PET technique, allowing estimation of receptor density in vivo (Zhang et al. 2010). However, the accuracy and interpretation of results depend on a number of parameters, including SRA. The latter was demonstrated to be an essential tool for optimization of imaging quality and correlation of radioactivity uptake and receptor expression (Velikyan et al. 2008; Velikyan et al. 2010). In particular, the quantification accuracy of receptor binding of [^{68}Ga]Ga-DOTA-TOC was investigated as a function of SRA in vitro on frozen sections of Rhesus monkey brain expressing SSTR. The dependence was described by a sigmoidal function with the region around the inflection point being the most sensitive to SRA variation (Fig. 3). The values of SRA corresponding to the top plateau provided stable target-to-nontarget ratio and thus high reproducibility of the in vitro biological assay and more accurate quantification (Velikyan et al. 2008). However, it should be mentioned that the correlation of the in vitro and in vivo uptake as a function of SRA might not be linear. Optimization of SRA is required, considering the losses of the tracer in vivo due to nonspecific adsorption, blood protein binding, and binding to physiologically expressed sites consuming tracer, thus demanding higher masses of vector and consequently lower SRA.

The short half-life of ^{68}Ga, allowing repetitive sequential examinations, in combination with fast target localization and blood clearance of SST analogs is of special interest for clinical use, providing a means for individual patient treatment design (Maecke et al. 2005; Velikyan et al. 2010). Modulation of [^{68}Ga]Ga-DOTA-TOC uptake in tumor and healthy organs was achieved by variation of the total amount of administered peptide. In particular, three sequential examinations of a patient were conducted on the same day, and the amount of octreotide administered immediately prior to [^{68}Ga]Ga-DOTA-TOC during the second and third examinations was escalated (Velikyan et al. 2010). The uptake increased in

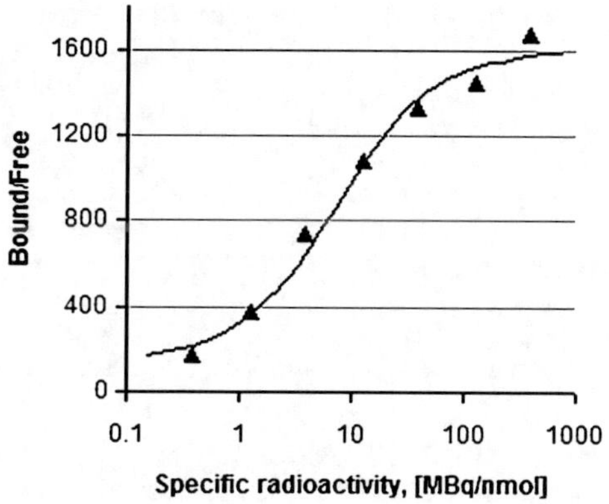

Fig. 3 Ratio of ligand bound to receptor and free ligand as a function of SRA, assuming constant radioactivity concentration. The ratio was obtained using the average of the uptake values for thalamus and cortex with relative standard deviation of 5–19%. The data were fitted to a sigmoid two-parameter Emax model. The optimization was done in MATLAB 7.0 using a least-squares method (LSQNONLIN, MATLAB, 2005, 7.0.4). Reproduced from Velikyan et al. (2008)

the tumor and metastases and at the same time decreased in the liver and spleen upon injection of 50 μg. Further enhancement to 250 and 500 μg resulted in a blocking effect in all tissues (Fig. 4, row 1) except for one patient (Fig. 4, row 2). The latter observation clearly demonstrates the importance of individualized patient diagnostic and therapeutic management.

[^{68}Ga]Ga-DOTA-TOC, [^{68}Ga]Ga-DOTA-TATE, and [^{68}Ga]Ga-DOTA-NOC have been extensively used in clinical studies, demonstrating fast pharmacokinetics, short scanning time, low radiation dose, and high sensitivity, resolution, detection rate, and image contrast, as well as the possibility for quantification (Kowalski et al. 2003; Baum et al. 2008; Henze et al. 2001; Hofmann et al. 2001; Velikyan et al. 2010; Hofmann et al. 2004; Koukouraki et al. 2006; Gabriel et al. 2007; Henze et al. 2004; Dimitrakopoulou-Strauss et al. 2006; Koukouraki et al. 2006; Kayani et al. 2008; Luboldt et al. 2010; Tan and Goh 2010; Ambrosini et al. 2010; Lincke et al. 2009; Rominger et al. 2010). Personalized diagnosis using these tracers is becoming a standard for selection of patient therapeutic management (Maecke et al. 2005; Henze et al. 2001; Gabriel et al. 2010; Putzer et al. 2010; Modlin et al. 2008; Win et al. 2007; Srirajaskanthan et al. 2010; Putzer et al. 2009; Milker-Zabel et al. 2006; Gehler et al. 2009; Prasad and Baum 2010; Ambrosini et al. 2010; Campana et al. 2010; Frilling et al. 2010; Versari et al. 2010; Van Riet et al. 2009; Ambrosini et al. 2008; Sainz-Esteban et al. 2010; Ambrosini et al. 2011; Traub-Weidinger et al. 2010; Boss et al. 2010; Henze et al. 2005; Conry et al. 2010). The vast experience of the clinical studies has been summarized in the form of guidelines for the assistance of nuclear medicine physicians in examination protocols as well as in interpretation and reporting of results (Virgolini et al. 2010; Janson et al. 2010).

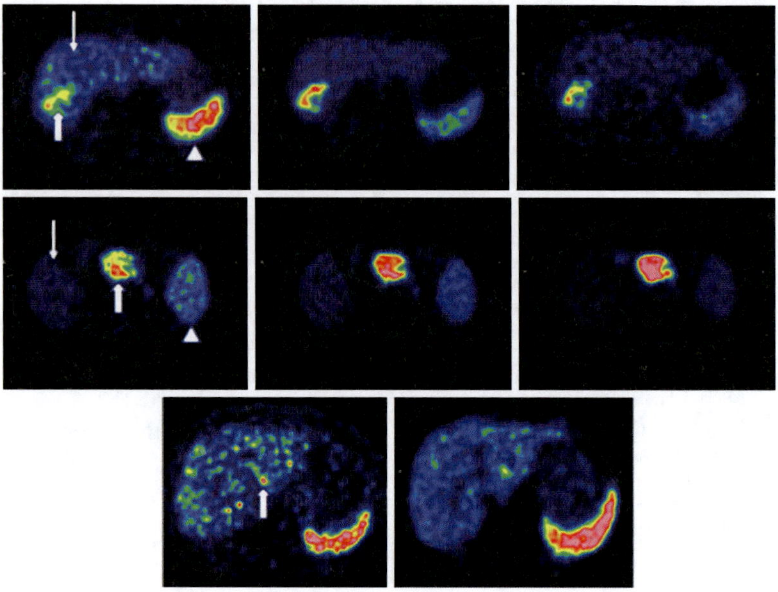

Fig. 4 *Row 1* : Transaxial [^{68}Ga]-DOTATOC-PET images of patient 1 with liver metastases from a colonic carcinoid who underwent three sequential PET-CT examinations. The tracer accumulation pattern in tumor tissue (*thick arrow*) increased in the second PET examination by pretreatment with 50 μg i.v. unlabeled octreotide but decreased again in the third examination that was proceeded by 500 μg i.v. octreotide. *Row 2* : Transaxial [^{68}Ga]-DOTATOC-PET images of patient 6 with a large endocrine pancreatic tumor who underwent three sequential PET-CT examinations. In contrast to the tumor uptake pattern in the other patients, as illustrated in *row 1*, the tumor accumulation (*thick arrow*) in this particular patient increased gradually over the three PET examinations. *Row 3* : Transaxial [^{68}Ga]-DOTATOC-PET images of patient 2, with multiple small liver metastases from a midgut carcinoid who was examined before and after interferon therapy. The [^{68}Ga]-DOTATOC accumulation decreased in the tumor tissue (*thick arrow*) in the second PET examination performed after 3 months of interferon therapy. In all patients, the [^{68}Ga]-DOTATOC PET accumulation in normal tissues, best appreciated in the spleen (*arrow head*) and liver (*thin arrow*), decreased gradually over the three examinations. Reproduced from Velikyan et al. (2010)

2.2 Imaging Human Epidermal Growth Factor Receptor (HER) Family

Various ^{68}Ga-labeled agents for imaging of the human epidermal growth factor receptor family overexpressed in malignant tumors such as breast, ovary, lung, colorectal, and urothelial have been developed and investigated (Yarden and Sliwkowski 2001; Walker and Dearing 1999; Witton et al. 2003; Hirsch et al. 2003; Neal and Mellon 1992; Vosjan et al. 2011). Thus, 53-amino-acid residue EGFR natural ligand (Velikyan et al. 2005; Sandstrom et al. 2011; Velikyan et al. 2006), 58-amino-acid residue Affibody® ligands (Tolmachev et al. 2010; Tolmachev and Orlova 2009; Ahlgren and Tolmachev 2010; Tolmachev et al. 2009), antibody

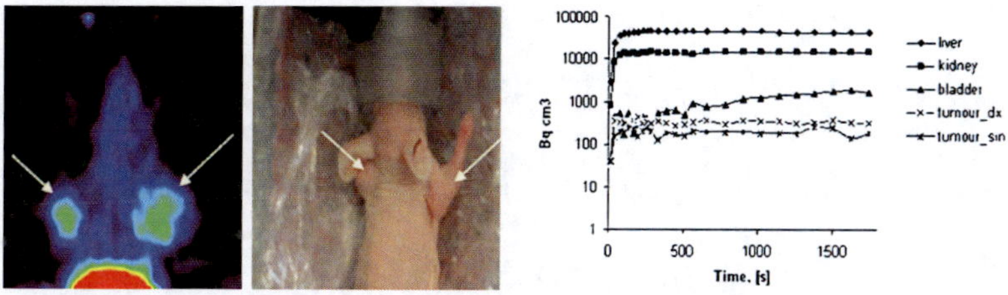

Fig. 5 (*Left*) Image showing a summation of frames 20–24 (20–30 min after injection) and photograph of the positioning of the mouse, in which the tumors (*arrows*) can clearly be seen at either side of the head. (*Right*) Pharmacokinetic curves showing the rapid distribution of [^{68}Ga]Ga-DOTA-hEGF (0.16 nmol injected) to liver, kidney, and tumors. Tumor_dx = right-side tumor; Tumor_sin = left-side tumor. Reproduced from Velikyan et al. (2005)

fragments (Vosjan et al. 2011; Smith-Jones et al. 2004; Smith-Jones et al. 2006), two-helix Affibody derivative (Ren et al. 2009), as well as tyrosine kinase inhibitor (Theeraladanon et al. 2010) have been thoroughly evaluated in vitro and in vivo in xenograft animal models.

The ligand hEGF was conjugated with DOTA (Velikyan et al. 2005; Velikyan et al. 2006) and NOTA (Sandstrom et al. 2011), and the resulting conjugates were labeled with ^{68}Ga and ^{67}Ga, respectively, under microwave heating and room temperature. The biological activity maintenance of the tracers was thoroughly studied by performing cell-binding assays, biodistribution studies, and microPET imaging in tumor-bearing mice (Fig. 5, left). [^{68}Ga]Ga-DOTA-hEGF demonstrated high affinity and fast pharmacokinetic (Fig. 5, right) compatible with application for in vivo imaging of breast or non-small cell lung cancer. However, imaging of head and neck squamous cell carcinoma would be challenging due to the high physiological expression of EGFRs particularly in salivary glands, thus resulting in high background uptake and masking of the signal from tumor cells. Blocking of uptake in healthy organs was necessary to decrease the background and improve the contrast. This could be achieved by pre-injection of nonlabeled EGF ligand. However, the required high amount of the latter would stimulate growth of cancer cells. To avoid the pharmacological effect, anti-EGFR Affibody® ligands [$Z_{EGFR:1907}$, $(Z_{EGFR:1907})_2$ or $(Z_{EGFR:955})_2$] were used for saturation of the physiologically expressed EGFR prior to administration of the tracer molecule based on hEGF ligand ([^{67}Ga]Ga-NOTA-Bn-NCS-hEGF) (Sandstrom et al. 2011). The dimeric Affibody molecule $(Z_{EGFR:1907})_2$ exhibited the best results, and the tumor-to-organ ratio in liver, salivary glands, and colon was improved in nude mice bearing UTSCC-7 cell xenograft.

^{68}Ga-labeling of DOTA-conjugated Affibody® molecules can be accomplished using either conventional or microwave heating without compromising the receptor binding capability (Velikyan 2005; Tolmachev et al. 2010). The influence of radiometal exchange on the ligand in vivo distribution was studied in a dual experiment, allowing direct comparison of ^{68}Ga- and ^{111}In-labeled DOTA-$Z_{HER2:342\text{-}pep2}$ (ABY-002). Co-injection of the tracers provided uniform conditions

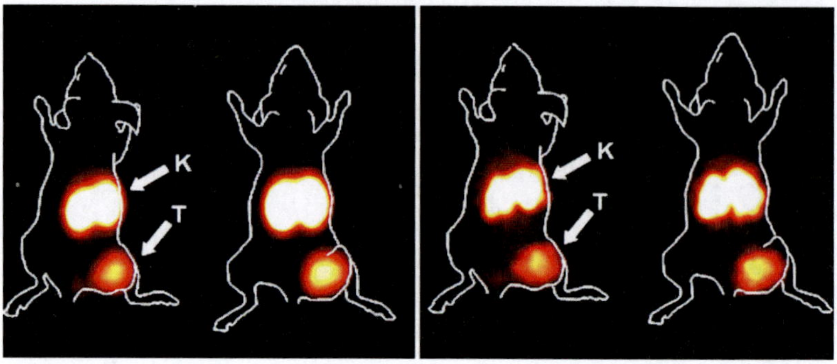

Fig. 6 Imaging of HER2 expression in SKOV-3 xenografts in BALB/c *nu/nu* mice using PET (*left*) and gamma-camera (*right*). Animals were injected with a mixture of ^{68}Ga-DOTA-$Z_{HER2:342}$ and ^{111}In-DOTA-$Z_{HER2:342}$. Animals were sacrificed 2 h p.i., and the PET image was acquired. Gamma-camera image was acquired 24 h later, after decay of ^{68}Ga. To facilitate interpretation, animal contours were derived from a digital photograph and superimposed over the PET and gamma-camera image. *Arrows* indicate tumor (T) and kidneys (K) in one representative animal. Reproduced from Tolmachev et al. (2010)

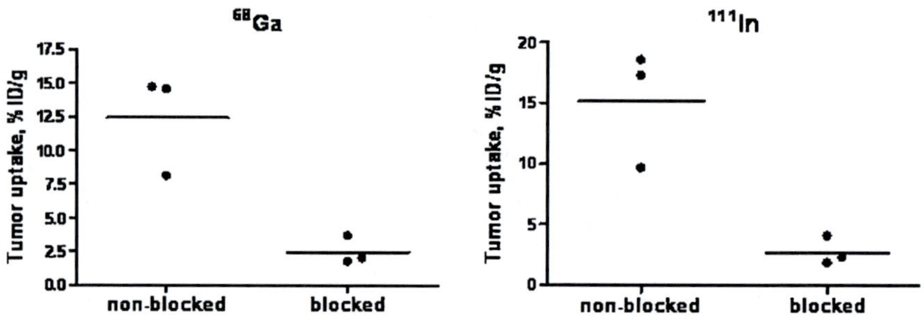

Fig. 7 In vivo binding specificity of ^{68}Ga-DOTA-$Z_{HER2:342}$ (*left panel*) and ^{111}In-DOTA-$Z_{HER2:342}$ (*right panel*), 2 h p.i. The blocked group was subcutaneously pre-injected with an excess amount of nonlabeled $Z_{HER2:342}$. Results are presented as percentage of injected dose per gram of tissue (% ID/g). Statistical significance in tumor uptake between the groups, according to Student's *t*-test, gave $p < 0.05$. Reproduced from Tolmachev et al. (2010)

for the biology validation experiments, eliminated the variation that might originate from individual differences amongst animals, and decreased the use of animals. Both tracers demonstrated specific uptake in vivo in SKOV-3 xenografts in mice (Figs. 6, 7). However, due to the faster fade of the ^{68}Ga-based counterpart from blood, lungs, gastrointestinal tract, and muscle, the tumor-to-organ ratio for this tracer was higher, thus resulting in better contrast (Tolmachev et al. 2010). Metastatic breast cancer was successfully visualized in clinical patient examination using [^{68}Ga]Ga-ABY-002 (Baum et al. 2010). The agent was well tolerated and rapidly cleared from blood, providing high image contrast. This was found to be valuable specifically for HER2 status of metastases not amenable to biopsy.

To accelerate clearance, the size of the Affibody® molecule was decreased to the two-helix molecule ([^{68}Ga]Ga-DOTA-MUT-DS) (Ren et al. 2009). Although the clearance became faster, this modification resulted in a drop of the affinity and tumor uptake in SKOV3 xenografts.

2.3 Imaging Angiogenesis

Imaging of integrin and vascular endothelial growth factor (VEGF) receptors overexpressed in tumors and ischemic injuries with extensive formation of new capillaries is an important means not only for diagnosis and monitoring response to therapy but also for antiangiogenic drug development. A ligand for VEGFR, single-chain VEGF (scVEGF), which is a functionally active single-chain version of VEGF (Backer et al. 2007, 2008), was conjugated to PEG linkers in order to adjust the pharmacokinetics and to couple to DOTA- or NOTA-based bifunctional chelators for efficient labeling with ^{68}Ga (Blom et al. 2011). The chelators were conjugated to Cys-tag in scVEGF via bifunctional PEG linkers of various lengths (2.0, 3.4, and 5.0 kDa), and the impact of these modifications on the radiolabeling efficiency and functional activity of the ligand was assessed. The labeling efficiency did not depend on the PEG linker length and was comparable for both DOTA and NOTA chelating moiety at elevated temperature provided by either conventional or microwave heating. However, NOTA offered the additional advantage of labeling at ambient temperature, providing mild labeling conditions for the relatively large sc-VEGF ($\sim$28 kDa) and the possibility for cold kit-type tracer production. An in vitro binding assay using multicellular spheroids of 293/KDR cell line confirmed the biological functionality of the scVEGF-based tracers. Accumulation of [^{68}Ga]Ga-NOTA-PEG-scVEGF could be detected in vivo in mouse 293/KDR xenografts. High kidney uptake was characteristic for all analogs.

An extensive number of peptide ligands with an exposed arginine-glycine-aspartic acid (RGD) sequence for binding to $\alpha_v\beta_3$ integrin receptors have been developed during the last two decades with the objective of visualizing angiogenesis and improving related drug development, diagnosis, and therapy monitoring (Dijkgraaf and Boerman 2009; Bergstrom et al. 2003; Garner and Lappin 2006; Chen et al. 2004; Haubner et al. 2004; Janssen et al. 2002; Liu 2006; Decristoforo et al. 2008; Indrevoll et al. 2006; Haukkala et al. 2009; Liu et al. 2009; Jeong et al. 2008; Li et al. 2008; Dijkgraaf et al. 2011). Specific radioactivity of a DOTA-containing analog could be increased considerably using microwave heating (Velikyan et al. 2004; Långström et al. 2008). Two bioconjugates with the same constitution but dislocation of a few amino acids with the aim of creating RGD sequence in one counterpart and DGF sequence in the other (negative control) were designed with the aim of demonstrating the necessity of the RGD motif for specific binding to $\alpha_v\beta_3$ integrin receptors. The distribution of these analogs was studied in primates using PET/CT imaging (unpublished data). Increased accumulation of the RGD counterpart was detected in the wall of the uterus, probably indicating neovascularization, and most importantly it could

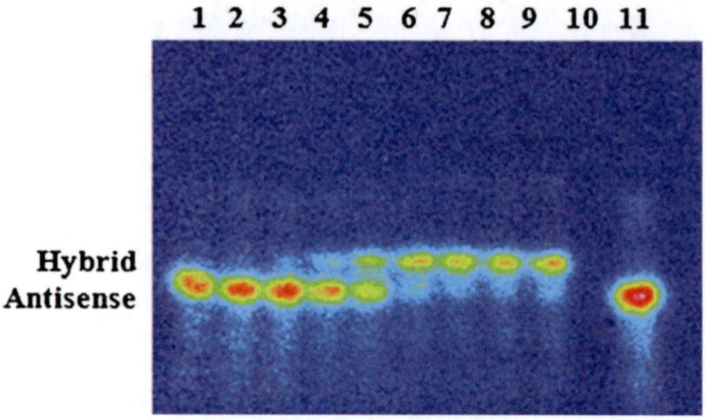

Fig. 8 Autoradiography of the polyacrylamide gel. Concentration-dependent hybridization of ^{68}Ga-labeled 17-mer antisense phosphorothioate oligonucleotide to the complementary 17-mer sense phosphodiester oligonucleotide in solution. The sense concentration was gradually increased (*lanes 1–9*); the references are sense oligonucleotide (*lane 10*), ^{68}Ga-labeled antisense oligonucleotide (*lane 11*), and molecular weight marker (*lane 12*)

partly be blocked by co-injection of excess cold analog, indicating binding specificity. Uptake of the analogs in other tissues was low.

2.4 Antisense Oligonucleotide-Based Tracers

Another class of biological macromolecules for targeted imaging is antisense oligonucleotides, which can be considered for in vivo imaging of gene expression and tumors that express ras oncogene point mutations (Tavitian 2005; Lendvai et al. 2009). An antisense oligonucleotide is a short, synthetic nucleic acid that may selectively hybridize with its complementary sequence in messenger RNA (mRNA). A number of various analogs with modifications in backbone, furanose ring moiety, as well as 3′- and 5′-end nucleotides for subsequent conjugation with bifunctional chelators were designed (Velikyan 2005; Lendvai et al. 2005, 2008; Velikyan et al. 2004). Labeling of oligonucleotides up to 9.8 kDa with ^{68}Ga was performed under microwave heating. Tracers based on phosphodiester, phosphorothioate, 2′-*O*-methyl phosphodiester, locked nucleic acid (LNA), LNA-DNA mixmer (LNA and DNA nucleotides in alternation along the sequence), and peptide nucleic acid were thoroughly assessed in vitro and in vivo in rat (Lendvai et al. 2005, 2008, 2009; Roivainen et al. 2004; Velikyan et al. 2004). The hybridization capability of the analogs was controlled in situ, where the concentration of the ^{68}Ga-labeled antisense oligonucleotide was kept constant while the concentration of sense was gradually increased, resulting in a gradual increase of hybrid formation (Fig. 8). The radioactivity organ distribution pattern varied considerably depending on the oligonucleotide modification. Uptake in nonhybridization specific tissue was most probably mediated by scavenger receptors (Lendvai et al. 2009). In vivo tumor accumulation of ^{68}Ga-labeled 17-mer

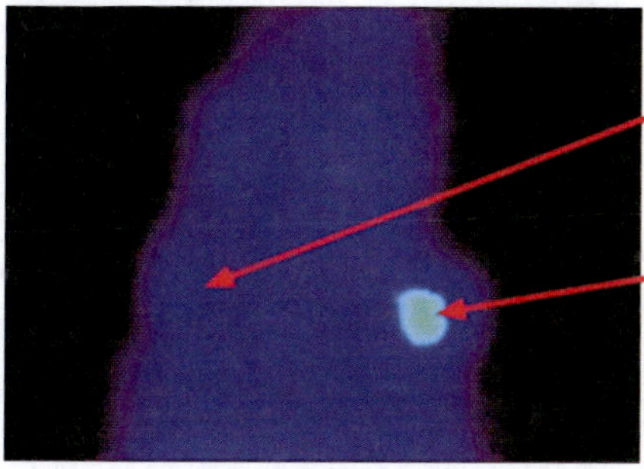

Fig. 9 PET image of an athymic rat bearing both A549 and BxPC-3 tumors, using ^{68}Ga-labeled PS antisense oligonucleotide specific to codon 12 mutated human K-ras oncogene. The human A549 cells (lung adenocarcinoma) contain K-ras point mutation in codon 12, and the human BxPC-3 cells (pancreatic adenocarcinoma, negative control) contain wild-type K-ras oncogene. Reproduced from Roivainen et al. (2004)

antisense phosphorothioate oligonucleotide was observed in rat model bearing xenografts with activated K-*ras* point mutation mRNA (Fig. 9) (Roivainen et al. 2004). Radioactivity accumulation was not detected in the negative control.

3 Pretargeted Imaging

The pretargeting concept has been introduced in order to overcome the problem in radioimmunotherapy and diagnostic imaging related to the slow pharmacokinetics and clearance of antibodies, leading, respectively, to high radiation dose to healthy tissue and poor image contrast (Hong et al. 2008; Frangioni 2009; Chang et al. 2002; Sharkey et al. 2010a, b; Goldenberg et al. 2006; Boerman et al. 2003). In the pretargeting process, bispecific antibody (bsmAb) or protein is first administered and given time for target localization and clearance from blood and healthy tissue. In the second step, a radiolabeled hapten or effector molecule with high affinity to the bispecific antibody or protein as well as fast pharmacokinetic and clearance properties is administered.

A bsmAb consists of two antigen-specific F(ab')$_2$ fragments covalently linked to a different F(ab) fragment for reaction with a hapten molecule (Fig. 10a). Various bsmAb constructs with mono- or divalent binding to tumor antigen as well as mono- and bivalent hapten molecules for imaging and therapy of breast cancer (anti-MUC1) (Schuhmacher et al. 2001a, b), melanoma (anti p97) (Somasundaram et al. 1993), lymphoma (anti-CD20, anti-HLA-DR) (Rossi et al. 2010; Sharkey et al. 2008), colorectal (anti-CEA) (Griffiths et al. 2004; Watine et al. 2001; Goldstein and Mitchell 2005), and pancreatic (anti-MUC1) (Gold et al. 2008; Forster et al. 2006) cancers have been investigated (Gold et al. 2008). The first pretargeting step may require several days, while the second step of radiolabeled hapten molecule administration and imaging may be accomplished within 1 h. A number of bivalent peptide hapten molecules containing histamine-succinyl-

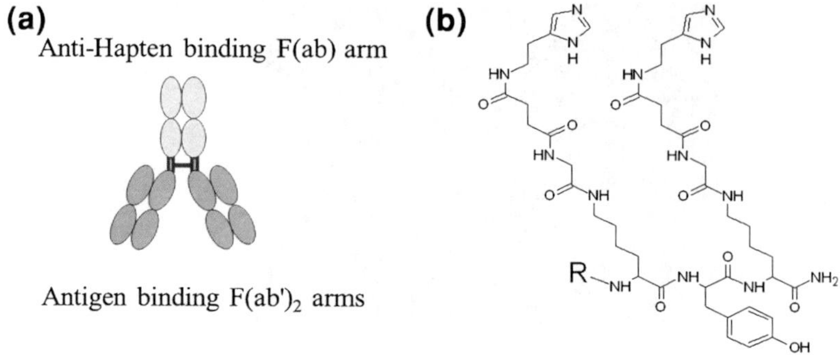

Fig. 10 **a** Schematic presentation of bsmAb. **b** Hapten molecule containing histamine-succinyl-glycine (HSG) residues, where R stands for the DOTA- or NOTA-based chelate moiety

glycine (HSG) residues and coupled to a chelate moiety (Fig. 10b) have been developed and used in combination with bsmAb specific to carcinoembryonic antigen (Griffiths et al. 2004; Sharkey et al. 2005; Goldenberg and Sharkey 2007; Goldenberg et al. 2008). Preclinical assessment in mice bearing human colon tumor xenografts revealed the superiority of pretargeted imaging using ^{67}Ga/^{68} Ga-labeled hapten peptide as compared with that of [^{18}F]-FDG in terms of uptake specificity and sensitivity (Schoffelen et al. 2010).

High affinity of an effector molecule such as biotin for avidin and streptavidin has also been employed in the pretargeting technique. In this setting, the target is first hit with a corresponding ligand, for example, antibody fragment (Forster et al. 2006) modified with avidin or streptavidin, then visualized by subsequent introduction of radiolabeled biotin.

Pretargeting can be utilized not only for imaging and therapy of cancer. It has also been explored to monitor the migration and survival of cells after transplantation of islets of Langerhans for treatment of type 1 diabetes mellitus. The influence of various modifications such as chelate moiety and linker on the binding capability of biotin to avidin was investigated (Blom et al. 2009). Introduction of DOTA and PEG or $(CH_2)_5$ chains (Fig. 11) did not deteriorate the binding specificity, but slightly decreased the binding efficiency as compared with the native biotin. The analog, [^{68}Ga]Ga-DOTA-$(PEG)_2$-biotin, demonstrated the highest stability in human serum, and its complex with avidin was even more stable (80% intact during 120 min). This tracer was further assessed preclinically using avidin-coated agarose resin microbeads (AARs) mimicking islets and avidin-coated islets of Langerhans isolated from human pancreata (Eriksson et al. 2011). The binding of the tracer to both systems was specific as confirmed by uptake blocking using excess native biotin in vitro. The tracer alone demonstrated fast distribution in vivo in mice, dominated by the partially blockable liver uptake and renal clearance. AARs were transplantated intraportally into diabetic C57BL/6 mice and showed increased uptake of the tracer in the liver as compared with baseline. These preliminary and promising results demonstrated that [^{68}Ga]Ga-DOTA-$(PEG)_2$-biotin has potential to become an imaging agent for monitoring survival of transplanted islets.

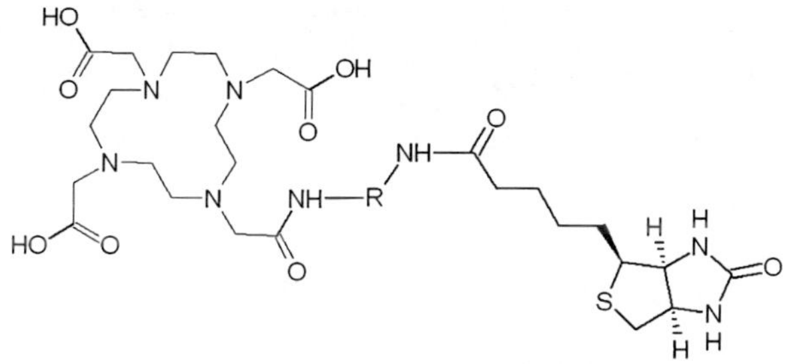

Fig. 11 Structure of biotin conjugate with DOTA moiety linked via spacer. R $= -(CH_2)_5-$
R $= -(CH_2)_2-O-(CH_2)_2-O-(CH_2)_2-$
R $= -(CH_2)_2-O-(CH_2)_2-O-(CH_2)_2-O-(CH_2)_2-$

4 Nontargeted Imaging

Particle-based imaging agents have been developed to deliver imaging reporters or therapeutic agents to the target, to assess blood flow and lung ventilation. Extensive work has been conducted on ^{68}Ga-labeling and preclinical assessment of nontoxic, nonantigenic, and biodegradable human serum albumin microspheres (HSAM), macroaggregated albumin (MAA), and albumin nanoparticles for examination of lung function by measuring pulmonary perfusion, cerebral blood flow, myocardial perfusion, vascular permeability, tumor perfusion, and blood pool by measuring angiogenesis as well as imaging and localization of sentinel lymph nodes for diagnosis, prognosis, as well as therapy and surgery planning (Schuster 1998; Wagner and Welch 1979; Yvert et al. 1979; Hayes et al. 1981; Steinling et al. 1985; Chesler et al. 1975; Mintun et al. 1986; Even and Green 1989; Mathias and Green 2008; Maziere et al. 1986; Maus et al. 2011; Wunderlich et al. 2010; Schiller et al. 2008; Richter et al. 2010; Beller et al. 1979; Schmidt et al. 2006; Hoffend et al. 2005; Mier et al. 2005; Schuster et al. 1995).

^{68}Ga-labeled carbon nanoparticle aerosol was developed for diagnosis of pulmonary emboli and assessment of lung ventilation distribution prior to lung resection. The agent was prepared using commercially available equipment (Technegas, Australia) wherein preconcentrated ^{68}Ga (Velikyan et al. 2004) was placed in a carbon crucible and exposed to high temperature, forming a pseudogas for inhalation (GallGas) (Borges et al. 2011). A comparative dual study was conducted in piglets wherein both [^{68}Ga]Ga-GallGas and [^{99m}Tc]-Technegas were inhaled by the same animal. There was equally homogeneous distribution of radioactivity in healthy control piglets (Fig. 12a). Absence of radioactivity and ventilation in obstructed lower lobe could be observed in both PET and SPECT images (Fig. 12b). However, the former exhibited larger variation in ventilation distribution, most probably related to diffuse bronchial constriction. The most prominent difference in the performance of the two imaging agents was observed

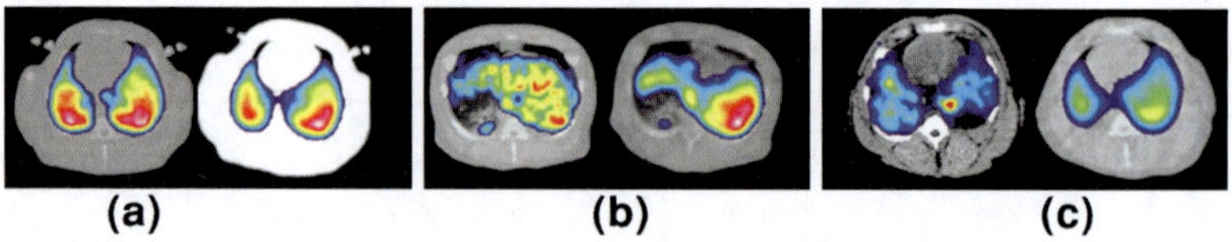

Fig. 12 Lung ventilation imaging using carbon particles behaving as a "pseudogas" for diagnosis of acute pulmonary emboli. Dual study using [^{68}Ga]Ga-GallGas (*left*) and [^{99m}Tc]-Technegas (*right*) in healthy piglets, demonstrating similarity in ventilation distribution (**a**), in piglets with lower lobar obstruction (**b**), and in piglets with diffuse airway obstruction induced by infusion of methacholine (**c**). (Borges et al. 2011)

in piglets with diffuse airway obstruction induced by infusion of methacholine (Fig. 12c). Poorly and well-ventilated regions could be distinguished by PET agent and correlated with measurement of end-expiratory lung volume by multiple-breath nitrogen washout. The superior performance of [^{68}Ga]Ga-GallGas in terms of better appreciation of heterogenecity of the airway response to bronchoconstrictive challenge was assigned to the higher resolution of PET as compared with SPECT. Distribution of similar ^{68}Ga-labeled aerosol was studied in two healthy volunteers (Kotzerke et al. 2010). Even uptake of radioactivity was observed in lung and without bronchial deposits. After inhalation, the radioactivity remained in the alveolar space, and no elimination via blood, urine, or feces could be observed within 3.5 h.

5 Low-Molecular-Weight Imaging Agents

Not only macromolecules have been tagged with ^{68}Ga but also small biologically active ones for visualization of cell proliferation, hypoxia, glycolysis, myocardium, and bone. Analogs comprising nitroimidazole and mercaptobenzynamine have been investigated for imaging of hypoxia, which is an important parameter in tumor and myocardial ischemia physiology (Chapman et al. 1983; Hoigebazar et al. 2010; Mukai et al. 2009). Detection of hypoxia is important for diagnosis, prognosis, treatment planning, and monitoring response to therapy. Lipophilic and cationic gallium complexes of N_4O_2, N_2S_2, and NS_3 have demonstrated myocardial uptake and retention in animal studies (Yang et al. 2010; Tsang et al. 1993; Hsiao et al. 2009; Plossl et al. 2008; Cutler et al. 1999; Zhang et al. 1992). Biphosphonates (Fellner et al. 2010) and ^{68}Ga-labeled ethylene diamino-*N,N,N',N'*-tetrakis-methylene phosphoric acid (Toegel et al. 2008; Mitterhauser et al. 2007) were found useful for early diagnosis of bone metastases. DOTA- and NOTA-coupled alanine and lysine analogs targeting transporters for cell proliferation visualization showed uptake in animal tumor models (Shetty et al. 2010a, b). [^{68}Ga]Ga-EC-guanine (Yang et al. 2006) and [^{68}Ga]Ga-EC-deoxyglucose (Yang and Kim 2005; Yang et al. 2005) have also demonstrated tumor uptake in animals.

6 Further Examples of Diverse Applications of ^{68}Ga

The list of examples of diverse applications of ^{68}Ga is rather extensive. ^{68}Ga-labeling of high-affinity urea-based inhibitors of prostate-specific membrane antigen (PSMA) for imaging of prostate cancer is an example of the translation of the ^{99m}Tc heritage to ^{68}Ga. *N,N'*-bis(diethylenetriamine pentaacetic acid)-pamoic acid bis-hydrazide was labeled with ^{68}Ga for visualization of necrosis that occurs in acute myocardial infarction, chronic heart failure, allograft rejection, stroke, neurodegenerative disorders, and inflammation (Prinsen et al. 2010). Substrates for overexpressed multidrug-resistance P-glycoprotein were developed for imaging and evaluation of tumor response to therapy (Sharma et al. 2005; Thews et al. 2010). ^{68}Ga-labeled ligand to vascular adhesion protein-1 (Lankinen et al. 2008; Autio et al. 2010; Silvola et al. 2010; Ujula et al. 2009), ionic ^{68}Ga (Makinen et al. 2005), ^{68}Ga-labeled siderophores (Petrik et al. 2010), and [^{68}Ga]Ga-citrate (Rizzello et al. 2009; Nanni et al. 2010) have been suggested for differentiation and diagnosis of inflammation and infection. Imaging of thrombosis and atherosclerosis (Welch et al. 1977; Yano et al. 1985) and pulmonary function (Mintun et al. 1987; Schuster et al. 2002) are further examples.

7 Conclusions

The diversity of ^{68}Ga-based imaging agents covers a broad range of vectors from small molecules to macromolecules, and further to particles. The advent of macrocyclic chelators, availability of ^{68}Ge/^{68}Ga generators, development of methods for ^{68}Ga preconcentration and purification, and breakthrough experience with somatostatin analogs have considerably contributed to the exponential growth of ^{68}Ga applications. The heritage of ^{99m}Tc plays an important role and influences the expansion of the ^{68}Ga-based tracer arsenal. ^{68}Ga-labeling chemistry is amenable to kit-type as well as automated radiopharmaceutical production, and is becoming a cost-effective complement to cyclotron-based tracers. It has the potential to facilitate development of clinically practical PET and may promote the PET technique worldwide for earlier and better diagnostics and beyond towards individualized medicine.

References

Ahlgren S, Tolmachev V (2010) Radionuclide molecular imaging using affibody molecules. Curr Pharm Biotechnol 11(6):581–589

Ambrosini V, Tomassetti P, Castellucci P, Campana D, Montini G, Rubello D, Nanni C, Rizzello A, Franchi R, Fanti S (2008) Comparison between 68 Ga-DOTA-NOC and 18F-DOPA PET for the detection of gastro-entero-pancreatic and lung neuro-endocrine tumours. Eur J Nucl Med Mol Imaging 35(8):1431

Ambrosini V, Zompatori M, De Luca F, Antonia DE, Allegri V, Nanni C, Malvi D, Tonveronachi E, Fasano L, Fabbri M, Fanti S (2010a) 68 Ga-DOTANOC PET/CT allows somatostatin receptor imaging in idiopathic pulmonary fibrosis: preliminary results. J Nucl Med 51(12):1950–1955

Ambrosini V, Nanni C, Zompatori M, Campana D, Tomassetti P, Castellucci P, Allegri V, Rubello D, Montini G, Franchi R, Fanti S (2010b) Ga-68-DOTA-NOC PET/CT in comparison with CT for the detection of bone metastasis in patients with neuroendocrine tumours. Eur J Nucl Med Mol Imaging 37(4):722–727

Ambrosini V, Campana D, Allegri V, Opocher G, Fanti S (2011) 68 Ga-DOTA-NOC PET/CT detects somatostatin receptors expression in von Hippel-Lindau cerebellar disease. Clin Nucl Med 36(1):64–65

Antunes P, Ginj M, Walter MA, Chen J, Reubi JC, Maecke HR (2007) Influence of different spacers on the biological profile of a DOTA-somatostatin analogue. Bioconjugate Chem 18(1):84–92

Asti M, De Pietri G, Fraternali A, Grassi E, Sghedoni R, Floroni F, Roesch F, Versari A, Salvo D (2008) Validation of Ge-68/Ga-68 generator processing by chemical purification for routine clinical application of Ga-68-DOTATOC. Nucl Med Biol 35(6):721–724

Autio A, Ujula T, Luoto P, Salomaki S, Jalkanen S, Roivainen A (2010) PET imaging of inflammation and adenocarcinoma xenografts using vascular adhesion protein 1 targeting peptide 68 Ga-DOTAVAP-P1: comparison with 18F-FDG. Eur J Nucl Med Mol Imaging 37(10):1918–1925

Backer MV, Levashova Z, Patel V, Jehning BT, Claffey K, Blankenberg FG, Backer JM (2007) Molecular imaging of VEGF receptors in angiogenic vasculature with single-chain VEGF-based probes. Nat Med 13(4):504–509

Backer MV, Levashova Z, Levenson R, Blankenberg FG, Backer JM (2008) Cysteine-containing fusion tag for site-specific conjugation of therapeutic and imaging agents to targeting proteins. Methods Mol Biol 494:275–294. Clifton, NJ

Barone R, Borson-Chazot F, Valkema R, Walrand S, Chauvin F, Gogou L, Kvols LK, Krenning EP, Jamar F, Pauwels S (2005) Patient-specific dosimetry in predicting renal toxicity with (90)Y-DOTATOC: relevance of kidney volume and dose rate in finding a dose-effect relationship. J Nucl Med 46(Suppl 1):99S–106S

Baum RP, Prasad V, Frischknecht M, Maecke H, Reubi J (2007) Bombesin receptor imaging in various tumors: first results of Ga-68 AMBA PET/CT. Eur J Nucl Med Mol Imaging 34:S193–S193

Baum RP, Prasad V, Hommann M, Horsch D (2008) Receptor PET/CT imaging of neuroendocrine tumors. Recent Results Cancer Res 170:225–242

Baum RP, Prasad V, Muller D, Schuchardt C, Orlova A, Wennborg A, Tolmachev V, Feldwisch J (2010) Molecular imaging of HER2-expressing malignant tumors in breast cancer patients using synthetic 111In- or 68 Ga-labeled affibody molecules. J Nucl Med 51(6):892–897

Bauwens M, Chekol R, Vanbilloen H, Bormans G, Verbruggen A (2010) Optimal buffer choice of the radiosynthesis of Ga-68-Dotatoc for clinical application. Nucl Med Commun 31(8):753–758

Behr TM, Behe M, Becker W (1999) Diagnostic applications of radiolabeled peptides in nuclear endocrinology. Q J Nucl Med 43(3):268–280

Beller GA, Alton WJ, Cochavi S, Hnatowich D, Brownell GL (1979) Assessment of regional myocardial perfusion by positron emission tomography after intra-coronary administration of Ga-68 labeled albumin microspheres. J Comput Assist Tomogr 3(4):447–452

Bergstrom M, Grahnen A, Langstrom B (2003) Positron emission tomography microdosing: a new concept with application in tracer and early clinical drug development. Eur J Clin Pharmacol 59(5–6):357–366

Bergstrom SK, Edenwall N, Laven M, Velikyan I, Langstrom B, Markides KE (2005) Polyamine deactivation of integrated poly(dimethylsiloxane) structures investigated by radionuclide imaging and capillary electrophoresis experiments. Anal Chem 77(3):938–942

Blom E, Langstrom B, Velikyan I (2009) (68)Ga-labeling of biotin analogues and their characterization. Bioconjug Chem 20:1146–1151

Blom E, Velikyan I, Monazzam A, Razifar P, Nair M, Razifar P, Vanderheyden J-L, Krivoshein AV, Backer M, Backer J, Långström B (2011) Synthesis and characterization of scVEGF-PEG-[68 Ga]NOTA and scVEGF-PEG-[68 Ga]DOTA PET tracers. J Labelled Compounds Radiopharm: n/a-n/a

Boerman OC, van Schaijk FG, Oyen WJG, Corstens FHM (2003) Pretargeted radioimmunotherapy of cancer: progress step by step. J Nucl Med 44(3):400–411

Borges JB, Velikyan I, Långström B, Sörensen J, Ulin J, Maripuu E, Sandström M, Widström C, Hedenstierna G (2011) Ventilation distribution studies comparing Technegas and Gallgas using 68 $GaCl_3$ as the label. J Nucl Med 52:206–209

Boss A, Bisdas S, Kolb A, Hofmann M, Ernemann U, Claussen CD, Pfannenberg C, Pichler BJ, Reimold M, Stegger L (2010) Hybrid PET/MRI of intracranial masses: initial experiences and comparison to PET/CT. J Nucl Med 51(8):1198–1205

Brom M, Oyen WJ, Joosten L, Gotthardt M, Boerman OC (2010) 68 Ga-labelled exendin-3, a new agent for the detection of insulinomas with PET. Eur J Nucl Med Mol Imaging 37(7):1345–1355

Cagnolini A, Chen J, Ramos K, Skedzielewski TM, Lantry LE, Nunn AD, Swenson RE, Linder KE (2010) Automated synthesis, characterization and biological evaluation of [(68)Ga]Ga-AMBA, and the synthesis and characterization of (nat)Ga-AMBA and [(67)Ga]Ga-AMBA. Appl Radiat Isot 68(12):2285–2292

Campana D, Ambrosini V, Pezzilli R, Fanti S, Labate AMM, Santini D, Ceccarelli C, Nori F, Franchi R, Corinaldesi R, Tomassetti P (2010) Standardized uptake values of 68 Ga-DOTANOC PET: a promising prognostic tool in neuroendocrine tumors. J Nucl Med 51(3):353–359

Cantorias MV, Figueroa SD, Quinn TP, Lever JR, Hoffman TJ, Watkinson LD, Carmack TL, Cutler CS (2009) Development of high-specific-activity Ga-68-labeled DOTA-rhenium-cyclized alpha-MSH peptide analog to target MC1 receptors overexpressed by melanoma tumors. Nucl Med Biol 36(5):505–513

Carlsson J, Forssell-Aronsson E, Glimelius B, Mattsson S (2002) Therapy with radiopharmaceuticals. Acta Oncol 41(7–8):623–628

Carlsson J, Forssell Aronsson E, Hietala SO, Stigbrand T, Tennvall J (2003) Tumour therapy with radionuclides: assessment of progress and problems. Radiother Oncol 66(2):107–117

Cescato R, Erchegyi J, Waser B, Piccand V, Maecke HR, Rivier JE, Reubi JC (2008) Design and in vitro characterization of highly sst2-selective somatostatin antagonists suitable for radiotargeting. J Med Chem 51(13):4030–4037

Chang C-H, Sharkey RM, Rossi EA, Karacay H, McBride W, Hansen HJ, Chatal J-F, Barbet J, Goldenberg DM (2002) Molecular advances in pretargeting radioimunotherapy with bispecific antibodies 1 supported in part by USPHS Grant R01-CA-84379 from the NIH and department of energy grant DE-FG01-00NE22941 (both to R. M. S.).1. Mol Cancer Ther 1(7):553–563

Chapman JD, Baer K, Lee J (1983) Characteristics of the metabolism-induced binding of misonidazole to hypoxic mammalian cells. Cancer Res 43(4):1523–1528

Chen X, Park R, Shahinian AH, Bading JR, Conti PS (2004) Pharmacokinetics and tumor retention of 125I-labeled RGD peptide are improved by PEGylation. Nucl Med Biol 31(1):11–19

Chesler DA, Hales C, Hnatowich DJ, Hoop B (1975) 3-dimensional reconstruction of lung perfusion image with positron detection. J Nucl Med 16(1):80–82

Conry BG, Papathanasiou ND, Prakash V, Kayani I, Caplin M, Mahmood S, Bomanji JB (2010) Comparison of Ga-68-DOTATATE and F-18-fluorodeoxyglucose PET/CT in the detection of recurrent medullary thyroid carcinoma. Eur J Nucl Med Mol Imaging 37(1):49–57

Cutler CS, Giron MC, Reichert DE, Snyder AZ, Herrero P, Anderson CJ, Quarless DA, Koch SA, Welch MJ (1999) Evaluation of gallium-68 tris(2-mercaptobenzyl)amine: a complex with brain and myocardial uptake. Nucl Med Biol 26(3):305–316 de Jong M, Bakker WH, Krenning EP, Breeman WA, van der Pluijm ME, Bernard BF, Visser TJ, Jermann E, Behe M, Powell P, Macke HR (1997) Yttrium-90 and indium-111 labelling, receptor binding and biodistribution of [DOTA0, d-Phe1, Tyr3]octreotide, a promising somatostatin analogue for radionuclide therapy. Eur J Nucl Med 24(4):368–371

De Jong M, Bakker WH, Breeman WA, Bernard BF, Hofland LJ, Visser TJ, Srinivasan A, Schmidt M, Behe M, Macke HR, Krenning EP (1998) Pre-clinical comparison of [DTPA0] octreotide, [DTPA0, Tyr3] octreotide and [DOTA0, Tyr3] octreotide as carriers for somatostatin receptor-targeted scintigraphy and radionuclide therapy. Int J Cancer 75(3):406–411

Decristoforo C, Hernandez Gonzalez I, Carlsen J, Rupprich M, Huisman M, Virgolini I, Wester HJ, Haubner R (2008) 68 Ga- and 111In-labelled DOTA-RGD peptides for imaging of alphavbeta3 integrin expression. Eur J Nucl Med Mol Imaging 35(8):1507–1515

Demmer O, Dijkgraaf I, Schottelius M, Wester HJ, Kessler H (2008) Introduction of functional groups into peptides via N-alkylation. Org Lett 10(10):2015–2018

Deshmukh MV, Voll G, Kuhlewein A, Macke H, Schmitt J, Kessler H, Gemmecker G (2005) NMR studies reveal structural differences between the gallium and yttrium complexes of DOTA-D-Phe1-Tyr3-octreotide. J Med Chem 48(5):1506–1514

Dijkgraaf I, Boerman OC (2009) Radionuclide imaging of tumor angiogenesis. Cancer Biother Radiopharm 24(6):637–647

Dijkgraaf I, Yim CB, Franssen GM, Schuit RC, Luurtsema G, Liu S, Oyen WJ, Boerman OC (2011) PET imaging of alphavbeta integrin expression in tumours with Ga-labelled mono-, di- and tetrameric RGD peptides. Eur J Nucl Med Mol Imaging 38(1):128–137

Dimitrakopoulou-Strauss A, Georgoulias V, Eisenhut M, Herth F, Koukouraki S, Macke HR, Haberkorn U, Strauss LG (2006) Quantitative assessment of SSTR2 expression in patients with non-small cell lung cancer using Ga-68-DOTATOC PET and comparison with F-18-FDG PET. Eur J Nucl Med Mol Imaging 33(7):823–830

Dimitrakopoulou-Strauss A, Hohenberger P, Haberkorn U, Macke HR, Eisenhut M, Strauss LG (2007) Ga-68-Labeled bombesin studies in patients with gastrointestinal stromal tumors: comparison with F-18-FDG. J Nucl Med 48(8):1245–1250

Eisenwiener KP, Prata MI, Buschmann I, Zhang HW, Santos AC, Wenger S, Reubi JC, Macke HR (2002) NODAGATOC, a new chelator-coupled somatostatin analogue labeled with [67/68 Ga] and [111In] for SPECT, PET, and targeted therapeutic applications of somatostatin receptor (hsst2) expressing tumors. Bioconjug Chem 13(3):530–541

Erchegyi J, Grace CR, Samant M, Cescato R, Piccand V, Riek R, Reubi JC, Rivier JE (2008) Ring size of somatostatin analogues (ODT-8) modulates receptor selectivity and binding affinity. J Med Chem 51(9):2668–2675

Eriksson O, Carlsson F, Blom E, Sundin A, Långström B, Korsgren O, Velikyan I (2011) Preclinical evaluation of a ^{68}Ga-labeled biotin analogue for applications in islet transplantation. Nucl Med Biol 38(6):827

Even GA, Green MA (1989) Gallium-68-labeled macroaggregated human serum albumin, 68 Ga-MAA. Int J Radiat Appl Instrum Part B Nucl Med Biol 16(3):319–321

Fani M, Mueller A, Tamma ML, Nicolas G, Rink HR, Cescato R, Reubi JC, Maecke HR (2010) Radiolabeled bicyclic somatostatin-based analogs: a novel class of potential radiotracers for SPECT/PET of neuroendocrine tumors. J Nucl Med 51(11):1771–1779

Fani M, Wang X, Nicolas G, Medina C, Raynal I, Port M, Maecke HR (2011) Development of new folate-based PET radiotracers: preclinical evaluation of Ga-DOTA-folate conjugates. Eur J Nucl Med Mol Imaging 38(1):108–119

Fellner M, Baum RP, Kubicek V, Hermann P, Lukes I, Prasad V, Rosch F (2010) PET/CT imaging of osteoblastic bone metastases with Ga-68-bisphosphonates: first human study. Eur J Nucl Med Mol Imaging 37(4):834

Forrer F, Uusijarvi H, Waldherr C, Cremonesi M, Bernhardt P, Mueller-Brand J, Maecke HR (2004) A comparison of (111)In-DOTATOC and (111)In-DOTATATE: biodistribution and dosimetry in the same patients with metastatic neuroendocrine tumours. Eur J Nucl Med Mol Imaging 31(9):1257–1262

Forssell-Aronsson E, Kjellen E, Mattsson S, Hellstrom M (2002) Medical imaging for improved tumour characterization, delineation and treatment verification. Acta Oncol 41(7–8):604–614

Forster GJ, Santos EB, Smith-Jones PM, Zanzonico P, Larson SM (2006) Pretargeted radioimmunotherapy with a single-chain antibody/streptavidin construct and radiolabeled DOTA-biotin: strategies for reduction of the renal dose. J Nucl Med 47(1):140–149

Frangioni JV (2009) The problem is background, not signal. Mol Imaging 8(6):303–304

Frilling A, Sotiropoulos GC, Radtke A, Malago M, Bockisch A, Kuehl H, Li J, Broelsch CE (2010) The impact of 68 Ga-DOTATOC positron emission tomography/computed tomography on the multimodal management of patients with neuroendocrine tumors. Ann Surg 252(5):850–856

Froidevaux S, Eberle AN (2002) Somatostatin analogs and radiopeptides in cancer therapy. Biopolymers 66(3):161–183

Froidevaux S, Eberle AN, Christe M, Sumanovski L, Heppeler A, Schmitt JS, Eisenwiener K, Beglinger C, Macke HR (2002) Neuroendocrine tumor targeting: study of novel gallium-labeled somatostatin radiopeptides in a rat pancreatic tumor model. Int J Cancer 98(6):930–937

Froidevaux S, Calame-Christe M, Schuhmacher J, Tanner H, Saffrich R, Henze M, Eberle AN (2004) A gallium-labeled DOTA-{alpha}-melanocyte-stimulating hormone analog for PET imaging of melanoma metastases. J Nucl Med 45(1):116–123

Gabriel M, Decristoforo C, Kendler D, Dobrozemsky G, Heute D, Uprimny C, Kovacs P, Von Guggenberg E, Bale R, Virgolini IJ (2007) 68 Ga-DOTA-Tyr3-octreotide PET in neuroendocrine tumors: comparison with somatostatin receptor scintigraphy and CT. J Nucl Med 48(4):508–518

Gabriel M, Andergassen U, Putzer D, Kroiss A, Waitz D, Von Guggenberg E, Kendler D, Virgolini IJ (2010) Individualized peptide-related-radionuclide-therapy concept using different radiolabelled somatostatin analogs in advanced cancer patients. Q J Nucl Med Mol Imaging 54(1):92–99

Gambhir SS (2002) Molecular imaging of cancer with positron emission tomography. Nat Rev Cancer 2(9):683–693

Garner RC, Lappin G (2006) The phase 0 microdosing concept. Br J Clin Pharmacol 61(4):367–370

Gebhardt P, Opfermann T, Saluz HP (2010) Computer controlled Ga-68 milking and concentration system. Appl Radiat Isot 68(6):1057–1059

Gehler B, Paulsen F, Oksuz MO, Hauser TK, Eschmann SM, Bares R, Pfannenberg C, Bamberg M, Bartenstein P, Belka C, Ganswindt U (2009) [68 Ga]-DOTATOC-PET/CT for meningioma IMRT treatment planning. Radiat Oncol 4:56

Ginj M, Chen J, Walter MA, Eltschinger V, Reubi JC, Maecke HR (2005) Preclinical evaluation of new and highly potent analogues of octreotide for predictive imaging and targeted radiotherapy. Clin Cancer Res 11(3):1136–1145

Gold DV, Goldenberg DM, Karacay H, Rossi EA, Chang CH, Cardillo TM, McBride WJ, Sharkey RM (2008) A novel bispecific, trivalent antibody construct for targeting pancreatic carcinoma. Cancer Res 68(12):4819–4826

Goldenberg DM, Sharkey RM (2007) Novel radiolabeled antibody conjugates. Oncogene 26(25):3734–3744

Goldenberg DM, Sharkey RM, Paganelli G, Barbet J, Chatal JF (2006) Antibody pretargeting advances cancer radioimmunodetection and radioimmunotherapy. J Clin Oncol 24(5):823–834

Goldenberg DM, Rossi EA, Sharkey RM, McBride WJ, Chang CH (2008) Multifunctional antibodies by the dock-and-lock method for improved cancer imaging and therapy by pretargeting. J Nucl Med 49(1):158–163

Goldstein MJ, Mitchell EP (2005) Carcinoembryonic antigen in the staging and follow-up of patients with colorectal cancer. Cancer Invest 23(4):338–351

Grace CR, Erchegyi J, Samant M, Cescato R, Piccand V, Riek R, Reubi JC, Rivier JE (2008a) Ring size in octreotide amide modulates differently agonist versus antagonist binding affinity and selectivity. J Med Chem 51(9):2676–2681

Grace CR, Erchegyi J, Reubi JC, Rivier JE, Riek R (2008b) Three-dimensional consensus structure of sst2-selective somatostatin (SRIF) antagonists by NMR. Biopolymers 89(12):1077–1087

Griffiths GL, Chang CH, McBride WJ, Rossi EA, Sheerin A, Tejada GR, Karacay H, Sharkey RM, Horak ID, Hansen HJ, Goldenberg DM (2004) Reagents and methods for PET using bispecific antibody pretargeting and 68 Ga-radiolabeled bivalent hapten-peptide-chelate conjugates. J Nucl Med 45(1):30–39

Haubner R, Kuhnast B, Mang C, Weber WA, Kessler H, Wester HJ, Schwaiger M (2004) [18F]Galacto-RGD: synthesis, radiolabeling, metabolic stability, and radiation dose estimates. Bioconjug Chem 15(1):61–69

Haukkala J, Laitinen I, Luoto P, Iveson P, Wilson I, Karlsen H, Cuthbertson A, Laine J, Leppanen P, Yla-Herttula S, Knuuti J, Roivainen A (2009) (68)Ga-DOTA-RGD peptide: biodistribution and binding into atherosclerotic plaques in mice. Eur J Nucl Med Mol Imaging

Hayes RL, Carlton JE, Kuniyasu Y (1981) A new method for labeling microspheres with 68 Ga. Eur J Nucl Med 6(11):531–533

Henze M, Schuhmacher J, Hipp P, Kowalski J, Becker DW, Doll J, Macke HR, Hofmann M, Debus J, Haberkorn U (2001) PET imaging of somatostatin receptors using [68GA]DOTA-D-Phe1-Tyr3-octreotide: first results in patients with meningiomas. J Nucl Med 42(7):1053–1056

Henze M, Schuhmacher J, Dimitrakopoulou-Strauss A, Strauss LG, Macke HR, Eisenhut M, Haberkorn U (2004) Exceptional increase in somatostatin receptor expression in pancreatic neuroendocrine tumour, visualised with Ga-68-DOTATOC PET. Eur J Nucl Med Mol Imaging 31(3):466

Henze M, Dimitrakopoulou-Strauss A, Milker-Zabel S, Schuhmacher J, Strauss LG, Doll J, Macke HR, Eisenhut M, Debus J, Haberkorn U (2005) Characterization of 68 Ga-DOTA-D-Phe1-Tyr3-octreotide kinetics in patients with meningiomas. J Nucl Med 46(5):763–769

Heppeler A, Froidevaux S, Macke HR, Jermann E, Behe M, Powell P, Hennig M (1999) Radiometal-labelled macrocyclic chelator-derivatised somatostatin analogue with superb tumour-targeting properties and potential for receptor-mediated internal radiotherapy. Chem Eur J 5(7):1974–1981

Heppeler A, Froidevaux S, Eberle AN, Maecke HR (2000) Receptor targeting for tumor localisation and therapy with radiopeptides. Curr Med Chem 7:971–994

Hirsch FR, Varella-Garcia M, Bunn PA Jr, Di Maria MV, Veve R, Bremmes RM, Baron AE, Zeng C, Franklin WA (2003) Epidermal growth factor receptor in non-small-cell lung carcinomas: correlation between gene copy number and protein expression and impact on prognosis. J Clin Oncol 21(20):3798–3807

Hoffend J, Mier W, Schuhmacher J, Schmidt K, Dimitrakopoulou-Strauss A, Strauss LG, Eisenhut M, Kinscherf R, Haberkorn U (2005) Gallium-68-DOTA-albumin as a PET blood-pool marker: experimental evaluation in vivo. Nucl Med Biol 32(3):287–292

Hofland LJ, Breeman WA, Krenning EP, de Jong M, Waaijers M, van Koetsveld PM, Macke HR, Lamberts SW (1999) Internalization of [DOTA degrees,125I-Tyr3]octreotide by somatostatin receptor-positive cells in vitro and in vivo: implications for somatostatin receptor-targeted radio-guided surgery. Proc Assoc Am Physicians 111(1):63–69

Hofmann M, Maecke H, Borner R, Weckesser E, Schoffski P, Oei L, Schumacher J, Henze M, Heppeler A, Meyer J, Knapp H (2001) Biokinetics and imaging with the somatostatin receptor PET radioligand (68)Ga-DOTATOC: preliminary data. Eur J Nucl Med 28(12):1751–1757

Hofmann M, Machtens S, Stief C, Langer F, Boerner AR, Maecke H, Knapp WH (2004a) Feasibility of Ga-68-DOTABOM PET in prostate carcinoma patients. Eur J Nucl Med Mol Imaging 31:S253–S253

Hofmann M, Beyer T, Boerner A, Mueller J, Frilling A, Maecke H, Muller S, Clauss R, Bockisch A, Knapp W (2004b) Improved imaging of SMS PET (Ga-68-DOTATOC) by PET/CT in carcinoids. Eur J Nucl Med Mol Imaging 31:S339

Hoigebazar L, Jeong JM, Choi SY, Choi JY, Shetty D, Lee YS, Lee DS, Chung JK, Lee MC, Chung YK (2010) Synthesis and characterization of nitroimidazole derivatives for 68 Ga-labeling and testing in tumor xenografted mice. J Med Chem 53(17):6378–6385

Hong H, Sun J, Cai W (2008) Radionuclide-based cancer imaging targeting the carcinoembryonic antigen. Biomark Insights 3:435–451

Hsiao YM, Mathias CJ, Wey SP, Fanwick PE, Green MA (2009) Synthesis and biodistribution of lipophilic and monocationic gallium radiopharmaceuticals derived from N,N'-bis(3-aminopropyl)-N,N'-dimethylethylenediamine: potential agents for PET myocardial imaging with Ga-68. Nucl Med Biol 36(1):39–45

Indrevoll B, Kindberg GM, Solbakken M, Bjurgert E, Johansen JH, Karlsen H, Mendizabal M, Cuthbertson A (2006) NC-100717: a versatile RGD peptide scaffold for angiogenesis imaging. Bioorg Med Chem Lett 16(24):6190–6193

Janson ET, Sorbye H, Welin S, Federspiel B, Gronbaek H, Hellman P, Mathisen O, Mortensen J, Sundin A, Thiis-Evensen E, Valimaki MJ, Oberg K, Knigge U (2010) Nordic Guidelines 2010 for diagnosis and treatment of gastroenteropancreatic neuroendocrine tumours. Acta Oncol 49(6):740–756

Janssen M, Oyen WJ, Massuger LF, Frielink C, Dijkgraaf I, Edwards DS, Radjopadhye M, Corstens FH, Boerman OC (2002) Comparison of a monomeric and dimeric radiolabeled RGD-peptide for tumor targeting. Cancer Biother Radiopharm 17(6):641–646

Jeong JM, Hong MK, Chang YS, Lee YS, Kim YJ, Cheon GJ, Lee DS, Chung JK, Lee MC (2008) Preparation of a promising angiogenesis PET imaging agent: Ga-68-labeled c(RGDyK)-isothiocyanatobenzyl-1,4,7-triazacyclononane-1,4,7-triacetic acid and feasibility studies in mice. J Nucl Med 49(5):830–836

Kayani I, Bomanji JB, Groves A, Conway G, Gacinovic S, Win T, Dickson J, Caplin M, Ell PJ (2008) Functional imaging of neuroendocrine tumors with combined PET/CT using 68 Ga-DOTATATE (DOTA-DPhe1, Tyr3-octreotate) and 18F-FDG. Cancer 112(11):2447–2455

Kotzerke J, Andreeff M, Wunderlich G (2010) PET aerosol lung scintigraphy using galligas. Eur J Nucl Med Mol Imaging 37(1):175–177

Koukouraki S, Strauss LG, Georgoulias V, Schuhmacher J, Haberkorn U, Karkavitsas N, Dimitrakopoulou-Strauss A (2006a) Evaluation of the pharmacokinetics of 68 Ga-DOTATOC in patients with metastatic neuroendocrine tumours scheduled for 90Y-DOTATOC therapy. Eur J Nucl Med Mol Imaging 33(4):460–466

Koukouraki S, Strauss LG, Georgoulias V, Eisenhut M, Haberkorn U, Dimitrakopoulou-Strauss A (2006b) Comparison of the pharmacokinetics of Ga-68-DOTATOC and F-18 FDG in patients with metastatic neuroendocrine tumours scheduled for Y-90-DOTATOC therapy. Eur J Nucl Med Mol Imaging 33(10):1115–1122

Kowalski J, Henze M, Schuhmacher J, Macke HR, Hofmann M, Haberkorn U (2003) Evaluation of positron emission tomography imaging using [68 Ga]-DOTA-D Phe(1)-Tyr(3)-Octreotide in comparison to [111In]-DTPAOC SPECT. First results in patients with neuroendocrine tumors. Mol Imaging Biol 5(1):42–48

Långström B, Velikyan I, Bergström M, Lindhe Ö (2008) ^{68}Ga-labeled peptide-based radiopharmaceuticals. WO/2008/026040

Lankinen P, Maekinen TJ, Poeyhoenen TA, Virsu P, Salomaeki S, Hakanen AJ, Jalkanen S, Aro HT, Roivainen A (2008) Ga-68-DOTAVAP-P1 PET imaging capable of demonstrating the phase of inflammation in healing bones and the progress of infection in osteomyelitic bones. Eur J Nucl Med Mol Imaging 35(2):352–364

Laven M, Velikyan I, Djodjic M, Ljung J, Berglund O, Markides K, Langstrom B, Wallenborg S (2005) Imaging of peptide adsorption to microfluidic channels in a plastic compact disc using a positron emitting radionuclide. Lab Chip 5(7):756–763

Lavén M, Wallenborg S, Velikyan I, Bergstrom S, Djodjic M, Ljung J, Berglund O, Edenwall N, Markides KE, Langstrom B (2004) Radionuclide imaging of miniaturized chemical analysis systems. Anal Chem 76(23):7102–7108

Lendvai G, Velikyan I, Bergstrom M, Estrada S, Laryea D, Valila M, Salomaki S, Langstrom B, Roivainen A (2005) Biodistribution of ^{68}Ga-labelled phosphodiester, phosphorothioate, and 2'-O-methyl phosphodiester oligonucleotides in normal rats. Eur J Pharm Sci 26(1):26–38
Lendvai G, Velikyan I, Estrada S, Eriksson B, Langstrom B, Bergstrom M (2008) Biodistribution of (68)Ga-labeled LNA-DNA mixmer antisense oligonucleotides for rat chromogranin-A. Oligonucleotides 18(1):33–49
Lendvai G, Monazzam A, Velikyan I, Eriksson B, Josephsson R, Langstrom B, Bergstrom M, Estrada S (2009a) Non-hybridization saturable mechanisms play a role in the uptake of (68)Ga-labeled LNA-DNA mixmer antisense oligonucleotides in rats. Oligonucleotides 19(3):223–232
Lendvai G, Estrada S, Bergstrom M (2009b) Radiolabelled oligonucleotides for imaging of gene expression with PET. Curr Med Chem 16(33):4445–4461
Li ZB, Chen K, Chen X (2008) (68)Ga-labeled multimeric RGD peptides for microPET imaging of integrin alpha(v)beta (3) expression. Eur J Nucl Med Mol Imaging 35(6):1100–1108
Lincke T, Singer J, Kluge R, Sabri O, Paschke R (2009) Relative quantification of indium-111 pentetreotide and gallium-68 DOTATOC uptake in the thyroid gland and association with thyroid pathologies. Thyroid 19(4):381–389
Liu S (2006) Radiolabeled multimeric cyclic RGD peptides as integrin alphavbeta3 targeted radiotracers for tumor imaging. Mol Pharm 3(5):472–487
Liu S, Edwards DS (1999) Tc-99 m-labeled small peptides as diagnostic radiopharmaceuticals. Chem Rev 99(9):2235–2268
Liu Z, Niu G, Shi J, Liu S, Wang F, Chen X (2009) (68)Ga-labeled cyclic RGD dimers with Gly3 and PEG4 linkers: promising agents for tumor integrin alphavbeta3 PET imaging. Eur J Nucl Med Mol Imaging 36(6):947–957
Luboldt W, Zophel K, Wunderlich G, Abramyuk A, Luboldt HJ, Kotzerke J (2010) Visualization of somatostatin receptors in prostate cancer and its bone metastases with Ga-68-DOTATOC PET/CT. Mol Imaging Biol 12(1):78–84
Lundqvist H, Tolmachev V (2002) Targeting peptides and positron emission tomography. Biopolymers 66(6):381–392
Maecke HR (2005) Radiolabeled peptides in nuclear oncology: influence of peptide structure and labeling strategy on pharmacology. Ernst Schering Res Found Workshop 49:43–72
Maecke HR, Hofmann M, Haberkorn U (2005) (68)Ga-Labeled peptides in tumor imaging. J Nucl Med 46(Suppl 1):172S–178S
Makinen TJ, Lankinen P, Poyhonen T, Jalava J, Aro HT, Roivainen A (2005) Comparison of F-18-FDG and Ga-68 PET imaging in the assessment of experimental osteomyelitis due to Staphylococcus aureus. Eur J Nucl Med Mol Imaging 32(11):1259–1268
Mansi R, Wang X, Forrer F, Waser B, Cescato R, Graham K, Borkowski S, Reubi JC, Maecke HR (2011) Development of a potent DOTA-conjugated bombesin antagonist for targeting GRPr-positive tumours. Eur J Nucl Med Mol Imaging 38(1):97–107
Maschauer S, Einsiedel J, Hocke C, Hubner H, Kuwert T, Gmeiner P, Prante O (2010) Synthesis of a Ga-68-labeled peptoid-peptide hybrid for imaging of neurotensin receptor expression in vivo. ACS Med Chem Lett 1(5):224–228
Mathias CJ, Green MA (2008) A convenient route to Ga-68 Ga-MAA for use as a particulate PET perfusion tracer. Appl Radiat Isot 66(12):1910–1912
Mathias CJ, Lewis MR, Reichert DE, Laforest R, Sharp TL, Lewis JS, Yang ZF, Waters DJ, Snyder PW, Low PS, Welch MJ, Green MA (2003) Preparation of 66 Ga- and 68 Ga-labeled Ga(III)-deferoxamine-folate as potential folate-receptor-targeted PET radiopharmaceuticals. Nucl Med Biol 30(7):725–731
Maus S, Buchholz H-G, Ament S, Brochhausen C, Bausbacher N, Schreckenberger M (2011) Labelling of commercially available human serum albumin kits with 68 Ga as surrogates for 99mTc-MAA microspheres. Appl Radiat Isot 69(1):171–175
Maziere B, Loc'h C, Steinling M, Comar D (1986) Stable labelling of serum albumin microspheres with gallium-68. Int J Rad Appl Instrum A 37(4):360–361

Meier G, Waldherr C, Herrmann R, Maecke H, Mueller-Brand J, Pless M (2004) Successful targeted radiotherapy with 90Y-DOTATOC in a patient with Merkel cell carcinoma. A case report. Oncology 66(2):160–163

Meyer GJ, Macke H, Schuhmacher J, Knapp WH, Hofmann M (2004) 68 Ga-Labelled DOTA-derivatised peptide ligands. Eur J Nucl Med Mol Imaging 31(8):1097–1104

Mier W, Hoffend J, Kramer S, Schuhmacher J, Hull WE, Eisenhut M, Haberkorn U (2005) Conjugation of DOTA using isolated phenolic active esters: the labeling and biodistribution of albumin as blood pool marker. Bioconjug Chem 16(1):237–240

Milker-Zabel S, Zabel-du Bois A, Henze M, Huber P, Schulz-Ertner D, Hoess A, Haberkorn U, Debus J (2006) Improved target volume definition for fractionated stereotactic radiotherapy in patients with intracranial meningiomas by correlation of CT, MRI, and [68 Ga]-DOTATOC-PET. Int J Radiat Oncol Biol Phys 65(1):222–227

Mintun MA, Terpogossian MM, Green MA, Lich LL, Schuster DP (1986) Quantitative measurement of regional pulmonary blood-flow with positron emission tomography. J Appl Physiol 60(1):317–326

Mintun MA, Dennis DR, Welch MJ, Mathias CJ, Schuster DP (1987) Measurements of pulmonary vascular permeability with pet and gallium-68 transferrin. J Nucl Med 28(11):1704–1716

Mitterhauser M, Toegel S, Wadsak W, Lanzenberger RR, Mien LK, Kuntner C, Wanek T, Eidherr H, Ettlinger DE, Viernstein H, Kluger R, Dudczak R, Kletter K (2007) Pre vivo, ex vivo and in vivo evaluations of Ga-68-EDTMP. Nucl Med Biol 34(4):391–397

Modlin IM, Oberg K, Chung DC, Jensen RT, de Herder WW, Thakker RV, Caplin M, Delle Fave G, Kaltsas GA, Krenning EP, Moss SF, Nilsson O, Rindi G, Salazar R, Ruszniewski P, Sundin A (2008) Gastroenteropancreatic neuroendocrine tumours. Lancet Oncol 9(1):61–72

Mukai T, Suwada J, Sano K, Okada M, Yamamoto F, Maeda M (2009) Design of Ga-DOTA-based bifunctional radiopharmaceuticals: Two functional moieties can be conjugated to radiogallium-DOTA without reducing the complex stability. Bioorg Med Chem 17(13):4285–4289

Mutic S, Malyapa RS, Grigsby PW, Dehdashti F, Miller TR, Zoberi I, Bosch WR, Esthappan J, Low DA (2003) PET-guided IMRT for cervical carcinoma with positive para-aortic lymph nodes-a dose-escalation treatment planning study. Int J Radiat Oncol Biol Phys 55(1):28–35

Nanni C, Errani C, Boriani L, Fantini L, Ambrosini V, Boschi S, Rubello D, Pettinato C, Mercuri M, Gasbarrini A, Fanti S (2010) 68 Ga-citrate PET/CT for evaluating patients with infections of the bone: preliminary results. J Nucl Med 51(12):1932–1936

Neal DE, Mellon K (1992) Epidermal growth factor receptor and bladder cancer: a review. Urol Int 48(4):365–371

Otte A, Jermann E, Behe M, Goetze M, Bucher HC, Roser HW, Heppeler A, Mueller-Brand J, Maecke HR (1997) DOTATOC: a powerful new tool for receptor-mediated radionuclide therapy. Eur J Nucl Med 24(7):792–795

Petrik M, Haas H, Dobrozemsky G, Lass-Florl C, Helbok A, Blatzer M, Dietrich H, Decristoforo C (2010) 68 Ga-siderophores for PET imaging of invasive pulmonary aspergillosis: proof of principle. J Nucl Med 51(4):639–645

Pettinato C, Sarnelli A, Di Donna M, Civollani S, Nanni C, Montini G, Di Pierro D, Ferrari M, Marengo M, Bergamini C (2008) (68)Ga-DOTANOC: biodistribution and dosimetry in patients affected by neuroendocrine tumors. Eur J Nucl Med Mol Imaging 35(1):72–79

Pless M, Waldherr C, Maecke H, Buitrago C, Herrmann R, Mueller-Brand J (2004) Targeted radiotherapy for small cell lung cancer using 90Yttrium-DOTATOC, an Yttrium-labelled somatostatin analogue: a pilot trial. Lung Cancer 45(3):365–371

Plossl K, Chandra R, Qua WC, Lieberman BP, Kung MP, Zhou R, Huang B, Kung HF (2008) A novel gallium bisaminothiolate complex as a myocardial perfusion imaging agent. Nucl Med Biol 35(1):83–90

Prasad V, Baum RP (2010) Biodistribution of the Ga-68 labeled somatostatin analogue DOTA-NOC in patients with neuroendocrine tumors: characterization of uptake in normal organs and tumor lesions. Q J Nucl Med Mol Imaging 54(1):61–67

Prinsen K, Li JJ, Vanbilloen H, Vermaelen P, Devos E, Mortelmans L, Bormans G, Ni YC, Verbruggen A (2010) Development and evaluation of a Ga-68 labeled pamoic acid derivative for in vivo visualization of necrosis using positron emission tomography. Bioorg Med Chem 18(14):5274–5281

Putzer D, Gabriel M, Henninger B, Kendler D, Uprimny C, Dobrozemsky G, Decristoforo C, Bale RJ, Jaschke W, Virgolini IJ (2009) Bone metastases in patients with neuroendocrine tumor: 68 Ga-DOTA-Tyr3-octreotide PET in comparison to CT and bone scintigraphy. J Nucl Med 50(8):1214–1221

Putzer D, Gabriel M, Kendler D, Henninger B, Knoflach M, Kroiss A, Vonguggenberg E, Warwitz B, Virgolini IJ (2010) Comparison of (68)Ga-DOTA-Tyr(3)-octreotide and (18)F-fluoro-L-dihydroxyphenylalanine positron emission tomography in neuroendocrine tumor patients. Q J Nucl Med Mol Imaging 54(1):68–75

Ren G, Zhang R, Liu Z, Webster JM, Miao Z, Gambhir SS, Syud FA, Cheng Z (2009) A 2-helix small protein labeled with 68 Ga for PET imaging of HER2 expression. J Nucl Med 50(9):1492–1499

Reubi JC (2001) Somatostatin receptor sst1-sst5 expression in normal and neoplastic human tissues using receptor autoradiography with subtype-selective ligands. Eur J Nucl Med 28(7):836–846

Reubi JC, Maecke HR (2008) Peptide-based probes for cancer imaging. J Nucl Med 49(11): 1735–1738

Reubi JC, Schär J-C, Waser B, Wenger S, Heppeler A, Schmitt JS, Mäcke HR (2000) Affinity profiles for human somatostatin receptor subtypes SST1-SST5 of somatostatin radiotracers selected for scintigraphic and radiotherapeutic use. Eur J Nucl Med Mol Imaging 27(3):273–282

Reubi JC, Macke HR, Krenning EP (2005) Candidates for peptide receptor radiotherapy today and in the future. J Nucl Med 46(Suppl 1):67S–75S

Richter T, Bergmann R, Pietzsch J, Kozle I, Hofheinz F, Schiller E, Ragaller M, van den Hoff J (2010) Effects of posture on regional pulmonary blood flow in rats as measured by PET. J Appl Physiol 108(2):422–429

Riss PJ, Kroll C, Nagel V, Rosch F (2008) NODAPA-OH and NODAPA-(NCS)n: synthesis, 68 Ga-radiolabelling and in vitro characterisation of novel versatile bifunctional chelators for molecular imaging. Bioorg Med Chem Lett 18(20):5364–5367

Rivier JE, Kirby DA, Erchegyi J, Waser B, Eltschinger V, Cescato R, Reubi JC (2005) Somatostatin receptor 1 selective analogues: 3 Dicyclic peptides. J Med Chem 48(2):515–522

Rizzello A, Di Pierro D, Lodi F, Trespidi S, Cicoria G, Pancaldi D, Nanni C, Marengo M, Marzola MC, Ai-Nahhas A, Rubello D, Boschi S (2009) Synthesis and quality control of Ga-68 citrate for routine clinical PET. Nucl Med Commun 30(7):542–545

Roivainen A, Tolvanen T, Salomaki S, Lendvai G, Velikyan I, Numminen P, Valila M, Sipila H, Bergstrom M, Harkonen P, Lonnberg H, Langstrom B (2004) 68 Ga-labeled oligonucleotides for in vivo imaging with PET. J Nucl Med 45(2):347–355

Rominger A, Saam T, Vogl E, Ubleis C, la Fougere C, Forster S, Haug A, Cumming P, Reiser MF, Nikolaou K, Bartenstein P, Hacker M (2010) In vivo imaging of macrophage activity in the coronary arteries using 68 Ga-DOTATATE PET/CT: correlation with coronary calcium burden and risk factors. J Nucl Med 51(2):193–197

Rossi EA, Rossi DL, Stein R, Goldenberg DM, Chang CH (2010) A bispecific antibody-IFNalpha2b immunocytokine targeting CD20 and HLA-DR is highly toxic to human lymphoma and multiple myeloma cells. Cancer Res 70(19):7600–7609

Sainz-Esteban A, Prasad V, Baum RP (2010) Pancreatic neuroendocrine tumor with involvement of the inferior mesenteric vein diagnosed by Ga-68 DOTA-TATE PET/CT. Clin Nucl Med 35(1):40–41

Sandstrom K, Haylock AK, Velikyan I, Spiegelberg D, Kareem H, Tolmachev V, Lundqvist H, Nestor M (2011) Improved Tumor-to-Organ Ratios of a novel (67)Ga-human epidermal growth factor radionuclide conjugate with preadministered antiepidermal growth factor receptor affibody molecules. Cancer Biother Radiopharm 26(5):593–600

Schiller E, Bergmann R, Pietzsch J, Noll B, Sterger A, Johannsen B, Wunderlich G, Pietzsch HJ (2008) Yttrium-86-labelled human serum albumin microspheres: relation of surface structure with in vivo stability. Nucl Med Biol 35(2):227–232

Schmidt K, Hoffend J, Altmann A, Strauss LG, Dimitrakopoulou-Strauss A, Engelhardt B, Koczan D, Peter J, Dengler TJ, Mier W, Eisenhut M, Haberkorn U, Kinscherf R (2006) Angiostatin overexpression in Morris hepatoma results in decreased tumor growth but increased perfusion and vascularization. J Nucl Med 47(3):543–551

Schmitt A, Bernhardt P, Nilsson O, Ahlman H, Kolby L, Maecke HR, Forssell-Aronsson E (2004) Radiation therapy of small cell lung cancer with 177Lu-DOTA-Tyr3-octreotate in an animal model. J Nucl Med 45(9):1542–1548

Schmitt A, Bernhardt P, Nilsson O, Ahlman H, Kolby L, Forssell-Aronsson E (2005) Differences in biodistribution between 99 mTc-depreotide, 111In-DTPA-octreotide, and 177Lu-DOTA-Tyr3-octreotate in a small cell lung cancer animal model. Cancer Biother Radiopharm 20(2): 231–236

Schoffelen R, Sharkey RM, Goldenberg DM, Franssen G, McBride WJ, Rossi EA, Chang CH, Laverman P, Disselhorst JA, Eek A, van der Graaf WT, Oyen WJ, Boerman OC (2010) Pretargeted immuno-positron emission tomography imaging of carcinoembryonic antigen-expressing tumors with a bispecific antibody and a 68 Ga- and 18F-labeled hapten peptide in mice with human tumor xenografts. Mol Cancer Ther 9(4):1019–1027

Schottelius M, Berger S, Poethko T, Schwaiger M, Wester HJ (2008) Development of novel Ga-68- and F-18-labeled GnRH-I analogues with high GnRHR-targeting efficiency. Bioconj Chem 19(6):1256–1268

Schuhmacher J, Kaul S, Klivenyi G, Junkermann H, Magener A, Henze M, Doll J, Haberkorn U, Amelung F, Bastert G (2001a) Immunoscintigraphy with positron emission tomography: gallium-68 chelate imaging of breast cancer pretargeted with bispecific anti-MUC1/anti-Ga chelate antibodies. Cancer Res 61(9):3712–3717

Schuhmacher J, Klivenyi G, Kaul S, Henze M, Matys R, Hauser H, Clorius J (2001b) Pretargeting of human mammary carcinoma xenografts with bispecific anti-MUC1/anti-Ga chelate antibodies and immunoscintigraphy with PET. Nucl Med Biol 28(7):821–828

Schuhmacher J, Zhang H, Doll J, Macke HR, Matys R, Hauser H, Henze M, Haberkorn U, Eisenhut M (2005) GRP receptor-targeted PET of a rat pancreas carcinoma xenograft in nude mice with a 68 Ga-labeled bombesin(6–14) analog. J Nucl Med 46(4):691–699

Schuster DP (1998) The evaluation of lung function with PET. Semin Nucl Med 28(4):341–351

Schuster DP, Kaplan JD, Gauvain K, Welch MJ, Markham J (1995) Measurement of regional pulmonary blood-flow with PET. J Nucl Med 36(3):371–377

Schuster DP, Stark T, Stephenson J, Royal H (2002) Detecting lung injury in patients with pulmonary edema. Intensive Care Med 28(9):1246–1253

Sharkey RM, Cardillo TM, Rossi EA, Chang CH, Karacay H, McBride WJ, Hansen HJ, Horak ID, Goldenberg DM (2005) Signal amplification in molecular imaging by pretargeting a multivalent, bispecific antibody. Nat Med 11(11):1250–1255

Sharkey RM, Karacay H, Litwin S, Rossi EA, McBride WJ, Chang CH, Goldenberg DM (2008) Improved therapeutic results by pretargeted radioimmunotherapy of non-Hodgkin's lymphoma with a new recombinant, trivalent, anti-CD20, bispecific antibody. Cancer Res 68(13):5282–5290

Sharkey RM, Rossi EA, McBride WJ, Chang CH, Goldenberg DM (2010a) Recombinant bispecific monoclonal antibodies prepared by the dock-and-lock strategy for pretargeted radioimmunotherapy. Semin Nucl Med 40(3):190–203

Sharkey RM, Rossi EA, Chang CH, Goldenberg DM (2010b) Improved cancer therapy and molecular imaging with multivalent, multispecific antibodies. Cancer Biother Radiopharm 25(1):1–12

Sharma V, Prior JL, Belinsky MG, Kruh GD, Piwnica-Worms D (2005) Characterization of a 67 Ga/68 Ga radiopharmaceutical for SPECT and PET of MDR1 P-glycoprotein transport

activity in vivo: validation in multidrug-resistant tumors and at the blood-brain barrier. J Nucl Med 46(2):354–364
Shetty D, Jeong JM, Ju CH, Lee YS, Jeong SY, Choi JY, Yang BY, Lee DS, Chung JK, Lee MC (2010a) Synthesis of novel 68 Ga-labeled amino acid derivatives for positron emission tomography of cancer cells. Nucl Med Biol 37(8):893–902
Shetty D, Jeong JM, Ju CH, Kim YJ, Lee JY, Lee YS, Lee DS, Chung JK, Lee MC (2010b) Synthesis and evaluation of macrocyclic amino acid derivatives for tumor imaging by gallium-68 positron emission tomography. Bioorg Med Chem 18(21):7338–7347
Silvola J, Autio A, Luoto P, Jalkanen S, Roivainen A (2010) Preliminary evaluation of novel 68 Ga-DOTAVAP-PEG-P2 peptide targeting vascular adhesion protein-1. Clin Physiol Funct Imaging 30(1):75–78
Smith-Jones PM, Stolz B, Burns C, Albert R, Reist HW, Fridrich R, Mäcke HM (1994) Gallium-67/gallium-68-[DFO]-octreotide- a potential radiopharmaceutical for PET imaging of somatostatin receptor-positive tumors: synthesis and radiolabeling in vitro and preliminary in vivo studies. J Nucl Med 35(2):317–325
Smith-Jones PM, Solit DB, Akhurst T, Afroze F, Rosen N, Larson SM (2004) Imaging the pharmacodynamics of HER2 degradation in response to Hsp90 inhibitors. Nat Biotechnol 22(6):701–706
Smith-Jones PM, Solit D, Afroze F, Rosen N, Larson SM (2006) Early tumor response to Hsp90 therapy using HER2 PET: comparison with 18F-FDG PET. J Nucl Med 47(5):793–796
Somasundaram C, Matzku S, Schuhmacher J, Zöller M (1993) Development of a bispecific monoclonal antibody against a gallium-67 chelate and the human melanoma-associated antigen p97 for potential use in pretargeted immunoscintigraphy. Cancer Immunol Immunother 36(5):337–345
Srirajaskanthan R, Kayani I, Quigley AM, Soh J, Caplin ME, Bomanji J (2010) The Role of 68 Ga-DOTATATE PET in patients with neuroendocrine tumors and negative or equivocal findings on 111In-DTPA-octreotide scintigraphy. J Nucl Med 51(6):875–882
Steinling M, Baron JC, Maziere B, Lasjaunias P, Loc'h C, Cabanis EA, Guillon B (1985) Tomographic measurement of cerebral blood flow by the ^{68}Ga-labelled-microsphere and continuous-$C^{15}O_2$-inhalation methods. Eur J Nucl Med Mol Imaging 11(1):29–32
Tan EH, Goh SW (2010) Exploring new frontiers in molecular imaging: emergence of Ga PET/CT. World J Radiol 2(2):55–67
Tavitian B (2005) Oligonucleotides as radiopharmaceuticals. Ernst Schering Res Found Workshop 49:1–34
Thakur ML (1995) Radiolabelled peptides: now and the future. Nucl Med Commun 16(9):724–732
Theeraladanon C, Takahashi N, Shiina M, Hamada K, Takada Y, Endo H, Tateishi U, Oka T, Ogata K, Inoue T (2010) Rational approach to the synthesis, evaluation, and 68 Ga labeling of a novel 4-anilinoquinoline epidermal growth factor receptor inhibitor as a new imaging agent that selectively targets the epidermal growth factor receptor tyrosine kinase. Cancer Biother Radiopharm 25(4):479–485
Thews O, Dillenburg W, Fellner M, Buchholz HG, Bausbacher N, Schreckenberger M, Rosch F (2010) Activation of P-glycoprotein (Pgp)-mediated drug efflux by extracellular acidosis: in vivo imaging with Ga-68-labelled PET tracer. Eur J Nucl Med Mol Imaging 37(10):1935–1942
Toegel S, Wadsak W, Mien LK, Viernstein H, Kluger R, Eidherr H, Haeusler D, Kletter K, Dudczak R, Mitterhauser M (2008) Preparation and pre-vivo evaluation of no-carrier-added, carrier-added and cross-complexed Ga-68-EDTMP formulations. Eur J Pharm Biopharm 68(2):406–412
Tofilon PJ, Saxman S, Coleman CN (2003) Molecular targets for radiation therapy: bringing preclinical data into clinical trials. Clin Cancer Res 9(10 Pt 1):3518–3520
Tolmachev V (1800) Stone-Elander S (2010) Radiolabelled proteins for positron emission tomography: pros and cons of labelling methods. Biochim Biophys Acta 5:487–510
Tolmachev V, Orlova A (2009) Update on affibody molecules for in vivo imaging of targets for cancer therapy. Minerva Biotecnologica 21(1):21–30

Tolmachev V, Friedman M, Sandstrom M, Eriksson TLJ, Rosik D, Hodik M, Stahl S, Frejd FY, Orlova A (2009) Affibody molecules for epidermal growth factor receptor targeting in vivo: aspects of dimerization and labeling chemistry. J Nucl Med 50(2):274–283

Tolmachev V, Velikyan I, Sandstrom M, Orlova A (2010) A HER2-binding Affibody molecule labelled with 68 Ga for PET imaging: direct in vivo comparison with the 111In-labelled analogue. Eur J Nucl Med Mol Imaging 37(7):1356–1367

Traub-Weidinger T, Von Guggenberg E, Dobrozemsky G, Kendler D, Eisterer W, Bale R, Putzer D, Gabriel M, Virgolini I (2010) Preliminary experience with Ga-68-DOTA-lanreotide positron emission tomography. Q J Nucl Med Mol Imaging 54(1):52–60

Tsang BW, Mathias CJ, Green MA (1993) A gallium-68 radiopharmaceutical that is retained in myocardium: $^{68}Ga[(4,6\text{-}MeO_2sal)_2BAPEN]^+$. J Nucl Med 34(7):1127–1131

Ujula T, Salomaki S, Virsu P, Lankinen P, Makinen TJ, Autio A, Yegutkin GG, Knuuti J, Jalkanen S, Roivainen A (2009) Synthesis, Ga-68 labeling and preliminary evaluation of DOTA peptide binding vascular adhesion protein-1: a potential PET imaging agent for diagnosing osteomyelitis. Nucl Med Biol 36(6):631–641

Van Riet J, Rattat D, Verbruggen A, Mortelmans L, Mottaghy FM (2009) Ga-68 DOTATOC PET/CT changed the therapeutic course of a patient with the sudden onset of vision problems. Clin Nucl Med 34(1):27–28

Velikyan I (2005) Synthesis, characterization and application of ^{68}Ga-Labelled Macromolecules http://urn.kb.se/resolve?urn=urn:nbn:se:uu:diva-5876. In: Doctoral Thesis from the Faculty of Sciences and Technology, Uppsala University, Swedened

Velikyan I (2011) Positron emitting [^{68}Ga]Ga-based imaging agents: chemistry and diversity. Med Chem 7:338–372

Velikyan I, Långström B (2004) Microwave method for preparing radiolabelled gallium complexes. WO/2004/089425

Velikyan I, Långström B (2006) ^{68}Ga-Labeling of a free and macromolecule conjugated macrocyclic chelator at room temperature. WO/2008/026051

Velikyan I, Beyer GJ, Langstrom B (2004a) Microwave-supported preparation of ^{68}Ga-bioconjugates with high specific radioactivity. Bioconj Chem 15(3):554–560

Velikyan I, Lendvai G, Valila M, Roivainen A, Yngve U, Bergstrom M, Langstrom B (2004b) Microwave accelerated ^{68}Ga-labelling of oligonucleotides. J Labelled Comp Radiopharm 47(1):79–89

Velikyan I, Långström B, Beyer G (2004) Method of obtaining gallium-68 and use thereof and device for carrying out said method. WO/2004/089517 A1, October 21

Velikyan I, Sundberg AL, Lindhe O, Hoglund AU, Eriksson O, Werner E, Carlsson J, Bergstrom M, Langstrom B, Tolmachev V (2005) Preparation and evaluation of (68)Ga-DOTA-hEGF for visualization of EGFR expression in malignant tumors. J Nucl Med 46(11):1881–1888

Velikyan I, Liljegren Sundberg Å, Långström B, Tolmachev V (2006) [^{68}Ga] DOTA hEGF for non-invasive measurement of EGFR expression in tumors using PET. WO/2006/090232

Velikyan I, Beyer GJ, Bergstrom-Pettermann E, Johansen P, Bergstrom M, Langstrom B (2008a) The importance of high specific radioactivity in the performance of (68)Ga-labeled peptide. Nucl Med Biol 35(5):529–536

Velikyan I, Maecke H, Langstrom B (2008b) Convenient preparation of 68 Ga-based PET-radiopharmaceuticals at room temperature. Bioconjug Chem 19(2):569–573

Velikyan I, Sundin A, Eriksson B, Lundqvist H, Sorensen J, Bergstrom M, Langstrom B (2010) In vivo binding of [68 Ga]-DOTATOC to somatostatin receptors in neuroendocrine tumours–impact of peptide mass. Nucl Med Biol 37(3):265–275

Versari A, Camellini L, Carlinfante G, Frasoldati A, Nicoli F, Grassi E, Gallo C, Giunta FP, Fraternali A, Salvo D, Asti M, Azzolini F, Iori V, Sassatelli R (2010) Ga-68 DOTATOC PET, endoscopic ultrasonography, and multidetector CT in the diagnosis of duodenopancreatic neuroendocrine tumors: a single-centre retrospective study. Clin Nucl Med 35(5):321–328

Virgolini I, Ambrosini V, Bomanji JB, Baum RP, Fanti S, Gabriel M, Papathanasiou ND, Pepe G, Oyen W, De Cristoforo C, Chiti A (2010) Procedure guidelines for PET/CT tumour imaging with 68 Ga-DOTA-conjugated peptides: 68 Ga-DOTA-TOC, 68 Ga-DOTA-NOC, 68 Ga-DOTA-TATE. Eur J Nucl Med Mol Imaging 37(10):2004–2010

Vosjan MJ, Perk LR, Roovers RC, Visser GW, Stigter-van Walsum M, van Bergen En Henegouwen PM, van Dongen GA (2011) Facile labelling of an anti-epidermal growth factor receptor nanobody with (68)Ga via a novel bifunctional desferal chelate for immuno-PET. Eur J Nucl Med Mol Imaging

Wagner SJ, Welch MJ (1979) Gallium-68 labeling of albumin and albumin microspheres. J Nucl Med 20(5):428–433

Walker RA, Dearing SJ (1999) Expression of epidermal growth factor receptor mRNA and protein in primary breast carcinomas. Breast Cancer Res Treat 53(2):167–176

Watine J, Miedouge M, Friedberg B (2001) Carcinoembryonic antigen as an independent prognostic factor of recurrence and survival in patients resected for colorectal liver metastases: a systematic review. Dis Colon Rectum 44(12):1791–1799

Wei L, Miao Y, Gallazzi F, Quinn TP, Welch MJ, Vavere AL, Lewis JS (2007) Gallium-68-labeled DOTA-rhenium-cyclized alpha-melanocyte-stimulating hormone analog for imaging of malignant melanoma. Nucl Med Biol 34(8):945–953

Welch MJ, Thakur ML, Coleman RE, Patel M, Siegel BA, Ter-Pogossian MM (1977) Gallium-68 labeled red cells and platelets new agents for positron tomography. J Nucl Med 18(6):558–562

Wild D, Schmitt JS, Ginj M, Macke HR, Bernard BF, Krenning E, De Jong M, Wenger S, Reubi JC (2003) DOTA-NOC, a high-affinity ligand of somatostatin receptor subtypes 2, 3 and 5 for labelling with various radiometals. Eur J Nucl Med Mol Imaging 30(10):1338–1347

Wild D, Macke HR, Waser B, Reubi JC, Ginj M, Rasch H, Muller-Brand J, Hofmann M (2005) 68 Ga-DOTANOC: a first compound for PET imaging with high affinity for somatostatin receptor subtypes 2 and 5. Eur J Nucl Med Mol Imaging 32(6):724

Wild D, Wicki A, Mansi R, Behe M, Keil B, Bernhardt P, Christofori G, Ell PJ, Macke HR (2010) Exendin-4-based radiopharmaceuticals for glucagonlike peptide-1 receptor PET/CT and SPECT/CT. J Nucl Med 51(7):1059–1067

Win Z, Al-Nahhas A, Towey D, Todd JF, Rubello D, Lewington V, Gishen P (2007) 68 Ga-DOTATATE PET in neuroectodermal tumours: first experience. Nucl Med Commun 28(5):359–363

Witton CJ, Reeves JR, Going JJ, Cooke TG, Bartlett JM (2003) Expression of the HER1-4 family of receptor tyrosine kinases in breast cancer. J Pathol 200(3):290–297

Wunderlich G, Schiller E, Bergmann R, Pietzsch H-J (2010) Comparison of the stability of Y-90-, Lu-177- and Ga-68- labeled human serum albumin microspheres (DOTA-HSAM). Nucl Med Biol 37(8):861–867

Yang DJ, Kim EE (2005) Tracer development and hybrid imaging. Eur J Nucl Med Mol Imaging 32(9):1001–1002

Yang DJ, Azhdarinia A, Kim EE (2005) Tumor Specific Imaging Using Tc-99 m and Ga-68 labeled radiopharmaceuticals. Curr Med Imaging Rev 1(1):25–34

Yang DJ, Kim EE, Inoue T (2006) Targeted molecular imaging in oncology. Ann Nucl Med 20(1):1–11

Yang BY, Jeong JM, Kim YJ, Choi JY, Lee YS, Lee DS, Chung JK, Lee MC (2010) Formulation of 68 Ga BAPEN kit for myocardial positron emission tomography imaging and biodistribution study. Nucl Med Biol 37(2):149–155

Yano Y, Budinger TF, Ebbe SN, Mathis CA, Singh M, Brennan KM, Moyer BR (1985) Gallium-68 lipophilic complexes for labeling platelets. J Nucl Med 26(12):1429–1437

Yarden Y, Sliwkowski MX (2001) Untangling the ErbB signalling network. Natl Rev Mol Cell Biol 2(2):127–137

Yvert JP, Maziere B, Verhas M, Comar D (1979) Simple, fast preparation of gallium-68-labeled human-serum albumin microspheres. Eur J Nucl Med 4(2):95–99

Zhang Z, Lyster DM, Webb GA, Orvig C (1992) Potential 67 Ga radiopharmaceuticals for myocardial imaging: tris(1-aryl-3-hydroxy-2-methyl-4-pyridinonato)gallium(III) complexes. Int J Rad Appl Instrum B 19(3):327–335

Zhang HW, Schuhmacher J, Waser B, Wild D, Eisenhut M, Reubi JC, Maecke HR (2007) DOTA-PESIN, a DOTA-conjugated bombesin derivative designed for the imaging and targeted radionuclide treatment of bombesin receptor-positive tumours. Eur J Nucl Med Mol Imaging 34(8):1198–1208

Zhang H, Moroz MA, Serganova I, Ku T, Huang R, Vider J, Maecke HR, Larson SM, Blasberg R, Smith-Jones PM (2010) Imaging expression of the human somatostatin receptor subtype-2 reporter gene with 68 Ga-DOTATOC. J Nucl Med: jnumed.110.079004

Zhernosekov KP, Filosofov DV, Baum RP, Aschoff P, Bihl H, Razbash AA, Jahn M, Jennewein M, Rosch F (2007) Processing of generator-produced 68 Ga for medical application. J Nucl Med 48(10):1741–1748

Nanoparticles and Phage Display Selected Peptides for Imaging and Therapy of Cancer

Cathy S. Cutler, Nripen Chanda, Ravi Shukla, Nebiat Sisay, Melchor Cantorias, Ajit Zambre, Mark McLaughlin, James Kelsey, Anandhi Upenandran, Dave Robertson, Susan Deutscher, Raghuraman Kannan and Kattesh Katti

Abstract

Molecular imaging probes are a special class of pharmaceuticals that target specific biochemical signatures associated with disease and allow for noninvasive imaging on the molecular level. Because changes in biochemistry occur before diseases reach an advanced stage, molecular imaging probes make it possible to locate and stage disease, track the effectiveness of drugs, treat disease, monitor response, and select patients to allow for more personalized diagnosis and treatment of disease. Targeting agents radiolabeled with positron emitters are of interest due to their ability to quantitatively measure biodistribution and receptor expression to allow for optimal dose determinations. ^{68}Ga is a positron emitter, which allows for quantitative imaging through positron emission chromatography (PET). The availability of ^{68}Ga from a generator and its ability to form stable complexes with a variety of chelates hold promise for expanding PET utilization to facilities unable to afford their own cyclotron. Nanoparticles conjugated with various proteins and peptides derived from phage display that can be selectively targeted are being developed and evaluated for guided imaging and therapy. Herein we highlight some initial efforts in combining the enhanced selectivity of nanoparticles and peptides with ^{68}Ga for use as molecular imaging probes.

C. S. Cutler (✉) · N. Chanda · R. Shukla · N. Sisay · M. Cantorias · A. Zambre · M. McLaughlin · J. Kelsey · A. Upenandran · D. Robertson · S. Deutscher · R. Kannan · K. Katti
Research Reactor Center, University of Missouri,
1513 Research Park Drive, Columbia, MO 65211-3400, USA
e-mail: cutlerc@missouri.edu

R. P. Baum and F. Rösch (eds.), *Theranostics, Gallium-68, and Other Radionuclides*,
Recent Results in Cancer Research 194, DOI: 10.1007/978-3-642-27994-2_8,

Contents

1 Introduction

Molecular imaging has shown its potential to noninvasively image both normal and abnormal biochemical pathways in individual patients. Molecular targets such as hypoxia, angiogenesis, receptor expression, and metabolism are just a few of the biochemical pathways that are of interest to evaluate as end-points in clinical trials. Preclinical imaging is becoming a key translational tool for proof of mechanism and concept studies. These combined with the new exploratory IND (eIND) and microdosing allow for determination of lead compounds in humans, and the development of theranostics for dual imaging and therapy holds promise for accelerated drug development and translation into the clinic.

1.1 Biomarkers

First, a clinical end-point is recognized. Then, a target is identified that represents a biological pathway that is capable of accurately assessing the clinical end-point. A probe or biomarker is then developed to interrogate the target. In addition to measuring function noninvasively, molecular imaging can provide quantified measurements of physiological parameters. Agents used for quantitative imaging can be categorized into four main groups: metabolic agents to measure in vivo pathways, trapped agents such as ^{18}F-labeled fluorodeoxyglucose (FDG) that is trapped in the first step of the glycolytic metabolism, perfusion agents to measure blood flow, and receptor-ligand agents to assess receptor expression. Imaging is increasingly being used in drug development: (a) to assess a drug's behavior in vivo, (b) to assess if the drug is reaching the target site, (c) to assess changes in function and structure that may occur as a consequence of treatment, and (d) to determine which patients will receive the most benefit as well as those who should be excluded due to toxicity. The aim is to evaluate the genetic and molecular profile of a patient's disease to determine which agents will result in the most

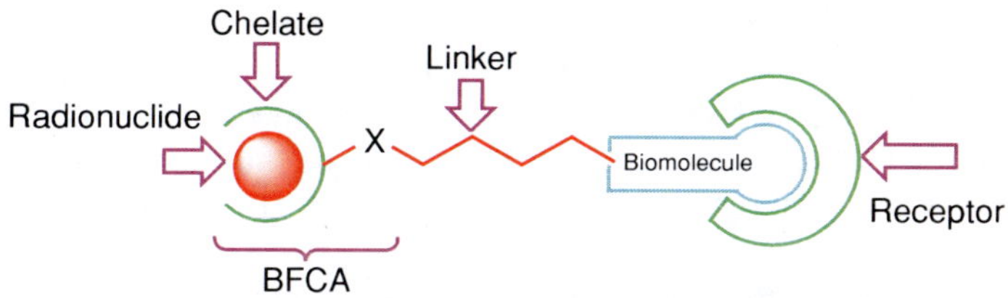

Fig. 1 Schematic illustrating traditional approach compared with receptor targeting

effective treatment for that patient with minimal toxicity. Probes or imaging agents used in drug development can be divided into four main utility types: target identification, proof of mechanism, proof of efficacy, and surrogate markers. Each provides different information and must be chosen and used appropriately to address the clinical question. Imaging markers for target identification are used to detect the presence of the target, quantitate the level of expression, and determine if they can be utilized as specific targets for therapeutic delivery. A biomarker for proof of mechanism assesses the modulation of the target by the therapeutic. Efficacy markers monitor the drug's action. Finally, surrogate markers are utilized when probe concentration is predictive of the effect of the therapeutic drug on clinical outcome. Use of such agents can dramatically improve treatment and are critical in developing treatments tailored to individual patients to deliver optimal dose.

A variety of platforms have been used to design imaging agents from radiolabeling small molecules, tracers that mimic the in vivo behavior of the natural substance, to the use of much more complex molecules such as antibodies and nanoparticles. The fundamental challenge for imaging is to have a high signal in the organ or function of interest, while maintaining a low signal in neighboring normal tissue, resulting in high image contrast. Therapy is far more stringent and requires delivering toxic doses selectively to diseased or cancer cells while sparing all normal tissues. Conventional agents have resulted in low therapeutic indices due to suboptimal biodistribution where only a minute portion of the intravenously administered drug reaches the target but large doses are delivered to normal tissues. Nanoparticles are being developed as an alternative due to their size and ability to circumvent some of the hurdles encountered with traditional agents. Nanoparticles have unique properties that can be optimized to allow for higher penetration and retention in tumor cells.

Traditional agents as shown in Fig. 1 consist of a biomolecule conjugated to a radiolabeled bifunctional chelator through a linker. The biomolecule acts as the guiding system to direct the radiolabel, the bifunctional chelator serves to stably complex the radioisotope, normally a metal, and the linker serves not only for stable conjugation but also as a pharmacodynamic modifier. Changes to the linker can be made to tune the uptake and clearance of the agent, such as increasing the hydrophobicity if the overall molecule proves to be too hydrophilic and clears too quickly. The length of the linker has been shown to enhance or decrease receptor uptake, such as being too short for the bulky chelator, interfering with binding, or too long, causing the peptide to fold around the linker and being unrecognized. Often the linker must be modified to meet the needs of each metal chelator to maximize uptake and clearance. Some linkers are designed to be cleavable to enhance uptake at the tumor site and reduce uptake in normal organs such as the kidneys.

A disadvantage of the conventional bifunctional chelating system is that only one radioactive molecule per targeting moiety at most is delivered. This is highly dependent on the specific activity of the radioisotope and on any metal contaminants, as many chelators are not selective but will bind to a number of common metals. A low specific activity and/or high presence of unwanted metal impurities can result in low labeling yields for the desired radioisotope and saturation of the receptor sites if they are present in low quantities. This has been recently demonstrated by Asti et al. (2010), who performed a systematic study evaluating the effect of specific activity and incorporation of a variety of metals on a typical DOTATOC clinical formulation.

2 Nanoparticles

Radioisotopes of gold and other coinage metals have nuclear properties that make them ideal for use in imaging and therapeutic applications. However, their biologically active redox chemistry and lack of stable chelating agents have to-date limited their utilization in vivo. They have experienced some use in the area of brachytherapy with the bare metal being encapsulated, but otherwise have been used sparingly, the major concern being the inherent toxicities observed for the free metals in vivo. In order to take advantage of their nuclear properties, we have been seeking alternative means of delivering radioisotopes more efficaciously. A novel approach is the development of metal nanoparticles that can be derivatized on their surface, allowing for optimization of biodistribution in vivo.

Once a metal nanoparticle is fabricated, its in vivo properties can be evaluated and altered by varying such properties as its size, charge, hydrodynamic size, organic surface layer, and shape. These can be optimized to enable more favorable uptake and clearance in vivo. Furthermore, due to their high surface area, they can be conjugated with a plethora of agents that can be used for selective targeting such as peptides and small molecules or agents either to enhance retention in the blood stream or to enhance clearance. These properties can be optimized through in vivo studies to develop lead compounds for imaging and therapy. A major advantage of nanoparticles over the commonly used bifunctional chelator approach is that the nanoparticle platform allows for much higher payload delivery, as more than one radioisotope can be incorporated into the nanoparticle and can result in a much higher dose delivery even with a low specific activity radionuclide.

Table 1 Properties of gold radioisotopes

Radionuclide	Half-life	Max β-energy (MeV)	Max γ-energy (keV)
Au-198	2.7 days	0.96 (99%), $E_{av} = 0.315$	411
Au-199	3.2 days	0.46, $E_{av} = 0.14$	158

2.1 Gold Radioisotope Properties

Radioisotopes of gold (Au) as shown in Table 1 have attractive nuclear properties that make them ideal for imaging and therapy. Two radioisotopes of gold stand out; one of which is ^{198}Au, which has a moderate-energy beta particle (0.96 keV β^- max), making it a good candidate for therapy, and more than 90% emission of a 412-keV gamma emission that allows for in vivo tracking and dosimetry calculation. These properties led to its initial use as a brachytherapy agent for prostate cancer. A second radioisotope, ^{199}Au, has a low-energy beta maximum (0.46 MeV) and emits a 158-keV gamma with 36% yield that is easily detected by SPECT cameras. Additionally, ^{199}Au can be produced carrier free by neutron irradiation of ^{198}Pt to produce ^{199}Pt that decays in 3.2 min to ^{199}Au.

Gold nanoparticles (AuNPs) have been around for quite some time, but their harsh production methods with toxic chemicals have prevented them from being attached easily to biomolecules for evaluation in vivo. A majority of metal nanoparticles are made with toxic chemicals that are not conducive for in vivo applications. Early on we evaluated safe, green methods to produce gold nanoparticles in aqueous solutions that would be amenable to use in biomolecular applications.

2.2 Gum Arabic Gold Nanoparticles

Our first synthesis consisted of using THPAL, a trimeric phosphino alanine, to reduce gold salts in water containing green organics, which would coat the surface of the gold nanoparticles and form 12–15 nm-sized gold nanoparticles with hydrodynamic diameter of 60–85 nm (Kannan et al. 2006). These methods have been shown to be robust and nontoxic in the nonradioactive form. The methods have been altered to allow for formation of both ^{198}Au and ^{199}Au nanoparticles and also have been shown amenable to formation with other coin metals such as palladium and silver. We have developed a library of such conjugates, three of which have been evaluated in induced tumor models and two are being translated into large animals for imaging and treatment of prostate cancer.

Gum arabic-coated gold nanoparticles (GA-^{198}AuNPs) were the first and most studied to date (Chanda et al. 2010). The reaction consists of heating water containing gum arabic, adding gold either as the $NaAuCl_4$ salt or the $H^{198}AuCl_4$ acid along with the THPAL, heating this solution briefly, which converts from a

Table 2 Comparison of uptake in selected tissues for GA-^{198}AuNP and EGCg-^{198}AuNP

Tissue	GA-^{198}AuNP	EGCg-^{198}AuNP
Liver	0.91 ± 0.26% ID	2.5 ± 1.7% ID
Kidney	0.13 ± 0.01% ID	Background
Small intestines	0.09 ± 0.00% ID	Background
Tumor	19.9 ± 4.2% ID	37.4 ± 1.8% ID
Carcass	18.5 ± 4.6% ID	17.8 ± 6.1% ID

pale-yellow solution to a red-burgundy one. Quality control has shown that this method results in 99% conversion of the radioactive gold to the nanoparticle form, which then can be brought to neutral pH and remains stable in the radioactive form for over 2 weeks. This formulation was initially evaluated for therapeutic efficacy in SCID mice bearing induced human prostate tumors. Different modes of injection were tried, with intratumoral injection resulting in the highest uptake and retention. These studies prompted us to evaluate their efficacy in tumor stabilization in the same tumor models. Tumors received a 70 Gy dose by administering 405 μCi. An overall 82% reduction in tumor volume was noted between the mice receiving GA ^{198}AuNP compared with controls receiving saline injections. Biodistributions at the end showed a reduction of gold nanoparticles in the tumor from 70% at 24 h to 19.9 ± 4.2% ID at 30 days post injection. Clearance was predominantly through the urinary track, and minimum uptake was observed in other organs as can be seen in Table 2. Based on these results, these nanoparticles are being evaluated for their therapeutic efficacy in canines with spontaneous prostate cancer. Prostate cancer in dogs has been shown to mimic that observed in humans on the functional level as well as in metastatic rate and occurrence. Studies to date have shown that dogs treated with the nanoconstructs tolerate the treatment well and that the disease is stabilized.

2.3 Epigallocatechin-Gallate Gold Nanoparticles

Another formulation was a receptor targeted approach which was developed using the Food and Drug Administration (FDA)-approved photochemical epigallocatechin-gallate (EGCg) (Shukla et al. 2011). EGCg is a major phytochemical component of green tea and has been used extensively as a food supplement because of its strong antioxidant properties. This method proved much simpler for two reasons: the nanoparticles could be formed at room temperature, and EGCg not only achieved reduction of the gold but also served as a stabilizing agent, resulting in an EGCg-conjugated gold nanoparticle (EGCg-^{198}AuNPs) formulation in a few minutes at room temperature in water. Additionally EGCg targets the LAMININ receptor (Lam 67R) which is overexpressed on human prostate cancer cells (Tachibana et al. 2004). Lam 67R is a 67-kDa cell surface protein, first isolated as a non-integrin high-affinity laminin binding protein from murine cancer cells in 1983 by two independent research groups (Rao et al. 1983; Malinoff and Wicha 1983). EGCg has been known to bind to Lam 67R with excellent specificity and selectivity (Tachibana et al. 2004). The in vivo biodistribution of EGCg-^{198}AuNPs was evaluated in SCID mice bearing human prostate cancer tumors and was shown to have an initial higher retention and to clear with time. Based on these results, they were evaluated in therapy trials with SCID mice bearing human prostate cancer. Due to the higher initial uptake, only a third of the dose activity (136 versus 405 μCi for the gold nanoparticles formed with gum arabic) needed to be injected to give a 70 Gy dose. The EGCg-^{198}AuNPs were shown to be more stable over time, remaining in solution far longer than their gum arabic analogs, and results showed similar reduction of tumor volumes (80% compared with 82%) with higher clearance from normal tissues except for the liver and the tumor, as can be seen in Table 2. From the data it is clear that selective targeting of the EGCg to the Lam 67R receptor results in an overall higher uptake and retention in the prostate tumor cells than GA-^{198}AuNP-treated ones. Due to the similar results with a smaller dose, these nanoparticles will also be evaluated in canine patients with spontaneous prostate cancer.

2.4 Bombesin Gold Nanoparticles

In addition to glycoprotein- and phytochemical-conjugated gold nanoparticles, we have also evaluated selective targeting by conjugating the 14-amino-acid peptide bombesin to the gold nanoparticle surface (McLaughlin et al. 2011a; Chanda et al. 2010). Bombesin (BBN) targets the gastrin-releasing peptide (GRP) receptors that are upregulated in a variety of cancers, predominantly breast, prostate, pancreatic, and lung cancers (Smith et al. 2003). The hypothesis was that attaching BBN to gold nanoparticles would result in selective uptake in prostate cancer, particularly metastases. Different formulations of gold nanoparticles conjugated to BBN (AuNP-BBN) with varying ratios of BBN to gold nanoparticles of 1:1, 2:1, and 3:1 were prepared and evaluated for their target specificity. AuNP-BBN conjugates evaluated through receptor binding assays demonstrated that the 1:3 AuNP-BBN conjugate showed the highest affinity and uptake (Chanda et al. 2010). This conjugate (BBN^{198}AuNP) was evaluated in SCID mice bearing human prostate PC-3 cells and in a spontaneous model of prostate cancer, the TRAMP mouse. Although the initial studies in PC-3 hinted at selective uptake, more thorough evaluation in which the uptake was compared with ^{64}Cu-NOTA-8-Aoc-BBN(7-14)NH_2 showed only nonselective uptake. Starch gold nanoparticles (S^{198}AuNP) were used as starting material to conjugate the BBN peptide. S^{198}Au-NPs were conjugated to BBN by use of BBN 7-14 conjugated to thioctic acid. ^{64}Cu-NOTA-8-Aoc-BBN(7-14)NH_2 was prepared as previously described (Prasanphanich et al. 2007). We used SCID mice bearing a flank model of human prostate cancer derived from a subcutaneous implant of PC-3 cells for pharmacokinetic studies. ^{64}Cu-NOTA-8-Aoc-BBN(7-14)NH_2 injected intravenously (i.v.) exhibited high uptake in the pancreas and tumor, similar to what has been previously reported; this uptake was reduced by pretreatment with cold BBN. The intraperitoneal (i.p.) route of administration of the agent showed similar accumulation in tissues except the tumor, which was lower and was not blocked by the cold BBN. However, other receptor-rich tissues such as the pancreas showed reduced uptake ($p \leq 0.05$). GA^{198}Au-NP when injected i.p. showed no tumor uptake and no differences when injected with the blocking dose of BBN. Starch ^{198}Au-NP showed no tumor uptake and no reduction in receptor-rich tissues when injected with cold BBN. The BBN-conjugated starch ^{198}Au-NP showed similar results with no uptake observed in the tumor and no significant difference in uptake in the receptor-rich pancreas.

In vitro receptor binding studies have shown a high affinity of BBN ^{198}Au-NP conjugates for the GRP receptor in PC-3 cells (Chanda et al. 2010). Studies in spontaneous models of prostate cancer have shown an accumulation of BBN^{198}Au-NP into tumor sites. Previously we reported that starch formulated BBN^{198}Au-NP conjugated showed selective targeted uptake in a tumor model of human prostate cancer (Chanda et al. 2010). To further test this hypothesis, we performed this more rigorous evaluation in the same model with the addition of cold BBN blocking studies and compared it with the high-affinity GRP receptor agent ^{64}Cu-NOTA-8-Aoc-BBN(7-14)NH_2. These studies indicate that the uptake observed in the pancreas is not due to receptor-mediated localization. Further, the i.p. route of administration appears to result in high nonselective uptake in the pancreas and other organs in the abdomen. Previous studies with BBN in our group have indicated that addition of linkers between the BBN peptide and the ^{198}Au-NPs may facilitate recognition of the receptor and mediate selective localization in the tumor. Future studies are planned to synthesize BBN^{198}Au-NP conjugated to BBN with different-sized linkers with the objective of increased receptor recognition. This result appears to differ from that observed in the TRAMP model, which demonstrated selective uptake in prostate tumor cells. Due to the less than optimal biodistribution, studies are ongoing to develop further analogs of these BBN-containing molecules with linkers that may aid in selective uptake of the agents.

2.5 DTDTPA Gold Nanoparticles for Molecular Imaging

We have investigated conjugation of ligands to gold nanoparticles to incorporate other metals to expand imaging beyond SPECT to PET/CT, MRI, and combinations. PET is of interest due to its increased sensitivity and resolution over SPECT and that it allows for quantitative imaging. Magnetic resonance imaging is growing in interest owing to its enhanced resolution over other imaging techniques, and it can be used in hybrid imaging with PET and SPECT. MRI is of great interest due to its ability to perform parametric imaging. We evaluated a formation of gold nanoparticles containing a dithiolated diethylene triamine pentaacetic acid ligand (DTDTPA). DTPA has been used to bind a variety of metals including gadolinium (Gd) for MRI imaging, indium (In) for SPECT imaging, and gallium (Ga) for SPECT with ^{67}Ga and PET with ^{68}Ga. As shown in Figs. 2–4, the DTDTPA-AuNPs were formed by a simple reduction of the gold salt in the presence of the DTDDTPA ligand (Debuttiere et al. 2006). These conjugates were easily labeled with ^{64}Cu at room temperature in 0.4 M ammonium acetate buffer at pH 4. Radio-TLC confirmed a 95% radiolabeling yield. Stability studies in rat serum indicated no aggregation over 4 days and no change in the plasmon resonance. DTDTPA-AuNPs were also easily labeled with ^{68}Ga. ^{68}Ga is a positron emitter with half-life of 68 min, and is an ideal isotope for PET imaging. It can be obtained for chemical synthesis via a ^{68}Ge/^{68}Ga generator. ^{68}Ga radiolabeling was performed at room temperature in 0.1 M ammonium acetate solution at pH 4.5 with vortexing. Radiolabeling yields of 97% were achieved, and the complex remained 95% intact at room temperature for over 6 h. Evaluation of pharmacokinetics of the ^{68}Ga and ^{64}Cu DTDTPA-AuNPs in normal mice is ongoing.

2.6 Alpha-Emitting Sequestering Nanoparticles

Recently, we have investigated nanoparticles with the alpha emitter ^{225}Ac, which hold much promise for targeted alpha therapies (McLaughlin et al. 2011b). The nuclear decay of ^{225}Ac (10-day half-life with emission of four alpha particles) holds the potential to become an ideal radiotherapy system. The 10 day half-life provides sufficient time for complex syntheses and attachment to targeting biomolecules, while the rapid decay and high LET of the daughters' alpha emissions ensures that the therapeutic payload is delivered in the vicinity of the target tissue. Despite the clear benefits of delivering multiple alpha particles from the decay of ^{225}Ac directly to tumor sites, the difficulty of sequestering the α-emitting daughters in traditional bifunctional-conjugated targeting modalities leads to release of the daughters and nonspecific uptake in nontarget organs. This nontarget dose negates the advantages of targeted alpha therapy, namely high tumor dose with minimal collateral damage to healthy tissue. To harness the potential of multiple α particles from ^{225}Ac, we have designed gold-coated lanthanum gadolinium phosphate nanoparticles (NPs) for the purpose of both retaining ^{225}Ac and its daughters and providing a versatile platform for attaching targeting agents for various tumor types within the body.

In order to retain ^{225}Ac and its daughters, we embedded ^{225}Ac into a binary mixture of $LaGdPO_4$ nanoparticles via hydrolysis of sodium tripolyphosphate in the presence of La^{3+} and Gd^{3+} ions. Next, citrate reduction of gold creates a shell of Au on the surface of the $LaGdPO_4$ particles. Magnetic $LaGdPO_4$-AuNPs are then separated from nonmagnetic AuNPs using a 0.5-T NdFeB magnet.

TEM analysis of these $LaGdPO_4$-AuNPs particles showed monodisperse particles with average diameters of 4–5 nm. Radiochemical analysis indicated that

$LaGdPO_4$-AuNPs without additional layers sequestered 60.2 ± 3.0% of the first decay daughter of ^{225}Ac, ^{221}Fr. Subsequent epitaxial growth with additional $LnPO_4$ layers increased daughter retention. The addition of two shells of $LaGdPO_4$ and one shell of Au increased ^{221}Fr retention to 69.2 ± 1.7%, while the addition of four shells of $GdPO_4$ and one shell of Au increased retention to 92 ± 1.0%. Retention of the first decay daughter is essential to minimize normal tissue toxicity. Daughter sequestration in these first-generation particles was high, but retention was improved by additional layers of Au and/or $LnPO_4$. Similar to the other AuNPs described above, we can attach biomolecules such as BBN or antibodies and plan to evaluate this in the future. The properties of low toxicity and favorable biodistribution make the $LaGdPO_4$-AuNP system a promising platform for targeted alpha therapy with ^{225}Ac.

3 Phage Display

Paul Ehrlich was the first to develop the concept of selective targeting of disease cells to minimize toxic side-effects. Ehrlich reasoned that, if a compound could be made that selectively targeted a diseased cell, then a toxin could be attached to that targeting moiety and delivered along with the agent of selectivity to the diseased cell. Hence, a "magic bullet" would be created that killed only the diseased cells. Antibodies, due to their high affinity, have been evaluated extensively for selective targeting and imaging of cancer. A few have actually been successfully translated into the clinic, such as ^{90}Y-labeled Zevalin and ^{131}I-labeled Bexxar for CD20-targeted radiolabeled monoclonal antibodies for treatment of follicular non-Hodgkin's lymphoma. However, antibodies suffer from long residence times in the blood, slow tumor penetration, and clearance rates through the hepatobiliary system and in some patients result in adverse hematological effects and resistance problems (Klatersky 2006; Goldenberg 2003). A variety of peptides are being evaluated for selective targeting due to their rapid blood clearance and faster uptake rates in target cells; they have increased tissue penetration and diffusion, clear primarily through the urinary tract, are nonimmunogenic, and can be easily and cost-effectively synthesized using solid-phase and solution-phase techniques. Most of the peptides in current development are either modifications of peptides found naturally or were derived from combinatorial libraries screened to find optimal candidates. A newer approach is the use of phage display, which links phenotype to genotype and offers the ability to develop peptides against any target, holding the promise of providing high-affinity targets for individualized patient treatments.

Phage display is a molecular tool that uses recombinant DNA technology to create bacteriophages with a desired peptide embedded in the surface of their protein shells. Agonists and antagonists of the target peptide can then be identified experimentally, enabling engineering of antibodies and peptides as possible new drugs. A recent development is the use of phage as nanoparticle imaging systems

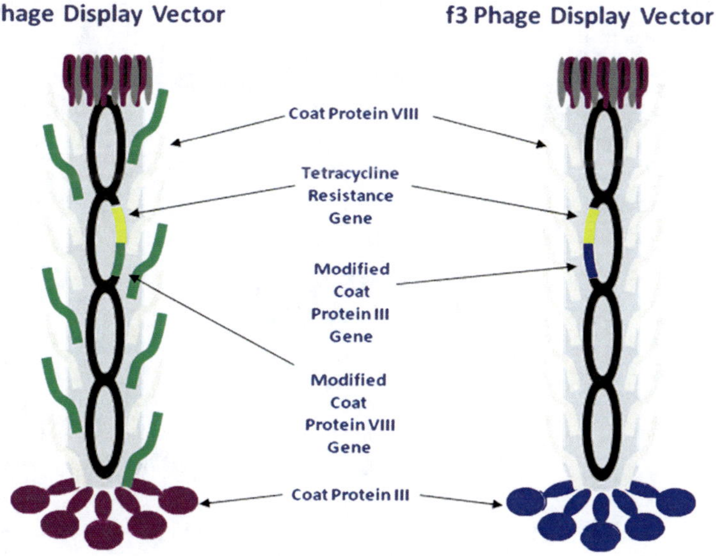

Fig. 2 Phage display vectors

(Newton-Northrup et al. 2009; Deutscher 2010). Phage display was invented in 1985 by George Smith at the University of Missouri when he demonstrated short peptides could be displayed by fusion onto phage coat proteins (Smith 1985). Advantages of phage display are the direct link from genotype to phenotype and that a library containing 10^9–10^{11} clones can be created in a couple of weeks. Illustrated in Fig. 5 is a phage display vector in which foreign small peptides are incorporated into the N-terminus of minor coat protein III (cpIII) of fd phage so that up to five copies of the peptide are displayed (Smith 1985). These libraries are then put through selection affinity methods to screen out unwanted nonspecific binders and to obtain peptides that bind with high affinity to the desired target. An in vivo screening method is illustrated in Fig. 6. The advantages of in vivo phage selection over in situ or in vitro methods is that selection occurs in the same complicated biological milieu where the selected peptide will be expected to selectively target, and it does not require knowledge of the target. Thus, libraries can be screened against induced human tumor cells to create peptides for individualized tumor cells. Once a desired peptide has been screened, its primary structure can be found by sequencing the peptide-coding sequence in the viral DNA. Each phage clone displays a single peptide.

Galectin-3 belongs to a family of β-galactoside-binding animal lectins which bind terminal galactopyranose residues on carbohydrates, most notably the Thomas–Friedenreich (TF) antigen. The TF antigen is a disaccharide Ga1β1-3Ga1NAc expressed on the surfaces of most adenocarcinomas including

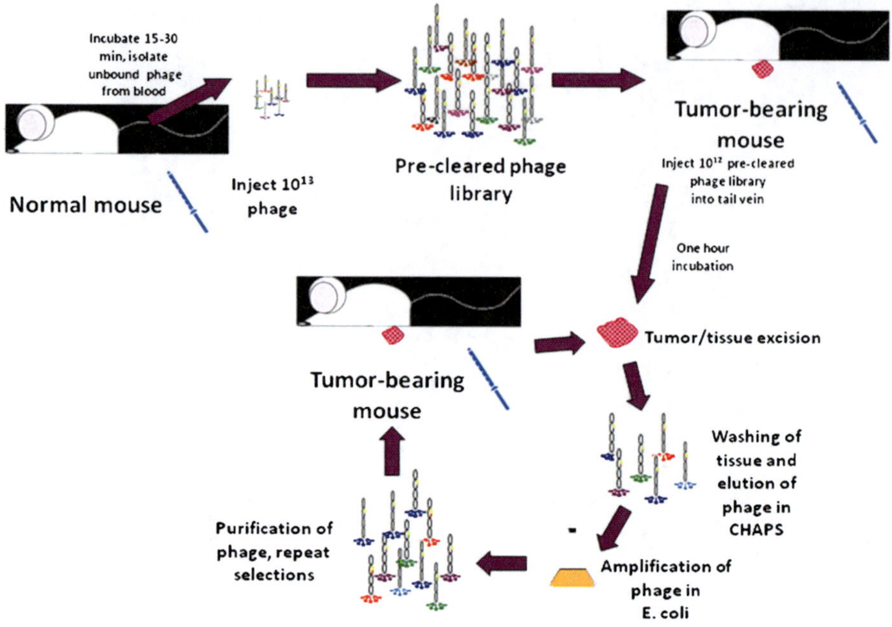

Fig. 3 In vivo selection of tumor phage

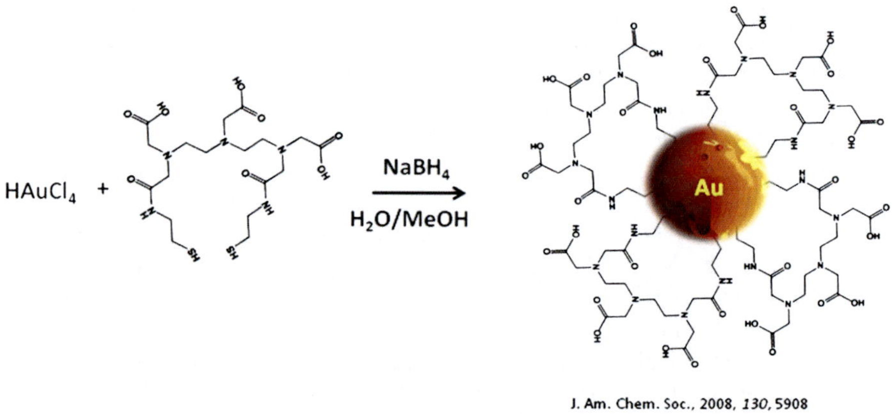

Fig. 4 Formation of DTDTPA gold nanoparticles for molecular imaging

breast and prostate cancer. A peptide that is avid to galectin-3 was identified from bacteriophage display (Zou et al. 2005). The peptide contains 16 amino acids with the following sequence: ANTPCGPYTHDCPVKR. Also known as G3-C12, the peptide was linked to the DOTA chelator using a tripeptide linker called Gly-Ser-Gly (GSG). Previously, DOTA(GSG)-G3-C12 was successfully labeled

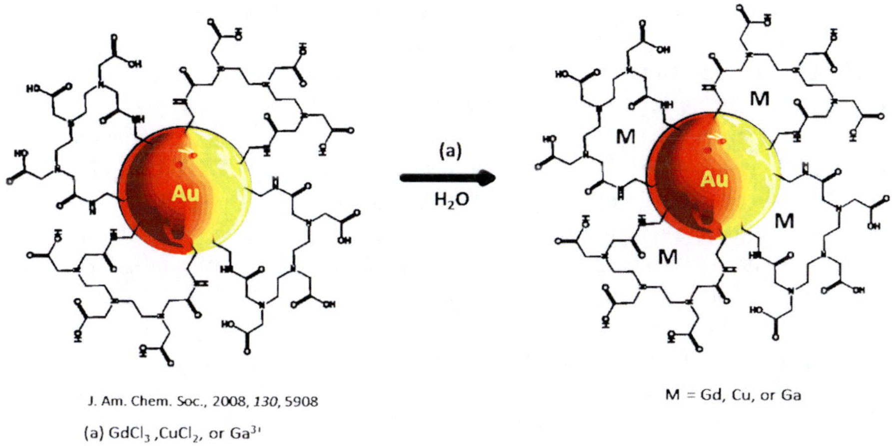

Fig. 5 Illustration of metal labeling of DTDTPA gold nanoparticles

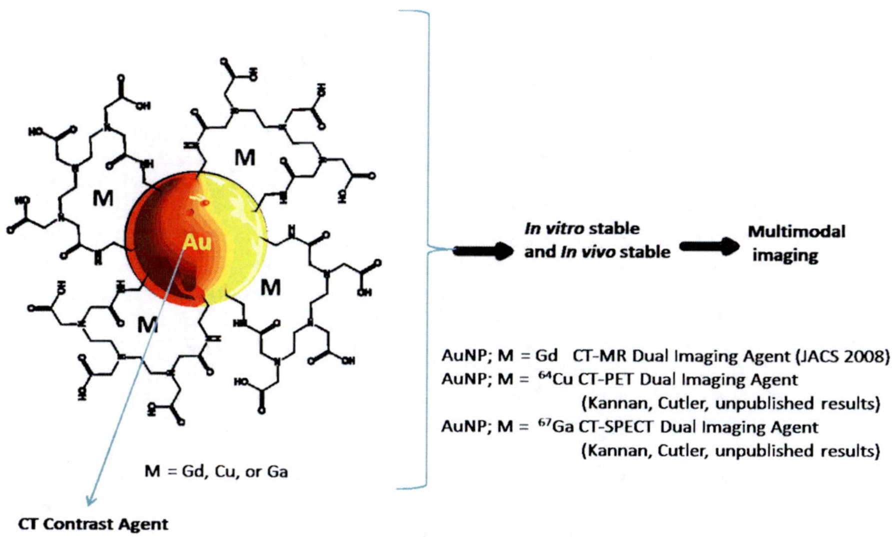

Fig. 6 DTDTPA gold nanoparticles for multimodality imaging

with ^{111}In, and the radiolabeled peptide evaluated in a human MDA-MB-435 breast tumor-bearing model (Kumar and Deutsher 2008). Results revealed tumor uptake of 1.2 ± 0.24%, 0.75 ± 0.05%, and 0.6 ± 0.04% ID/g at 0.5, 1.0, and 2 h post injection. Blocking studies with the nonradiolabeled peptide resulted in a 52% reduction at 2 h post injection. A major drawback was the high kidney uptake of 22%

ID/g at 2 h. Results indicated that ^{111}In-DOTA(GSG)-G3-C12 is a potential SPECT imaging agent for breast tumors that are positive for galectin-3 (Figs. 4, 5, 6).

PET imaging using ^{68}Ga can provide quantitative measurements of small tumors that can hardly be detected by SPECT. In another study, we explored the ability to label DOTA(GSG)-G3-C12 with ^{68}Ga as an alternative approach to ^{111}In SPECT imaging. Preliminary results indicated that ^{68}Ga-DOTA(GSG)-G3-C12 could be successfully prepared in 0.1 M ammonium acetate (pH 5) at 100°C for 30 min. The labeling efficiency was 52% with an impure peptide mixture. Additionally, microwave labeling techniques were developed, similar to those reported previously (Cantorias et al. 2009) Yields were similar, but the reaction could be accomplished in 1 min with additional time being required for HPLC, normally 15 min. The HPLC-purified peptide was further tested for stability at room temperature, and challenged in rat serum. Radio-TLC and HPLC confirmed that the ^{68}Ga-labeled peptide remained intact up to 85% out to 4 h. Based on these results, future evaluation in tumor models is planned.

References

Asti M, Farioli D, Murray L, Guidotti C, Cutler CS, Mayer P, Salvo D (2010) Influence of cations on the coordination reaction of DOTATATE with yttrium and lutetium technetium and other metals in chemistry and medicine. In: Mazzi U, Eckelmann WC, Volkert WA (eds) SGEditoriali. Padova, Italy, pp 249–250

Cantorias M, Figueroa SD, Quinn TP, Lever JR, Hoffman TJ, Watkinson LD, Carmack TL, Cutler CS (2009) Development of a high specific activity ^{68}Ga-labeled DOTA-Rhenium-cyclized α-MSH peptide peptide analog to target MC1 receptors overexpressed by melanoma tumors. Nucl Med Biol 36(5):505–513

Chanda N, Kattumuri K, Shukla R, Zambre A, Katti K, Upendran A, Kulkarni RR, Kan P, Fent GM, Casteel SW, Smith CJ, Boote E, Robertson JD, Cutler CS, Lever JR, Katti KV, Kannan R (2010) Bombesin functionalized gold nanoparticles show in vitro and in vivo cancer receptor specificity. PNAS 107(19):8760–8765

Chandra N, Kan P, Watkinson LD, Carmack TL, Shukla R, Engelbrecht H, Lever JR, Katti K, Fent GM, Casteel SW, Zambre A, Smith CJ, Miller WH, Jurisson SS, Boote E, Robertson DR, Cutler CS, Dobrovolskaia M, Kannan R, Katti KV (2010) Radioactive gold nanoparticles in cancer therapy: therapeutic efficacy studies of GA-198AuNP nano construct in prostate tumor–bearing mice. Nanomed: NMB 6(2):201–209

Debuttiere P-J, Roux S, Vocanson F, Billotey C, Beuf O, Favre-Réguillon A, Lin Y, Pellet-Rostaing S, Lamartine R, Perriat P, Tillement O (2006) Design of gold nanoparticles for magnetic resonance imaging. Adv Funct Mater 16(18):2330–2339

Deutscher SL (2010) Phage display in molecular imaging and diagnosis of cancer. Chem Rev 110:3196–3211. doi:10.1021/cr900317f

Goldenberg DM (2003) Targeted therapy of cancer with radiolabeled antibodies. *J Nucl Med* 43(5):309, 693–713

Kannan R, Rahing V, Cutler C, Pandrapragada R, Katti KK, Kattumuri V, Robertson JD, Casteel SJ, Jurisson S, Smith C, Boote E, Katti KV (2006) Nano compatible chemistry toward fabrication of target-specific gold nanoparticles. J Am Chem Soc (Communication) 128(35):11342–11343. doi:10.1021/ja63280c

Klatersky J (2006) Adverse effects of the humanized antibodies used as cancer therapeutics. J Curr Opin Oncol 18:316

Kumar SR, Deutsher SL (2008) ^{111}In-labeled galectin-3 targeting peptide as a SPECT agent for imaging breast tumors. J Nucl Med 49:796–803
Malinoff HL, Wicha MS (1983) Isolation of a cell surface receptor protein for laminin from murine fibrosarcoma cells (trans from eng). J Cell Biol 96(5):1475–1479 (in eng)
McLaughlin M, Chanda N, Lever JR, Smith CJ, Kannan R, Katti K, Katti K, Cutler CS (2011a) Evaluation of receptor affinity of Au-198-starch-nanoparticles conjugated to bombesin. J Labelled Compd Radiopharm 54:S549
McLaughlin M, Woodward J, Broderick M, Standaert R, Rondinone A, Robertson DR, Mirzadeh S, Kennel SJ (2011b) Synthesis and characterization of a novel gold coated $LaGdPO_4$ nanoparticles containing actinium-225. In: 7th symposium on targeted alpha therapy. Berlin, Germany, 17–19 July 2011
Newton-Northrup JR, Figueroa SD, Quinn TP, Deutscher SL (2009) Bifunctional-phage based pre targeted imaging of human prostate cancer. Nucl Med Biol 36:789–800
Prasanphanich A et al (2007) [64Cu-NOTA-8-Aoc-BBN-(7–14)NH2] targeting vector for positron-emission tomography imaging of gastrin-releasing peptide receptor-expressing tissues. *PNAS* 104:12462–12467
Rao NC, Barsky SH, Terranova VP, Liotta LA (1983) Isolation of a tumor cell laminin receptor (translated from eng). Biochem Biophys Res Commun 111(3):804–808 (in eng)
Shukla R, Zambre A, Nripen C, Kan P, Engelbrecht H, Cutler CS, Lever JR, Smith CJ, Caldwell CW, Katti K, Upendran A, Kannan R, Katti KV (2011a) Clinical translation of radioactive gold nano particle-based nano ceutical (EGCG-198AuNP) for prostate tumor therapy. J Labelled Compd Radiopharm 54:S89
Shukla R, Chanda N, Zambre A, Katti K, Upendran A, Kulkarni RR, Nune S, Casteel SW, Smith CJ, Boote E, Robertson JD, Lever JR, Cutler CS, Caldwell C, Kannan R, Katti KV (2011b) Green nanotechnology approach generates biocompatible gold nanoparticles: inherently therapeutic radioactive 198AuNP-EGCg shows efficacy in treating prostate cancer via Laminin 67 receptor mediated endocytosis. *PNAS* submitted
Smith GP (1985) Flamentous fusion phage: novel expression vectors that display cloned antigens on the virion surface. Science 228:1315
Smith CJ, Volkert WA, Hoffman TJ (2003) Gastrin releasing peptide (GRP) receptor targeted radiopharmaceuticals: a concise update. Nucl Med Biol 30:861–868
Tachibana H, Koga K, Fujimura Y, Yamada K (2004) A receptor for green tea polyphenol EGCG (translated from eng). Nat Struct Mol Biol 11(4):380–381 (in eng)
Zou J, Glinsky VV, Landon LA, Matthews L, Deutscher SL (2005) Peptides specific to the galatin-3carbohydrate recognition domain inhibit metastasis-associated cancer cell adhesion. Carcinogenesis 26:309–318

"Click"-Cyclized ^{68}Ga-Labeled Peptides for Molecular Imaging and Therapy: Synthesis and Preliminary In Vitro and In Vivo Evaluation in a Melanoma Model System

Molly E. Martin, M. Sue O'Dorisio, Whitney M. Leverich, Kyle C. Kloepping, Susan A. Walsh and Michael K. Schultz

Abstract

Cyclization techniques are used often to impart higher in vivo stability and binding affinity to peptide targeting vectors for molecular imaging and therapy. The two most often used techniques to impart these qualities are lactam bridge construction and disulfide bond formation. While these techniques have been demonstrated to be effective, orthogonal protection/deprotection steps can limit achievable product yields. In the work described in this chapter, new α-melanocyte stimulating hormone (α-MSH) peptide analogs were synthesized and cyclized by copper-catalyzed terminal azide-alkyne cycloaddition "click" chemistry techniques. The α-MSH peptide and its cognate receptor (melanocortin receptor subtype 1, MC1R) represent a well-characterized model system to examine the effect of the triazole linkage for peptide cyclization on receptor binding in vitro and in vivo. Four new DOTA-conjugated α-MSH analogs were cyclized and evaluated by in vitro competitive binding assays, serum stability testing, and in vivo imaging by positron emission tomography (PET) of tumor-bearing mice. These new DOTA-conjugated click-cyclized analogs exhibited selective high binding affinity (<2 nM) for MC1R on melanoma cells in vitro, high stability in human serum, and produced high-contrast PET/CT images of tumor xenografts. ^{68}Ga-labeled DOTA bioconjugates displayed rapid

M. E. Martin · M. Sue O'Dorisio · W. M. Leverich
Department of Pediatric Hematology/Oncology, Carver College of Medicine, The University of Iowa, ML B180, 500 Newton Road, Iowa City, IA 52242, USA

K. C. Kloepping · S. A. Walsh · M. K. Schultz (✉)
Departments of Radiology and Radiation Oncology (Free Radical Radiation Biology Program), Carver College of Medicine, The University of Iowa, ML B180, 500 Newton Road, Iowa City, IA 52242, USA
e-mail: michael-schultz@uiowa.edu

R. P. Baum and F. Rösch (eds.), *Theranostics, Gallium-68, and Other Radionuclides*, Recent Results in Cancer Research 194, DOI: 10.1007/978-3-642-27994-2_9,

pharmacokinetics with receptor-mediated tumor accumulation of up to 16 ± 5% ID/g. The results indicate that the triazole ring is an effective bioisosteric replacement for the standard lactam bridge assemblage for peptide cyclization. Radiolabeling results confirm that Cu catalyst is sufficiently removed prior to DOTA chelator addition to enable insertion of radio metals or stable metals for molecular imaging and therapy. Thus, these click-chemistry-cyclized variants show promise as agents for melanocortin receptor-targeted imaging and radionuclide therapy.

Contents

1 Introduction

1.1 Targeted Peptides for Molecular Imaging and Therapy

Peptides are emerging as potent and selective ligands that can be designed to bind with high affinity and specificity to cell surface receptors for a wide range of in vitro and in vivo biomedical applications. One area of research that has seen considerable proliferation is the use of peptide bioconjugates for targeted molecular imaging and therapy of cancer. For this application, peptide analogs are developed to bind selectively to specific cell surface receptors that are upregulated on malignant tumors. The peptide sequences employed are either based on the native cognate binding ligand or can be selected using peptide library approaches

(Heppeler et al. 2000; Zwanziger and Beck-Sickinger 2008). To enable the use of the identified sequences for molecular imaging and therapy of cancer, molecular modifications are made to improve binding to cognate receptors, stabilize the bioconjugates to in vivo degradation, and install chelator moieties for radiolabeling. In this way, these same peptide ligands can be used to exploit receptor overexpression in tumor tissues for diagnosis, staging, targeted radionuclide therapy, and measurement of therapeutic response (Heppeler et al. 2000; Eberle and Froidevaux 2003).

While the potential of radiolabeled peptides for molecular targeting of cell surface receptors has been demonstrated, identified native peptide sequences often are degraded rapidly in vivo. Thus, investigators have devised numerous structural modifications that impart improved pharmacodynamic properties over the native peptide sequences, while preserving (and even enhancing) the molecular targeting characteristics of the peptide analogs (Vlieghe et al. 2010; Nestor 2009); For example, *N*-terminal acylation and *C*-terminal amidation help to prevent degradation by exoproteases. Substitution of D-amino acids at positions susceptible to endoproteases can also add stability to peptide-based diagnostics and therapeutics (Vlieghe et al. 2010). One particularly powerful approach to inhibit proteolysis of peptides is cyclization. Cyclization can not only provide added in vivo stability to peptide-based targeting vectors; it can also enhance receptor affinity and biological potency by restricting the peptide to an active conformation (Okarvi 2004; Turner et al. 2007; Nestor 2009). Several approaches to cyclization have been advanced, including disulfide coupling, lactam bridge assembly, and metal coordination strategies (Raposinho et al. 2010). The receptor affinity and in vivo stability advantages of the cyclized variants of peptides prepared using these techniques have been demonstrated (Fani et al. 2010; Froidevaux et al. 2004; Miao et al. 2008; Cantorias et al. 2009; Guo et al. 2010). On the other hand, potential drawbacks of these approaches may include reversibility (disulfide bridges), multiple protection and deprotection steps (lactam assembly), and restriction in radionuclides that can be employed for imaging and therapy (technetium/rhenium cyclizations). Here, cyclization of peptides by copper-catalyzed "click" chemistry for molecular imaging is presented. While click chemistry has been used previously for a number of peptide cyclization bioconjugate chemistry applications, few investigators have implemented this strategy for targeted molecular imaging and therapy. To highlight the potential advantages of click cyclization for radiopharmaceutical synthesis applications, a well-characterized peptide/receptor model was chosen to facilitate comparison of standard lactam-bridge-cyclized variants to click-cyclized variants. Thus, DOTA-modified α-melanocyte stimulating hormone (α-MSH) derivatives were cyclized using the lactam bridge and click triazole formation techniques. The resulting bioconjugates were evaluated in vitro by receptor binding assays to cells expressing cognate receptor melanocortin receptor subtype 1 (MC1R) and serum stability tests. Select click-cyclized derivatives were radiolabeled with positron-emitting radionuclide ^{68}Ga for in vivo evaluation of pharmacodynamics and PET/CT imaging characteristics in tumor-bearing mice.

1.2 Cyclized Melanocyte Stimulating Hormone

α-MSH is a peptide hormone that is the endogenous ligand for melanocortin receptor subtype 1 (MC1R), which is upregulated in malignant melanoma, along with other receptors in the MC family (Ghanem et al. 1988; Siegrist et al. 1988; Tatro et al. 1990; Eberle et al. 1991; Lunec et al. 1992). The native sequence is a linear 13-amino-acid peptide (Ac-Ser-Tyr-Ser-Met-Glu-His-Phe-Arg-Trp-Gly-Lys-Pro-Val-NH_2) (Harris and Lerner 1957). α-MSH binds the MC1R with high affinity, but it has a biological half-life of less than 3 min in vivo (Cowell et al. 2002). Thus, for targeted molecular imaging and therapy, modifications to the native peptide sequence are required to impart sufficient in vivo stability to promote accumulation of the radiolabeled tracer in malignant tissue of interest. To enable the use of α-MSH for this application, several modified analogs have been synthesized and tested in an effort to add biological stability and improve targeting (Hruby et al. 2003). One particularly promising conformation that has proven effective in protecting the peptide from enzymatic degradation has replaced the Met at position 4 with Nle, while L-Phe has been exchanged with D-Phe. The resulting analog, [Nle^4, D-Phe^7]-α-MSH (NDP-α-MSH), is a more potent peptide ligand with extended biological activity resulting from resistance to degradation by serum proteases (Sawyer et al. 1980).

Further developments in α-MSH analogs included structure–function experiments that have helped to elucidate the amino acid residues necessary for receptor binding affinity of α-MSH for melanocortin receptors. These experiments have identified the "essential core" of native α-MSH peptide as His^6-Phe^7-Arg^8-Trp^9 (Hruby et al. 1987). From the identification of this four-amino-acid core, a highly potent cyclic analog, MTII, was constructed from only seven residues of the native α-MSH sequence with cyclization to restrict the conformation—adding further stability to the structure—while maintaining targeting affinity (Al-Obeidi et al. 1989a, b; Bednarek et al. 1999a, b). Structurally, the sequence of MTII, Ac-Nle-cyclo(Asp-His-D-Phe-Arg-Trp-Lys)-NH_2, retains the core residues, while forming a lactam bridge through cyclization of the aspartic acid and lysine side-chains. This cyclic analog is over 100-fold more potent than the linear α-MSH peptide in lizard skin assays (Sugg et al. 1988; Al-Obeidi et al. 1989a, b). Several analogs of MTII have been prepared in an effort to increase biological activity and impart receptor subtype specificity (Bednarek et al. 1999a, b, 2000; Cai et al. 2004; Mayorov et al. 2006a, b; Ying et al. 2006; Bednarek et al. 2007a, b; Grieco et al. 2008).

Although the reported efficacy of the lactam-bridge-cyclized variants sparked our interest in extending the use of these derivatives for our investigations, the synthetic strategy proved somewhat problematic. Cyclization by lactam bridge required orthogonal protecting strategies to keep the *N*-terminus protected while cyclization occurred through the side-chains of aspartic acid and lysine. In our hands, deprotection of the allyl/alloc groups also partially removed the *N*-terminal Fmoc, leaving the *N*-terminus unprotected and available for reaction (Fig. 1; analytical data not shown). These observations prompted us to examine alternative

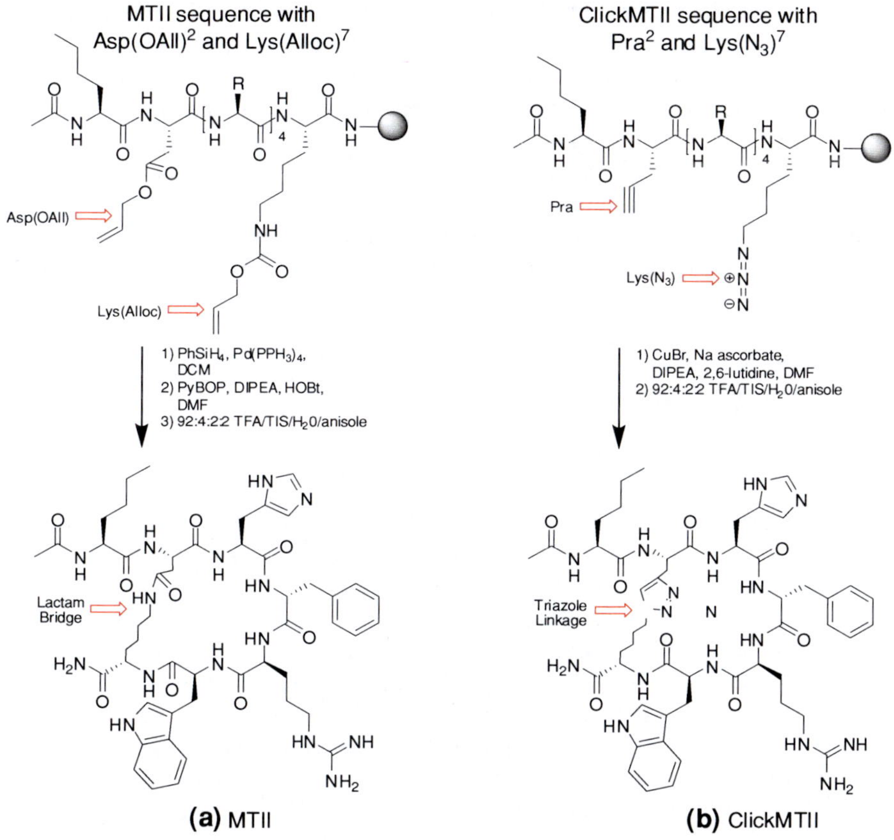

Fig. 1 Cyclized α-MSH analogs: **a** MTII, a seven-amino-acid derivative of α-MSH cyclized through lactamization of Asp^2 and Lys^7, and **b** ClickMTII, where the aspartic acid has been replaced by propargylglycine and the side-chain moiety of lysine has been changed to an azide, cyclized utilizing click chemistry between the terminal alkyne and azide to form a triazole

strategies to cyclization that could reduce the use of protective and deprotective strategies—and perhaps improve overall synthetic yields. Our assessment of the optimum characteristics of a bioconjugate strategy for the cyclization reaction included rapid kinetics, reactive selectivity that could minimize (or simplify) protection/deprotection steps, and mild reaction conditions that would be amenable to our standard automated peptide synthesis. Investigations along these lines led us to examine the use of copper-catalyzed "click" chemistry as an approach that appears to combine these optimum reaction characteristics. In the present study, new cyclic analogs of MTII were designed and constructed utilizing cyclization via copper-catalyzed "click" chemistry. The MTII sequence was modified to contain propargylglycine and terminal-azide-modified Lys [Lys(N_3)] to afford efficient cyclization of the peptide within the framework of standard automated peptide synthesis—through a triazole ring formation between the alkyne-modified Gly and Lys(N_3) in high yield. In addition, the approach enabled facile manipulation of the synthetic positioning of the metal chelator DOTA insertion to determine its effect on receptor affinity and peptide stability. The resulting compounds were labeled with positron-emitting radionuclide ^{64}Cu to perform in vitro stability testing in human serum and ^{68}Ga to produce bioconjugates for targeted molecular imaging by positron emission tomography (PET). Thus, in this chapter we present synthesis of several derivatives prepared in this manner, in vitro competitive cell binding assays, stability evaluations in serum, and preliminary evaluations of in vivo behavior by biodistribution studies and PET imaging.

2 Experimental

2.1 Chemicals and Reagents

Fmoc-protected amino acids, 2-(7-aza-1*H*-benzotriazole-1-yl)-1,1,3,3-tetramethyluronium hexafluorophosphate, 1-hydroxybenzotriazole, benzotriazole-1-ly-oxy-tris-pyrrolidinophosphonium hexafluorophosphate, and Rink amide resin for peptide synthesis were obtained from Advanced ChemTech (Louisville, KY). DOTA-tris (*t*-Bu ester) was purchased from Macrocyclics (Dallas, TX). *N*,*N*-Dimethylformamide, *N*,*N*-diisopropylethylamine, methanol, trifluoroacetic acid, anisole, acetonitrile, $PhSiH_3$, $Pd(PPH_3)_4$, and 2,6-lutidine were purchased from Thermo Fisher Scientific (Waltham, MA). Dichloromethane, triisopropylsilane, sodium ascorbate, copper(I) bromide, bovine serum albumin (BSA), 1,10-phenanthroline, HEPES, human serum, and citric acid were from Sigma Aldrich (St. Louis, MO). Dulbecco's modified Eagle's medium (DMEM), minimum essential medium (MEM), fetal bovine serum (FBS), and penicillin/streptomycin were from Invitrogen Life Technologies (Carlsbad, CA). B16/F10 murine melanoma cells were a gift from Dr. Michael Anderson at the University of Iowa (Iowa City, IA).

2.2 Peptide Synthesis

A total of ten linear and cyclized α-MSH peptide analogs were prepared, characterized, and tested in this study (Table 1). Four linear peptides, including α-MSH (Ac-SYSMEHFRWGKPV-NH_2) and NDP-α-MSH (Ac-SYS-Nle-EHfRWGKPV-NH_2), and their DOTA-conjugated variants, were synthesized on Rink amide resin at 0.1 mmol scale following standard Fmoc procedures on an AAPPTEC Apex 396 automated multiple peptide synthesizer. DOTA-tris (*t*-Bu ester) was coupled to the *N*-terminus of the protected linear peptides on-resin. Each peptide-resin (1 equiv peptide) was suspended in *N*,*N*-dimethylformamide (DMF), and DOTA-tris (*t*-Bu ester) (5 equiv), 2-(7-aza-1*H*-benzotriazole-1-yl)-1,1,3,3-tetramethyluronium hexafluorophosphate (HATU; 5 equiv), 1-hydroxybenzotriazole (HOBt; 5 equiv),

Table 1 α-MSH peptide analogs with competitive binding assay and stability data

Peptide	Sequence	Mass (obs/calc)	IC_{50} (nM)	24-h stability (% remaining)
α-MSH	Ac-SYSMEHFRWGKPV-NH_2	1,664.7/ 1,664.9	2.1 ± 0.4	N.D.
DOTA-α-MSH	DOTA-SYSMEHFRWGKPV-NH_2	2,009.0/ 2,009.3	1.8 ± 0.3	7.4
NDP-α-MSH	Ac-SYS-Nle-EHfRWGKPV-NH_2	1,646.6/ 1,646.9	0.21 ± 0.03	N.D.
DOTA-NDP-α-MSH	DOTA-SYS-Nle-EHfRWGKPV-NH_2	1,990.6/ 1,991.2	0.59 ± 0.11	41
MTII	Ac-Nle-cyclo[DHfRWK]-NH_2	1,024.6/ 1,024.2	0.26 ± 0.08	N.D.
ClickMTII	Ac-Nle-cyclo[Pra-HfRW-Lys(N_3)]-NH_2	1,048.3/ 1,048.2	0.39 ± 0.06	N.D.
DOTA-ClickMTII	DOTA-Nle-cyclo[Pra-HfRW-Lys(N_3)]-NH_2	1,392.3/ 1,392.6	25 ± 1	100
DOTA-GG-ClickMTII	DOTA-GG-Nle-cyclo[Pra-HfRW-Lys(N_3)]-NH_2	1,506.1/ 1,506.7	2.7 ± 0.8	99
ClickMTII-K-DOTA	Ac-Nle-cyclo[Pra-HfRW-Lys(N_3)]-K(DOTA)-NH_2	1,562.4/ 1,562.8	1.4 ± 0.2	99
ClickMTII-GGK-DOTA	Ac-Nle-cyclo[Pra-HfRW-Lys(N_3)]-GGK(DOTA)-NH_2	1,676.6/ 1,676.9	1.1 ± 0.2	100

and *N*,*N*-diisopropylethylamine (DIPEA; 10 equiv) were added and the reaction mixed at 37°C overnight. Completeness of coupling was checked by the Kaiser test for free amines (Kaiser et al. 1970). The peptide-resin was filtered, washed with DMF, dichloromethane (DCM), and methanol, and allowed to dry. Peptides were cleaved and deprotected with 95:2.5:2.5 trifluoroacetic acid (TFA)/triisopropylsilane (TIS)/water for 2 h at room temperature, then precipitated with ice-cold ether. The peptides were purified on reversed-phase high-performance liquid chromatography (RP-HPLC) by injection onto a Vydac C_{18} semipreparative column (10 × 250 mm, 10 μm, 300 Å; Grace, Deerfield, IL) eluted at 5 ml/min with 0.1% TFA and a 20–30% gradient of acetonitrile over 30 min while monitoring absorbance at 280 nm. The peak of interest was collected, concentrated by rotary evaporation, and lyophilized. Purified peptides were characterized on an Agilent 1100 LC-ESI-ion trap mass spectrometer (Table 1).

A single lactam-bridge-cyclized peptide (MTII, Ac-Nle-cyclo[DHfRWK]-NH_2) was synthesized as described above, with the exception that Fmoc-Asp(Allyl)-OH and Fmoc-Lys(Alloc)-OH residues were inserted for selective deprotection to facilitate cyclization of the Fmoc-protected peptide on-resin (Fig. 1). Following synthesis, according to published procedures, the Allyl and Alloc groups were to be removed selectively by adding $PhSiH_3$ (24 equiv) and $Pd(PPH_3)_4$ (0.10 equiv) in DCM and mixing for 10 min at room temperature (Thieriet et al. 1997). The peptide-resin was filtered and washed with DCM, and the deprotection was repeated. Complete removal of the Alloc group was tested by running the Kaiser test to detect free amine of the lysine side-chain. Peptide cyclization between the acid group of the aspartic acid and the primary amine of the lysine was achieved by addition of benzotriazole-1-ly-oxy-tris-pyrrolidinophosphonium hexafluorophosphate (PyBOP; 1.1 equiv), DIPEA (2.2 equiv), and HOBt (0.5 equiv) in DMF. The reaction was mixed overnight at room temperature, and the resin was filtered and washed with DMF, DCM, and methanol. The cyclized peptide was cleaved and deprotected with 92:4:2:2 TFA/TIS/water/anisole for 2 h at room temperature, then precipitated with ice-cold ether. The cyclic MTII peptide was purified by semipreparative HPLC as described above using a 20–35% gradient of acetonitrile, and the purified peptide was characterized on an Agilent 1100 LC-ESI-ion trap mass spectrometer.

Five click-cyclized MTII analogs were synthesized by similar methods (Table 1; Fig. 1). In this case, the internal amino acid sequences for these five MTII analogs differed, with the insertion of of Pra and $Lys(N_3)$ residues to facilitate cyclization through triazole ring formation via "click" chemistry. In addition, an Fmoc-Lys(Dde)-OH was added for peptides with a *C*-terminal lysine residue. Following synthesis, peptides containing a Lys(Dde) were selectively deprotected by treatment with 2% hydrazine for 15 min. Peptides were cyclized by modification of methods by Turner et al. (2007). Briefly, the peptide-resin was swelled in DMF and DIPEA prior to addition of 2,6-lutidine (10 equiv each). Sodium ascorbate was added as 1% solution in 1:4 water/DMF (v/v; 3 equiv) followed by copper(I) bromide as 1% solution in acetonitrile (1 equiv). Sodium ascorbate was added to maintain copper as the monovalent, catalytically active cationic form. The reaction mixture was stirred at 37°C overnight, and the peptide-resin was filtered and washed with DMF, DCM, and methanol. DOTA-tris (*t*-Bu ester) was coupled to the primary amine (either *N*-terminus or lysine side-chain), and peptides were cleaved/deprotected as described above. To examine the effect of DOTA conjugation on binding affinity and stability, four ClickMTII variants were constructed with DOTA conjugated to either the *N*- or *C*-terminus of the peptide: (1) DOTA coupled directly to the free amine of the *N*-terminus, (2) DOTA coupled through a glycine–glycine (GG) spacer added to the *N*-terminus of the peptide sequence, (3) DOTA attached to the *C*-terminus via the ε-amine side-chain of a lysine residue added to the *C*-terminal end of the peptide, or (4) through the lysine side-chain of a glycine–glycine–lysine spacer. The click-cyclized peptides were purified by semipreparative HPLC using a 20–30% or 20–35% gradient of acetonitrile, and the purified peptides were characterized on an Agilent 1100 LC-ESI-ion trap mass spectrometer (Table 1).

2.3 In Vitro Competitive Binding Assay

B16/F10 murine melanoma cells were cultured in high-glucose DMEM supplemented with 10% (v/v) FBS, 100 U/mL penicillin, and 100 μg/mL streptomycin in 150-cm^3 culture flasks at 37°C in a humidified 5% CO_2 incubator; cells were grown to 70% confluency and used in competitive binding assays similar to the methods developed by Siegrist et al. (1988). Cells were scraped from the culture flasks, counted on a Beckman Coulter cell counter, and resuspended in binding media (MEM containing 25 mM HEPES, 0.2% BSA, and 0.3 mM 1,10-phenanthroline). For binding assays, a total volume of 500 μL was used in 1.5-mL Eppendorf tubes. The cell suspension (50 μL containing approximately 4 million cells) was incubated with approximately 30,000 cpm of [^{125}I]-[Nle^4,D-Phe^7]-α-MSH and increasing concentrations of α-MSH or peptide analog ranging from 10^{-6} to 10^{-11} M. The tubes were mixed at 25°C, 600 rpm on an Eppendorf Thermomixer for 1.5 h. Following incubation, cells were pelleted by centrifugation, the media was aspirated, pellets were transferred to 12 × 75 mm glass tubes, and the radioactivity of the cell pellet was determined using a PerkinElmer Cobra II gamma counter (PerkinElmer, Freemont, CA). All handling of radioactive materials was conducted using procedures and protocols approved through the University of Iowa Environmental Health and Safety Committee and Health Protection Office, adhering to as low as reasonably achievable (ALARA) principles. Each experiment was performed in quadruplicate, and binding curves were plotted; 50% inhibition concentration (IC_{50}) values and their associated standard errors were calculated with GraphPad Prism 5 curve-fitting software (GraphPad Prism version 5.01 for Windows; GraphPad Software, San Diego, CA).

2.4 Radiochemistry

^{64}Cu was obtained as $^{64}CuCl_2$ solution from the College of Medicine, Washington University in Saint Louis (WashU, St. Louis, MO, USA). Radiolabeling of DOTA-peptides with ^{64}Cu was carried out as described previously (Anderson et al. 2008; Boswell et al. 2008; Brechbiel 2008; Hausner et al. 2009). Briefly, ^{64}Cu was received from WashU in approximately 10–40 μl of mildly acidic solution in a screw-top plastic "v-vial," enclosed within appropriate lead shielding. To this vial was added ultrapure water or pH 6 sodium acetate buffer solution to final volume of 200 μl, and the solution was mixed. The 200 μl solution was withdrawn and transferred to a 1.5-ml plastic v-vial (SealRite, natural microcentrifuge tube, Cat# 1615-5500, USA Scientific), and a measurement of the total activity was determined by dose calibrator (CRC-25R, Capintech, Ramsey, NJ). Aliquots of appropriate radioactivity amounts could then be transferred volumetrically to appropriate radiolabeling solutions. Generally, 10 nmoles peptide was suspended in 50 μl pH 6 acetate buffer. To this solution was added an appropriate aliquot of ^{64}Cu master solution, and the solution was incubated for 45 min at 70°C. This solution was used without further purification for in vitro stability testing. The identity of radiolabeled species was confirmed by radioHPLC retention time comparison with UV traces of the unlabeled species at 280 nm.

Radiolabeling with ^{68}Ga was carried out through the use of a ^{68}Ge/^{68}Ga generator system (IGG100; Eckert Ziegler GmbH, Berlin, Germany) with total ^{68}Ge activity of approximately 600 MBq at the time of experiments presented here. The system was aged between 5–10 months for experiments conducted for this investigation. The methodology employed involves a single-step purification of ^{68}Ga eluted from the generator with 10 ml 0.1 M HCl at flow rate of approximately 2 ml/min directly to a cation exchange (Strata^{TM}-XC, 33 μm, Strong Cation, 30 mg/ml #8B-S029-TAK, Phenomenex) column mounted by supports fabricated in house. Following generator elution, the generator outflow line is disconnected and the Strata-XC column is air-dried using a 20-ml plastic syringe (2x). Once dry, pure ^{68}Ga is eluted from the Strata-XC column with 400 μl of 98% acetone/0.05 M HCl (prepared weekly and stored at 4°C) directly to a glass vial containing 5–10 nmoles DOTA-peptide conjugate dissolved in 5 mL pure water that had been preheated to approximately 80°C. This solution was then heated (open vessel) to 100°C and ^{68}Ga (with the DOTA-peptide) are incubated for 15 m. Acetone is evaporated to less than 300 ppm in the final purified drug product by this method. Following the radiolabeling incubation period, the reaction mixture containing the [^{68}Ga]-peptide and a small amount of free ^{68}Ga was drawn up through a Strata^{TM}-X cartridge (33 μm Polymeric Reversed Phase C-18, 30 mg/1ml, #8B-S100-TAK, Phenomenex® Inc., Torrance, CA, USA) that had been preconditioned by passing 1 mL 95% ethanol (USP for injection) and 2.5 ml pure water. The cartridge was then rinsed with 2 ml water to remove any residual free ^{68}Ga, and finally the purified ^{68}Ga-peptide conjugate was eluted in 500 μl of 1:1 ethanol (95%):isotonic saline solution. Radiochemical purity was determined by radioHPLC as described for ^{64}Cu.

2.5 Serum Stability Assay

Stability of chelator-modified peptide bioconjugates was determined by radioTLC (^{64}Cu labeled) using iTLC-SG glass microfiber chromatography paper impregnated with silica gel (Varian, Lake Forest, CA, USA) as described in detail previously.(Rockey et al. 2011) Briefly, iTLC paper was cut into 5 × 25 cm^2 strips and heated at 100°C for at least 30 min prior to measurements. Radiolabeled peptides were added to human serum and allowed to incubate at 37°C. At specified time points, 2 μl of the labeled peptide/serum mixture was spotted at a predetermined origin on the strips, and the iTLC strips were developed for about 3 min with a mobile phase of 0.1 M citric acid. Under these conditions, it was determined in advance that stable (intact) peptide remains at the origin, while free ^{64}Cu migrates with the mobile phase and peptide fragmentation can be observed by intermediately dispersed retention times. The strips were then dried with a common hairdryer. Possible fragmentation of the radiolabeled chelator-modified bioconjugates was determined through exposure of the iTLC strips to a storage phosphor screen (Fujifilm, Minamiashigara, Kanagawa, Japan) and subsequent screen imaging with a Typhoon^{TM} FLA 7000 PhosphorImager (GE Healthcare Bio-sciences AB, Uppsala, Sweden). Data analysis of the phosphor images was performed using ImageQuant^{TM} Analysis Toolbox software (TL 7.0; GE Healthcare Bio-sciences AB, Uppsala, Sweden). The percent intact radiolabeled chelator-modified peptides was calculated by dividing the integrated signal intensity over the bottom half of the TLC strips by the total integrated signal intensity over the entire length of the TLC strips. The technique was confirmed by radioHPLC. The pH of solutions was confirmed by use of an Horiba Compact pH-meter (model B-213; Horiba Scientific Instruments, Ann Arbor, MI, USA), calibrated daily at pH 4 and pH 7 using standard buffers or colorpHast pH paper (0–14 range; Merck KGaA, Darmstadt, Germany).

2.6 In Vivo PET Imaging and Biodistribution Studies

All animal experiments were performed according to approved protocols that were compliant to all rules and regulations of federal regulatory bodies and the University of Iowa Animal Care and Use Committee.

Female SCID hairless mice (6–8 weeks old) were implanted subcutaneously with three million MC1R-expressing cells (B16-F10 murine melanoma). Five to seven days after inoculation, tumors had grown to approximately 100–200 mg and the tumor-bearing mice were subjected to in vivo biodistribution and imaging studies using ^{68}Ga-labeled MTII variants. For biodistribution studies, approximately 7.5 MBq (200 μCi) of [^{68}Ga]DOTA-MTII variants (specific activity 30–50 MBq nmole^{-1} and radiochemical purity >98%) was injected intravenously into the lateral tail vein using tuberculin insulin-type syringes (Becton Dickinson; 8 mm (5/16"), 500 μl, 31G Ultra-Fine^{TM} needle) (Guo et al. 2010). Following injection of the radiolabeled tracer, animals were placed back in cages that were lined with absorbent material to sequester excretion for measurement at the conclusion of the uptake period (1.5 h). The uptake period for the comparison was determined by consideration of the radionuclide half-life of ^{68}Ga, as well as preliminary pharmacokinetic studies using [^{68}Ga]DOTA-Amide-NDP-α-MSH and literature reviews of other cyclized α-MSH analogs. At the conclusion of the uptake period, animals were sacrificed by approved procedures. Blood, tissues, and organs of interest (heart, liver, kidneys, lung, brain, muscle, and tumors) were resected, dabbed on blotter paper to remove excess blood, transferred to preweighed snap-cap v-vials, weighed, and assayed for radioactivity by scintillation counting. The radioactivity in excretion (urine and feces) was determined by the total activity that could be wiped from the floor of wire-bottom cages using the inserted absorbent pads and urine extracted from the bladder. Following resections and removal of urine from the bladder, the carcass was also counted by dose calibrator measurement to complete a measure of radioactivity balance. The radioactivity measurements were normalized to percent injected dose per gram (% ID/g) of tissue for each tissue sample with appropriate decay corrections applied. An evaluation of the biodistribution of "free" $^{68}Ga^{3+}$ was conducted to determine the possible contribution of free radio metal to tumor accumulation of injected dose. Finally, receptor-mediated tumor accumulation to xenograft tumors was confirmed by co-injection of 50–750 μg unlabeled NDP-α-MSH together with ^{68}Ga DOTA-peptide conjugates.

In vivo imaging studies were conducted to complete the preliminary evaluation of the click-cyclized peptides. For imaging, animals were anesthetized and injected with approximately 25 MBq [^{68}Ga]-peptide (specific activity 30–50 MBq $nmole^{-1}$) suspended in approximately 100 μl saline solution. Animals were allowed access to food and water at all times. Imaging of the biodistribution of the radiolabeled peptide was conducted at 1.5 h post injection (p.i.) using an Inveon™ small-animal PET/CT (Siemens, Inc., Knoxville, TN, USA). A 15-min static scan was employed for imaging. Immediately prior to scanning, the bladder contents were carefully expunged and collected in an absorbent pad for quantification of urine radioactivity and to prevent urinary contamination of the imaging bed.

3 Results

3.1 Peptide Synthesis

The lactam-bridge-cyclized α-MSH peptide analog MTII and click-cyclized variant ClickMTII were synthesized utilizing similar Fmoc procedures (Rink amide resin) and final Fmoc removal and *N*-terminal acylation. Thus, the molecular compositions were identical, with the exception of the linkage used for cyclization (Fig. 1). For lactam bridge formation of MTII, removal of allyl/alloc protecting groups was required to prepare the peptide for cyclization by amide bond formation via the acid moiety of the aspartic acid and the primary amine of lysine (lactam bridge formation). While much of the synthetic strategy for preparation of the ClickMTII derivative was the same, the cyclization strategy in this case was achieved through cycloaddition of the alkyne group of propargylglycine and the azide of an azido-modified lysine residue to form the triazole ring (Fig. 1). Following cyclization, peptides were deprotected and cleaved from the resin, purified by semipreparative HPLC, and characterized by LC–MS (data not shown).

To facilitate radiolabeling with ^{64}Cu and ^{68}Ga, a DOTA chelator was conjugated to the MTII and ClickMTII variants by standard methods. To conjugate DOTA to the *N*-terminus of MTII, the *N*-terminal Fmoc was left in place at the end of the peptide synthesis. The peptide was then treated with palladium catalyst and phenyltrihydrosilane for removal of the allyl and alloc protecting groups and cyclized as previously described (see Sect. 2.2, "Peptide Synthesis"). However, HPLC analysis of the *N*-terminal Fmoc-protected MTII peptide before cyclization by HPLC showed the presence of two major peaks, corresponding to the peptide with and without the *N*-terminal Fmoc (data not shown). Thus, difficulty in synthesizing an *N*-terminal Fmoc-protected MTII prevented smooth attachment of DOTA to this peptide, and alternative click chemistry strategies were pursued.

On the other hand, ClickMTII was synthesized smoothly without *N*-terminal acylation, facilitating DOTA addition to the free amine of the *N*-terminus. In this case, *N*-terminal Fmoc protection was not necessary as cyclization was carried out by click chemistry, which does not involve a primary amine. DOTA was then coupled to the peptide by formation of an amide bond between a carboxylic acid on DOTA and the primary amine of the *N*-terminus. DOTA-ClickMTII was finally deprotected and cleaved from the resin, purified by semipreparative HPLC, and characterized by LC–MS (Table 1).

In addition to the MTII and ClickMTII peptides, native α-MSH, NDP-α-MSH, and their *N*-terminal DOTA derivatives were prepared for use in in vitro experiments for structure–activity comparisons (Table 1). Preparative HPLC-purified peptides were rechromatographed on analytical RP-HPLC to establish structure on the basis of retention time and mass determined by LC–MS. For each purified peptide, a single major peak demonstrated >95% purity that also produced a singly charged positive ion in the ESI–MS corresponding to the calculated mass of the desired peptide (Table 1).

3.2 Radiolabeling

DOTA-GG-ClickMTII and ClickMTII-GGK-DOTA were radiolabeled with ^{64}Cu in acetate buffer (pH 6) for 45 min at 70°C. For ^{64}Cu, no further purification was required to obtain radiochemical purity of >98% with specific activity of >35 MBq nmole^{-1} peptide conjugate (FIG). Similar results were obtained for radiolabeling with ^{68}Ga. In this case, radiolabeling was conducted by elution of ^{68}Ga from a manual generator system. Following a radiolabeling step (5 ml water, pH 3.5, 15 min, 100°C), final purification of the ^{68}Ga-labeled peptides was performed using a disposable C_{18} reverse-phase cartridge. Radiochemical purity was routinely >98% with specific activities up to 45 MBq nmole^{-1} of peptide conjugate.

3.3 In Vitro Competitive Binding Assays

The ClickMTII peptide analogs, without and with DOTA, were evaluated for their binding affinity to melanocortin receptors in B16/F10 murine melanoma cells. Competitive binding assays were carried out using the radiolabeled ligand [^{125}I]-NDP-α-MSH and increasing amounts of α-MSH analog. Experiments were carried out in quadruplicate, and binding curves were plotted as the mean and standard error of the four sets of data (Fig. 2; Table 1). The uncertainties of these results are based on the standard deviation of the regression curve fit-derived affinity results of the quadruplicate measurements. MTII (closed circles) and ClickMTII (open circles) give similar curves, with IC_{50} values of 0.26 and 0.39 nM, respectively.

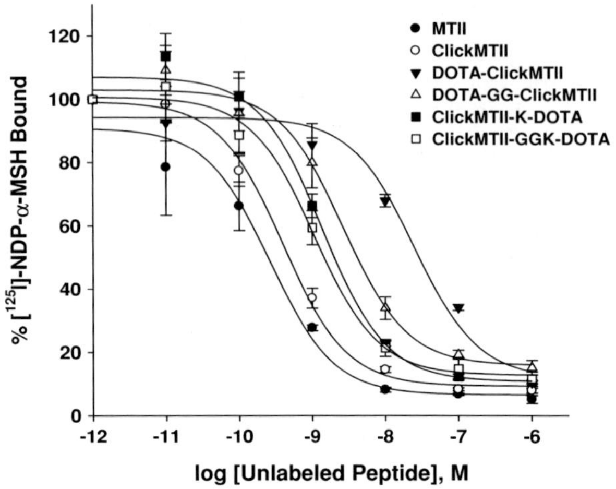

Fig. 2 Competitive inhibition of ^{125}I-NDP-α-MSH binding to B16/F10 murine melanocytes by α-MSH analogs. Competitive binding curves are the mean and standard error of quadruplicate experiments

Addition of DOTA to the *N*-terminus of ClickMTII (DOTA-ClickMTII; closed triangles) results in a 64-fold decrease in binding affinity and an IC_{50} of 25 nM. Due to the large increase in the IC_{50} with the addition of DOTA, three other analogs were synthesized to optimize the placement of DOTA. DOTA was conjugated to the *C*-terminus through the side-chain of an added lysine residue (ClickMTII-K-DOTA; $IC_{50} = 1.4$ nM). Two peptides were also synthesized with glycine spacers to see if the added distance between the DOTA and the peptide would increase binding affinity (DOTA-GG-ClickMTII and ClickMTII-GGK-DOTA; $IC_{50} = 2.7$ and 1.1 nM, respectively). Binding affinity data are summarized in Table 1.

3.4 Serum Stability

DOTA-conjugated peptides were radiolabeled with ^{64}Cu in pH 6.0 acetate buffer and used without further purification. Labeled peptides were added to human serum and incubated at 37°C to determine both the stability of the radionuclide within the DOTA complex and the stability of the peptide to serum proteases. At specified time points, samples were removed and analyzed by radioTLC as described in the experimental procedures. When spotted on the iTLC strip, intact [^{64}Cu]-DOTA-peptide remained where initially spotted, while free ^{64}Cu and peptide fragments migrated with variable retention characteristics with the solvent. Immediately upon addition of the peptides to the serum, a reference sample was taken of each peptide. At this zero time point, all [^{64}Cu]-DOTA-peptides remained intact and did not migrate with the solvent (Fig. 3). Analysis of the iTLC strips at

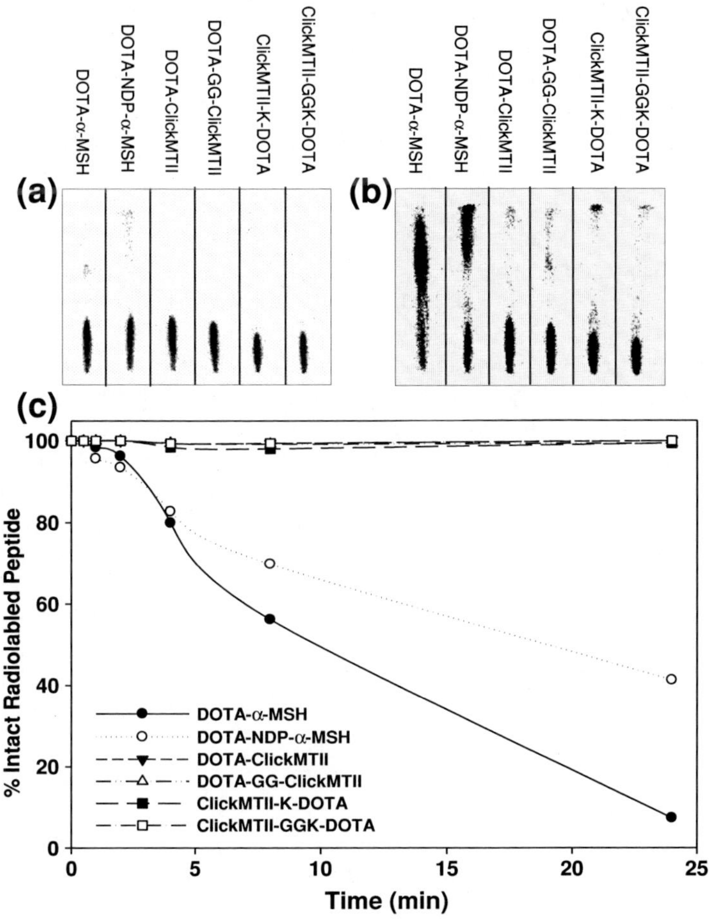

Fig. 3 Stability of [^{64}Cu]-DOTA-peptide analogs in human serum. Radiolabeled peptides were incubated in human serum at 37°C, and at specified time points samples were spotted on iTLC paper and developed with 0.1 M citric acid. **a** shows the peptides in serum at $t = 0$ min; all of the radiolabeled peptide remains at the bottom of the plate. By 24 h, the linear peptides α-MSH and NDP-α-MSH are degraded by the serum while the cyclic ClickMTII analogs remain intact (**b**). **c** graphically represents the degradation data over the 24 h time period for all peptides

24 h showed that a significant amount of both linear test peptides (DOTA-α-MSH and DOTA-NDP-α-MSH) were degraded by the serum, while the cyclized DOTA-ClickMTII analogs were intact (Fig. 3). The four DOTA-ClickMTII peptides remained stable throughout the entire 24-h experiment, while the linear DOTA-α-MSH and DOTA-NDP-α-MSH begin to degrade after 1 h in serum. By 24 h, only 7.4% of DOTA-α-MSH and 41% of NDP-α-MSH remained, while >99% of all four DOTA-conjugated cyclized ClickMTII analogs remained stable (Fig. 3; Table 1).

3.5 In Vivo Biodistribution and Imaging

The tumor targeting properties of the click-cyclized peptides for targeted molecular imaging were evaluated in tumor-bearing female SCID hairless mice. The in vivo biodistribution of DOTA-GG-ClickMTII and ClickMTII-GGK-DOTA were examined at 90 min post injection of 25–33 MBq ^{68}Ga-labeled DOTA-peptide conjugate. Receptor blocking studies were conducted for the DOTA-GG-Click-MTII derivative by co-injection of unlabeled NDP-α-MSH peptide to confirm receptor-mediated tumor accumulation of the tracers in vivo. The tumor accumulation was 16.0 $\pm$ 5.7% ID/g for DOTA-GG-ClickMTII and 10.2 $\pm$ 1.3% ID/g for ClickMTII-GGK-DOTA at 90 min post injection. Urinary excretion of the radiolabeled peptides was assessed by collection of urine in an absorbent pad during the uptake period. These results demonstrated fast pharmacokinetics with 78.8 $\pm$ 8.6% of the injected dose voided within the 90-min uptake period. Blocking studies reduced tumor uptake to 5 $\pm$ 0.9% ID/g of tumor tissue. Normal organ uptake of the tracers was low, with the highest values observed in kidney (5% ID/g), lung (5% ID/g), and heart (5% ID/g), with tumor:kidney ratio >3 for each DOTA-peptide conjugate at 90 min post injection. The tumor:blood ratios were 5.0 $\pm$ 3.4 for the DOTA-GG-MTII variant and 3.2 $\pm$ 1.1 for the MTII-GGK-DOTA derivative at 90 min post injection. Low liver retention was observed for both variants (1.1 $\pm$ 0.7% ID/g and 1.3 $\pm$ 0.1% ID/g respectively). Injection of $^{68}Ga^{3+}$ in saline produced a completely different biodistribution pattern indicative of relatively stable radiometal–DOTA coupling (Table 2).

4 Discussion

4.1 Click Cyclizations and Peptide Synthesis

We have prepared five cyclic α-MSH analogs with high affinity for MC1R and prolonged stability in human serum using copper-catalyzed click chemistry. Upregulation of cell surface receptor expression, such as melanocortin receptors, in cancer cells has been identified as a promising target for the development of targeted molecular imaging agents and tumor-targeting drugs. Many of the endogenous ligands of these receptors are peptides, such as α-MSH, which is the native peptide ligand for the melanocortin receptors. In its native form, a linear 13-amino-acid peptide, α-MSH is rapidly degraded and not very useful in the clinical realm. Alanine replacement scans led to the discovery of the "essential core" needed for receptor binding and bioactivity, along with replacements of Nle^4 and D-Phe^7 to give NDP-α-MSH with very high bioactivity combined with increased stability (Sawyer et al. 1980; Sahm et al. 1994; Cone 2000). The design of cyclic α-MSH analogs has further increased receptor binding affinities and biological stability (Al-Obeidi et al. 1989a, b). A variety of techniques have been utilized for cyclization of α-MSH peptides, the most common strategies being the

Table 2 In vivo biodistribution summary of ^{68}Ga-labeled DOTA-conjugated click-cyclized peptides[a]

	DOTA-GG-ClickMTII	DOTA-GG-ClickMTII (blocked)	ClickMTII-GGK-DOTA	Free $^{68}Ga^{3+}$
Tissue	% ID/g[b]	% ID/g	% ID/g	% ID/g
Blood	3.2 ± 1.0	3.6 ± 0.6	3.2 ± 1.0	12.5 ± 3.2
Heart	4.6 ± 2.5	1.8 ± 0.3	5.0 ± 0.2	5.4 ± 0.5
Liver	1.1 ± 0.7	2.5 ± 1.2	1.3 ± 0.1	2.0 ± 0.8
Kidney	4.7 ± 0.9	11.7 ± 2.1	5.4 ± 0.1	5.0 ± 0.6
Brain	2.3 ± 1.1	0.4 ± 0.1	1.3 ± 0.0	0.6 ± 0.0
Muscle	3.1 ± 1.8	1.7 ± 0.4	2.9 ± 0.4	2.6 ± 0.9
Lung	4.9 ± 1.3	3.8 ± 0.9	4.2 ± 0.5	6.9 ± 4.4
Tumor	16.0 ± 5.7	5.0 ± 0.9	10.2 ± 1.3	11.0 ± 2.2
Tumor:blood	5.0 ± 3.4	1.4 ± 0.7	3.2 ± 1.1	0.9 ± 2.7
Tumor:kidney	3.4 ± 3.3	0.4 ± 1.5	1.9 ± 0.7	2.2 ± 1.4
Tumor:liver	14.0 ± 3.2	2.0 ± 1.0	7.9 ± 0.7	5.4 ± 1.5
	% ID	% ID	% ID	% ID
Excretion	78.8 ± 8.6	61.7 ± 9.0	ND[c]	12.9 ± 1.7

Animals were injected via tail vein with approximately 25 MBq ^{68}Ga-labeled compound with specific activity >35 MBq nmole^{-1} and >98% radiochemical purity. Animals were sacrificed at 90 min post injection

[a] Mean ± S.D. ($n = 3$)

[b] % ID/g = percent injected dose per gram

[c] not determined

lactam bridge, disulfide coupling, and metal coordination (Miao et al. 2008; Cantorius et al. 2009; Guo et al. 2010, 2011). Cyclization restricts the peptide to a secondary structure designed to better fit the binding pocket of the receptor in hope of enhancing binding affinity, stability, and potentially even receptor selectivity (Raposinho et al. 2010).

In the present study, a novel class of cyclic α-MSH analogs has been synthesized utilizing cyclization by copper-catalyzed click chemistry. The aspartic acid has been substituted with propargylglycine, while the terminal-primary amine on the side-chain of the internal lysine has been replaced by an azide function. The Cu(I)-catalyzed Huisgen 1,3-dipolar cycloaddition of the alkyne and azide is a mild and selective bioconjugation reaction that forms a 1,4-disubstituted 1,2,3-triazole (Huisgen 1963). The triazole moiety has been described as an isosteric replacement for the amide bond (Brik et al. 2005; Bock et al. 2007). This study not only describes the potential advantages of the click chemistry approach for the cyclization reaction of a specific peptide molecular targeting vector, but also examines the effect of the triazole ring on binding of the small peptide to the melanocortin receptors as an alternative to lactam, disulfide, and other compositional cyclization constructs for molecular imaging and radionuclide therapy.

Based on the sequence of the cyclic peptide MTII, five ClickMTII analogs were prepared and tested for their binding affinity and serum stability as compared with the original MTII peptide (Table 1). MTII, a seven-amino-acid peptide containing the core residues His-D-Phe-Arg-Trp for receptor binding, was cyclized by a lactam bridge through the side-chains of aspartic acid and lysine. This required orthogonal protection of the peptide so that the Asp and Lys could be deprotected and cyclized while the rest of the peptide (side-chains and *N*-terminus) remained protected on the resin (Fig. 1). Following synthesis, the peptide was acylated on the *N*-terminus, the allyl/alloc groups were deprotected, the lactam bridge was formed on-resin, and the peptide was deprotected and cleaved from the resin. For cyclization by the click reaction, propargylglycine and azido-modified lysine were substituted for aspartic acid and lysine, respectively. As expected, the click chemistry approach did not require protection and subsequent deprotection at this step, greatly simplifying our synthetic strategy and potentially increasing our overall synthetic yields.

After solid-phase synthesis of the peptide, the *N*-terminus was acylated, the peptide was directly cyclized by addition of Cu(I) bromide (with ascorbate), and then deprotected and cleaved from the resin by standard techniques. In our hands, the alkyne and azide moieties are stable (unreactive) to all steps of the peptide synthesis and cyclization may be performed at any point in the reaction scheme without involving protecting group chemistry. For lactam bridge formation, cyclization was only possible on-resin prior to deprotection and cleavage so that cyclization occurred between the selected acid and amine groups. Cyclization of the *N*-terminal acylated MTII peptide by click reaction also proved more efficient than lactamization (Fig. 1). This means that the peptide could also be synthesized and then deprotected and cleaved from the resin with cyclization performed as a final step under mild aqueous conditions. It is expected that dilution could be used at this step to minimize dimerization if required.

In order to be useful as an in vivo imaging agent, a metal chelator was incorporated into the peptide sequence. DOTA is a 12-membered macrocyclic compound that is a prototype chelation moiety used for coupling of a variety of di- and trivalent metals (including ^{64}Cu) for both imaging and therapy. Numerous bifunctional derivatives are available for facile conjugation to peptides through the formation of an amide bond (as well as other potential bioconjugate strategies). DOTA positioning has been described previously to have a profound effect on the tumor targeting and kidney uptake characteristics of linear and cyclized α-MSH analogs (Froidevaux et al. 2004; Guo et al. 2009). For our investigation, we initially utilized the free amine of the *N*-terminus as an efficient connection point for MTII and ClickMTII analogs. Thus, both the lactam-bridge-cyclized MTII and click-cyclized ClickMTII peptides were synthesized without acylation of the *N*-terminus so that the free amine could serve as the point of attachment for

DOTA. In the case of MTII, to enable efficient cyclization, the *N*-terminus should remain Fmoc-protected during the allyl/alloc deprotection and subsequent lactam bridge cyclization. Based on previous studies, we expected that these orthogonal protecting groups would allow for the selective deprotection and cyclization to occur—through the side-chains of the aspartic acid and lysine—while preserving the *N*-terminal amine Fmoc protection (Bloomberg et al. 1993; Dessolin et al. 1995; Thieriet et al. 1997). However, in our hands, during the allyl/alloc deprotection step, a fraction of the Fmoc was removed from the *N*-terminus of peptide, exposing the terminal amine for potential reaction with the aspartic acid side-chain at the cyclization step (data not shown). This observation indicated the potential for reduced selectivity of the technique. This behavior was observed despite numerous minor modifications to our synthetic strategy, and the results prompted us to examine alternative strategies.

With this knowledge, our efforts turned solely to the more selective click chemistry approach to cyclization of DOTA-conjugated ClickMTII peptides. As mentioned above, the ClickMTII peptide sequence was prepared without *N*-terminal acylation. In addition, the *N*-terminus was left as a free amine as protection was not needed for cyclization by the click reaction. Following peptide synthesis, ClickMTII was cyclized by introduction of CuBr and sodium ascorbate (to preserve the catalytic monovalent Cu^{+} state), which is selective for the cycloaddition reaction of terminal alkynes with azide moieties. DOTA was then coupled to the *N*-terminus and the peptide was purified by semipreparative RP-HPLC, followed by characterization by LC–MS. When analyzed by RP-HPLC, the crude peptide (data not shown) had a major peak corresponding to the DOTA-conjugated cyclized peptide, with a greatly simplified synthetic process. The propargyl and azido amino acids required for cyclization of the peptide were stable to the solid-phase peptide synthesis reagents and are selective for the click cyclization and did not require orthogonal protecting groups. In addition, because the click reaction utilizes an internal azide (rather than an amine), the *N*-terminus could be Fmoc-deprotected following peptide synthesis without interfering with subsequent steps. Following synthesis, the crude peptide was purified by standard semipreparative RP-HPLC techniques in high purity (>95%). Overall, the synthesis of DOTA-ClickMTII required fewer steps and provided a more efficient pathway to formation of the cyclized peptide. These characteristics opened efficient avenues for synthesis of three other novel peptides based on the click cyclization (Table 1). Studies to optimize this process for the highest possible chemical yields are underway in our laboratories.

Previous reports demonstrate not only the profound effect of DOTA positioning on molecular targeting, but also the significant effect of the composition of chelator–amino acid linkers on the binding affinity and pharmacodynamic properties of peptide targeting vectors for molecular imaging (Garrison et al. 2008; Fragogeorgi et al. 2009; Guo et al. 2011). Three unique DOTA conjugates were prepared based on these findings. In an effort to increase the spacing between the DOTA and the peptide, a glycine spacer was added to afford *N*-terminal conjugated DOTA-GG-ClickMTII. A *C*-terminal end DOTA conjugate of the click-cyclized peptide was achieved by attachment to the ε-amine of a lysine residue placed at the *C*-terminus, ClickMTII-K-DOTA. Finally, a glycine spacer was added to the *C*-terminal DOTA derivative resulting in the conjugate ClickMTII-GGK-DOTA (Table 1). These conjugates were evaluated by in vitro cell binding assays, and the most promising candidates were further evaluated by in vivo biodistribution studies and finally by PET/CT imaging.

4.2 In Vitro Evaluation

4.2.1 Binding Affinity Assays

The lactam-cyclized MTII peptide and ClickMTII α-MSH analogs, along with DOTA-conjugated ClickMTII variants described above, were evaluated for selective binding to MC1R on B16/F10 murine melanoma cells in competitive binding assays (Fig. 2). While the affinity figure of merit IC_{50} was observed to be slightly elevated (lower affinity) for the click-cyclized ClickMTII peptide in comparison with the lactam-bridge-cyclized MTII (ClickMTII $IC_{50} = 0.39$ nM; MTII $IC_{50} = 0.26$ nM), the results were not statistically significant based on the uncertainty derived from $n = 4$ experimental runs for each peptide. These data suggest that replacement of the lactam bridge by a triazole ring does not significantly affect binding of the peptide to the receptors in B16/F10 cells. On the other hand, conjugation of DOTA directly to the *N*-terminus, DOTA-ClickMTII, resulted in a 64-fold increase in the IC_{50} over the ClickMTII peptide without DOTA (25 nM). This decrease in binding affinity indicated that DOTA was interfering with binding, possibly as a result of being too close to the core amino acids that interact with the binding pocket of the receptors, thereby impeding the docking reaction by steric hindrance. To test this hypothesis, a glycine spacer was added to increase the distance between the binding domain of the peptide and the DOTA moiety. The effect on binding for the resulting derivative (DOTA-GG-ClickMTII) was a reduction in the observed IC_{50} by a factor of 9 to a value of 2.7 nM, which is comparable to previously reported values for lactam-bridge-cyclized DOTA-conjugated α-MSH analogs (1.77 nM, Guo et al. 2010; 2.1 nM, Guo et al. 2011). Attachment at the *C*-terminus, ClickMTII-K-DOTA, gave an IC_{50} of 1.4 nM, which was lowered to 1.1 nM in ClickMTII-GGK-DOTA with the addition of a glycine spacer. These binding measurements compare favorably with high-affinity linear peptide derivatives DOTA-α-MSH and DOTA-NDP-α-MSH (IC_{50} 2.1 and 0.59 nM, respectively) and are similar to binding affinities of linear variants reported by Froidevaux et al. (1.37 nM, Froidevaux et al. 2004; see Table 1). Thus, the three novel analogs DOTA-GG-ClickMTII, ClickMTII-K-DOTA, and Click-MTII-GGK-DOTA show promise as potential imaging agents with comparable binding affinities based on in vitro competitive receptor affinity assessment.

4.2.2 Serum Stability Comparisons

DOTA-conjugated peptides were also tested for their stability in human serum (Fig. 3). A method was developed that enabled efficient qualitative examination of the stability of the peptide constructs in serum—with operationally defined quantitative information about the stability of the ^{64}Cu-DOTA complexation and fragmentation of the peptide obtained by examining the migration of radioactivity signal on iTLC strips. Further experimental details of the method development can be obtained in Rockey et al. (2011). Peptides were radiolabeled with ^{64}Cu and incubated with human serum to test for stability of the radionuclide within the DOTA chelator and the stability of the peptide to serum proteases. As expected and based on the migration of apparent peptide fragments, the linear-peptide forms DOTA-α-MSH and DOTA-NDP-α-MSH were relatively unstable in serum, with only 7.4% and 41% of the radioactivity signal remaining at iTLC strip origin at the 24-h sampling timepoint, respectively. α-MSH is known to have a half-life of less than 3 min in vivo, so while the DOTA may stabilize it from some proteases, relatively rapid degradation in serum is expected. DOTA-NDP-α-MSH, while more biologically stabile due to the amino acid substitutions and DOTA conjugation, as a linear peptide is expected to be susceptible to serum proteases and with enough time is expected to be degraded, albeit at a slower rate. In contrast, but in agreement with previously reported lactam-bridge-cyclized α-MSH analogs (Guo et al. 2010), all four click-cyclized DOTA-conjugated (ClickMTII) analogs appeared to remain stable for at least 24 h in human serum (>99% intact radiolabeled peptides), and the ^{64}Cu-DOTA complex remained stable as well. Thus, from analysis of the iTLC strips, the DOTA-conjugated ClickMTII peptides were not significantly degraded by serum proteases within 24 h, and they were also able to retain the ^{64}Cu within the DOTA chelator. This is in contrast to linear DOTA-α-MSH and DOTA-NDP-α-MSH, which appear as a degraded "smear" on the iTLC strip at 24 h (Fig. 3).

4.3 In Vivo Biodistributions and PET Imaging

The tumor targeting properties of the click-cyclized peptides for targeted molecular imaging were evaluated in tumor-bearing female SCID mice. The in vivo biodistribution of DOTA-GG-ClickMTII and ClickMTII-GGK-DOTA were examined at 90 min post injection of 25–33 MBq ^{68}Ga-labeled DOTA-peptide conjugate. Receptor blocking studies were conducted for the DOTA-GG-ClickMTII derivative by co-injection of unlabeled NDP-α-MSH peptide to confirm receptor-mediated tumor accumulation of the tracers in vivo. The results are comparable to previous investigations of similar lactam-bridge and stable-metal-cyclized α-MSH analogs (Miao et al. 2008; Guo et al. 2009, 2010, 2011; Cantorias et al. 2009), indicating that the triazole linkage is an effective replacement for the lactam bridge for peptide cyclization. The tumor accumulation was 16.0 ± 5.7% ID/g for *N*-terminal DOTA-conjugate DOTA-GG-ClickMTII and 10.2 ± 1.3% ID/g for *C*-terminal DOTA-modified ClickMTII-GGK-DOTA at 90 min post injection. A reduced-ring-size lactam-bridge variant presented by Guo et al. (2010) appears to have advantages over all other such cyclized derivatives, with tumor accumulation of greater than 24% ID/g of tumor tissue reported. These results and our findings suggest that further modifications to the click cyclization approach could result in improved tumor targeting characteristics, which is the subject of continued investigation in our laboratories. Urinary excretion of the radiolabeled peptides was assessed by collection of urine during the uptake period. These results demonstrated fast pharmacokinetics, with $78.8 \pm 8.6\%$ of the injected dose voided by urinary excretion within the 90-min uptake period, which is comparable to previously reported pharmacokinetic behavior of cyclized α-MSH analogs (Miao et al. 2008; Guo et al. 2009, 2010, 2011; Cantorias et al. 2009). Blocking studies reduced tumor uptake to $5 \pm 0.9\%$ ID/g, demonstrating that tumor accumulation of the examined peptide derivatives is receptor mediated. Interestingly, blocking to 5% ID/g required co-injection of nearly 500 μg cold NDP-α-MSH. Based on a comparison of our blocking results with other studies reported, it appears that the B16/F10 cell line cultured in our laboratory possesses higher receptor density than the B16/F1 cell line used for studies presented by others, which is the subject of further investigation. Normal organ uptake of the tracers was low and similar to recent reports of other DOTA-modified cyclized α-MSH analogs, with the highest values observed in kidney (5% ID/g), lung (5% ID/g), and heart (5% ID/g) with tumor:kidney ratio >3 for each DOTA-peptide conjugate at 90 min post injection. The tumor:blood ratios were 5.0 ± 3.4 for the DOTA-GG-MTII variant and 3.2 ± 1.1 for the MTII-GGK-DOTA derivative at 90 min post injection. Low liver retention was observed for both variants ($1.1 \pm 0.7\%$ ID/g and $1.3 \pm 0.1\%$ ID/g, respectively) labeled with ^{68}Ga. Injection of $^{68}Ga^{3+}$ in saline produced a completely different biodistribution pattern, indicative of relatively stable radiometal–DOTA coupling. The two most similar lactam-bridge-cyclized DOTA conjugates examined for comparison (Guo et al. 2010, 2011) were evaluated at 30 min and 120 min post injection, while our results were evaluated in this preliminary investigation at 90 min post injection. Interestingly, the tumor:normal ratios reported here are roughly intermediate to the time points presented elsewhere, suggesting that the click-cyclized variants display similar behavior to lactam-bridge-cyclized derivatives of α-MSH.

Good tumor accumulation properties observed for the DOTA-GG-ClickMTII variant prompted us to examine the potential of this α-MSH analog for in vivo PET imaging. These studies were carried out by tail vein injection of approximately 18.5 MBq ^{68}Ga-labeled DOTA-GG-ClickMTII and imaging at 90 min post injection. Excellent tumor contrast was observed with clear tumor visualization of MC1R-positive B16/F10 tumor xenograft (Fig. 4). The PET/CT image reveals rapid tumor accumulation and renal excretion of the click-cyclized peptide with only tumor, kidneys, and bladder apparent in the whole-body field of view of the PET/CT image (Fig. 4). Tumor contrast observed for this investigation is excellent and comparable to previously reported findings for lactam-bridge-cyclized α-MSH (Miao et al. 2008; Guo et al. 2009, 2010, 2011; Cantorias et al. 2009).

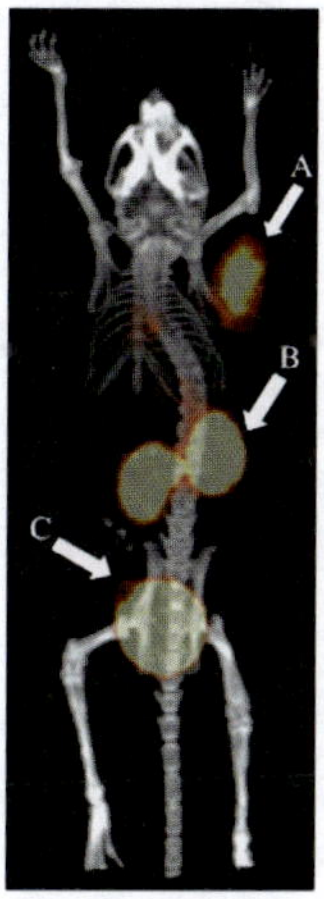

Fig. 4 PET/CT image of the biodistribution of [^{68}Ga]DOTA-GG-MTII; 35 MBq radiolabeled peptide; tail vein injection; 90 min accumulation period; 15 min static acquisition: **a** xenograft B16-F10 mouse melanoma tumor, **b** kidney accumulation and retention, and **c** bladder accumulation and retention. The average and standard deviation of the biodistribution of [^{68}Ga]DOTA-GG-MTII are given in Table 2

5 Summary and Conclusions

A novel class of cyclized MTII-type α-MSH peptide analogs have been synthesized and cyclized by Cu(I)-catalyzed terminal azide-alkyne cycloaddition "click" chemistry techniques. Three new DOTA-conjugated analogs—DOTA-GG-Click-MTII, ClickMTII-K-DOTA, and ClickMTII-GGK-DOTA—have exhibited <2 nM affinity for MC1R receptor-positive malignant cells in vitro and high stability in human serum. The DOTA-GG-ClickMTII variant was further evaluated by PET imaging in a xenograft mouse model of melanoma. Thus, these click-chemistry-cyclized variants show promise as agents for melanocortin receptor-targeted imaging and radionuclide therapy. These results indicate that the triazole ring is an effective bioisosteric replacement for the lactam bridge in cyclization of the MTII peptide, as ClickMTII has affinity for receptor-positive cells comparable to that of MTII (cyclized by lactamization). Radiolabeling results confirm that Cu catalyst is sufficiently removed prior to DOTA chelator addition to enable preparation with sufficient radiochemical purity (>98%) and high specific activity (>35 MBq nmole^{-1}) for molecular imaging applications. Cyclization by this click chemistry strategy is advantageous for this application because it obviates the need for protecting groups required for standard lactam bridge formation used in previous approaches to cyclizing α-MSH analogs. Both the propargylglycine and azido-lysine residues are stabile to all steps of the peptide synthesis and selective for the click cyclization, so side-chain protection/deprotection is not necessary. The click cyclization approach is a valuable tool for preparation of DOTA-conjugated peptides for molecular imaging and radionuclide therapy.

Acknowledgments Support for this work was provided by the American Cancer Society (IRG-77004-31; M.K.S.), the Holden Comprehensive Cancer Center (M.E.M., M.K.S.), Neuroendocrine Tumor Fund (M.S.O.), and University of Iowa Dance Marathon (M.E.M.). M.E.M. is supported by T32 University of Iowa Institutional Training Grant in Hematologic and Oncologic Childhood Diseases (HL080070). The authors thank Dr. Kevin Rice, Dr. Lynn Teesch, and Vic Parcell for spirited assistance with mass spectral analyses.

References

Al-Obeidi F, Castrucci AMDL, Hadley ME, Hruby VJ (1989a) Potent and prolonged-acting cyclic lactam analogs of α-melanotropin: design based on molecular dynamics. J Med Chem 32(12):2555–2561. doi:10.1021/jm00132a010

Al-Obeidi F, Hadley ME, Pettitt BM, Hruby VJ (1989b) Design of a new class of superpotent cyclic α-melanotropins based on quenched dynamic simulations. J Am Chem Soc 111(9):3413–3416. doi:10.1021/ja00191a044

Anderson CJ, Wadas TJ, Wong EH, Weisman GR (2008) Cross-bridged macrocyclic chelators for stable complexation of copper radionuclides for PET imaging. Q J Nucl Med Mol Imag 52(2):185–192. doi:R39072063

Bednarek MA, Macneil T, Kalyani RN, Tang R, Van der Ploeg LHT, Weinberg DH (1999a) Analogs of MTII, lactam derivatives of α-melanotropin, modified at the N-terminus and their selectivity at human melanocortin receptors 3, 4, and 5. Biochem Biophys Res Commun 261(1):209–213

Bednarek MA, MacNeil T, Kalyani RN, Tang R, Van der Ploeg LHT, Weinberg DH (2000) Analogs of lactam derivatives of α-melanotropin with basic and acidic residues. Biochem Biophys Res Commun 272(1):23–28

Bednarek MA, MacNeil T, Tang R, Fong TM, Angeles Cabello M, Maroto M, Teran A (2007a) Potent and selective peptide agonists of α-melanocyte stimulating hormone (αMSH) action at human melanocortin receptor 5; their synthesis and biological evaluation in vitro. Chem Biol Drug Des 69(5):350–355. doi:10.1111/j.1747-0285.2007.00513.x

Bednarek MA, MacNeil T, Tang R, Fong TM, Cabello MA, Maroto M, Teran A (2007b) Potent and selective agonists of human melanocortin receptor 5: cyclic analogues of α-melanocyte-stimulating hormone. J Med Chem 50(10):2520–2526. doi:10.1021/jm0614275

Bednarek MA, Silva MV, Arison B, MacNeil T, Kalyani RN, Huang RR, Weinberg DH (1999b) Structure-function studies on the cyclic peptide MT-II, lactam derivative of alpha-melanotropin. Peptides 20(3):401–409. doi:10.1016/S0196-9781(99)00048-0

Bloomberg GB, Askin D, Gargaro AR, Tanner MJA (1993) Synthesis of a branched cyclic peptide using a strategy employing Fmoc chemistry and two additional orthogonal protecting groups. Tetrahedron Lett 34(29):4709–4712

Bock VD, Speijer D, Hiemstra H, van Maarseveen JH (2007) 1,2,3-Triazoles as peptide bond isosteres: synthesis and biological evaluation of cyclotetrapeptide mimics. Org Biomol Chem 5(6):971–975

Boswell CA, Regino CA, Baidoo KE, Wong KJ, Bumb A, Xu H, Milenic DE, Kelley JA, Lai CC, Brechbiel MW (2008) Synthesis of a cross-bridged cyclam derivative for peptide conjugation and ^{64}Cu radiolabeling. Bioconjugate Chem 19(7):1476–1484. doi:10.1021/bc800039e

Brechbiel MW (2008) Bifunctional chelates for metal nuclides. Q J Nucl Med Mol Imag 52(2):166–173

Brik A, Alexandratos J, Lin Y-C, Elder JH, Olson AJ, Wlodawer A, Goodsell DS, Wong C-H (2005) 1,2,3-Triazole as a peptide surrogate in the rapid synthesis of HIV-1 protease inhibitors. Chem BioChem 6(7):1167–1169. doi:10.1002/cbic.200500101

Cai M, Cai C, Mayorov AV, Xiong C, Cabello CM, Soloshonok VA, Swift JR, Trivedi D, Hruby VJ (2004) Biological and conformational study of β-substituted prolines in MT-II template: steric effects leading to human MC5 receptor selectivity*. J Pept Res 63(2):116–131. doi:10.1111/j.1399-3011.2003.00105.x

Cantorias MV, Figueroa SD, Quinn TP, Lever JR, Hoffman TJ, Watkinson LD, Carmack TL, Cutler CS (2009) Development of high-specific-activity ^{68}Ga-labeled DOTA-rhenium-cyclized α-MSH peptide analog to target MC1 receptors overexpressed by melanoma tumors. Nucl Med Biol 36(5):505–513

Cone RD (ed) (2000) The melanocortin receptors. Humana, Totowa

Cowell SM, Balse-Srinivasan PM, Ahn JM, Hruby VJ (2002) Design and synthesis of peptide antagonists and inverse agonists for G protein-coupled receptors. Methods Enzymol 343:49–72

Dessolin M, Guillerez M-G, Thieriet N, Guibé F, Loffet A (1995) New allyl group acceptors for palladium catalyzed removal of allylic protections and transacylation of allyl carbamates. Tetrahedron Lett 36(32):5741–5744

Eberle AN, Froidevaux S (2003) Radiolabeled α-melanocyte-stimulating hormone analogs for receptor-mediated targeting of melanoma: from tritium to indium. J Mol Recognit 16(5): 248–254. doi:10.1002/jmr.633

Eberle AN, Verin VJ, Solca F, Siegrist W, Kuenlin C, Bagutti C, Stutz S, Girard J (1991) Biologically active monoiodinated α-MSH derivatives for receptor binding studies using human melanoma cells. J Recept Res 11(1–4):311–322

Fani M, Mueller A, Tamma M-L, Nicolas G, Rink HR, Cescato R, Reubi JC, Maecke HR (2010) Radiolabeled bicyclic somatostatin-based analogs: a novel class of potential radiotracers for SPECT/PET of neuroendocrine tumors. J Nucl Med 51(11):1771–1779. doi:10.2967/jnumed.110.076695

Fragogeorgi EA, Zikos C, Gourni E, Bouziotis P, Paravatou-Petsotas M, Loudos G, Mitsokapas N, Xanthopoulos S, Mavri-Vavayanni M, Livaniou E, Varvarigou AD, Archimandritis SC (2009) Spacer site modifications for the improvement of the in vitro and in vivo binding properties of 99 mTc-N3S-X-Bombesin[2–14] derivatives. Bioconjugate Chem 20:856–867

Froidevaux S, Calame-Christe M, Schuhmacher J, Tanner H, Saffrich R, Henze M, Eberle AN (2004) A gallium-labeled DOTA-α-melanocyte- stimulating hormone analog for PET imaging of melanoma metastases. J Nucl Med 45(1):116–123

Garrison JC, Rold TL, Sieckman GL, Naz F, Sublett SV, Figueroa AD, Volkert WA, Hoffman TJ (2008) Evaluation of the pharmacokinetic effects of various linking groups using the ^{111}In-DOTA-X-BBN(7–14)NH_2 structural paradigm in prostate cancer model. Bioconjugate Chem 19:1803–1812

Ghanem GE, Comunale G, Libert A, Vercammen-Grandjean A, Lejeune FJ (1988) Evidence for alpha-melanocyte-stimulating hormone (α-MSH) receptors on human malignant melanoma cells. Int J Cancer 41(2):248–255. doi:10.1002/ijc.2910410216

Grieco P, Cai M, Liu L, Mayorov A, Chandler K, Trivedi D, Lin G, Campiglia P, Novellino E, Hruby VJ (2008) Design and microwave-assisted synthesis of novel macrocyclic peptides active at melanocortin receptors: discovery of potent and selective hMC5R receptor antagonists. J Med Chem 51(9):2701–2707. doi:10.1021/jm701181n

Guo H, Yang J, Gallazzi F, Prosnitz ER, Sklar LA, Miao Y (2009) Effect of DOTA position on melanoma targeting and pharmacokinetic properties of ^{111}In-labeled lactam bridge-cyclized α-MSH peptide. Bioconjugate Chem 20:2162–2168

Guo H, Yang J, Gallazzi F, Miao Y (2010) Reduction of the ring size of radiolabeled lactam bridge-cyclized α-MSH peptide, resulting in enhanced melanoma uptake. J Nucl Med 51(3):418–426. doi:10.2967/jnumed.109.071787

Guo H, Yang J, Gallazzi F, Miao Y (2011) Effects of the amino acid linkers on the melanoma-targeting and pharmacokinetic properties of ^{111}In-labeled lactam bridge-cyclized α-MSH peptide. J Nucl Med 52:608–616. doi:10.2967/jnumed.110.086009

Harris JI, Lerner AB (1957) Amino-acid sequence of the [alpha]-melanocyte-stimulating hormone. Nature 179(4574):1346–1347

Hausner SH, Kukis DL, Gagnon MK, Stanecki CE, Ferdani R, Marshall JF, Anderson CJ, Sutcliffe JL (2009) Evaluation of [^{64}Cu]Cu-DOTA and [^{64}Cu]Cu-CB-TE2A chelates for targeted positron emission tomography with an alphavbeta6-specific peptide. Mol Imaging 8(2):111–121

Heppeler A, Froidevaux S, Eberle AN, Maecke HR (2000) Receptor targeting for tumor localisation and therapy with radiopeptides. Curr Med Chem 7:971–994

Hruby VJ, Cai M, Grieco P, Han G, Kavarana M, Trivedi DEV (2003) Exploring the stereostructural requirements of peptide ligands for the melanocortin receptors. Ann N Y Acad Sci 994(1):12–20. doi:10.1111/j.1749-6632.2003.tb03157.x

Hruby VJ, Wilkes BC, Hadley ME, Al-Obeidi F, Sawyer TK, Staples DJ, DeVaux AE, Dym O, Castrucci AMdL (1987) α-Melanotropin: the minimal active sequence in the frog skin bioassay. J Med Chem 30(11):2126–2130. doi:10.1021/jm00394a033

Huisgen R (1963) 1,3-Dipolar cycloadditions. Past and future. Angew Chem Int Ed 2(10): 565–598. doi:10.1002/anie.196305651 (in English)

Kaiser E, Colescott RL, Bossinger CD, Cook PI (1970) Color test for detection of free terminal amino groups in the solid-phase synthesis of peptides. Anal Biochem 34(2):595–598

Lunec J, Pieron C, Thody AJ (1992) MSH receptor expression and the relationship to melanogenesis and metastatic activity in B16 melanoma. Melanoma Res May 2(1):5–12

Mayorov AV, Cai M, Chandler KB, Petrov RR, Van Scoy AR, Yu Z, Tanaka DK, Trivedi D, Hruby VJ (2006a) Development of cyclic Î^{3}-MSH analogues with selective hMC3R agonist and hMC3R/hMC5R antagonist activities. J Med Chem 49(6):1946–1952. doi:10.1021/jm0510326

Mayorov AV, Han S-Y, Cai M, Hammer MR, Trivedi D, Hruby VJ (2006b) Effects of macrocycle size and rigidity on melanocortin receptor-1 and -5 selectivity in cyclic lactam α-melanocyte-stimulating hormone analogs. Chem Biol Drug Des 67(5):329–335. doi: 10.1111/j.1747-0285.2006.00383.x

Miao Y, Gallazzi F, Guo H, Quinn TP (2008) ^{111}In-labeled lactam bridge-cyclized α-melanocyte stimulating hormone peptide analogues for melanoma imaging. Bioconjugate Chem 19(2):539–547. doi:10.1021/bc700317w

Nestor JJ Jr (2009) The medicinal chemistry of peptides. Curr Med Chem 16:4399–4418

Okarvi SM (2004) Synthesis, radiolabeling and in vitro and in vivo characterization of a technetium-99 m-labeled alpha-M2 peptide as a tumor imaging agent. J Pept Res 63(6): 460–468. doi:10.1111/j.1399-3011.2004.00160.x

Raposinho PD, Correia JDG, Oliveira MC, Santos I (2010) Melanocortin-1 receptor-targeting with radiolabeled cyclic α-melanocyte-stimulating hormone analogs for melanoma imaging. Pept Sci 94(6):820–829. doi:10.1002/bip.21490

Rockey WM, Huang L, Kloepping KC, Baumhover NJ, Giangrande PH, Schultz MK (2011) Synthesis and radiolabeling of chelator-RNA aptamer bioconjugates with copper-64 for targeted molecular imaging. Bioorg Med Chem 19(13):4080–4090 (July 1)

Sahm UG, Olivier GWJ, Branch SK, Moss SH, Pouton CW (1994) Synthesis and biological evaluation of [alpha]-MSH analogues substituted with alanine. Peptides 15(7):1297–1302

Sawyer TK, Sanfilippo PJ, Hruby VJ, Engel MH, Heward CB, Burnett JB, Hadley ME (1980) 4-Norleucine, 7-d-phenylalanine-alpha-melanocyte-stimulating hormone: a highly potent alpha-melanotropin with ultra long biological activity. Proc Natl Acad Sci U S A 77(10): 5754–5758

Siegrist W, Oestreicher M, Stutz S, Girard J, Eberle AN (1988) Radioreceptor assay for α-MSH using mouse B16 melanoma cells. J Recept Res 8(1–4):323–343

Sugg EE, De L, Castrucci AM, Hadley ME, Van Binst G, Hruby VJ (1988) Cyclic lactam analogs of Ac-[Nle4].alpha.-MSH4-11-NH_2. Biochemistry 27(21):8181–8188. doi:10.1021/bi00421a029

Tatro JB, Entwistle ML, Lester BR, Reichlin S (1990) Melanotropin receptors of murine melanoma characterized in cultured cells and demonstrated in experimental tumors in situ. Cancer Res 50(4):1237–1242

Thieriet N, Alsina J, Giralt E, Guibé F, Albericio F (1997) Use of alloc-amino acids in solid-phase peptide synthesis. Tandem deprotection-coupling reactions using neutral conditions. Tetrahedron Lett 38(41):7275–7278

Turner RA, Oliver AG, Lokey RS (2007) Click chemistry as a macrocyclization tool in the solid-phase synthesis of small cyclic peptides. Org Lett 9(24):5011–5014. doi:10.1021/ol702228u

Vlieghe P, Lisowski V, Martinez J, Khrestchatisky M (2010) Synthetic therapeutic peptides: science and market. Drug Discovery Today 15(1–2):40–56

Ying J, Gu X, Cai M, Dedek M, Vagner J, Trivedi DB, Hruby VJ (2006) Design, synthesis, and biological evaluation of new cyclic melanotropin peptide analogues selective for the human melanocortin-4 receptor. J Med Chem 49(23):6888–6896. doi:10.1021/jm060768f

Zwanziger D, Beck-Sickinger AG (2008) Radiometal targeted tumor diagnosis and therapy with peptide hormones. Curr Pharm Des 14:2385–2400

Early Experience with ^{68}Ga-DOTATATE Preparation

Maung Maung Saw

Abstract

Neuroendocrine tumors (NETs) are a rare form of cancer. NETs frequently express cell membrane-specific peptide receptors, such as somatostatin receptors (SSTRs). Radiolabeled peptides bind to SSTR and provide in vivo histopathological information for diagnostic purposes. ^{68}Ga-DOTATATE has higher sensitivity for low-grade tumors and greater avidity to well-differentiated NETs than ^{18}F-FDG, being superior to ^{111}In-DTPA-octreotide and ^{18}F-DOPA in evaluation of well-differentiated metastatic NETs. The feasibility of ^{68}Ga-DOTATATE application in routine clinical practice for PET imaging of NETs was determined in a limited number of known cases ($n = 6$). ^{68}Ga-DOTATATE scan could detect all known sites of NETs and in one case previously unknown peritoneal metastasis. Early regulatory consideration is important for routine clinical use.

Contents

M. M. Saw (✉)
Clinical Imaging Research Centre, National University of Singapore,
14 Medical Drive, #B1 01/02, 117599 Singapore, Singapore
e-mail: medmms@nus.edu.sg

R. P. Baum and F. Rösch (eds.), *Theranostics, Gallium-68, and Other Radionuclides*,
Recent Results in Cancer Research 194, DOI: 10.1007/978-3-642-27994-2_10,

1 Introduction

Cancer is the second major cause of death in Singapore. The crude annual cancer death rate was 103.9 per 100,000 in 2003–2007. Neuroendocrine tumors (NETs) are not in the top 10 cancer killers in Singapore. For the age group of 0–14 years, endocrine tumors constitute 5.4% of male cancers and 3.3% of cancers in females. NETs constitute 1.2% of the endocrine tumor incidence rate for all age groups (Trends in Cancer Incidence in Singapore 1968). The number of histologically proven NET cases in Singapore from the period 1998–2007 is presented in Table 1.

NETs are defined as epithelial neoplasms with predominant neuroendocrine differentiation, arising in most organs of the body (Modlin et al. 2008). NETs constitute a heterogeneous group of tumors that frequently express cell membrane-specific peptide receptors, such as somatostatin receptors (SSTRs) (Kaltsas et al. 2005). At least five SSTR subtypes have been identified (SSTRs 1–5) (Reisine and Bell 1995). Of NETs, 70–90% express SSTR-2 and SSTR-5 (Papotti et al. 2002). Diagnosis of NET primaries and metastases is challenging, as these lesions are small in size with variation in many anatomical locations. Radiolabeled peptides bind to SSTR and provide in vivo histopathological information for diagnostic purposes (Signore et al. 2001). Peptides have fast clearance, rapid tissue penetration, and low antigenicity, features making them suitable as good targeting molecules for radiopharmaceuticals.

The commonest tracer for SPECT imaging is commercially available ^{111}In-DTPA-octreotide (^{111}In-Octreoscan®) with detection sensitivity of 67–100% (Kaltsas et al. 2001, 2004). Diagnostic sensitivity of ^{18}F-FDG is low for tumors with low proliferation index, slow growth rate, and low glucose consumption such as NETs (Adams et al. 1998; Belhocine et al. 2002). Many ^{68}Ga radiopharmaceuticals have been used for SSTR imaging. The efficiency of PET tracer ^{68}Ga-DOTATOC for detecting NETs is better than that of ^{111}In-Octreoscan® (Buchmann et al. 2007). ^{68}Ga-DOTATOC is superior to ^{111}In-DTPA-octreotide in detecting small tumors and tumors with low-density SSTR expression (Kowalski et al. 2003). Superior imaging quality of PET is attributed to improved detection by ^{68}Ga-DOTATOC (Hofmann et al. 2001).

Table 1 Number of NET cases by anatomic site (1998–2007)

Site	Number of cases (histology–neuroendocrine cancer)			
	1998–2002	2003–2007	1998–2007	Percentage of tumor of the site
Nasopharynx (ICD-9 147)	3	3	6	0.2
Esophagus (ICD-9 150)	3	3	6	0.7
Stomach (ICD-9 151)	19	20	39	0.9
Small intestine (ICD-9 152)	13	21	34	12.6
Colon (ICD-9 153)	39	46	85	1.1
Rectum and anus (ICD-9 154)	65	101	166	3.2
Liver (ICD-9 155)	3	1	4	0.3
Gall blabber and extrahepatic bile duct (ICD-9 156)	2	3	5	0.8
Pancreas (ICD-9 157)	8	22	30	2.8
Retroperitoneum and peritoneum (ICD-9 158)	1	0	1	0.7
Nasal cavities and sinuses (ICD-9 160)	5	3	8	3.4
Larynx (ICD-9 161)	1	2	3	0.4
Lung (ICD-9 162)	59	51	110	1.2
Thymus and mediastinum (ICD-9 164)	6	3	9	4
Skin excluding melanoma (ICD-9 173)	2	0	2	0.1
Female breast (ICD-9 174)	4	8	12	0.1
Cervix uteri (ICD-9 180)	11	8	19	0.9
Corpus uteri (ICD-9 182)	3	2	5	0.2
Ovary and uterine adnexa (ICD-9 183)	1	4	5	0.2
Vagina and vulva (ICD-9 184)	0	1	1	0.5
Prostate (ICD-9 185)	0	4	4	0.1
Bladder (ICD-9 188)	6	1	7	0.4
Other endocrine glands (ICD-9 194)	1	1	2	1.2

ICD International Classification of Disease

There is great interest in use of ^{68}Ga radiopharmaceuticals due to:

1. The availability of ^{68}Ga from a ^{68}Ge/^{68}Ga generator
2. Superior imaging quality of ^{68}Ga–SSTR analogs over ^{111}In-DTPA-octreotide
3. Potential to switch to therapy with ^{177}Lu and ^{90}Y (theranostics)
4. Possibility of the availability of cold kits

5. As an alternative PET radioisotope to cyclotron-based $^{18}F^{-}$
6. As a PET equivalent to ^{99m}Tc radiopharmaceuticals for SPECT.

The parent, ^{68}Ge with half-life of 270.8 days, is produced by accelerator. ^{68}Ga has half-life of 68 min and decays by β^{+}_{max} of 1.92 MeV (89%) and electron capture (11%) (Maecke et al. 2005). A number of $^{68}Ge/^{68}Ga$ generator systems have been developed, with their unique advantages and disadvantages. The ^{68}Ga generator with calcinated hydrous tin dioxide column has been in use for many years with average yield of 65%. ^{68}Ge breakthrough was reported to be 6.1×10^{-4}% (Aardaneh and van der Walt 2006).

^{68}Ga-DOTATATE has higher sensitivity for low-grade tumors and greater avidity to well-differentiated NETs than ^{18}F-FDG, which shows greater avidity to poorly differentiated NETs (Kayani et al. 2008). ^{68}Ga-DOTATATE can identify additional lesions in patients with negative or equivocal ^{111}In-DTPA-octreotide scans. It shows good lesion recognition in low-grade tumors and changes clinical management in 70.6% of patients (Srirajaskanthan et al. 2010). ^{68}Ga-DOTATATE is superior to ^{18}F-DOPA PET in evaluation of well-differentiated metastatic NETs (Haug et al. 2009).

The aim of this study is to determine feasibility of ^{68}Ga-DOTATATE application in routine clinical practice for PET imaging of NETs in a limited number of patients ($n = 6$).

2 Materials and Methods

2.1 DOTA-Tyr^3-Octreotate

DOTA-Tyr^3-octreotate was purchased commercially (DOTA-dPhe-Cys-Tyr-dTrp-Lys-Thr-Cys-Thr-OH; molecular formula: $C_{65}H_{90}N_{14}O_{19}S_2$; molecular weight: 1,435.6; purity (HPLC): >99%; peptide content: 86.8%). DOTATATE vials were prepared in house. A peptide vial contained 62.5 μg peptide, 0.25 mg gentisic acid, and 25 μL glacial acetic acid.

2.2 $^{68}Ge/^{68}Ga$ Generator

Gallium generator (30 mCi) was purchased from iThamba and eluted with 0.6 M HCl (ultrapure). The elution profile was determined with 0.5 mL fractions of 0.6 M HCl for 10 mL, upon receipt of the generator. The generator was pre-eluted 2 h prior to the radiolabeling process with 5 mL 0.6 M HCl to flush impurities. The generator was eluted with three fractions of 0.6 M HCl (first 1 mL, second 1.5 mL, third 7.5 mL; fractionation method). The second, 1.5 mL fraction was collected for radiolabeling, whereas the first and third fractions were discarded.

2.3 ^{68}Ga Radiolabeling

Generator eluate (second 1.5 mL, pH 1) was added to a peptide vial, and the pH of the solution was immediately adjusted to 3.8–4.0 by adding 1 M sodium acetate solution. The vial was heated to 95–100°C for 10 min. The reaction mixture was cooled down to room temperature, and the purification was completed with C18 Sep-Pak cartridge, eluted with 2 mL 99.7% ethanol. It was reformulated with 1 mL 4.4% EDTA plus 9 mL sterile water for injection and filtered through 0.22-μM Millipore filter. Quality control was performed by radio-TLC with 0.1 M sodium citrate as mobile phase and silica gel as stationary phase with RCP >95%. Synthesis was done manually.

2.4 Scan Procedure

^{68}Ga-DOTATATE (111–185 MBq, 3–5 mCi) was injected into patients with proven NET ($n = 6$), and 1 h post-injection scan was performed with 64-Slice GEMINI TF PET/CT. Patient studies were performed under a "name-patient permit" issued by the relevant regulatory authority.

3 Results and Discussion

3.1 Generator Elution Profile

The elution profile of the generator showed that the majority of activity was in the second, 1.5 mL fraction, while the first, 1.0 mL and third, 7.5 mL fractions contained negligible amounts of radioactivity (Fig. 1). This second, 1.5 mL fraction which contained the bulk of radioactivity was used for radiolabeling.

3.2 Post-Elution Processing

Metallic impurities in the generator eluate such as Zn^{II} from decay, Fe^{III} from the eluent, and metal ions from the generator column can greatly influence ^{68}Ga radiolabeling. Post-elution processing of generator eluate can be achieved by cation exchange column, anion exchange column, combination of cation and anion exchange columns, and fractionation method (Zhernosekov et al. 2007; Roesch and Riss 2010). A fractionation method reported in literature was used in this study (Breeman et al. 2005). Though this method cannot chemically remove the metallic impurities, it can minimize the impurity content.

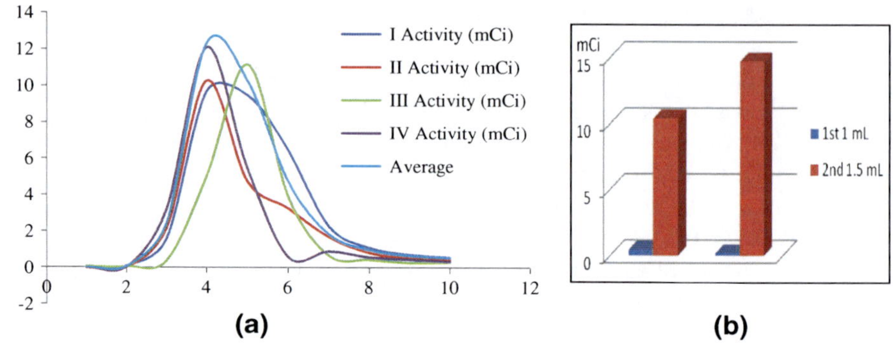

Fig. 1 **a** Elution profile of ^{68}Ge/^{68}Ga generator (*x*-axis, number of 0.5 mL fractions), **b** radioactivity contained in the first and second fractions

3.3 Radiolabeling

Rapid adjustment of pH of ^{68}Ga solution to 3.8–4 immediately after generator elution (within a few minutes) is the most critical step for efficient and successful labeling. Due to its low redox potential, the 3+ oxidation state of gallium is the most stable form in aqueous solution. Gallium has a strong tendency to form strong complexes (both soluble and insoluble) with hydroxyl ions. Fully hydrated (hexaaquo) Ga^{3+} ions are stable only at acidic conditions, while at pH above 4.5, gallium forms insoluble hydroxides [$Ga(OH)_3$]. At physiologic pH, gallium exists predominantly as soluble species, $[Ga(OH)_4]^-$ (gallate) (Green and Welch 1989). Total solubility of gallium at physiologic pH is limited, and thus very high specific activity is needed to keep it soluble in water. Radiolabeling has to be carried out in a pH range of 3–4.5 (Nayak and Brechbiel 2009). Hydrolysis and formation of insoluble complex can be avoided by ligand-exchange reaction in the presence of weak, stabilizing ligands such as citrate, acetate, or oxalate.

To achieve high-quality imaging, the radiolabeling method should not alter or degrade the peptide biological properties. This can be achieved by simple and mild radiolabeling conditions affording high purity, high specific activity, stable compounds which can provide high target-to-nontarget ratio and the ability to achieve imaging at 1–2 h post injection (Ferreira et al. 2010). 1,4,7,10-Tetraazacyclododecane-1,4,7,10-tetraacetic acid (DOTA) is the most commonly used bifunctional chelator (BFC) for ^{68}Ga, but radiolabeling requires elevated temperature (e.g., 100°C) or microwaving to obtain adequate yields and specific activities within a short period of time (e.g., 10 min) (Velikyan et al. 2004). In this study, DOTA-conjugated peptide was efficiently labeled with ^{68}Ga, showing sufficient in vivo stability.

3.4 Loss of Radioactivity During Radiolabeling

A variable amount of radioactivity (20–50%) was lost after heating of the reaction mixture by adsorption to the glass wall of the vial, which could not be retrieved by repeated washing. Considering the facts that the molar sensitivity of PET imaging equipment is 10^{-11}–10^{-12} mol/L with required molecular probe mass of 1–100 ng (Levin 2005) and mass-dependent uptake of radiolabeled SSTR analog by NETs (de Jong et al. 1999), the loss of radiolabeled compound by adsorption to the glass vial wall may have significant impact on the quality of the scan.

Radiometals are available in very low concentrations (10^{-6}–10^{-9} mol/L); sorption of radioisotope on container can be pronounced depending on the type of container. Chemisorption is also very pronounced for radioisotopes which can react with the surface, e.g., sorption of hydroxo complexes of tri- and tetravalent elements by silanol groups on glass surfaces. The ion-exchange capacity of glass surface is on the order of 10^{-10} mol/cm^2 ($\sim 10^{14}$ ions/cm^2). Ion exchange or chemisorption can be prevented by (a) using high concentration of H^+ to suppress ion exchange and hydrolysis, (b) high concentration of nonisotopic cations, anions, or other substances, and (c) hydrophobization of the glass surface (e.g., by treating with silicones) (Lieser 1997). Use of specially treated glass vials and routine measurement of container for leftover activity after radiolabeling will be useful for manual synthesis.

3.5 Clinical Imaging

^{68}Ga-DOTATATE scans showed physiologic uptakes and accumulation in the known sites of NET in all patients. In one patient, previously unknown peritoneal metastasis was detected (Fig. 2). SSTR is expressed in many normal tissues such as the pituitary gland, salivary glands, thyroid, gastric mucosa, duodenum, ileum, colon, pancreas, etc. (Reubi et al. 2001). Physiological uptakes such as uptakes by the pituitary gland and spleen were observed in all cases.

3.6 Patient Complaints

Four out of six patients felt varying degree of burning sensation along the vein of injection and one patient developed phlebitis, which might be attributable to ethanol content in the final formulation. The severity of pain was significantly reduced by slow injection and diluting the final volume of injection to 20 mL. Intravenous injection of ethanol is known to cause pain on injection (Mahdi and McBride 1999; Serdons et al. 2008). Ethanol is a class three residual solvent which cannot produce human health hazard at levels normally accepted in pharmaceuticals. Permitted daily exposure of 50 mg per day or less (corresponding to 5,000 ppm) would be acceptable without justification.[1] Content of residual

[1] (a) United States Pharmacopoeia 33-NF28, (b) European Pharmacopoeia 7.0

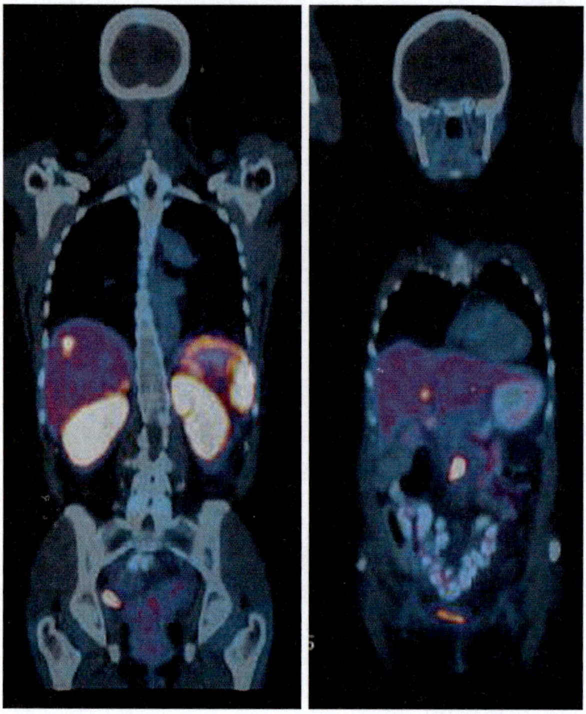

Fig. 2 ^{68}Ga-DOTATATE scans in a patient with proven case of NET with liver lesions, showing previously unknown peritoneal metastasis

solvents such as ethanol and acetone should be measured by gas chromatography (GC) routinely or at least for initial 10 validation runs with subsequent revalidation whenever there is a change in radiolabeling method. For routine clinical use of ^{68}Ga-labeled SSTR analogs, impurities contained in the final formulation should be determined regularly (Milos Petrik et al. 2010).

3.7 Regulatory Requirement for Routine Clinical Use

Radiopharmaceuticals are classified as pharmaceutical products, and routine clinical use of radiopharmaceuticals requires a regulatory license, permit, or special exemption. Obtaining a product license or marketing authorization requires many years of effort and cost. Synthesis of new investigational products should meet good manufacturing practices (GMP) conditions, and the establishment of a GMP-compliant cleanroom facility needs major renovation with significant incurred cost. Obtaining a Medicines and Healthcare Products Regulatory Agency MHRA-style special permit also needs special regulatory considerations or amendment of legislation in certain geographical areas.

Due to the rapid success of ^{68}Ga radiopharmaceuticals for use in many clinical conditions, the pace of clinical success surpasses the linked issue of industrial and regulatory development, unlike in the case of the technetium story, which evolved over decades with the availability of regulatory-approved ^{99}Mo/^{99m}Tc generators, regulatory-approved cold kits, and reconstitution of ^{99m}Tc radiopharmaceuticals as hospital radiopharmacy-based aseptic compounding under current Good Radiopharmaceuticals Practice (cGRPP) (Breeman and Verbruggen 2007).

In the absence of pharmacopoeia monographs on ^{68}Ga radiopharmaceuticals, preparation of these radiopharmaceuticals cannot be regarded as compendia formulation or magistral preparation. A draft monograph on gallium (^{68}Ga) edotreotide was released recently for comment, and adoption of this monograph might assist in obtaining regulatory permission for routine clinical use [Gallium (^{68}Ga) 2011].

3.8 Number of Cases

According to the Singapore Cancer Registry Report No. 7, the number of cases of NET was 563 in the period 1998–2007 (Table 1). One can assume 51 local cases per year, or four local cases per month. Equal or larger number of patients can be expected from oversea referrals. ^{18}F-FDG is the only reimbursed PET procedure, whilst ^{68}Ga radiopharmaceuticals are not. Due to the (1) significant cost of the ^{68}Ge/^{68}Ga generator, (2) cost of peptide and other consumables, (3) absence of reimbursement procedure, (4) relatively low number of scans per month (estimated to be 4–8 per month), and (5) significant cost of setting up ^{68}Ga laboratory consisting of radio-HPLC, radio-TLC, etc., the financial viability of provision of routine clinical services for ^{68}Ga radiopharmaceuticals may need careful consideration. Financial support such as research grants or other forms of special financial support may be required.

3.9 Future Directions

The thermodynamic stability constant of Ga^{III}-DOTA complex ($\log K = 21.33$) is comparable to that of the Fe^{III}-transferrin complex ($\log K = 20.3$) with a possibility of in vivo transmetalation (Clarke and Martell 1991a; Decristoforo et al. 2008). The small ionic radius of Ga^{III} of 76 pm is a perfect match for the cavity formed by the nine-membered triazamacrocyclic chelator 1,4,7-triazacyclononane-1,4,7-triacetic acid (NOTA). The thermodynamic stability constant of the Ga^{III}-NOTA complex ($\log K = 30.98$) is approximately 10 orders of magnitude higher than that of the DOTA counterpart (Clarke and Martell 1991b). NOTA incorporates efficiently with ^{68}Ga and affords high in vivo stability (Singh et al. 2011). ^{68}Ga can form complexes with NODAGATATE ([NODAGA^0, Tyr^3]octreotate) at room temperature within 10 min in near-quantitative yield without requirement for purification (Velikyan et al. 2008). This method becomes very attractive for development of efficient, robust, room-temperature ^{68}Ga labeling of peptides with the possibility of kit formulation.

3.10 Lessons Learnt

Though the number of patients in this study is small, it has generated many factors to be considered for successful introduction of ^{68}Ga radiopharmaceuticals for routine clinical use, as follows:

1. Ga^{III} aqueous chemistry has to be considered seriously for efficient labeling, especially for manual synthesis;
2. Generator performance should be monitored throughout its life cycle;
3. Robust and efficient radiolabeling method is required;
4. Contents of the final formulation should be well defined, including residual solvents;
5. Purification procedures such as post-elution purification versus final purification should be considered;
6. Validation should be performed for the synthesis process, quality control procedures, and quality assurance procedures;
7. Use of validated semi-automated or automatic synthesizers may be preferable;
8. All relevant procedures should be recorded according to good documentation practice, for potential regulatory submission;
9. Pharmacopoeia monograph should be adopted as magistral preparation with compendia method;
10. Regulatory requirements or possibly GMP should be considered early;
11. Gallium generator should be used for multiple applications such as ^{68}Ga-citrate, ^{68}Ga-DOTA-bisphosphonate, etc., together with ^{68}Ga-DOTATATE;
12. Sharing of ^{68}Ga generator among many centers can be considered for cost-effectiveness.

4 Conclusion

The feasibility of ^{68}Ga-DOTATATE application in routine clinical practice for PET imaging of NETs was determined in a limited number of known cases ($n = 6$). ^{68}Ga-DOTATATE scan could detect all known sites of NETs and in one case previously unknown peritoneal metastasis. Early regulatory consideration will be required for successful provision of clinical service with ^{68}Ga-DOTATATE.

Acknowledgments The author thanks RadLink Diagnostic Imaging Pte Ltd, Radlink PET and Cardiac Imaging Centre for the generous support, and the late Dr. Shahid Mahmood for his leadership and vision.

References

Aardaneh K, van der Walt TN (2006) Ga_2O for target, solvent extraction for radiochemical separation and SnO_2 for the preparation of a 68Ge/68Ga generator. J Radioanal Nucl Chem 268:25–32

Adams S, Baum RP, Hertel A et al (1998) Metabolic (PET) and receptor (SPET) imaging of well- and less well differentiated tumors: comparison with the expression of the Ki-67 antigen. Nucl Med Commun 19:641–647

Belhocine T, Foidart J, Rigo P et al (2002) Fluorodeoxyglucose positron emission tomography and somatostatin receptor scintigraphy for diagnosing and staging carcinoid tumors: correlations with the pathological indexes p53 and Ki-67. Nucl Med Commun 23:727–734
Breeman WAP, Verbruggen AF (2007) The 68Ge/68Ga generator has high potential, but when can we use 68Ga-labelled tracers in clinical routine? Eur J Nucl Med Mol Imaging 34:978–981
Breeman WAP, de Jong M, de Blois E et al (2005) Radiolabelling DOTA-peptides with 68Ga. Eur J Nucl Med 32:478–1104
Buchmann I, Henze M, Engelbrecht S et al (2007) Comparison of 68Ga-DOTATOC PET and 111In-DTPAOC (octreoscan) SPECT in patients with neuroendocrine tumors. Eur J Nucl Med Mol Imaging 34:1617–1626
Clarke ET, Martell AE (1991a) Stabilities of trivalent metal ion complexes of the tetraacetate derivatives of 12-, 13- and 14-membered tetraazamacrocycles. Inorg Chim Acta 190:37–46
Clarke ET, Martell AE (1991b) Stabilities of the Fe(III), Ga(III), and In(III) chelates of N,N', N''-triazacyclononanetriacetic acid. Inorg Chim Acta 181:273–280
de Jong M, Breeman WAP, Bernard BF et al (1999) Tumour uptake of the radiolabelled somatostatin analogue [DOTA0, TYR3]octreotide is dependent on the peptide amount. Eur J Nucl Med 26:693–698
Decristoforo C, Gonzalez HI, Carlsen J et al (2008) 68Ga- and 111In-labelled DOTA-RGD peptides for imaging of Rvβ3 integrin expression. Eur J Nucl Med Mol Imaging 35:1507–1515
Ferreira CL, Lamsa E, Woods M (2010) Evaluation of bifunctional chelates for the development of gallium-based radiopharmaceuticals. Bioconjugate Chem 21:531–536
Gallium (68Ga) edotreotide (2011) Draft monographs and general texts for comment Pharmaeuropa 23: 297–313
Green MS, Welch MJ (1989) Gallium radiopharmaceutical chemistry. Int J Rad Appl Instrum B 16:435–448
Haug A, Christoph J, Auernhammer CJ, Wängler B et al (2009) Intraindividual comparison of 68Ga-DOTA-TATE and 18F-DOPA PET in patients with well-differentiated metastatic neuroendocrine tumors. Eur J Nucl Med Mol Imaging 36:765–770
Hofmann M, Maecke H, Börner AR et al (2001) Biokinetics and imaging with the somatostatin receptor PET radioligand ^{68}Ga-DOTATOC: preliminary data. Eur J Nucl Med 28:1751–1757
Kaltsas G, Mukherjee JJ, Grossman AB (2001) The value of radiolabelled MIBG and octreotide in the diagnosis and management of neuroendocrine tumors. Clin Endocrinol 55:575–587
Kaltsas G, Rockall A, Papadogias D et al (2004) Recent advances in radiological and radionuclide imaging and therapy of neuroendocrine tumors. Eur J Endocrinol 151:15–27
Kaltsas GA, Papadogias D, Makras P et al (2005) Treatment of advanced neuroendocrine tumors with radiolabelled somatostatin analogues. Endocr Relat Cancer 12:683–699
Kayani I, Bomanji JB, Groves A et al (2008) Functional imaging of neuroendocrine tumors with combined PET/CT using 68Ga-DOTATATE (Dota-DPhe1, Tyr3-octreotate) and 18F-FDG. Cancer 112:2447–2455
Kowalski J, Henze M, Schuhmacher J et al (2003) Evaluation of positron emission tomography imaging using [^{68}Ga]-DOTA-D Phe^{1}-Tyr^{3}-octreotide in comparison to [^{111}In]-DTPAOC SPECT. First results in patients with neuroendocrine tumors. Mole Imaging Biol 5:42–48
Levin CS (2005) Primer on molecular imaging technology. Eur J Nucl Med Mol Imaging 32: S-325–S-345
Lieser KH (1997) Nuclear and radiochemistry: fundamentals and applications. VCH Wiley, Weinheim
Maecke HR, Hofmann M, Haberkorn U (2005) 68Ga-labeled peptides in tumor imaging. J Nucl Med 46:172S–178S
Mahdi AS, McBride AJ (1999) Intravenous injection of alcohol by drug injectors: report of three cases. Alcohol Alcohol 34:918–919
Milos Petrik M, Ocak M, Rupprich M, et al (2010) Impurity in 68Ga-peptide preparation using processed generator eluate. doi:10.2967/jnumed.109.070953
Modlin IM, Oberg K, Chung DC et al (2008) Gastroenteropancreatic neuroendocrine tumors. Lancet Oncol 9:61–72

Nayak TK, Brechbiel MW (2009) Radioimmunoimaging with longer-lived positron-emitting radionuclides: potentials and challenges. Bioconjugate Chem 20:825–841
Papotti M, Bongiovanni M, Volante M et al (2002) Expression of somatostatin receptor types 1–5 in 81 cases of gastrointestinal and pancreatic endocrine tumors: a correlative immunohistochemical and reverse-transcriptase polymerase chain reaction analysis. Virchows Arch 440:461–475
Reisine T, Bell GI (1995) Molecular biology of somatostatin receptors. Endocr Rev 16:427–442
Reubi JC, Waser B, Schaer JC, Laissue JA (2001) Somatostatin receptor sst1–sst5 expression in normal and neoplastic human tissues using receptor autoradiography with subtype-selective ligands. Eur J Nucl Med 28:836–846
Roesch F, Riss PJ (2010) The renaissance of the 68Ge/68Ga radionuclide generator initiates new developments in 68Ga radiopharmaceutical chemistry. Cur Top Med Chem 10:1633–1668
Serdons K, Verbruggen A, Bormans G (2008) The presence of ethanol in radiopharmaceutical injections. J Nucl Med 49:2071
Signore A, Annovazzi A, Chianelli M, Corsetti F et al (2001) Peptide radiopharmaceuticals for diagnosis and therapy. Eur J Nucl Med 28:1555–1565
Singh AN, Liu W, Hao G et al (2011) Multivalent bifunctional chelator scaffolds for gallium-68 based positron emission tomography imaging probe design: signal amplification via multivalency. Bioconjugate Chem 22:1650–1662
Srirajaskanthan R, Kayani I, Quigley AM et al (2010) The role of 68Ga-DOTATATE PET in patients with neuroendocrine tumors and negative or equivocal findings on 111In-DTPA-octreotide scintigraphy. J Nucl Med 51:875–882
Trends in Cancer Incidence in Singapore (1968–2007). Singapore Cancer Registry Report No. 7
Velikyan I, Beyer GJ, Langstrom B (2004) Microwave supported preparation of 68Ga bioconjugates with high specific radioactivity. Bioconjugate Chem 15:554–560
Velikyan I, Maecke H, Langstrom B (2008) Convenient preparation of 68Ga-based PET-radiopharmaceuticals at room temperature. Bioconjugate Chem 19:569–573
Zhernosekov KP, Filosofov DV, Baum RP et al (2007) Processing of generator-produced 68Ga for medical application. J Nucl Med 48:1741–1748

^{68}Ga-Radiopharmaceuticals for PET Imaging of Infection and Inflammation

Vijay Kumar and Dilip K. Boddeti

Abstract

Infection imaging has been challenging over the past four decades, which provided an excellent playing field for researchers working in this area, and till date the quest continues to find an ideal imaging agent. Labelled leukocytes were first developed in the 1970s for imaging infection lesions such as osteomyelitis, cellulitis, diabetic foot, Crohn's disease, inflammatory bowel disease, fever of unknown origin, etc. Subsequently labelled antibiotics such as ^{99m}Tc-labelled ciprofloxacin have emerged for directly identifying live bacterial infections. From the early 1970s through the mid-1980s, ^{67}Ga-Citrate was the prime radionuclide for imaging of inflammation and infection of musculoskeletal origin. Although ^{68}Ga-PET was described in 1960s for tumour imaging, recent reports described ^{68}Ga-Citrate and ^{68}Ga-transferrin as possible agents for PET-imaging of infection due to successful application of ^{67}Ga-Citrate SPECT in the past, despite its limitations. It is important to establish a faster imaging method for ^{68}Ga, as its half-life is 68 min compared to 78.3 hrs

V. Kumar (✉) · D. K. Boddeti
Department of Nuclear Medicine & PET,
Westmead Hospital and The Children's Hospital at Westmead,
Westmead, NSW 2145, Australia
e-mail: Vijay.Kumar@swahs.health.nsw.gov.au

D. K. Boddeti
e-mail: dilip.boddeti@health.nsw.gov.an

V. Kumar · D. K. Boddeti
Department of Nuclear Medicine, The Children's Hospital at Westmead,
Sydney, NSW, Australia

V. Kumar
Sydney Medical School, University of Sydney, Sydney, Australia

R. P. Baum and F. Rösch (eds.), *Theranostics, Gallium-68, and Other Radionuclides*, Recent Results in Cancer Research 194, DOI: 10.1007/978-3-642-27994-2_11,

for ^{67}Ga. Preparation of ^{68}Ga-Citrate and ^{68}Ga-transferrin is described, with very high yield and high radiochemical purity (RCP), which is ideally suited for routine clinical studies. Biodistribution of ^{68}Ga-Citrate-PET images were characterised with high blood pool, high liver and bone (growth plate) uptake with low soft-tissue activity. ^{68}Ga-Citrate or ^{68}Ga-transferrin was able to detect infected lesions in rats within 5–10 min post injection but a focal intense uptake at the lesion (SUV_{max}) was visualized only at 30 min, which increased for up to 6 hrs post injection with concomitant decrease in the cardiac blood pool activity. The liver and bowel activity decreased after 90 min then stabilised. In the patient studies, infection lesions were detected within 30 min post injection of ^{68}Ga-Citrate. Cardiac blood pool and liver activities decreased during the period of study. Interestingly, there was persistent high vascular activity in the thigh region. One of the major limitations of ^{67}Ga-Citrate SPECT is the delayed post injection waiting time of 48 hrs, in contrast to 60 min post injection waiting with ^{68}Ga-Citrate. The distinct difference in imaging time is intriguing, although there is no chemical difference between ^{67}Ga-Citrate and ^{68}Ga-Citrate, except for the radiolabel. No literature is available on early imaging times using ^{67}Ga-SPECT. When compared ^{68}Ga/^{67}Ga-Citrate images at 60 min post injection in normal rats, ^{68}Ga-PET showed better images with low background activity than ^{67}Ga-SPECT agent. This may be due to short half-life of ^{68}Ga (68 min), as it would have decayed one half-life at 60 min post-imaging time, compared to the SPECT agent (^{67}Ga), which would require 76 hrs to undergo one half-life. Therefore, the visual difference in background can be attributed to the difference in the half-lives of these two agents. Similarly, uptake of ^{68}Ga by liver, cardiac blood pool activity is much lower than ^{67}Ga at 60 min post injection period, may be attributed to the faster decay of ^{68}Ga than ^{67}Ga. High background activity of ^{68}Ga-Citrate in the thorax and upper abdomen at 60 min post-injection may interfere with detecting lesions in these regions; therefore, ^{68}Ga-PET is more suitable for imaging lesions in the lower abdomen and the extremities. The short half-life of ^{68}Ga (68 min) may be advantageous from low dosimetry to the patients, but disadvantageous for longer periods of study. Since ^{68}Ga-Citrate was capable of detecting infection within 60 min, the need for imaging for longer periods may not be warranted. The functional imaging was not limited to diagnosing infection but it could be extended to surgical planning and antibiotic therapy monitoring of osteomyelitis and in distinguishing prosthetic infection from loosening of prosthesis. ^{18}F-FDG is sensitive but has the limitation of giving false positive results in patients with bone prosthesis, even if there is no infection or mobilisation. But the available literature clearly indicated ^{68}Ga-Citrate was positive only in cases of infection. In summary, preliminary reports suggest ^{68}Ga-Citrate PET/CT is useful in the diagnosis of suspected bone infections with reliable sensitivity, specificity, positive predictive value, negative predictive value and overall accuracy. Preliminary reports with ^{68}Ga-Transferrin showed it is capable of detecting both Gram-positive *Staphylococcus aureus* (*Staph A*) and Gram-negative *Proteus mirobilis*. This is an incidental finding but gives an insight into the potential of this agent to detect more than one bacterial infection.

Contents

1 Introduction

Infection imaging is complicated due to the multitude of intervening factors influencing the process of infection. The task is further complicated with superimposing factors associated with inflammation and infection. The ideal imaging agent should detect infection lesions with high sensitivity and high specificity and be cost-effective. Since a large number of radiopharmaceuticals have emerged continually for infection imaging, certain criteria are defined to characterize an ideal agent (Tulchinsky and Peters 2005). In the first place, a high percentage of the agent should localize at the target lesion very rapidly. Secondly it should reside long enough at the target to allow optimal imaging. Nontarget organs and tissues should have low uptake. The agent should be cleared from blood pool rapidly to improve the target-to-blood ratio. The uptake of the agent should be proportional to the degree of infection. Labeling should be simple and uncomplicated with long shelf-life for the cold kit. It should not be expensive. Radiation dosimetry should be reasonable, and immunological response should be minimal.

Labeled leukocytes have been developed for imaging infection, pioneered by McAfee and Thakur (1976a, b) over four decades ago, holding the center stage in this area to date, as it has been very effective in diagnosing various lesions such as osteomyelitis, cellulitis, diabetic foot, Crohn's disease, inflammatory bowel disease (Allan et al. 1993), fever of unknown origin (FUO), etc. Functional imaging was not limited to diagnosis of infection but extended also to surgical planning and monitoring of antibiotic therapy for infection (Nanni et al. 2010) and in distinguishing prosthetic infection from loosening of prosthesis (Merkel et al. 1986; Palestro et al. 1991; Palestero 1994, 2003). The role of leukocytes in infection imaging opened up many approaches based on targeting specific receptors present on leukocytes such as interleukins, cytokines, etc. Subsequently, many new agents have emerged on a regular basis over the last four decades. Antibiotics such as ^{99m}Tc-labeled ciprofloxacin have emerged for directly identifying live bacterial infections (Vinjamuri et al. 1996).

From the early 1970s through the mid-1980s, ^{67}Ga-citrate was the prime radionuclide for imaging of inflammation and infection of musculoskeletal origin (along with ^{99m}Tc-methylene diphosphonate), and even today among the myriad of techniques currently available, this tracer is still an important tool in the diagnostic armamentarium of nuclear medicine (Edwards and Hayes 1969; Lavender et al. 1971; Hoffer 1980; Silberstein et al. 1981; Kelly et al. 1990). However, the clinical utility of this agent is compromised due to several limitations such as poor image quality of ^{67}Ga single-photon emission computed tomography (SPECT), high background activity and interference from liver and bowel activity, delayed post-injection waiting time of at least 48–72 h, the associated high radiation exposure, and high cost of the radionuclide. Nevertheless, ^{67}Ga-citrate is used currently in many centers around the world for specific conditions such as FUO (Littenberg et al. 1973; Hopkins and Mende 1975) and osteomyelitis (Modic et al. 1985; Lisbona et al. 1993), and in immunocompromised patients (Bitran et al. 1987; Tatsch et al. 1990; Moser et al. 1990). Although imaging infection and inflammation has been a major research focus for a long time, to date no single radiopharmaceutical has emerged which can clearly distinguish infection from inflammation.

Infection imaging has been challenging, and the quest continues to find an ideal imaging agent (Ito et al. 1971; Ma et al. 1997; Boerman et al. 2001; Bombardieri et al. 2003; Hughes 2003; El-Maghraby et al. 2006). ^{68}Ga-citrate was investigated by our group and others for PET imaging of infection due to successful application of ^{67}Ga-citrate SPECT in the past, despite its limitations (Hopkins and Mende 1975; Henkin 1978; Weiner et al. 1981; Tsan 1985). It is important to establish a faster imaging method for ^{68}Ga, as its half-life is 68 min compared with 78.3 h for ^{67}Ga. ^{68}Ga PET was described in the 1960s for tumor uptake studies, but ^{68}Ge/^{68}Ga generator chemistry was investigated only in the late 1970s (Ehrhardt and Welch 1978; Zhernosekov et al. 2007; Asti et al. 2008). Recent studies indicated a possible role for ^{68}Ga-chloride to monitor bone healing in experimental osteomyelitis (Makinen et al. 2005) and for pancreatic adenocarcinoma xenografts in rats (Ujula et al. 2009). We have previously demonstrated the ability of ^{68}Ga-apo-transferrin and ^{68}Ga-citrate to detect *Staphylococcus aureus* (*Staph A*) infection (Kumar et al. 2009, 2012). More recently, ^{68}Ga-citrate was described for PET imaging of *Staph A* infection (Rizzello et al. 2009; Kumar et al. 2012) and osteomyelitis (Nanni et al. 2010). The prime focus of the current chapter is to establish the capability and clinical utility of ^{68}Ga-labeled agents in general for PET imaging of infection in patient studies, including osteomyelitis, cellulitis, abscess detection, and antibiotic therapy monitoring. The chapter also explores the potential of other agents for imaging inflammation.

2 Overview on Infection Imaging

2.1 Labeled Leukocytes for Imaging Infection

No review on infection imaging would be complete unless the historical development of labeled leukocytes is reviewed briefly. Labeled leukocyte studies, by in vitro method, using ^{111}In-oxine, hexamethylpropyleneamine oxime (^{99m}Tc-HMPAO), and ^{99m}Tc-stannous colloid have paved the way for extensive research and clinical studies on infection imaging. However, the technique had the inherent limitation of personnel safety risks of infection and cross-contamination, as it involved isolating leukocytes, labeling them with a suitable agent, and reinjecting them into the patient. To overcome this problem, attempts were made to directly target leukocytes by in vivo labeling technique. There are several receptors present on leukocytes and granulocytes which can be targeted with suitable ligands such as monoclonal antibodies (MoAb), antibody fragments (Fab'), or peptides. It is beyond the scope of this chapter to describe every radiopharmaceutical under these categories; rather, we mention a few agents such as anti-NCA90-Fab (Leukoscan) (Becker et al. 1995; Barron et al. 1999), murine MoAb IgG1 (Granuloscient; CIS Bio International) (Thakur et al. 1988, 1996)—cross reactive to antigen 95 on neutrophils, and anti-CD15 antigen (Neutrospect, ^{99m}Tc-fanolesomab, Leu Tech) (Mozley et al. 1999; Rypins et al. 2002; Skehan et al. 2003), in terms of their design and clinical utility. Leukotriene B4 receptor is abundantly expressed on granulocyte cell surface, and the receptor-binding agent DPC-11870 is described (van Eerd et al. 2003), having potential to detect infection and inflammation.

2.2 Labeled Antibiotics for Infection Imaging

Broad-spectrum antibiotic such as ciprofloxacin is taken up and retained by bacteria but not by mammalian cells. Based on this principle, ^{99m}Tc-labeled ciprofloxacin was used to directly target "live bacteria" (Vinjamuri et al. 1996) to detect infection by "in vivo" method with considerable promise, although this did not materialize in clinical trials. Analogs of a natural mammalian antimicrobial agent such as ubiquicidin and its shorter fragments emerged later (Iqbal et al. 2004; Akhtar et al. 2005) and were used in animal studies, entering clinical trials recently. Although a large number of bacterial infection imaging agents have been described, fungal infection agents have been relatively fewer due to difficulties associated with the design. ^{99m}Tc-labeled fluconazole (a fungal antibiotic) has been reported in animal studies but did not progress beyond that due to limitations of the agent (Welling et al. 2000, 2002; Lupetti et al. 2002, 2003). Chitin is specifically expressed in fungal cell wall but not in bacterial or human cell wall. Based on this concept, a new fungal imaging agent, labeled chitinase (^{123}I-ChiB_E144Q), has been developed to detect fungal infection (Siaens et al. 2004). A recent report described use of ^{68}Ga-RP for imaging fungal infection (Petrik et al. 2010). The emergence of newer agents and newer trends points to better understanding to distinguish fungal from bacterial infection.

2.3 ^{67}Ga-Citrate for Infection Imaging

Diagnosis of infection has long been an issue and has been approached with several imaging methods, but the optimal diagnostic procedure or a standard diagnostic flow chart has not yet been identified (Ichiya et al. 1996). Biopsy of the infected area is an invasive procedure and not always diagnostic (50% sensitivity has been reported) (Sugawara et al. 1999; Einhorn 1998; de Winter et al. 2002). MRI is a sensitive but nonspecific technique and is contraindicated in patients with prosthesis or bone implant (Koort et al. 2004; Ma et al. 1997). Morphologic imaging procedures are not specific and may present significant artifacts in patients with prosthesis. Furthermore, these tests are not reliable for diagnosis of response to antibiotic therapy (Palestro 1994; Chianelli et al. 1997). White blood cell (WBC) scintigraphy is generally sensitive and specific for the nonaxial skeleton, but the procedure is long and complicated (Peters 1994).

The role of gallium for infection imaging has changed considerably during the past several years. It was the frontline option for radionuclide imaging of infection, but it has been overtaken to a very great extent by labeled leukocyte imaging. Despite the success of the labeled white-cell technique, gallium still plays an important role in radionuclide evaluation of infection. It is not possible, for a variety of reasons, to perform white-cell imaging on all patients, and gallium imaging is certainly an acceptable substitute. In certain circumstances, rather than merely being a substitute, gallium is an important complement to leukocyte imaging (Palestro 1994). This is best illustrated by the patient with FUO. Although a negative leukocyte study effectively excludes acute infection, it fails to identify the source of the patient's fever, a not uncommon situation in view of the fact that only approximately 25% of all FUOs are caused by infection. A complementary gallium study under these circumstances may identify either a chronic infectious process or even a neoplasm, conditions for which white-cell imaging is relatively insensitive. Although leukocyte imaging is probably superior to gallium for most infections of the musculoskeletal system, this technique is of limited value in patients with suspected vertebral osteomyelitis. There are data that suggest that sequential bone gallium imaging may be a better way to diagnose this entity. Finally, in immunocompromised patients (Kramer et al. 1989), gallium imaging is clearly the procedure of choice for detecting the opportunistic respiratory infections and lymph node abnormalities that are so prevalent in this population (Palestro 1994).

3 Difference Between ^{67}Ga-SPECT and ^{68}Ga-PET

3.1 Production of ^{67}Ga and Pure ^{68}Ga

^{67}Ga-citrate was a well-established SPECT agent for infection imaging, but required 48–72 h post-injection imaging time. However, ^{68}Ga-citrate was shown to be effective within 60 min post-injection imaging time. Faster kinetics indicated a lot of potential for clinical application. The striking difference in post-injection imaging time between these two radiopharmaceuticals is intriguing and very difficult to comprehend. Therefore, production of ^{67}Ga and ^{68}Ga is reviewed in detail to gain possible insight into understanding the aforementioned difference in behavior between these two radionuclides.

^{67}Ga is a cyclotron-generated radiopharmaceutical that can be produced from targets of enriched, stable zinc isotopes by a variety of nuclear reactions using either deuterons or protons. It emits gamma-rays over a broad range of 93–880 keV, with the following four principal energy peaks suitable for imaging: 93, 184, 296, and 388 keV. It has no beta emissions. ^{67}Ga is a group IIIb transition metal, similar to the ferric ion in terms of its charge, atomic radius, and the inorganic complexes it forms. Unlike iron, however, it cannot be reduced in vivo and does not react with protoporphyrin IX to form heme. Approximately 10–25% of the tracer dose is excreted via the kidneys during the first 24 h after intravenous injection, after which time the principal route of excretion is the colon. By 48 h after injection, approximately 75% of the injected dose remains in the body and is equally distributed among the liver, bone and bone marrow, and soft tissues (Palestro 1994). This normal distribution can, however, be very variable and may confound image interpretation.

The cost-effective production, easy availability, and versatile linker-based chemistry system has opened up enormous research interest in the development of ^{68}Ga-labeled pharmaceuticals. ^{68}Ga is produced by ^{68}Ge/^{68}Ga generator (Kopecky et al. 1973; Kopecky and Mudrová 1974; Aardaneh and van der Walt 2006; Zhernosekov et al. 2007), unlike ^{67}Ga, which is produced by cyclotron. The generator eluate is contaminated with radioactive and metallic impurities ($^{68}Zn^{II}$, Ti^{IV}, and Fe^{III}), which could greatly influence the utility of the product. Besides, the eluate contains measurable amounts of long-lived ^{68}Ge and high concentration of hydrochloric acid, which in many cases prevent direct use of the eluate for labeling peptides and organic compounds. Three different approaches were recently described in the literature for processing generator-derived $^{68}Ga^{III}$: anion exchange, cation exchange, and fractionation methods. Comprehensive information on this aspect is reviewed by Roesch and Riss (2010).

Anion Exchange Method: The anion exchange method was first published in 1961, based on adsorption of ^{68}Ge by Al_20_3 column and subsequent elution of ^{68}Ga with 5.5 M HCl, which was later revised in 2004 (Hofmann et al. 2001; Velikyan et al. 2004). The ^{68}Ge/^{68}Ga generator was eluted with HCl (5.5 M), and the mixture passed through an anion exchange column where the anionic

$(GaCl_6)^{3-}$ and $(GaCl_4)^{-}$ complexes were strongly absorbed, whilst Ge^{IV}, Al^{III}, Ti^{IV}, Zn^{II}, Fe^{III}, and In(III) were practically not retained. ^{68}Ga was then eluted with <200 μL pure water. However, this strategy was not efficient for removing Fe(III) and Zn(II), as these cations also formed strong anionic chlorocomplexes. The processes of eluting the generator, synthesis, and purification of the labeled product are time-consuming and invariably lead to reduction of the overall yields to around 46 ± 5% of the product (Velikyan et al. 2004).

Fractionation Method: Fractionation was another way to purify generator-produced ^{68}Ga, described by Breeman et al. (2004), to overcome problems such as eluate volume, acidic pH, and content of ^{68}Ge and chemical impurities. The concept utilizes the fact that the eluted ^{68}Ga activity peaks within 1–2 mL, representing about 2/3 of the total activity. In the context of synthesizing ^{68}Ga-labeled compounds, decay-corrected yields of ^{68}Ga radiopharmaceuticals thus could not exceed 60–70%. Contents of ^{68}Ge and metallic impurities were minimized because of the lower eluate volume used, but principally not chemically removed prior to the ^{68}Ga labeling steps.

Cation Exchange Method: This method was developed by Zhernosekov et al. (2007) using a ^{68}Ge/^{68}Ga generator from Cyclotron Co., Ltd., Obninsk, Russia. The key step in this procedure consists of direct transfer of the initial ^{68}Ge/^{68}Ga eluate (in 0.1 M HCl) to a cation exchange resin. Due to high distribution coefficients, ^{68}Ga was quantitatively adsorbed on cation exchange resin (50 mg) directly from the generator eluate. A small volume (1.0 mL) of 80% acetone/0.15 N HCl mixture was applied to elute impurities such as Ge^{IV}, Ti^{IV}, Zn^{II}, and Fe^{III}. Subsequently, 0.4 mL 98% acetone/0.05 N HCl mixture was used to completely desorb pure ^{68}Ga from the resin for transfer online to a labeling vial. Post-processing purified the generator eluate of impurities, reduced the volume to 0.4 mL, and took 4 min, with overall ^{68}Ga recovery yields of 97 ± 2%. Production, radiochemical processing, and quality evaluation of ^{68}Ge suitable for use in ^{68}Ge/^{68}Ga generator were elaborated by Rösch and Knapp (Russ) (2003) and Rösch and Filosofov (2010).

3.2 Development of ^{68}Ga Chemistry

Although ^{68}Ga PET was described in the 1960s for tumor uptake studies, ^{68}Ge/^{68}Ga generator chemistry was investigated only in the late 1970s, and no further work was described for nearly four decades. Over the last decade, ^{68}Ge/^{68}Ga generators were available commercially, and sophisticated online eluate post-processing was established (Zhernosekov et al. 2007). In parallel, ^{68}Ga radiopharmaceutical chemistry was reintroduced (Maecke and Andre 2007; Roesch and Riss 2010).

Even clinically, applications of ^{68}Ga-labeled peptides with the macrocyclic chelating agent 1,4,7,10-tetraazacyclododecane-*N–N*',*N*'',*N*''-tetraacetic acid (DOTA) have been successfully introduced by Frank Rösch and colleagues (Henze et al. 2001; Breeman et al. 2004; Gabriel et al. 2007), and novel versatile bifunctional chelators, e.g., NODAPA-OH (Riss et al. 2008), have been developed to target tumor imaging by positron emission tomography (PET). Subsequently, several potential ^{68}Ga-labeled somatostatin analogs such as ^{68}Ga-DOTA-NOC and ^{68}Ga-DOTA-TATE were described and clinically utilized by Baum et al. (2008, 2010) and others (Rufini et al. 2006; Antunes et al. 2007; Conry et al. 2010). Other agents such as ^{68}Ga-DOTA-bombesin and ^{68}Ga-DOTA-Glu-gastrin, which bind to their respective G-peptide coupled transmembrane tumor receptors, have emerged continually (Dimitrakopoulou-Strauss et al. 2007; Jeong et al. 2008).

3.3 Mechanism of Cellular Uptake of Ga-Citrate

The cellular uptake of ^{67}Ga is a complex mechanism which is not fully understood. Earlier concepts suggested that ^{67}Ga uptake was mediated exclusively by neutrophils (Burleson et al. 1973, 1974; Arseneau et al. 1974; Gelrud et al. 1974; Larson 1978), which is no longer acceptable. Several theories support that ^{67}Ga uptake is dependent on multiple factors: adequate blood supply, increased capillary permeability (Tzen et al. 1980), uptake by leukocytes, and direct uptake by bacteria (Menon et al. 1978). The most generally accepted theory is that ^{67}Ga is delivered to infected or inflammatory lesions primarily by binding to plasma transferrin and to some extent by lactoferrin and bacterial siderophores (Weiner et al. 1981; Shongwe et al. 1992). All these factors may contribute to accumulation and retention of gallium radioactivity at the site of infection and inflammation.

Transferrin is a glycoprotein with high affinity for binding iron on its domain. This domain belongs to the "transferrin superfamily" including other iron-binding molecules such as lactoferrin, melanotransferrin, and ovotransferrin. Ferric iron binding with transferrin requires the presence of an anion such as carbonate, which facilitates binding by excluding water from the two coordination sites (Aisen and Listowsky 1980; Huebers and Finch 1987; Harris and Aisen 1989). Available evidence suggests that anion binding is a prerequisite prior to iron binding (Bailey et al. 1988). In our experiments we prepared the ^{68}Ga-*apo*-transferrin complex in the presence of carbonate ions, similar to iron-binding experiments. The percentage of complex formed was very high (>98%). On the other hand, when we prepared ^{68}Ga-*apo*-transferrin in saline, without carbonate ion, the percentage of complex formed was low (<15%). These observations clearly indicate that the binding of ^{68}Ga to *apo*-transferrin in vitro is carbonate ion dependent, which is comparable to iron binding to transferrin.

When leukocytes localize at sites of inflammation, they excrete at least some of their intracellular lactoferrin, which remains localized and bound to macrophages. Gallium, transported either in ionic form or bound to transferrin, may leak through the vascular epithelium at the site of infection, where it is then bound to the lactoferrin. Another uptake mechanism may involve direct uptake of gallium by infective organisms themselves, an occurrence that has been shown in vitro. Microorganisms grown in a low-iron environment produce siderophores that have an extraordinary binding affinity for gallium as well as iron. Because there is very little free iron present in most tissues, it is assumed that pathogenic microorganisms produce siderophores, and the siderophore–gallium complex is presumably then transported directly into the cell (Lim et al. 1998).

4 Application of ^{68}Ga-Radiopharmaceuticals for Infection Imaging

4.1 Biodistribution of ^{67}Ga/^{68}Ga-Citrate in Normal Rats and Humans

^{67}Ga-citrate was obtained from commercial supplier (ANSTO, Australia). ^{68}Ga-citrate was prepared by mixing post-processed pure $^{68}GaCl_3$ (150–200 MBq/2.0 mL saline) with 0.25 mL sodium citrate (0.1 M). It was incubated for 5 min at room temperature and sterilized by final filtering with 0.22-μ filter. The radiochemical purity (RCP) of ^{68}Ga-citrate was >99% as determined by ITLC-SG/methanol:glacial acetic acid (9:1 v/v) (free ^{68}Ga, $R_f = 0$; bound ^{68}Ga, $R_f = 1$) (Rizzello et al. 2009). This method of preparation is much simpler than other methods described in literature (Rizzello et al. 2009), which are time consuming and gave lower yields. Stability was >98% over the 6-h period when the study was performed by mixing 0.3 mL ^{68}Ga-citrate solution with 1.5 mL human serum at 37°C. RCP was measured at 1 h interval.

It was hypothesized that commercially available ^{67}Ga-citrate may contain some impurities (e.g., heavy-metal ions Ge, Ti), which interfered with the uptake process. To substantiate this hypothesis, the biodistribution of ^{67}Ga-citrate, before and after purification, was studied in normal rats at 60 min post-injection period (Fig. 1). ^{67}Ga-citrate was purified with cation exchange resin, similar to preparing pure ^{68}Ga (Zhernosekov et al. 2007; Kumar et al. 2012). Animal studies showed that ^{67}Ga-citrate SPECT images were characterized by uptake of the agent in blood pool, liver, and bone (growth plate), with low soft tissue activity both before (Fig. 1a) and after purification (Fig. 1b). Since our results indicated no distinct difference in biodistribution of ^{67}Ga-citrate before and after purification, it is reasonable to conclude that the commercially supplied ^{67}Ga is free of any contamination, and that this is not a factor in the observed difference in biodistribution.

No literature is available on early imaging times using ^{67}Ga SPECT. In our study we compared ^{68}Ga-citrate PET and ^{67}Ga-citrate SPECT images at 60 min post injection in normal rats, and the results showed relatively lower background activity for the PET agent compared with the SPECT agent (Fig. 1c). This may be due to the short half-life of ^{68}Ga (68 min), as it would have undergone nearly one half-life decay within the 60 min imaging time, compared with the SPECT agent (^{67}Ga), which has half-life of 76 h. Therefore, the visual difference in background can be attributed to the difference in half-life between these two agents. Similarly, uptake of ^{68}Ga by liver, cardiac blood-pool activity is much lower than for ^{67}Ga,

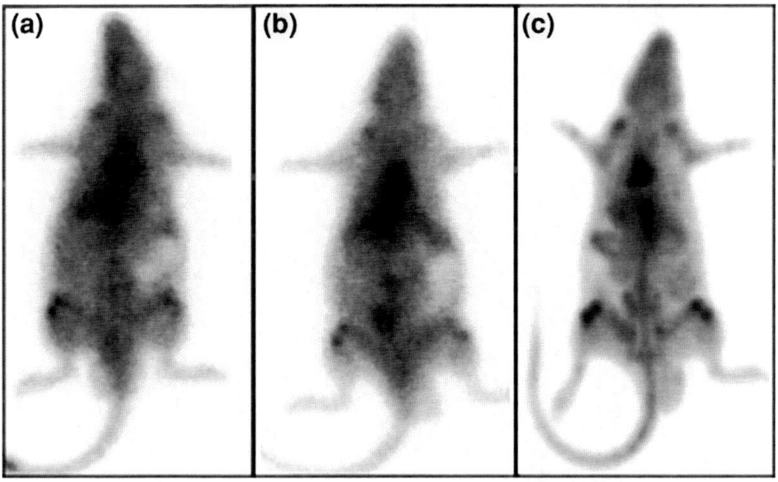

Fig. 1 Biodistribution of Ga-citrate in normal rats. Ga-citrate (40 MBq) was injected into rats, and images were acquired at 60 min post-injection. ^{67}Ga-citrate SPECT images are shown in **a** (before purification) and **b** (after purification). ^{68}Ga-citrate PET image is shown in **c**. Reproduced from Kumar et al. (2012)

which may be attributed to the faster decay of ^{68}Ga than ^{67}Ga. The lack of uptake by the kidneys and bladder is comparable in both cases, which might explain the high vascular retention of activity in the patient study. High vascular retention may be due to high protein binding of the agent, which is to be substantiated with experimental evidence.

At our institution, the radiotracer is not routinely used except in pediatric patients for selected indications such as FUO. To obtain diagnostically useful images, a multipeak gamma camera equipped with a suitable medium-energy collimator is mandatory for imaging with ^{67}Ga-citrate (Palestro 1994). ^{67}Ga was prepared as ^{67}Ga-citrate to facilitate solubilization, and approximately 150–200 MBq (5 mCi) was injected in patient studies; images were acquired 60 min after injection. The images indicated normal distribution of the radiotracer in liver, bone, bone marrow, and soft tissues. Bowel activity was minimal (Fig. 2a). On the other hand, biodistribution of ^{68}Ga-citrate shows distinct high vascular activity, which is not typical of ^{67}Ga-citrate images. ^{68}Ga-citrate showed moderate hepatic uptake and mild bone marrow activity. Bowel activity was absent (Fig. 2b) (Nanni et al. 2010).

Background activity of ^{68}Ga-citrate in the thorax and upper abdomen at 60 min post injection suggests possible interference with detecting lesions in these regions but may also indicate suitability for imaging the lower abdomen and the extremities. The short half-life of ^{68}Ga (68 min) may be advantageous in terms of low dose to patients, but is disadvantageous for use of this radionuclide for longer periods of study. In our institution, we are performing clinical evaluation of this agent for imaging cellulitis and abscesses.

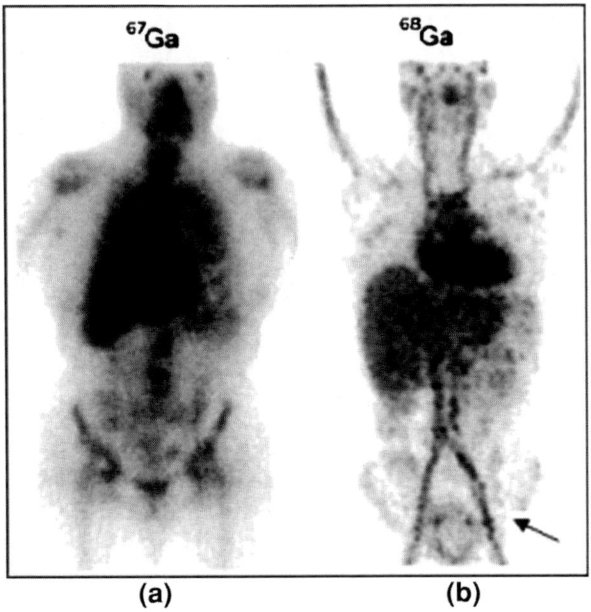

Fig. 2 Physiologic biodistribution of ^{67}Ga-citrate whole-body scintigraphy and ^{68}Ga-citrate PET/CT. Intense uptake of ^{67}Ga-citrate is seen in the liver, blood pool, and kidneys (**a**). Significantly less uptake of ^{68}Ga-citrate is seen in the liver, and kidneys but very high vascular activity (*arrow*) (**b**). Reproduced with permission (Nanni et al. 2010)

4.2 ^{68}Ga-Citrate PET for Imaging *Staph A* Infection in an Animal Model

In experimentally induced *Staph A* infection in an animal model, Kumar et al. (2009, 2012) demonstrated avid uptake of ^{68}Ga-citrate at infected lesions within 10 min post injection, but focal intense uptake (SUV_{max}) at 30 min (Fig. 3a). They also demonstrated that the SUV_{max} at the target increased in a time-dependent manner for up to 6 h post injection, with concomitant decrease in cardiac blood pool activity (Fig. 3b). Liver and bowel activity decreased up to 90 min, then stabilized. Bone marrow and growth plate uptake at joints showed moderately high uptake over the period of study. Muscular uptake decreased steadily with increased Target/Muscle (T/M) ratios over the entire period of the study from 3.7 to 8.5.

4.3 ^{68}Ga-Citrate for Diagnostic PET Imaging of Osteomyelitis and Follow-Up Treatment

Available literature indicates a number of parameters for imaging infection using different imaging modalities such as bone scanning, labeled white blood cell scanning, and MRI with sensitivity and specificity of 82–25%, 84–80% (21–60%

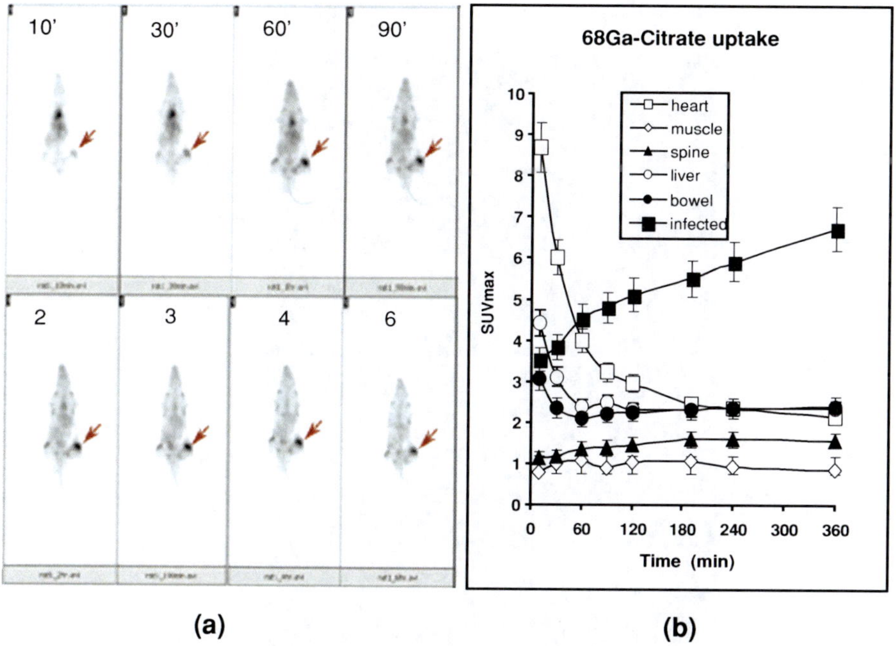

Fig. 3 ^{68}Ga-citrate uptake by *Staph A* infection in a rat model. ^{68}Ga-citrate (15 MBq) was injected into an anesthetized rat, and images were acquired at different time intervals (**a**). Infection lesions are shown by the *arrows*. SUV_{max} was calculated for each time point over infected lesions and different organs, and the values are plotted in **b**. Mean ± SD was calculated ($n = 5$) and plotted in the graph. Reproduced from Kumar et al. (2012)

for axial skeleton), and 84–60%, respectively (Ma et al. 1997; Termaat et al. 2005). According to results presented by Nanni et al. (2010), the performance of ^{68}Ga-citrate PET/CT was not really superior to that of a conventional imaging diagnostic flow chart (reporting slightly higher sensitivity and comparable specificity, but with data from limited evaluation). Nevertheless, the following advantages were clearly indicated: simple and fast diagnostic procedure, no false positivity in cases of bone implants, and low dosimetry due to short half-life. The short half-life of ^{68}Ga-citrate, although an advantage from a dosimetric point of view, could be considered a drawback at the same time, because it does not allow the long uptake time typical of ^{67}Ga-citrate scintigraphy. However, their final results showed that a short uptake time was long enough to visualize a pathologic process, although a longer time would have guaranteed higher contrast due to reduction of background (Gelrud et al. 1974). In most patients with bone infection, they reported relatively low SUV_{max}, in comparison with background. Positive ^{68}Ga PET/CT scans presented mean SUV_{max} of 4.4 ± 1.8. SUV_{max} was 3.9 ± 1.8 (range 1.7–8.0) for acute osteomyelitis, 5.5 ± 2.0 (range 4.0–7.0) for chronic osteomyelitis, and 5.8 ± 2.0 (range 3.7–8.6) for diskitis (Nanni et al. 2010).

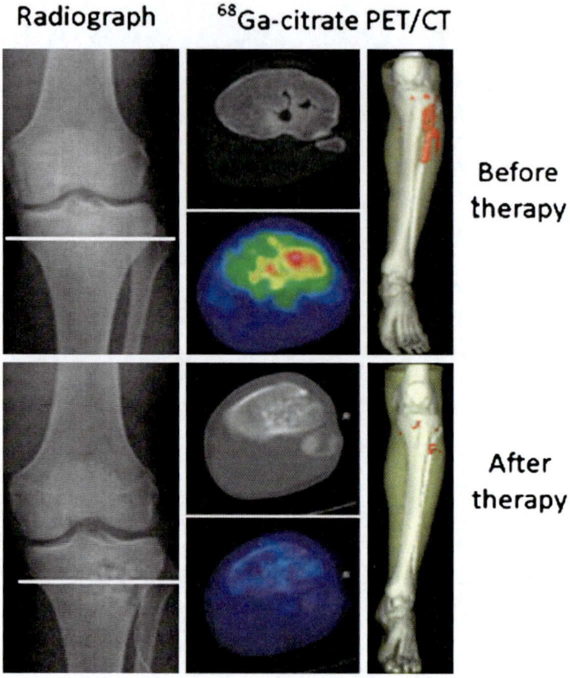

Fig. 4 Comparison of ^{68}Ga-citrate PET/CT before and after surgical curettage in a patient affected by acute osteomyelitis. On *right*, three-dimensional reconstruction shows bone infection (*red* area) also involving surrounding soft tissue. After therapy, no uptake is evident, confirming complete response. Reproduced from Nanni et al. (2010)

Although they used visual criteria to decide on all positive findings (tracer uptake significantly higher than background), most patients had SUV_{max} between 2 and 4, a value that certainly does not clearly highlight the infected area at first glance on the maximum intensity projection image. Therefore, they reviewed each scan carefully, slice by slice, and had one false-positive result from study of a total of 31 patients, which on further examination turned out to be a tumor lesion. This event was predictable because ^{67}Ga-citrate has long been used as a marker for imaging tumors (Bombardieri et al. 2003).

The importance of functional imaging is not limited to diagnosis of infection but extends also to surgical planning. Three-dimensional reconstruction images obtained with ^{68}Ga-citrate PET/CT was shown to be very useful in a patient affected by acute osteomyelitis before and after surgical curettage, confirming complete response to antibiotic therapy (Fig. 4). Similarly, ^{68}Ga-citrate PET/CT has shown avid uptake of the agent before surgery, which resolved completely after surgical curettage and local antibiotic therapy in a patient affected by acute osteomyelitis of left tibial implant (Fig. 5). Fusion of ^{68}Ga-citrate PET images and CT images provides the surgeon with an accurate and detailed basis to better plan

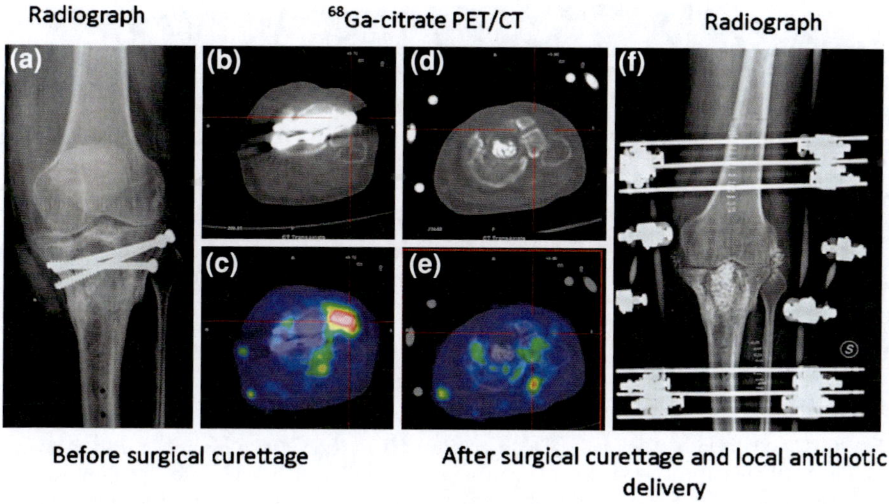

Fig. 5 Comparison of ^{68}Ga-citrate PET/CT before and after surgical curettage in patient affected by acute osteomyelitis of left tibial implant. Radiograph before therapy (**a**), CT scan before therapy (**b**), ^{68}Ga-citrate PET/CT scan before therapy (**c**), CT scan after therapy (**d**), ^{68}Ga -citrate PET/CT scan after therapy (**e**), and radiograph after therapy (**f**). **c** Focus of increased ^{68}Ga-citrate uptake in lateral side of left tibial plate close to metal implant is consistent with acute osteomyelitis (SUV_{max} 3.1). **e** After surgical curettage and local antibiotic delivery, tracer uptake completely normalizes. After 1 year of follow-up, patient was still free from pain. Reproduced from Nanni et al. (2010)

the operation and possibly improve patient outcome. They studied biopsy samples in all patients, but reported that only 11 of 30 biopsy samples (37%) were diagnostic. They found 4 false-positive scans, 23 true-positive scans, 13 true-negative scans, and no false-negative scans, resulting in sensitivity of 100%, specificity of 76%, positive predictive value of 85%, negative predictive value of 100%, with overall accuracy of 90%. They did not find significant tracer uptake in uninfected bone implants (Nanni et al. 2010).

It is widely believed that ^{18}F-FDG is the more standard in vivo marker of bone infection. ^{18}F-FDG is sensitive but has the great limitation of giving positive results in patients with bone prosthesis, even if there is no infection or mobilization (Gravius et al. 2010). In the population study by Nanni et al. (2010), many patients had different types of prostheses or bone implants, but ^{68}Ga-citrate was positive only in cases of infection. However, direct comparison of the performance of the two tracers is important, and no more comments can be made without such a comparison.

In summary, their preliminary work with ^{68}Ga-citrate PET/CT evaluated the sensitivity, specificity, positive predictive value, negative predictive value, and overall accuracy of ^{68}Ga-citrate PET/CT in a population of patients with suspected bone infection. Their study did not include recently operated patients or patients with recent bone fractures. Patients with bone implants showed significant artifacts

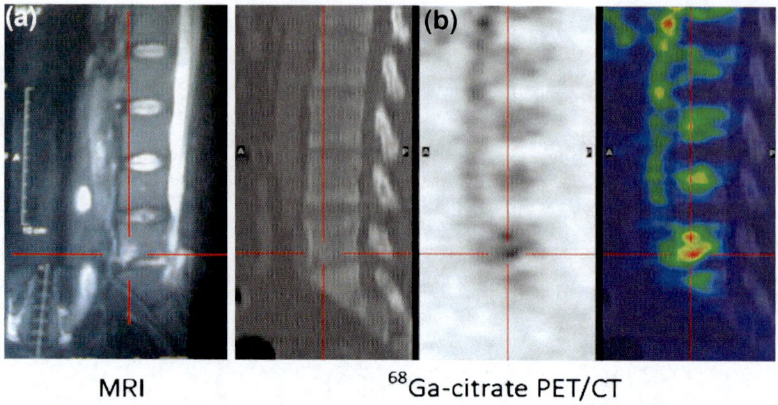

Fig. 6 Comparison of MRI and ^{68}Ga-citrate PET/CT in patient with discitis. **a** MRI shows area of abnormal signal in L5–S1 that is not unequivocally consistent with infective discitis (MRI). **b** ^{68}Ga-citrate PET/CT shows focal area of increased tracer uptake consistent with inflammation (SUV_{max} 5.3). Reproduced from Nanni et al. (2010)

on CT images but no false-positive results in the corresponding PET series, which they attributed to a correction of the View-Point iterative algorithm. Interestingly, no false-negative results were found and the negative predictive value of ^{68}Ga-citrate PET/CT was therefore quite high. This finding was confirmed by a previous preclinical publication (Makinen et al. 2005), but they indicated that the main limitation of this study is the lack of a gold standard to validate the PET/CT results—a long follow-up—which is the only reliable approach due to the cited limitations of other diagnostic procedures. They concluded "^{68}Ga-Citrate PET/CT is a new diagnostic tool that can be considered in the flow chart of patients with bone infection. However, more experience is required to further validate these results" (Nanni et al. 2010).

4.4 ^{68}Ga-Citrate PET/CT for Imaging of Discitis, Cellulitis, and Abscess

Diagnosing discitis has been a challenge for a long time. However, vertebral lesions are diagnosed more distinctly as an intense focal uptake of ^{18}F-FDG than any other agent (Stumpe et al. 2000), although this is expensive to perform. MRI has shown considerable success in diagnosing discitis, as shown by the area of abnormal signal in L5–S1, equivocally consistent with infective discitis, in Fig. 6. However, it is again very expensive to perform on a routine basis. ^{68}Ga-citrate PET/CT, which is very cost-effective and uses an easily available agent, has been shown to define discitis as focal area of increased tracer uptake consistent with inflammation (Fig. 6b). In the past, ^{99m}Tc-labeled ciprofloxacin (Infecton) has been successful, as it defined the lesions associated with discitis as hot area with

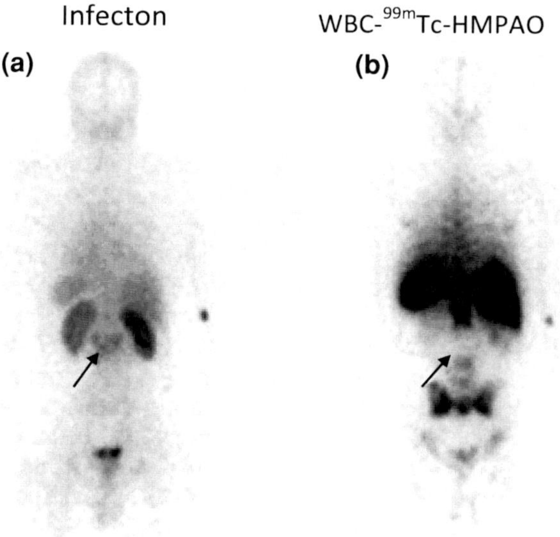

Fig. 7 Ability of Infecton (^{99m}Tc-ciprofloxacin) and ^{99m}Tc-HMPAO leukocytes in detecting spinal bone lesions. Infecton images reveal hot area with soft tissue extension in L2 and L3 (**a**). ^{99m}Tc-HMPAO-labeled leukocyte study shows a large photopenic area of defect (**b**). Defects are indicated by *arrows*. Reproduced from Kumar (2005)

soft tissue extension in L2 and L3 in Fig. 7a. Conventional imaging agents such as ^{99m}Tc-HMPAO-labeled leukocyte study had limited value in imaging discitis, as it defines a large photopenic area of defect which is hard to diagnose (Fig. 7b).

Preliminary findings from our institution in patients with cellulitis and abscess indicated the potential for ^{68}Ga-citrate PET/CT for imaging infection. We have performed a preliminary study in 12 patients using this agent, and the results indicated that infection could be identified within 60 min after injecting ^{68}Ga-citrate, which is a considerable improvement over ^{67}Ga-citrate studies which required 48–72 h post-injection time. However, whether this agent could be used as a first-line agent for imaging infection requires further substantiation. In a patient study, an infected area in the abdomen at the site of recent appendectomy was detected within 30 min post injection of ^{68}Ga-citrate (Fig. 8), which was consistent with CT, and subsequently the abscess (43 mL volume) was drained from the corresponding lesion and microbiology results further confirmed the findings. The SUV_{max} of the lesion increased from 3.3 to 6.7 from 30 to 60 min (Fig. 8a–c) post-injection period. Cardiac blood pool and liver activities decreased during the period of study. Interestingly, there was persistent high vascular activity in the thigh region. The prolonged vascular retention is consistent with low renal and bladder activity. No bowel activity was seen (Kumar et al. 2012). As the biodistribution of the agent was high in thorax and abdominal region, it has limited but meaningful application (low SUV_{max}) for imaging infection in these areas but may be ideally suited for imaging infection in the extremities (high SUV_{max}).

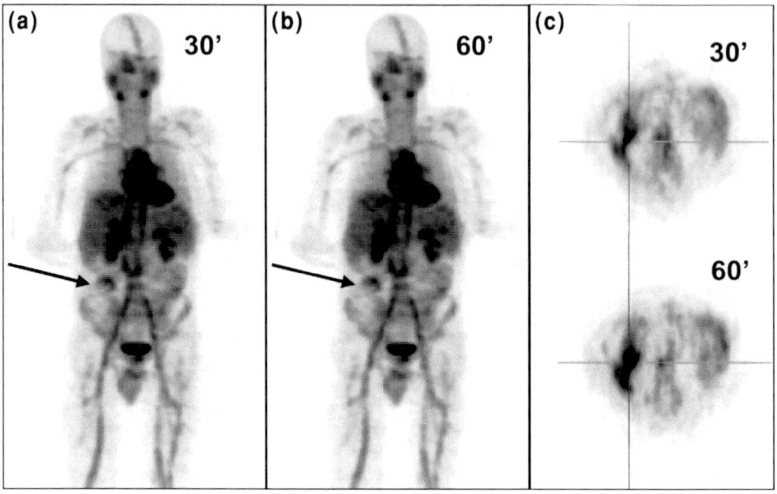

Fig. 8 ^{68}Ga-citrate PET imaging of a patient with intra-abdominal infection. ^{68}Ga-citrate (150 MBq) was injected into a patient, and images were acquired at 30 and 60 min intervals. Intra-abdominal infection lesions are shown by *arrows*. Transverse images are shown in **c**. High vascular activity and high activity in parotid and salivary glands can be seen in **a** and **b**. Reproduced from Kumar et al. (2012)

4.5 ^{68}Ga-Apo-Transferrin (^{68}Ga-TF) for PET Imaging of Bacterial Infection

The clinical utility of ^{67}Ga SPECT is somehow compromised due to the delayed post-injection waiting time of at least 24–48 h. In this context, one of the concerns related to ^{68}Ga imaging was the short half-life of ^{68}Ga ($t_{1/2} = 68$ min), which may question the fundamental concept of using this PET radionuclide for longer periods of study. We examined whether the ^{68}Ga-TF complex, once prepared in vitro, is capable of detecting infection faster than ^{68}Ga-citrate (Kumar et al. 2011). This approach might provide circumstantial experimental evidence if the delayed imaging time associated with ^{67}Ga-citrate is due to a longer time required for in vivo binding of Ga^{3+} to plasma transferrin. TF is a glycoprotein with high affinity for binding iron on its domain. The capability of TF to bind Ga^{3+} is similar to iron-binding mechanisms (Martinez et al. 1990). Therefore, we prepared $^{68}Ga^{3+}$-TF complex in vitro and examined whether this new PET tracer is capable of detecting bacterial infection much faster than ^{68}Ga-citrate. It is important to establish a faster imaging method for ^{68}Ga as its half-life is 68 min compared with 78.3 h for ^{67}Ga.

^{68}Ga-TF was prepared by mixing post-processed pure $^{68}GaCl_3$ (180 MBq/ 0.5 mL) with a solution containing 2.0 mg TF in 1.5 mL sodium carbonate (0.1 M, pH 7.0). The reaction vial was incubated in a water bath at 40°C for 1 h. TF used in the experiments was capable of binding up to 1.0 GBq $^{68}GaCl_3$ under the reaction conditions described. The RCP was >99%. When ^{68}Ga-TF was

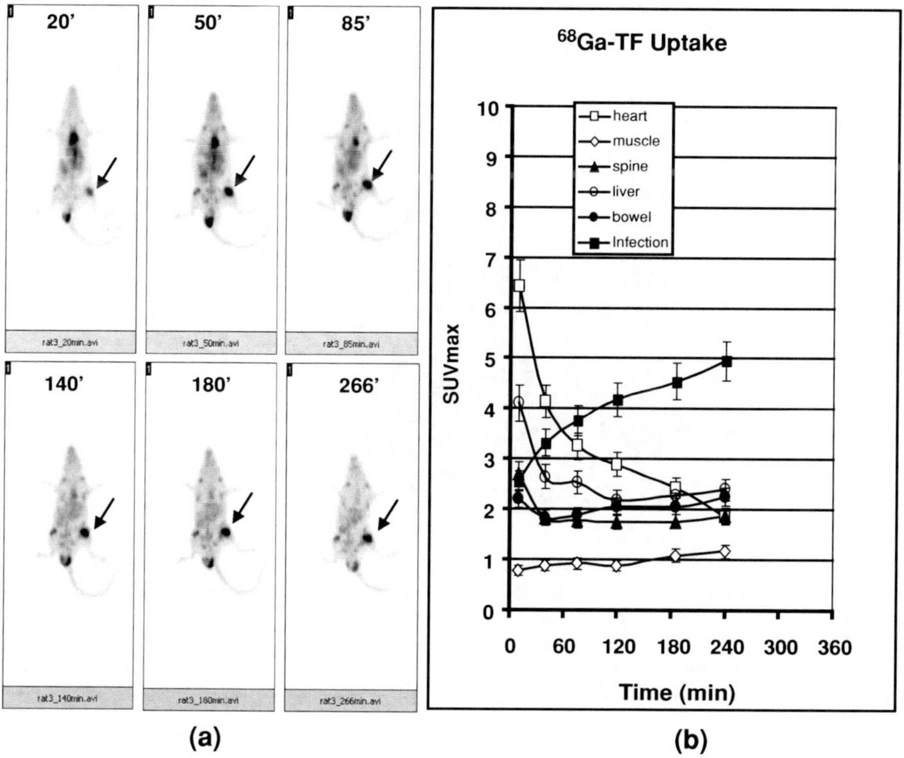

Fig. 9 ^{68}Ga-TF uptake by *Staph A* infection in a rat model. ^{68}Ga-TF (10-15 MBq/0.2 mL) was injected into an anesthetized rat, and images were acquired at different time intervals (up to 4 h). Infection site is indicated by *arrows* (**a**). SUV_{max} was calculated for each time point over different organs and plotted in **b**. Progressive increase of SUV_{max} at the target and the concomitant decrease in cardiac blood pool activity could be visualized. Mean ± SD was calculated and plotted. Reproduced from Kumar et al. (2011)

prepared under identical conditions, except saline was used instead of sodium carbonate solution, the RCP was <15% (Kumar et al. 2011). Therefore, it is mandatory to use sodium bicarbonate instead of saline for preparing ^{68}Ga-TF. The solutions were sterilized for animal injection by final filtering with 0.22-μ filter. The RCP of ^{68}Ga-TF was determined by TLC/alumina chromatography, using sodium citrate (0.1 M) as solvent (free ^{68}Ga, $R_f = 1$; bound ^{68}Ga, $R_f = 0$). Stability study was performed by mixing 0.3 mL ^{68}Ga-TF solution with 1.5 mL human serum at 37°C. RCP was measured at 1 h interval.

When ^{68}Ga-TF (10–15 MBq/0.2 mL) was injected into infected rats, the lesion was detectable within 20 min post injection, although intense, focal uptake was seen only after 50 min post injection (Fig. 9a). The accumulation of activity at the lesion increased with time, as shown by significantly increased SUV_{max} at the target from 20 min for up to 4 h post injection (Fig. 9b). There was a considerable

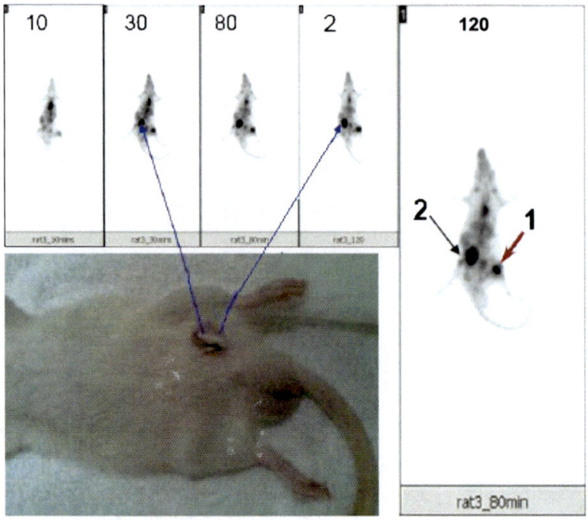

Fig. 10 ^{68}Ga-TF uptake by *Staph A* and an additional infection lesion. ^{68}Ga-TF (10–15 MBq/ 0.2 mL) was injected into an anesthetized rat, and images were acquired at different time intervals as shown in the figure. Intense uptake was seen at or after 30 min post-injection images at the site corresponding to *Staph A* injection (*arrow* 1). An additional intense, focal uptake was seen in the lower right abdominal area, which was identified to be infection due to *Proteus mirabilis* (*arrow* 2). Reproduced from Kumar et al. (2011)

decrease in cardiac activity during the initial 90 min post-injection period, but a small percentage of activity was measurable for up to 4 h post injection of the study. The activity associated with liver and bowel decreased rapidly up to 90 min of the post-injection period. The low level of activity then persisted for up to 4 h post-injection time. There was marginal increase in the activity associated with the spine over the entire period of the study, whereas muscular uptake increased marginally during the initial 60 min post-injection time but then decreased steadily over the period of the study. Since the background activity was washed out in a time-dependent manner, the T/M ratio increased progressively over the entire period of the study from 2.2 to 7.5 from 10 min to 4 h post injection (Fig. 9b) (Kumar et al. 2011).

The results in one particular rat showed avid uptake of the agent, as expected at the site corresponding to *Staph A*-induced infection in the right thigh. It also showed an additional lesion, with clearly defined intense focal uptake in the lower abdominal area, which was persistent during the entire period of study (Fig. 10). Physical examination of the additional lesion site indicated an infected wound and an abscess on the skin. When biopsied, microbiology identified the organism as *Proteus mirabilis*. Therefore, the study indicated that ^{68}Ga-TF is capable of detecting both Gram-positive and Gram-negative infection caused by both *Staph A* and *Proteus mirabilis*, and may be extrapolated to all anaerobic bacteria.

Therefore, with the circumstantial experimental evidence, it may be reasonable to conclude that ^{68}Ga-TF complex is able to accumulate at bacterial and inflammatory lesions (Henkin 1978; Tsan 1985). Available literature suggests that the total amount of TF in humans is approximately 240 mg/kg (Bernstein 1998). Therefore, it is reasonable to assume in our study that the mass of injected TF (0.2 mg/rat) in ^{68}Ga-apo-transferrin is too small to induce any unexpected pharmacological effect to influence the biodistribution of the agent.

4.6 Comparison of ^{68}Ga-Chloride and ^{18}F-FDG for PET Imaging of Osteomyelitis and Human Pancreatic Adenocarcinoma Xenografts in Rats

PET using ^{18}F-FDG is ideal for imaging infection, inflammation, and tumor, which are typically characterized by increased glucose metabolism and increased expression of glucose transporters (Ichiya et al. 1996; Sugawara et al. 1999; Stumpe et al. 2000). ^{18}F-FDG uptake is elevated in activated inflammatory cells such as leukocytes, granulocytes, and macrophages because of the above phenomenon. Early bone healing also mimics infection, as it involves an inflammatory phase, which represents a highly activated state of cell metabolism and glucose consumption (Einhorn 1998), and therefore findings with ^{18}F-FDG PET imaging may be complicated by not differentiating inflammation, infection, and bone healing. It has been proposed that an interval of 3–6 months should be allowed to minimize the risk of false-positive findings in patients with postsurgical and traumatic bone healing (de Winter et al. 2002). Recent studies in a rabbit osteomyelitis model indicated that bone infection could be distinguished from bone healing by means of ^{18}F-FDG PET after only an interval of 3 weeks (Koort et al. 2004). However, the transient ^{18}F-FDG uptake by healing bones could still create problems in differential diagnosis under these clinical conditions.

The clinical utility of the two agents ^{18}F-FDG and ^{68}Ga-chloride was compared for monitoring normal bone healing and osteomyelitis in rat tibia (Fig. 11). Quantitative uptake of these agents was also estimated to verify the uptake of ^{18}F-FDG and ^{68}Ga, in normal bone healing and osteomyelitis. The results showed, based on 120-min dynamic imaging, that accumulation of ^{68}Ga was slower (70 min post injection) than that of ^{18}F-FDG (40 min post injection) in the infected bone. On the other hand, they showed increased uptake of both tracers (^{18}F-FDG and ^{68}Ga) in osteomyelitic tibia compared with contralateral normal tibia. Control animals with healing bone defects showed slightly increased uptake of ^{18}F-FDG, but no apparent increase in ^{68}Ga uptake was seen as compared with contralateral intact tibia (Makinen et al. 2005).

They also correlated the intensity of tracer uptake to pathological changes in the infected cortical bone. Interestingly, their initial observation suggests that ^{68}Ga did not accumulate in healing bones without infection (compared with contralateral intact tibia), in contrast to the avid uptake of ^{18}F-FDG. Further studies are needed to clarify the value of ^{68}Ga-chloride PET for healing bones, but greater potential is demonstrated than for ^{18}F-FDG. Stability and clinical utility of ^{68}Ga-chloride are

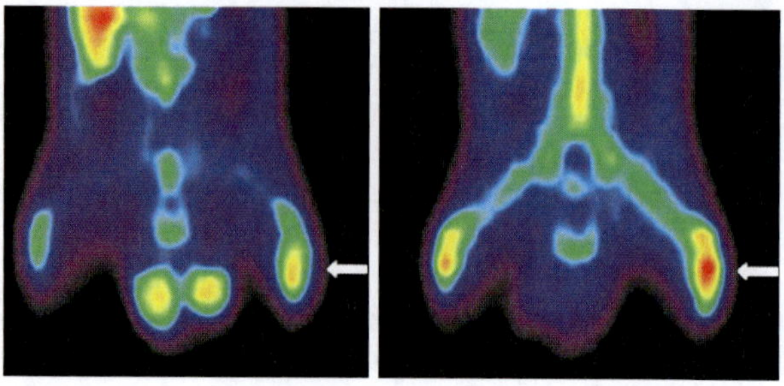

Fig. 11 Comparative ^{18}F-FDG (*left*) and ^{68}Ga (*right*) PET coronal images of the lower body in an osteomyelitic animal at 2 weeks. The left infected tibia (*white arrow*) shows increased tracer uptake for ^{18}F-FDG (SUV ratio 1.8) and ^{68}Ga (SUV ratio 1.6) compared with the intact right tibia. Reproduced from Makinen et al. 2005

not well established, whereas ^{68}Ga-citrate is a more stable agent than the former, as discussed in the earlier chapters.

Ujula et al. (2009) investigated the value of ^{68}Ga-chloride for PET imaging of tumors, comparing it against ^{18}F-FDG. They used human pancreatic adenocarcinoma xenograft in rat as an experimental tumor model, as imaging and early diagnosis of pancreatic cancer still remain a challenge (Nakao et al. 2006; Saif et al. 2008). In the past, ^{18}F-FDG and ^{67}Ga-citrate were widely used for imaging tumors, but not ^{68}Ga-chloride. Their results revealed that ^{68}Ga-chloride was able to differentiate experimental tumors from surrounding normal tissues. They also presented data showing that tumor uptake of ^{68}Ga-chloride was lower than that of ^{18}F-FDG. Both tracers were capable of visualizing subcutaneous tumors; however, they clearly demonstrated using dynamic PET imaging that tumor uptake of ^{68}Ga-chloride was much faster than that of ^{18}F-FDG. Blood clearance of ^{68}Ga radioactivity from heart was slower compared with ^{18}F-FDG, which is in accordance with Ga^{3+} binding to transferrin, consistent with our observation (Kumar et al. 2011). The slow clearance was consistent with the low tumor-to-blood ratio of ^{68}Ga-chloride as noticed by ex vivo studies.

They concluded "^{68}Ga-Chloride delineated subcutaneously implanted pancreatic adenocarcinoma xenografts by PET, but the uptake was lower than FDG. Further studies to clarify the value of ^{68}Ga-Chloride for PET imaging of tumors are warranted" (Ujula et al. 2009).

As the focus of this review is on ^{68}Ga-radiopharmaceuticals for imaging infection and inflammation, examination of the clinical utility of other radiopharmaceuticals such as proteins, liposomes, and activated adhesion molecules would lie beyond the scope of this chapter. ^{68}Ga-labeled siderophores for fungal imaging were shown to have excellent potential to specifically identify fungal infections (Petrik et al. 2010), which is an enormous advantage in patients undergoing chemotherapy who are prone to fungal infection.

5 Evaluation of ^{99m}Tc- and ^{68}Ga-Glucosamine for Imaging Inflammatory Arthritis

^{18}F-FDG has been the most widely used PET agent for more than two decades for imaging a variety of tumors, infection, and inflammation. Localization is based on increased glucose utilization (Shulkin 1997; Coleman 2000; Weber et al. 2000). PET imaging usually shows better sensitivity and resolution than SPECT imaging. However, use of PET is still limited by factors such as limited availability and high cost. Besides, PET radiopharmaceuticals are expensive, cumbersome to prepare, and often have ultrashort half-life. Therefore, ^{99m}Tc-labeled glucosamine, a glucose analog, has been explored to identify similar pathology with potentially greater utility.

Glucosamine has been used for treating inflammatory arthritis, although the underlying mechanism is not clearly established. It was suggested that glucosamine might serve as the "building block" to form the polymers, glycosaminoglycans, which are involved with formation and repair of cartilage. It was also envisaged that glucosamine uptake, similar to FDG, is enhanced during increased glycolysis associated with inflammatory arthritis. Therefore, deoxyglucosamine was labeled with ^{99m}Tc-pertechnetate (^{99m}Tc-ECDG), and its utility in detecting inflammatory arthritis in patients was explored (Kumar et al. 2007).

5.1 Chemical Structures of Glucose Analogs and Synthesis of ^{99m}Tc-Labeled Deoxyglucosamine

The molecular structures of the three compounds are presented in Fig. 12. When the hydroxyl group of 2-deoxyglucose is substituted with –NH_2 group, it becomes 2-deoxyglucosamine, and when ^{18}F is substituted it becomes ^{18}F-FDG (Fig. 12). Glucosamine was linked with a N_2S_2 chelator [ethylene dicysteine (EC)] as described by Yang et al. (2003, 2004) to form ECDG. ^{99m}Tc-labeling was achieved by mixing freshly eluted ^{99m}Tc-pertechnetate (1.5 GBq/2.5 mL saline for injection) to a N_2 vial containing 1.0 mg ECDG and 0.1 mg stannous chloride. Radiolabeling occurred within minutes, and the RCP of the labeled compound was >98% when tested by Whatman-31/acetone chromatography (Kumar et al. 2007).

Studies were performed to demonstrate the potential imaging capability of ^{99m}Tc-ECDG in detecting inflammatory arthritis. Experimental arthritis was induced by subcutaneously injecting 0.1 mL *Mycobacterium tuberculosis* (10 mg/mL squalene) at the base of the tail of the rats. The rats developed arthritis at the joints within 8–10 days after injection. SPECT imaging studies showed focal uptake of ^{99m}Tc-ECDG at the arthritic inflammatory lesions within 30 min post injection (Kumar et al. 2007).

Based on the encouraging results from the preclinical studies, a preliminary study was performed with ^{99m}Tc-ECDG in a human volunteer with clinical symptoms of inflammatory arthritis at the left knee and pain-free normal right

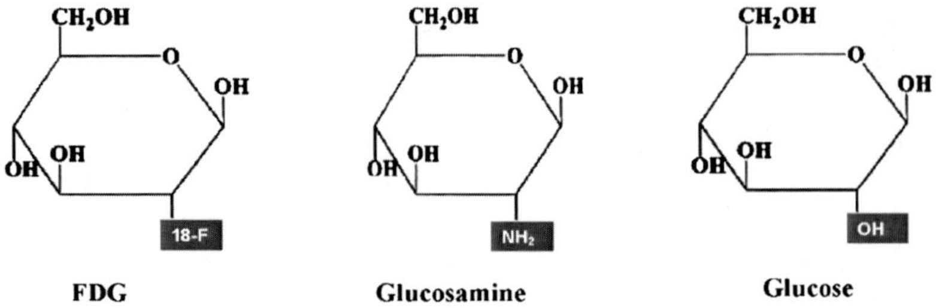

Fig. 12 Chemical structures of ^{18}F-FDG, d-glucosamine, and glucose. The molecular structure of glucose analogs are indicated in this figure. When the hydroxyl group of 2-deoxyglucose is substituted with $-NH_2$ group, it becomes 2-deoxyglucosamine, and when ^{18}F is substituted it becomes ^{18}F-FDG (^{18}F- fluorodeoxyglucose)

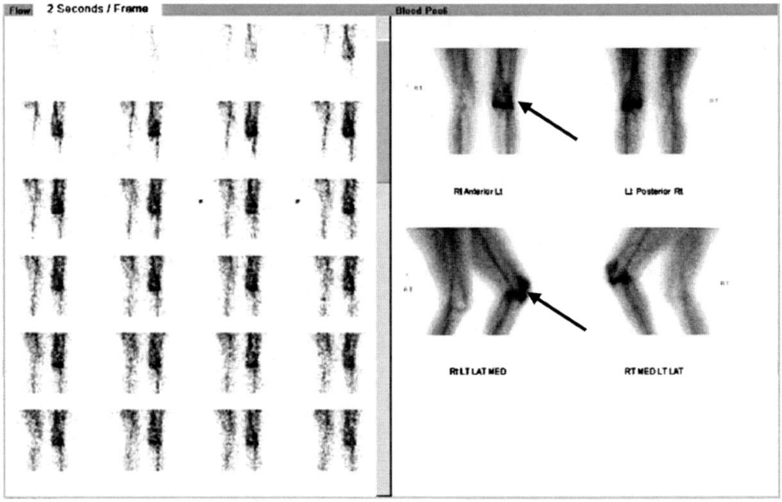

Fig. 13 Imaging of inflammatory arthritis with ^{99m}Tc-glucosamine (^{99m}Tc-ECDG). ^{99m}Tc-ECDG was injected intravenously (about 10 MBq/0.2 mL saline) in arthritic rats, and images were obtained at the indicated times after injection. The focal uptake of the agents is indicated at the left knees by the *arrows* at the arthritic lesions. Reproduced from Kumar et al. (2007)

knee. The initial blood pool images were consistent with significantly increased blood flow at the arthritic lesions at the left side compared with the contralateral normal joints (Fig. 13). The delayed images at 3 h clearly confirmed focal uptake of the agent at the left knee without remarkable uptake at the right knee. We have investigated more than 100 patients with inflammatory arthritis, and our results are encouraging and strongly suggest a role for ^{99m}Tc-ECDG as a potential biomarker for imaging arthritic patients using this agent.

5.2 Synthesis of ^{68}Ga-Glucosamine and Preliminary Results

Future work is planned to prepare ^{68}Ga-labeled glucosamine to take advantage of higher resolution and image quality of ^{68}Ga PET than ^{99m}Tc–ECDG. DO2A-glucosamine was synthesised by Riss et al. (2011) We radiolabeled DO2A with post-processed pure $^{68}Ga^{3+}$ by boiling for at least 10 min at 100°C. Our results have shown that the labeled product had high RCP (>98%) and was stable for longer than 6 h without compromising stability (>95%), and the stability was not compromised when challenged with citrate (Rinne et al. 2010).

Biodistribution of ^{68}Ga-labeled glucosamine (^{68}Ga-DO2A) in normal animal study indicated rapid uptake of the agent by the kidneys, blood pool, and growth plates of the bones. Interestingly, there was no uptake of the agent by brain, which is consistent with ^{99m}Tc-ECDG but distinctly different from ^{18}F-FDG, which accumulates in brain. This differential uptake by the brain may be usefully exploited by using ^{68}Ga-labeled glucosamine for imaging brain tumors, as the absence of interfering brain uptake would be a major advantage over ^{18}F-FDG. Further work is being undertaken to explore the full potential of this agent for inflammatory arthritis and brain tumor imaging.

6 Conclusion

A simple method is described to prepare ^{68}Ga-citrate with high yield (>99%) and high RCP (>99%), being ideal for routine clinical preparation (Kumar et al. 2012). The results show that ^{68}Ga-citrate is capable of detecting *Staph A* infection in the rat model within 1 h after intravenous injection. As a proof of concept, intra-abdominal infection in a patient was detected as focal uptake within 30 min after ^{68}Ga-citrate administration. ^{18}F-FDG is sensitive but has the great limitation of giving positive results in patients with bone prosthesis, even if there is no infection or mobilization (Gravius et al. 2010). On the other hand, ^{68}Ga-citrate was positive only in cases of infection in many patients with different types of prostheses or bone implants (Nanni et al. 2010). Therefore, ^{68}Ga-citrate PET/CT is a new diagnostic tool that can be considered in the flow chart of patients with bone infection. However, more experience is required to further validate these results. Both ^{18}F-FDG and ^{68}Ga were shown to accumulate in *Staphylococcus aureus*-induced osteomyelitis. However, ^{68}Ga, in contrast to ^{18}F-FDG, did not accumulate in healing bones without infection, indicating its potential clinical utility to distinguish the two conditions. ^{68}Ga-chloride and ^{18}F-FDG PET imaging were able to delineate subcutaneously implanted human pancreatic adenocarcinoma xenografts in rats, where ^{18}F-FDG was clearly shown to be superior (Ujula et al. 2009). It was also reported that $^{68}GaCl_3$ can bind TF to give a high specific activity preparation in small volume, with preliminary results suggesting that ^{68}Ga-TF is capable of detecting *Staphylococcus aureus*-induced infection in the rat model, within 1 h after intravenous injection, indicating its high potential for clinical utility.

^{99m}Tc-labeled glucosamine is shown to be a potential biomarker for inflammatory arthritis, and it could be extended to explore the clinical value of ^{68}Ga-labeled glucosamine in this context. ^{68}Ga-labeled glucosamine may have very high potential for imaging brain tumors, as the absence of interfering brain uptake would be a major advantage over ^{18}F-FDG.

Acknowledgments We express sincere thanks to several authors for allowing us to reproduce figures and information from their published articles as acknowledged in the respective sections.

References

Aardaneh K, van der Walt K (2006) Ga_2O for target, solvent extraction for radiochemical separation and SnO_2 for the preparation of a ^{68}Ge/^{68}Ga generator. J Radioanal Nucl Chem 268:25–32

Aisen P, Listowsky I (1980) Iron transport and storage proteins. Annu Rev Biochem 49:357–393

Akhtar MS, Qaisar A, Irfanullah J et al (2005) Antimicrobial peptide ^{99m}Tc-ubiquicidin 29–41 as human infectionimaging agent: clinical trial. J Nucl Med 46:567–573

Allan RA, Sladen GE, Bassingham S et al (1993) Comparison of simultaneous ^{99m}Tc-HMPAO and ^{111}In oxine labelled white cell scans in the assessment of inflammatory bowel disease. Eur J Nucl Med 20:195–200

Antunes P, Ginj M, Zhang H et al (2007) Are radiogallium-labelled DOTA-conjugated somatostatin analogues superior to those labelled with other radiometals. Eur J Nucl Med Mol Imaging 34:982–993

Arseneau JC, Aamodt R, Johnston GS et al (1974) Evidence for granutocytic incorporation of 67gallium in chronic granulocytic leukemia. J Lab Clin Med 83:496–503

Asti S et al (2008) Validation of ^{68}Ge/^{68}Ga generator processing by chemical purification for routine clinical application of ^{68}Ga-DOTATOC. Nucl Med Biol 35:721–724

Barron B, Hanna C, Passalaqua AM, Lamki L, Wegener WA, Goldenberg DM (1999) Rapid diagnostic imaging of acute, nonclassic appendicitis by leukoscintigraphy with sulesomab, a technetium 99 m-labeled antigranulocyte antibody Fab' fragment. LeukoScan Appendicitis Clinical Trial Group. Surgery 125:288–296

Bailey S, Evans RW, Garratt RC et al (1988) Molecular structure of serum transferrin at 3.3 Å resolution. Biochemistry 27:5804–5812

Baum RP, Prasad V, Hommann M et al (2008) Receptor PET/CT imaging of neuroendocrine tumors. Recent Results Cancer Res 170:225–242

Baum RP, Prasad V et al (2010) Molecular imaging of HER2-expressing malignant tumors in breast cancer patients using synthetic ^{111}In- or ^{68}Ga-labeled affibody molecules. J Nucl Med 51(6):892–897

Bernstein L (1998) Mechanisms of therapeutic activity for Gallium. Pharmacol Rev 50:665–682

Becker W, Repp R, Hansen HJ et al (1995) Binding characteristics and kinetics of a new Tc-99 m-antigranulocyte Fab' fragment (Leukoscan TM). J Nucl Med 36(Suppl):208P

Bitran J, Bekerman C, Weinstein R et al (1987) Patterns of gallium-67 scintigraphy in patients with acquired immunodeficiency syndrome and the AIDS related complex. J Nucl Med 28: 1103–1106

Boerman OC, Dams ETM, Oyen WJG, Corstens FHM, Storm G (2001) Radiopharmaceuticals for scintigraphic imaging of infection and inflammations. Inflamm Res 50:55–64

Bombardieri E, Aktolun C, Baum RP, Bishof-Delaloye A, Buscombe J, Chatal JF (2003) ^{67}Ga scintigraphy: procedure guidelines for tumor imaging. Eur J Nucl Med Mol Imaging 30: BP125–BP131

Breeman WAP, de Jong M, de Blois E et al (2004) Radiolabelling DOTA-peptides with ^{68}Ga. Eur J Nucl Med 32:478–485

Burleson R, Johnson M, Head H (1973) Scintigraphic demonstration of experimental abscesses with intravenous ^{67}Ga-citrate and ^{67}Ga labeled blood leukocytes. Ann Surg 178:446–451

Burleson RL, Johnson MC, Head H (1974) In vitro and in vivo labeling of rabbit blood leukocytes with ^{67}Ga-citrate. J Nucl Med 15:98–101

Chianelli M, Mather SJ, Martin-Comin J, Signore A (1997) Radiopharmaceuticals for the study of inflammatory processes: a review. Nucl Med Commun 18:437–455

Conry BG, Papathanasiou ND, Prakash V et al (2010) Comparison of ^{68}Ga-DOTATATE and ^{18}F-fluorodeoxyglucose PET/CT in the detection of recurrent medullary thyroid carcinoma. Eur J Nucl Med Mol Imaging 37:49–57

Coleman RE (2000) FDG imaging. Nucl Med Biol 27(7):689–690

de Winter F, Vogelaers D, Gemmel F, Dierckx RA (2002) Promising role of ^{18}F-fluoro-D-deoxyglucose positron emission tomography in clinical infectious diseases. Eur J Clin Microbiol Infect Dis 21:247–257

Dimitrakopoulou-Strauss A, Hohenberger P, Haberkorn U, Macke HR, Eisenhut M (2007) ^{68}Ga-labeled bombesin studies in patients with gastrointestinal stromal tumours: comparison with ^{18}F-FDG. J Nucl Med 48:1245–1250

Edwards CL, Hayes RL (1969) Tumor scanning with ^{67}Ga-citrate. J Nucl Med 10:103–105

Ehrhardt GJ, Welch MJ (1978) A new germanium-68/gallium-68 generator. J Nucl Med 19: 925–929

Einhorn TA (1998) The cell and molecular biology of fracture healing. Clin Orthop 355S:7–21

El-Maghraby TA, Moustafa HM, Pauwels EK (2006) Nuclear medicine methods for evaluation of skeletal infection among other diagnostic modalities. Q J Nucl Med Mol Imaging 50:167–192

Gabriel M, Decristoforo C, Kendler D et al (2007) ^{68}Ga-DOTA-Tyr3-octreotide PET in neuroendocrine tumors: comparison with somatostatin receptor scintigraphy and CT. J Nucl Med 48:508–518

Gelrud LG, Arseneau JC, Milder MS et al (1974) The kinetic of 67-gallium incorporation into inflammatory lesions: experimental and clinical studies. J Lab Clin Med 85:489–495

Gravius S, Gebhard M, Ackermann D et al (2010) Analysis of ^{18}F-FDG uptake pattern in PET for diagnosis of aseptic loosening versus prosthesis infection after total knee arthroplasty: a prospective pilot study. Nuklearmedizin 49:115–123

Harris DC, Aisen P (1989) In: Loehr TM et al (ed) Iron carriers and iron proteins. VCH, Weinheim, pp 239–351

Henkin RE (1978) Gallium-67 in the diagnosis of inflammatory disease. In: Hoffer PB, Bekerman C, Henkin RE (eds) Gallium-67 imaging. Wiley, New York, pp 65–92

Henze M, Schuhmacher J, Hipp P et al (2001) PET imaging of somatostatin receptors using ^{68}Ga-DOTA-D-Phel-Tyr3-octreotide: first results in patients with meningiomas. J Nucl Med 42:1053–1056

Hofmann M, Mäcke HR, Börner AR et al (2001) Biokinetics and imaging with the somatostatin receptor PET radioligand ^{68}Ga-DOTA TOC: preliminary data. Eur J Nucl Med 28:1751–1757

Hopkins GB, Mende CW (1975) Gallium-67 and subphrenic abscesses—is delayed scintigraphy necessary? J Nucl Med 16:609–611

Hoffer P (1980) Gallium: mechanisms. J Nucl Med 21:282–285

Hughes DK (2003) Nuclear medicine and infection detection: the relative effectiveness of imaging with ^{111}In-oxine–, ^{99m}Tc-HMPAO–, and ^{99m}Tc-stannous fluoride colloid-labeled leukocytes and with ^{67}Ga-citrate. J Nucl Med Technol 31:196–201

Huebers HA, Finch CA (1987) The physiology of transferrin and transferring receptors. Physiol Rev 67:520–582

Ichiya Y, Kuwabara Y, Sasaki M et al (1996) FDG-PET in infectious lesions: the detection and assessment of lesion activity. Ann Nucl Med 10:185–191

Iqbal MS, Khan J, Irfanullah MA et al (2004) 99mTc-labeled antimicrobial peptide ubiquicidin (29–41) accumulates less in Escherichia coli infection than in Staphlococcus aureus infection. J Nucl Med 45:849–856

Ito Y, Okuyama S, Awano T, Takahashi K, Sato T (1971) Diagnostic evaluation of Ga-67 scanning of lung cancer and other diseases. Radiology 101:355–362

Jeong JM, Hong MK, Chang YS et al (2008) Preparation of a promising angiogenesis PET imaging agent: ^{68}Ga-labeled c(RGDyK)-isothiocyanatobenzyl-1,4,7-triaza-cyclononane-1,4,7-triacetic acid and feasibility studies in mice. J Nucl Med 49(5):830–836

Kelly MJ, Kalff V, Hicks RJ et al (1990) ^{111}In-oxine labelled leukocyte scintigraphy in the detection and localization of active inflammation and sepsis. Med J Aust 152:352–357

Kopecky P, Mudrová B, Svoboda K (1973) The study of conditions for the preparation and utilization of ^{68}Ge–^{68}Ga generator. Int J Appl Radiat Isot 24:73–80

Kopecky P, Mudrová B (1974) ^{68}Ge–^{68}Ga generator for the production of ^{68}Ga in an ionic form. Int J Appl Radiat Isot 25:263–268

Koort JK, Mäkinen TJ, Knuuti J, Jalava J, Aro HT (2004) Comparative ^{18}F-FDG-PET imaging of experimental Staphylococcus aureus osteomyelitis and normal bone healing. J Nucl Med 45:1406–1411

Kramer EL, Sanger JH, Garay SM et al (1989) Diagnostic implications of Ga-67 chest scan patterns in human immunodeficiency virus-seropositive patients. Radiology 170:671–676

Kumar V (2005) Radiolabeled white blood cells and direct targeting of micro-organisms for infection imaging. Q J Nucl Med Mol Imaging 49:325–338

Kumar V, Ali M, Angelides S et al (2007) Synthesis and characterisation of ^{99m}Tc-glucosamine and ^{99m}Tc-His-CP and evaluation of their utility in imaging inflammatory arthritis. J ANZ Nucl Med 38(3):10–13

Kumar V, Boddeti DK, Evans SG, Roesch F, Howman-Giles R (2009) Is ^{68}Ga-citrate a novel agent for PET-imaging of Staphylococcus aureus infection? Eur J Nucl Med Mol Imaging 36(Suppl 2):S194–S233

Kumar V, Boddeti DK, Evans SG, Roesch F, Howman-Giles R (2011) Potential use of ^{68}Ga-apo-transferrin as a PET imaging agent for detecting Staphylococcus aureus infection. Nucl Med Biol 38:393–398

Kumar V, Boddeti DK, Evans SG, Angelides S (2012) ^{68}Ga-citrate-PET for diagnostic imaging of infection in rats and for intra abdominal infection in a patient. Current radiopharmaceuticals 5:71–75

Larson SM (1978) Mechanisms of localization of gallium-67 in tumors. Semin Nucl Med 8:193–203

Lavender JP, Lowe J, Baker JR et al (1971) Gallium-67 citrate scanning in neoplastic and inflammatory lesions. Br J Radiol 44:361–366

Lisbona R, Derbekyan V, Novales-Diaz J et al (1993) Gallium-67 scintigraphy in tuberculous and nontuberculousn infectious spondylitis. J Nucl Med 34:853–859

Littenberg RL, Taketa RM, Alazraki NP et al (1973) Gallium-67 for localization of septic lesions. Ann Intern Med 79:403–406

Lim Y, Shin SH, Lee SI, Kim IS, Rhec JH (1998) Iron-repressibility of siderophore and transferrin-binding protein Staphylococcus aureus. FEMS Microbiol Lett 163:19–24

Lupetti A, Welling MM, Mazzi U et al (2002) Technetium-99m labelled fluconazole and antimicrobial peptides for imaging of Candida albicans and aspergillus fumigatus infections. Eur J Nucl Med Mol Imaging 29:674–679

Lupetti A, Nibbering PH, Welling MM, Pauwels EK (2003) Radiopharmaceuticals: new antimicrobial agents. Trends Biotechnol 21:70–73

Maecke HR, Andre JP (2007) ^{68}Ga-PET radiopharmacy: a generator-based alternative to ^{18}F-radiopharmacy. In: Schubiger PA, Lehmann L, Friebe M (eds) PET chemistry, the driving force in molecular imaging. Springer, New York, pp 215–241

Martinez JL, Delgado-Iribarren A, Baquero F (1990) Mechanisms of iron acquisition and bacterial virulence. FEMS Microbiol Rev 75:45–56

Makinen TJ, Lankinen P, Poyhonen T et al (2005) Comparison of ^{18}F-FDG and ^{68}Ga PET imaging in the assessment of experimental osteomyelitis due to Staphylococcus aureus. Eur J Nucl Med Mol Imaging 32:1259–1268

Ma LD, Frassica FJ, Bluemke DA, Fishman EK (1997) CT and MRI evaluation of musculoskeletal infection. Crit Rev Diagn Imaging 38:535–568

McAfee JG, Thakur ML (1976a) Survey of radioactive agents for in vitro labelling of phagocytic leukocytes I. Soluble agents. J Nucl Med 17:480–487

McAfee JG, Thakur ML (1976b) Survey of radioactive agents for in vitro labelling of phagocytic leukocytes II. Particles. J Nucl Med 17:488–492

Merkel KD, Brown ML, Fitzgerald RH Jr (1986) Sequential technetium-99m HMDP gallium-67 citrate imaging for the evaluation of infection in the painful prosthesis. J Nucl Med 27: 1413–1417

Menon S, Wagner HN Jr, Tsan MF (1978) Studies on gallium-accumulation in inflammatory lesions II. Uptake by Staphylococcus aureus: concise communication. J Nucl Med 19:44–47

Mozley PD, Thakur ML, Alavi A et al (1999) Effects of a ^{99m}Tc-labeled murine immunoglobulin M antibody to CD15 antigens on human granulocyte membranes in healthy volunteers. J Nucl Med 40:2107–2114

Modic MT, Feiglin DH, Piraino DW et al (1985) Vertebral osteomyelitis: assessment using MR. Radiology 157:157–166

Moser E, Tatsch K, Kirsch C-M et al (1990) Value of ^{67}gallium scintigraphy in primary diagnosis and follow-up of opportunistic pneumonia in patients with AIDS. Lung 168(suppl):692–703

Nakao A, Fujii T, Sugimoto H et al (2006) Oncological problems in pancreatic cancer surgery. World J Gastroenterol 12:4466–4472

Nanni C et al (2010) ^{68}Ga-Citrate PET/CT for Evaluating Patients with Infections of the Bone. Preliminary results. J Nucl Med 51(12):1932–1936

Palestro CJ, Swyer AJ, Kim CK, Goldsmith SJ (1991) Infected knee prosthesis: diagnosis with In-Ill-leukocyte, Tc-99m sulfur colloid, and Tc-99m MDP imaging. Radiology 179:645–648

Palestro CJ (1994) The current role of gallium imaging in infection. Semin Nucl Med 24:128–141

Palestero CJ (2003) Nuclear medicine, the painful prosthetic joint, and orthopaedic infection. J Nucl Med 44:927–929

Peters AM (1994) The utility of ^{99m}Tc HMPAO-leukocytes for imaging infection. Semin Nucl Med 24:110–127

Petrik M, Haas H, Dobrozemsky G et al (2010) ^{68}Ga-Siderophores for PET imaging of invasive pulmonary aspergillosis: proof of principle. J Nucl Med 51(4):639–645

Rinne J, Boddeti DK, Burchardt C, Kumar V, Angelides S, Roesch F (2010) Preparation of ^{68}Ga-labelled glucosamine. Int Med J 40(Suppl 2):1–39 (Abstract)

Rizzello A, Di Pierro D, Lodi F et al (2009) Synthesis and quality control of ^{68}Ga citrate for routine clinical PET. Nucl Med Comm 30:542–545

Riss PJ, Kroll C, Nagel V, Roesch F (2008) NODAPA-OH and NODAPA-(NCS)n: Synthesis, ^{68}Ga-radiolabelling and in vitro characterisation of novel versatile bifunctional chelators for molecular imaging. Bioorg Med Chem Lett 18:5364–5367

Riss PJ, Burchrdt c, Roesch F (2011) A methodical ^{68}Ga labeling study of DO2A-(butyl-L-tyrosine) 2 with cation-exchanger post-processed ^{68}Ga: practical aspects of radiolabelling. Contrast Media Mol Imag 6:492–498

Roesch F, Riss PJ (2010) The renaissance of the ^{68}Ge/^{68}Ga radionuclide generator initiates new developments in ^{68}Ga radiopharmaceutical chemistry. Curr Top Med Chem 10:1–35

Rösch F, Filosofov DV (2010) Production, radiochemical processing and quality evaluation of Ge-68 suitable for production of a ^{68}Ge/^{68}Ga generator. In: IAEA-TEC-DOC radioisotopes and radiopharmaceuticals, series 2: production and processing of parent radionuclides for generators: ^{68}Ga, ^{82}Sr, ^{90}Sr, ^{188}W for nuclear medicine applications, Int Atomic Energy Agency, Vienna ISBN 978-92-0-101110-7

Rösch F, Knapp FF (Russ) (2003) Radionuclide generators. In: Vértes A, Nagy S, Klencsár Z (eds) Handbook of nuclear chemistry. Kluwer Academic, Dordrecht, The Netherlands

Rufini V, Calcagni ML, Baum RP (2006) Imaging of neuroendocrine tumors. Semin Nucl Med 36:228–247

Rypins EB, Kipper SL, Weiland F et al (2002) ^{99m}Tc anti-CD 15 monoclonal antibody (LeuTech) imaging improves diagnostic accuracy and clinical management in patients with equivocal presentation of appendicitis. Ann Surg 235:232–239

Saif MW, Cornfeld D, Modarresifar H, Ojha B (2008) FDG positron emission tomography CT (FDG-PET-CT) in the management of pancreatic cancer: initial experience in 12 patients. J Gastrointest Liver Dis 17:173–178

Silberstein EB, Fernandez-Ulloa M, Hall J (1981) Are oral cathartics of value in optimizing the gallium scan? concise communication. J Nucl Med 22:424–427

Shulkin BL (1997) PET applications in pediatrics. Q J Nucl Med 41(4):281–291

Shongwe MS, Smith CA, Ainscough EW et al (1992) Anion binding by human lactoferrin: results from crystallographic and physicochemical studies. Biochemistry 31:4451–4458

Siaens R, Eijsink VG, Dierckx R, Slegers G (2004) ^{123}I-Labeled chitinase as specific radioligand for in vivo detection of fungal infections in mice. J Nucl Med 45:1209–1216

Skehan SJ, White JF, Evans JW et al (2003) Mechanism of accumulation of ^{99m}Tc-sulesomab in inflammation. J Nucl Med 44:11–18

Stumpe KD, Dazzi H, Schaffner A, von Schulthess GK (2000) Infection imaging using whole-body FDG-PET. Eur J Nucl Med 27:822–832

Sugawara Y, Gutowski TD, Fisher SJ et al (1999) Uptake of positron emission tomography tracers in experimental bacterial infections: a comparative biodistribution study of radiolabeled FDG, thymidine, L-methionine, ^{67}Ga-citrate, and ^{125}I-HSA. Eur J Nucl Med 26:333–341

Tatsch K, Knesewitsch P, Matuschke A et al (1990) ^{67}Ga-scintigraphy for evaluation of AIDS-related intestinal infections. Nucl Med Commun 11:649–655

Termaat MF, Raijmakers PG, Scholten HJ et al (2005) The accuracy of diagnostic imaging for the assessment of chronic osteomyelitis: a systematic review and meta-analysis. J Bone Jt Surg Am 87:2464–2471

Thakur ML, Richard MD, White FW III (1988) Monoclonal antibodies as agents for selective radiolabeling of human neutrophils. J Nucl Med 29:1817–1825

Thakur ML, Marcus CS, Henneman P et al (1996) Imaging inflammatory diseases with neutrophil-specific technetium-99m-labeled monoclonal antibody anti-SSEA-1. J Nucl Med 37:1789–1795

Tsan MF (1985) Mechanism of gallium-67 accumulation in inflammatory lesions. J Nucl Med 26:88–92

Tulchinsky M, Peters AM (2005) Leukocyte receptor-binding radiopharmaceuticals for infection and inflammation scintigraphy. J Nucl Med 46:718–721

Tzen KY, Oster ZH, Wagner HN Jr, Tsan MF (1980) Role of iron-binding proteins and enhanced capillary permeability on the accumulation of gallium-67. J Nucl Med 21:31–35

Ujula T, Salomäki S, Autio A et al (2009) ^{68}Ga-chloride PET reveals human pancreatic adenocarcinoma xenografts in rats—comparison with FDG. Mol Imaging Biol 12:259–268

van Eerd JE, Oyen WJ, Harris TD et al (2003) A bivalent leukotriene B(4) antagonist for scintigraphic imaging of infectious foci. J Nucl Med 44:1087–1091

Velikyan I et al (2004) Microwave-supported preparation of ^{68}Ga bioconjugates with high specific radioactivity. Bioconjugate Chem 15:554–560

Vinjamuri S, Hall AV, Solanki KK, Bomanji J, Siraj Q, O'Shaughnessy E et al (1996) Comparison of ^{99m}Tc infecton imaging with radiolabelled white-cell imaging in the evaluation of bacterial infection. Lancet 347:233–235

Weber WA, Schwaiger M, Avril N (2000) Quantitative assessment of tumor metabolism using FDG-PET imaging. Nucl Med Biol 27(7):683–687

Weiner R, Hoffer PB, Thakur ML (1981) Lactoferrin: its role as a ^{67}Ga-binding protein in polymorphonuclear leukocytes. J Nucl Med 22:32–37

Welling MM, Paulusma-Annema A, Balter HS et al (2000) Technetium-99m labelled antimicrobial peptides discriminate between bacterial infections and sterile inflammations. Eur J Nucl Med 27:292–301

Welling MM, Mongera S, Lupetti A et al (2002) Radiochemical and biological characteristics of ^{99m}Tc-UBI 29–41 for imaging of bacterial infections. Nucl Med Biol 29:413–422

Yang DJ, Kim CG, Schechter NR, Azhdarinia A et al (2003) Imaging with ^{99m}Tc-ECDG targeted at the multifunctional glucose transport system: feasibility study with rodents. Radiology 226:465–473

Yang DJ, Yukihiro M, Podoloff DA et al (2004) Assessment of therapeutic tumor response using ^{99m}Tc-ethylenedicysteine-glucosamine. Cancer Biother Radiopharm 19:443–456

Zhernosekov KP, Filosofov DV, Baum RP et al (2007) Processing of generator produced ^{68}Ga for medical application. J Nucl Med 48:1741–1748

^{68}Ga-Labeled Bombesin Analogs for Receptor-Mediated Imaging

Raunak Varshney, Puja P. Hazari, P. Fernandez, J. Schulz, M. Allard and Anil K. Mishra

Abstract

Targeted receptor-mediated imaging techniques have become crucial tools in present targeted diagnosis and radiotherapy as they provide accurate and specific diagnosis of disease information. Peptide-based pharmaceuticals are gaining popularity, and there has been vast interest in developing ^{68}Ga-labeled bombesin (Bn) analogs. The gastrin-releasing peptide (GRP) family and its Bn analog have been implicated in the biology of several human cancers. The three bombesin receptors GRP, NMB, and BRS-3 receptor are most frequently ectopically expressed by common, important malignancies. The low expression of Bn/GRP receptors in normal tissue and relatively high expression in a variety of human tumors can be of biological importance and form a molecular basis for Bn/GRP receptor-mediated imaging. To develop a Bn-like peptide with favorable tumor targeting and pharmacokinetic characteristics for possible clinical use, several modifications in the Bn-like peptides, such as the use of a variety of chelating agents, i.e., acyclic and macrocyclic agents with different spacer groups and with different metal ions (gallium), have been performed in recent years without significant disturbance of the vital binding scaffold. The favorable physical properties of ^{68}Ga, i.e., short half-life, and the fast localization of small peptides make this an ideal combination to study receptor-mediated imaging in patients.

R. Varshney · P. P. Hazari · A. K.Mishra (✉)
DCRS, INMAS, DRDO, Brig. S.K. Mazumdar Road, Delhi 110054, India
e-mail: akmishra63@gmail.com

R. Varshney
e-mail: raunak_varshney@yahoo.com

P. Fernandez · J. Schulz · M. Allard
University of Bordeaux, CNRS, INCIA, UMR 5287, F-33400, Talence, France

R. P. Baum and F. Rösch (eds.), *Theranostics, Gallium-68, and Other Radionuclides*, 221
Recent Results in Cancer Research 194, DOI: 10.1007/978-3-642-27994-2_12,

Abbreviations

Ac	Acetyl
Aca	Aminohexanoic acid
ACMpip	4-Aminocarboxymethylpiperidine
AMBA	Aminobenzoyl
Bn/BBN	Bombesin
BRS-3	Bombesin receptor subtype 3
Bzdig	p-aminobenzyldiglycolic acid
BZH_3	[DTyr^{6},βAla^{11},Thi^{13},Nle^{14}]Bn(6–14)
Cha	Cyclohexylalanine
DOTA	1,4,7,10-Triazacyclododecanetetraacetic acid
DTPA	Diethylenetriaminepentaacetic acid
Des-Met	Methionine removed
FA01010	(4*R*,5*S*)-4-Amino-5-methylheptanoic acid
GRP	Gastrin-releasing peptide
GRP-R/GRPR	Gastrin-releasing peptide receptor
Ga	Gallium
GI	Gastrointestinal
mIP	*meta*-phenylalanine
MBq	Megabecquerel
NHEt	Et = ethyl
NMB	Neuromedin B
NMBR	Neuromedin B receptor
NOTA	1,4,7-Triazacyclononanetriacetic acid
PEG2	(2-Aminoethyl)-carboxymethyl ether
PEG4	15-Amino-4,7,10,13-tetraoxapentadecanoic acid
PET	Positron emission tomography
RM1	H-DPhe-Gln-Trp-Ala-Val-Gly-His-Sta-Leu-NH_2
RGD	(Arginine-glycine-aspartic acid)
SPECT	Single-photon emission computed tomography
Sta	Statine: (3*S*,4*S*)-4-amino-3-hydroxy-6-methylheptanoic acid
Tha	β-(2-Thienyl) alanine
Thi	3-(2-Thienyl) alanine
Tpi	2,3,4,9-Tetrahydro-1*H*-pyridol[3,4-*b*]indol-3-carboxylic acid

Contents

1 Introduction

Advances in cancer medicine have occurred due to the ease of use and availability of artificial radionuclides, providing the opportunity to label specific biological molecules using well-defined chelating systems to develop novel radiopharmaceuticals. In parallel, novel imaging modalities provide better understanding of the biological process of the disease. It is convenient to define radiodiagnosis and radiotherapy solely on the basis of the radiophysical properties of the radionuclide. The principle of targeting tumoral receptors with radiolabeled vector conjugates for diagnostic oncology is that the modified radiolabeled vector identifies receptor-positive tumors not only at presumed sites but also at unforeseen sites. It has high sensitivity, because lesions as small as 5–10 mm can be detected. However, to achieve this, it requires a substantial concentration of tumoral receptors and a high tumor-to-background ratio. The receptor has to bind the radioligand with high affinity and eventually internalize it. Accordingly, this strategy relies primarily on the presence of tumoral receptors able to bind with high affinity to vector conjugates, and not on a receptor-mediated physiological or pathophysiological action of the peptides. Successful clinical applications of this principle include diagnostic and therapeutic targeting of peptide receptors with radiolabeled peptides (Krenning et al. 1993; Li et al. 2002). The ideal imaging compound would have high binding affinity for the target, specific uptake and retention in the target, rapid clearance from nontarget tissue, adequate capillary permeability, and high stability and integrity in vivo, and would be easy to prepare and safe to use. Considering these criteria, peptides have been increasingly considered as imaging probes, given their distinct advantages over other small molecules (Aloj and Morelli 2004; Okarvi 2004; Reubi and Maecke 2008).

Radiolabeled peptides have been the focus of research due to their potential as molecular imaging probes and therapeutic agents (Okarvi 2004). Peptides are more important than any other class of molecules for stimulating, inhibiting, or regulating numerous biological functions through their respective receptors. The molecular basis for use of radiopeptides was found to be that peptide receptors are overexpressed by certain tumors (Reubi 2003). Peptide receptors are located on the plasma membrane and allow internalization of the receptor–ligand complex, upon binding of a ligand. Positron-emitting radionuclide-labeled peptides are used to make an accurate tumor diagnosis, to quantify the radiation dose to tumors and critical organs, so allowing dose planning and dose monitoring for successful radiotherapy, and to follow tumor response to chemo- and radiotherapy (Lundqvist and Tolmchev 2002; Kowalski et al. 2003; Mutic et al. 2003). Failure to estimate patient dosimetry might be one of the reasons why radioimmunotherapy has advanced slowly during the last 20 years (Eary 2001). The new approach in radionuclide therapy based on radiolabeled peptides enables individualized imaging protocols (Gambhir 2002; Carlsson et al. 2003; Tofilon et al. 2003; Maecke et al. 2005; Reubi et al. 2005). Radionuclides coupled to tumor-specific peptides are currently under development, in preclinical investigations and clinical trials. Weiner and Thakur (2002) presented a selected list of peptides, their functions, and target cells that are presently under investigation using radiopeptides. Among the peptides for tumor targeting, Bn and its analogs have received significant interest as they exhibit high affinity and specificity for the gastrin-releasing peptide receptor (GRP-R) (Smith et al. 2003e, 2005), which is known to be overexpressed in cancer tissues.

A peptide has to be modified to carry radioisotopes to the target, and at the same time, still maintain its high biological activity to be used in nuclear medicine. The clinical impact of radiolabeled peptides is at the diagnostic level: in vivo receptor scintigraphy for localization of tumors and their metastases; and at the therapeutic level: peptide receptor-mediated radiotherapy of tumors is emerging as an important treatment option. Investigation of radiopeptides appeared to be a small niche in the large field of oncology. The most outstanding example is the analogs of somatostatin. Commercially available, FDA-approved drugs (Krenning et al. 2004; Okarvi 2004) include ^{111}In-DTPA-OctreoScan, a somatostatin receptor binder that is well established for diagnosis of neuroendocrine tumors. NeoTect, another approved somatostatin-receptor-binding analog labeled with ^{99m}Tc, shows good specificity for lung cancer detection. The short half-life of ^{68}Ga in combination with the fast target localization and blood clearance of DOTATOC is of special interest for clinical use (Maecke et al. 2005). These results have led to a growth in the development of radiolabeled peptides for diagnostic and therapeutic applications. Comparative studies of imaging the somatostatin receptor in neuroendocrine tumor using ^{111}In-octreotide (SPECT detection) versus ^{68}Ga-DOTA-TOC (Hofmann et al. 2001; Kowalski et al. 2003) and ^{68}Ga-DOTA-1-NAI^{3}-octreotide (Wild et al. 2005) (PET detection) have also been conducted, revealing better performance of the PET tracers. It has been the intent of many researchers to develop Bn-conjugated radioligands (^{68}Ga) for Bn receptors (Krenning et al. 2004), because Bn and its receptors are associated with many types of human cancer (Preston et al. 1996; Reubi et al. 2002).

The development of Bn derivatives for imaging and therapy, involving the peptide sequences, labeling moieties, and radionuclides, is an important area of research. Research efforts have been made to optimize the peptide sequences, leading to improved binding affinity and metabolic stability. The C-terminus of bombesin is essential for high-affinity binding and biological potency (Moody et al. 1982), so the N-terminus of bombesin is modified in order to allow labeling with radioisotopes. A number of ^{99m}Tc- and ^{111}In-labeled Bn analogs have been developed as diagnostic probes for SPECT (Varvarigou et al. 2004). ^{90}Y-, ^{177}Lu-, and ^{188}Re-labeled Bn conjugates have been evaluated (Smith et al. 2003d; Zhang et al. 2004), and metallic PET nuclides such as ^{64}Cu, ^{68}Ga, and ^{86}Y (Schuhmacher et al. 2005;

Biddlecombe et al. 2007) has been limited for bombesin conjugates for PET imaging.

2 Bombesin Receptors and Their Ligands

Bombesin receptors are normally present in the central nervous system, endocrine and exocrine glands (Kiehne et al. 2002; Matsumoto et al. 2003; Pazos-Moura et al. 2003), epithelia, and smooth muscle, where their stimulation regulates or modulates different functions from feeding, sleep–awake rhythm, and release of hormones to peristalsis or morphogenesis (Severi et al. 1989; Lommel 2001; Mollet et al. 2003).

The bombesin receptor family consists of four receptor subtypes, of which three have been identified from mammalian origin. These subtypes are classified as the neuromedin B (NMB) preferring receptor (NMB-R or BB1) found in esophageal and intestinal smooth muscle (Battey et al. 1992), the GRP preferring receptor (GRP-R or BB2) whose density in human cancer is very high, and the orphan Bn receptor subtype 3 (BRS-3 or BB3) found in the testis and in lung carcinoma cells (Fathi et al. 1993). A naturally occurring high-affinity ligand for BRS-3 has not been identified. Bombesin, NMB, and GRP activate BRS-3 only at micromolar concentrations, and the Bn receptor subtype 4 (BRS-4 or BB4), which was found in frog brain (Akeson et al. 1997), may exist in mammals as well (Table 1). In mammals, the bombesin-like peptides (BLPs) are thought to play important roles in various physiological and pathologic processes. GRP receptor subtypes bind GRP and bombesin with high affinity (K_d 10 nM) and neuromedin B with lower affinity (K_d 350 nM; Jensen and Coy 1991). In contrast, the neuromedin B receptor subtype has higher affinity for neuromedin B (K_d 0.3 nM) than for GRP or bombesin (K_d 2 nM; Jensen and Coy 1991). A GRP receptor subtype is present in the jejunum, antrum, and pancreas (Fischer and Schonbrunn 1988; Von Schrenck et al. 1989; Seybold et al. 1990; Vigna et al. 1990; Gugger and Reubi 1999; Markwalder and Reubi 1999; Whitley et al. 1999; Reubi et al. 2002; Reubi 2003; Krenning et al. 2004; Cornelio et al. 2007; Jensen et al. 2008), whereas a neuromedin B receptor subtype is expressed in the esophagus (Von Schrenck et al. 1989).

The bombesin receptor family is receiving increased attention as a means of localizing tumors or other disease processes by receptor-mediated imaging (Okarvi 2008; Gonzalez et al. 2008; Tweedle 2009; Schroeder et al. 2010). Anastasi et al. (1971) initiated research into the 14-amino-acid peptide bombesin receptor system with the isolation of the liner amidated tetradecapeptide bombesin from the skin of the European frogs *Bombina bombina, Bombina variegate*, and *Bombina orientalis* (Erspamer et al. 1970; Erspamer 1988; La Bella et al. 2002; Jensen et al. 2008). Amphibian bombesin has various effects in mammals, and bombesin-like immunoreactivity has been noticed in mammalian brain, lung, and gastrointestinal (GI) tract including the pancreas (Ghatei et al. 1984). McDonald et al. isolated a 27-amino-acid peptide, using antisera developed against bombesin, from porcine stomach, homologous to the C-terminus of bombesin, which was named GRP after its first known activity of inducing gastrin

Table 1 Bombesin and its receptor subtypes

SN	Receptor subtype	Native peptide	Origin
1	NMB-R or BB1	Neuromedin B	Mammalian
2	GRP-R or BB2	Gastrin-releasing peptide	Mammalian
3	BRS-3 or BB3	Bombesin	Mammalian
4	BRS-4 or BB4	Bombesin	Amphibian

secretion from G cells in the gastric antrum. GRP peptide shares the seven -COOH terminal amino acids with Bn (McDonald et al. 1979). The second mammalian bombesin-like decapeptide NMB was isolated by Minamino et al. (1983), from porcine spinal cord (McDonald et al. 1979). NMB is widely distributed in the brain and GI tract, and like GRP, shares six of the seven -COOH terminal amino acids with litorin (Minamino et al. 1983). A third bombesin-like peptide, neuromedin C (NMC or GRP-10), is identical to the carboxy-terminal subsequence (Jensen 1994; Ladenhein et al. 1994; Hajri et al. 1996; Kane et al. 1996; Kim et al. 1996; Koh et al. 1999) of GRP and has a potent contractile action on rat uterus in the characteristic manner of bombesin (Minamino et al. 1984).

Bombesin and GRP are known as brain–gut peptides and exert a variety of physiological actions in the nervous system and the gut. The normal physiological role of GRP in the human body is to stimulate secretions of gastrointestinal hormones and by the exocrine pancreas and to modulate gastrointestinal motility. Bombesin response appears to be central nervous system mediated, and its expression is not dependent on the vagus nerves or adrenal glands and does not rely on gastric secretion. The demonstrated central nervous system-mediated effects (Tachf et al. 1980) of bombesin include development of sustained hyperglycemia (Brown et al. 1979; Moore 1973) and hyperglucagonemia (Nemeroff et al. 1979), which is adrenal dependent through an increase in sympathetic outflux (Brown et al. 1979). It has been shown that hyperglycemia (Brown et al. 1979; Tachf et al. 1980), hyperglucagonemia (Lin and Warrick 1974; Christiansen et al. 1976), and increased sympathetic outflux (Osumi et al. 1977; Yamaguchi et al. 1977) singly decrease gastric acid secretion in experimental animals and in humans. Both peptides are good carriers for radiometals to target cancer, since their receptors are overexpressed in a number of cancer types. Since Bn is assumed to be more stable than GRP, developments have mainly been focused on Bn analogs. Cuttitta et al. (1985) demonstrated that Bn and GRP can stimulate small cell lung cancer growth (Reubi 2003), and the same were shown by the group of Rozengurt et al. (1990) to be mitogenic in Swiss 3T3 cells. They reported that Bn-like peptides could function as autocrine growth factors in small cell lung cancer (SCLC) (Cuttitta et al. 1985; Rozengurt 1990). It is known that SCLC cells produce BLPs and overexpress Bn/GRP (Cuttitta et al. 1985), forming an autocrine or paracrine loop to promote SCLC growth and invasion. A number of researchers using different methodologies to block either the BLPs or GRP-R have reported significant growth inhibition of SCLC in vitro as well

Bombesins

pGlu-Gln-Arg-Leu-Gly-Asn-Gln-Trp-Ala-Val-

Gly-His-**Leu**-Met-$CONH_2$

Ranatensins

pGlu-Gln-Arg-Leu-Gly-Asn-Gln-Trp-Ala-Val-

Gly-His-**Phe**-Met-$CONH_2$

Phyllolitorins

pGlu-Gln-Arg-Leu-Gly-Asn-Gln-Trp-Ala-Val-

Gly-**Ser**-Leu-Met-$CONH_2$

Fig. 1 Bombesin and related peptides

as in vivo (Avis et al. 1991; Halmos and Schally 1997). GRP acts mainly in the central and enteric nervous systems, and it regulates several physiological processes including satiety, thermoregulation, and circadian rhythm, as well as release of other peptide hormones.

Bn and GRP share a seven-amino-acid sequence in their C-terminal regions that is essential for receptor binding and biological activity (Shipp et al. 1991; Cai et al. 1994; Faintuch et al. 2008). Since GRP mimics every effect of bombesin, GRP was initially considered to be mammalian bombesin, but GRP and bombesin are distinct peptides (Nagalla et al. 1992). Based on the fact that both GRP and bombesin are found in frog and on phylogenetic examination, it is suggested that the two peptides separated before the vertebrate radiation. The similar biological activity of the peptides is explained by the difference in only 1 of the 10 carboxy-terminal residues. The peptides were divided into three groups on the basis of the amino group: the bombesin-related peptides, the ranatesin peptide, and the phyllolitorin peptide (Erspamer et al. 1970; Erspamer 1988; Jensen et al. 2008) (Fig. 1).

Ranatesin, an undecapeptide isolated from the skin of *Rana pipiens*, was also isolated from porcine spinal cord by using stimulation of rat uterine contractility as a bioassay by Minamino et al. (1983). The other analog is alytesin, isolated from *Alytes obstetricians* (Erspamer et al. 1970; Preston et al. 1996). All peptides are associated in sequence and share an amidated methionine at their carboxyl termini (C-termini), which characterizes the bombesin subfamilies and exhibits similar side-effects in pharmacological assays (Erspamer et al. 1970; Anastasi et al. 1971). The bombesins and ranatensins have leucine and phenylalanine as the penultimate residue, respectively, and the phyllolitorins have a serine as the third residue from the carboxyl terminus.

BLPs are neuropeptides found in both the central and peripheral nervous systems as well as in endocrine-like cells in several tissues including lung and thyroid (Lebacq-Verheyden et al. 1990; Sunday et al. 1988). They play important physiologic roles in regulating smooth muscle contraction, modulation of neuron firing rate (Lebacq-Verheyden et al. 1990; Spindel 1986), release of hormones in the gastrointestinal tract, and secretion of pancreatic enzymes, and serve as neurotransmitters in the central nervous systems (Bunnett 1994). Nerve fibers containing bombesin-like immunoreactivity are distributed in the intrinsic neurons of the stomach, pancreas, small intestine, and colon (Moran et al. 1988). BLPs have also been shown to stimulate proliferation of some GI tumors (Narayan et al. 1990), suggesting that these peptides may play a role in the development of cancers. However, it is not clear to what extent the growth-promoting effects of bombesin are due to a direct action on target cells or to the release of other growth factors (Upp et al. 1988; Liehr et al. 1992; Bunnett 1994). Bn/GRP-Rs are tied to G-protein through their intracellular domain and belong to the G-protein receptor (GPR-R/GPRR) superfamily. Bn/GRP-R multiple cellular signal transduction pathways are activated on binding, including protein kinase C (PKC), mitogen-activated protein kinase (MAPK), tyrosine phosphorylation of focal adhesion kinase (FAK), paxillin, p130cas, and calcium mobilization, resulting in cell proliferation and growth (Aprikian et al. 1997; Hellmich et al. 1999).

BLPs have also been shown to have mitogenic effects in a number of cancer cell lines (Bunnett 1994). Of these four receptors, three (BRS-3, NMB-R, and GRP-R) have been shown to be expressed to varying degrees in a variety of human tumors and human cancer cell lines (Reubi et al. 2002; Cornelio et al. 2007). For prostate and breast carcinomas, the GRP-R subtype has received the most attention from the research community due to the high expression density of the receptor relative to the NMB-R and BRS-3 subtypes (Gugger and Reubi 1999; Markwalder and Reubi 1999; Reubi et al. 2002). In normal human tissues, the pancreas has the highest degree of GPR-R gene expression, while the stomach, brain, and adrenal glands have notably lower levels (Jensen et al. 2008). The low expression of GPR-R in normal tissue relative to the increased expression in many cancers has validated GPR-R as a target for cancer detection and treatment. So far, a native peptide ligand showing high binding affinity to the BRS-3 subtype has not yet been identified. The Bn receptor family consists of three hepta-helical, guanine-nucleotide-binding regulatory protein (G-protein) coupled receptors, which are situated at the outer membrane of target cells and comprise three members in mammals: the 384-amino-acid GRP receptor (GRP-R) with high affinity for GRP, which has 55% amino acid identity to the 390-amino-acid neuromedin B receptor (NMBR) with high affinity for NMB, and the 399-amino-acid orphan BB3 receptor (BB3-R), bombesin receptor subtype 3 (BRS-3) (Okarvi 1999). The BRS-3 receptor is included in the mammalian Bn receptor family because it has 47–52% homology to GRPR and NMBR even though its natural ligand is still unknown (Bunnett 1994; Reubi 2003; Krenning et al. 2004). BRS-3 has a more limited distribution than GRPR and NMBR, but is found in both the central nervous system (CNS) and peripheral tissues, especially the GI tract (Okarvi 1999). The BRS-3 receptor has been replicate from human, mouse, and sheep, and tissue-specific expression has been reported (Whitley et al. 1999).

Bombesin initiates many of its biological effects by binding to and activating specific cell surface receptors which are coupled to phospholipase C signaling cascades via pertussis toxin-insensitive G-proteins (Fischer and Schonbrunn 1988; Rozengurt 1991; Bunnett 1994) and also activates a number of tyrosine kinase cascades (Okarvi 1999; Reubi 2003; Krenning et al. 2004). Many of the effects of bombesin are produced by the second messengers inositol 1,4,5-trisphosphate and diacylglycerol (Swope and Schonbrunn 1988; Rozengurt 1991; Bunnett 1994) leading to intracellular calcium mobilization (Kroog et al. 1995; Ryan et al. 1998). Amphibian bombesin exhibits high affinity for all the receptor subtypes (Erspamer 1988; Kroog et al. 1995). More specifically, GRP, which is an agonist, is endocytosed following receptor binding. The receptors are either recycled to the cell surface or degraded, while the ligand remains in the perinuclear space.

3 Targeted Approach to Receptor-Mediated Imaging

The identification of various Bn receptors and their receptor-mediated imaging have prompted the development of a wide variety of GPR-R targeted diagnostic imaging, chemotherapy, and radiotherapy agents. Radiolabeled GRP remains in the target tissue for longer periods of time, compared with radiolabeled antagonists, resulting in higher accumulation of radioactivity in GRP-R-positive tissues (Van de Wiele et al. 2001). Upon binding of the agonist bombesin analog to the GPR-R, the peptide and the attached chemotherapy agent and/or radionuclide are internalized and thereby retained in the cell. The bifunctional chelate design has primarily been used in the development of GPR-R-targeted Bn analogs for nuclear diagnostic imaging and radiotherapy. This approach has four distinctive components: a targeting vector, a radiometal, a chelation system, and a linking group (Fig. 2).

3.1 Why Bombesin Receptor-Mediated Imaging?

3.1.1 A Targeting Vector

The choice of targeting vectors for bombesin analogs has varied from the use of the entire 14-amino-acid bombesin peptide to truncated portions of the peptide, with the latter being most prevalent in the literature. In any event, the targeting vector must employ the Bn (8–14)NH_2 or a GPR-R-targeted derivative of this amino acid sequence in order to achieve uptake in GPR-R-expressing tissues. Novel pharmacological insights regarding bombesin-like peptides and the interaction with their respective receptors have been elucidated to aid future treatment and imaging of epithelial cell-derived tumors. The presence of Bn receptors on tumor tissues is receiving amplified attention, both for tumor imaging as well as to target cytotoxic agents by using either radiolabeled Bn analogs or other cytotoxic agents formed by coupling various Bn receptor ligands using various linkers to

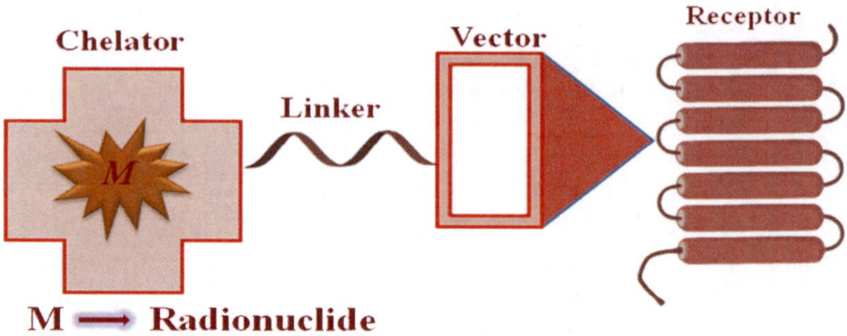

Fig. 2 Schematic representation of receptor-mediated approach

various cytotoxic agents (Okarvi 2004; Zhou et al. 2004; Schroeder et al. 2010; Tweedle 2009; Okarvi 2008; Gonzalez et al. 2008) (Table 2). This receptor-mediated targeting approach is being used with many peptides (Okarvi 2004; Gonzalez et al. 2008; Okarvi 2008; Tweedle 2009; Schroeder et al. 2010). There is particularly interest in this receptor family for a number of reasons. Bn receptors are overexpressed in various major human cancers such as prostate, breast, and small cell lung cancer (Nanda et al. 2010). The Bn family of receptors, particularly GRPR, has been shown to be one of most overexpressed or ectopically expressed family of G protein-coupled receptors by small lung cancer cells (GRPR: 85–100%, NMBR: 55%, BRS: 3–25%), non-small cell lung cancer (GRPR: 74–78%, NMBR: 67%, BRS: 3–8%), pancreatic pancreatic cancer (GRPR: 75%, NMBR: 100%), prostate cancer (GRPR: 60–100%, 0%-NMBR, BRS-3), head and neck squamous cell cancers (GRPR: 100%), glioblastomas (GRPR: 85%), neuroblastomas (GRPR: 72%, NMBR: 46%, 0%, BRS: 3), breast cancer (GRPR: 40–70%, NMBR: 0%, BRS: 3), intestinal carcinoids (NMBR: 46%, 0%, GRPR, BRS: 3), and bronchial carcinoids (35%-BRS: 3, 4%-NMBR, GRPR: 0%) (Anderson and Welch 1999; Reubi et al. 2002; Moody et al. 2003; Jensen and Moody 2006; Sancho et al. 2011). These data illustrate that each Bn receptor subtype may be overexpressed on different types of tumors, and the same type of tumor may coexpress more than one Bn receptor subtype, indicating that universal bombesin analogs have the potential (Weiner and Thakur 2002) to visualize these tumors with high incidence. Mantey et al. (1997) and Pradhan et al. (1998) developed a common ligand, [DTyrP6P, βAla11P, PheP13P, NleP14P]Bn (Reubi 1995; Heasley 2001; Signore et al. 2001; Weiner and Thakur 2002; Laskin and Sandler 2004; Okarvi 2004) having high affinity to all receptor subtypes. A novel GRP variant, GRP1–46, isolated from pregnant ovine endometrium, was characterized and shown to have low affinity for both GRP-R and NMB-R in rodent and human cell lines and mobilized inositol phosphate in cell lines expressing GRP-R and NMB-R but not BRS-3 (Giraud et al. 2010). Owing to frequent aberrant expression in epithelial cancers, GRP-R has been explored for receptor-mediated targeting of imaging and therapeutic agents in human malignancies (Nanda et al. 2010).

Table 2 Bn analogs used in various imaging studies[218]

SN	Bombesin analog	Amino acid position relative to Bn sequence in bold														References
		1	2	3	4	5	6	7	8	9	10	11	12	13	14	
1	Bombesin	Pyr	Gln	Arg	Leu	Gly	Asn	Gln	Trp	Ala	Val	Gly	His	Leu	Met-NH_2	Varvarigou et al. (2002), Okarvi and Al-Jammaz (2003)
2	GRP (13–27)	**Tyr**	**Pro**	Arg	Leu	Gly	Asn	His	Trp	Ala	Val	Gly	His	Leu	Met-NH_2	Breeman et al. (1999)
3	Litorin [pGlu^6,Phe^{13}] Bn(6–14)	–	–	–	–	–	**pGlu**	Gln	Trp	Ala	Val	Gly	His	**Phe**	Met-NH_2	Durkan et al. (2007)
4	(a) Demobesin 3 [N_4^0,Pro^1,Tyr^4]Bn, (b) Demobesin 4 [N_4^0,Pro^1,Tyr^4,Nle^{14}]Bn	**N_4-Pro**	Gln	Arg	Tyr	Gly	Asn	Gln	Trp	Ala	Val	Gly	His	Leu	(a) Met-NH_2, (b) Nle-NH_2	Nock et al. (2005)
5	[Lys^3]Bn	Pyr	Gln	Lys	Leu	Gly	Asn	Gln	Trp	Ala	Val	Gly	His	Leu	Met-NH_2	Chen et al. (2004), Dimitrakopoulou-Strauss et al. (2006), Yang et al. (2006), Zhang et al. (2006), Abiraj et al. (2008), Santos-Cuevas et al. (2008, 2009)
6	(a) [Tyr^4]Bn, (b) [εLys^3,Tyr^4]Bn	Pyr	Gln	(a) Arg, (b) εLys	Tyr	Gly	Asn	Gln	Trp	Ala	Val	Gly	His	Leu	Met-NH_2	Rogers et al. (1997), Breeman et al. (1999, 2002)
7	[Gln^1,Tyr^4]Bn	**Gln**	Gln	Arg	**Tyr**	Gly	Asn	Gln	Trp	Ala	Val	Gly	His	Leu	Met-NH_2	Achilefu et al. (2002)

(continued)

Table 2 (continued)

SN	Bombesin analog	Amino acid position relative to Bn sequence in bold														References
		1	2	3	4	5	6	7	8	9	10	11	12	13	14	
8	[Gly^1]Bn	**Gly**	Gln	Arg	Leu	Gly	Asn	Gln	Trp	Ala	Val	Gly	His	Leu	Met-NH_2	Lantry et al. (2006), Montet et al. (2006)
9	(a) [Pro^1,Tyr^4]Bn (MP2346), (b) [Pro^1,Tyr^4,Nle^{14}]Bn	**Pro**	Gln	Arg	Tyr	Gly	Asn	Gln	Trp	Ala	Val	Gly	His	Leu	(a) Met-NH_2, (b) Nle-NH_2	Breeman et al. (1999, 2002), Cescato et al. (2008), Schroeder et al. (2010)
10	[Cys^0,Aca^1]Bn(2–14)	**Cys-Aca**	Gln	Arg	Leu	Gly	Asn	Gln	Trp	Ala	Val	Gly	His	Leu	Met-NH_2	Scopinaro et al. (2002, 2004)
11	Bn(2–14)	_	Gln	Arg	Leu	Gly	Asn	Gln	Trp	Ala	Val	Gly	His	Leu	Met-NH_2	Ferro-Flores et al. (2006), Gourni et al. (2006), Abiraj et al. (2008), Fragogeorgi et al. (2009), Koumaria nou et al. (2009)
12	(a) [Lys^{14}]Bn(2–14), (b) [Lys^3,Tyr^4] Bn(2–14)	_	Gln	Arg	(a) Leu, (b) Tyr	Gly	Asn	Gln	Trp	Ala	Val	Gly	His	Leu	(a) Lys-NH_2 (b) Met-NH_2	Scopinaro et al. (2007), Hohne et al. (2008), Ho et al. (2009)
13	[mIP]Bn(2–14)	**mIP**	Gln	Arg	Leu	Gly	Asn	Gln	Trp	Ala	Val	Gly	His	Leu	Met-NH_2	Rogers et al. (1997)
14	Bn(4–14)	_	_	_	Leu	Gly	Asn	Gln	Trp	Ala	Val	Gly	His	Leu	Met-NH_2	Abiraj et al. (2008)
15	[$Ser^{4,5,6}$]Bn(4–14)	_	_	_	**Ser**	**Ser**	Ser	Gln	Trp	Ala	Val	Gly	His	Leu	Met-NH_2	Smith et al. (2003c)

(continued)

Table 2 (continued)

SN	Bombesin analog	Amino acid position relative to Bn sequence in bold														References
		1	2	3	4	5	6	7	8	9	10	11	12	13	14	
16	[ACMpip^{5},Tha^{6},βAla^{11}, Tha^{13},Nle^{14}]Bn(5–14) (MP2653)	_	_	_	_	**AC Mpip**	**Tha**	Gln	Trp	Ala	Val	**βAla**	His	**Tha**	Met-NH_2	Biddlecombe et al. (2007), Schroeder et al. (2010)
17	(a) [Tyr^{5},DPhe^{6},ψPhe^{14}] Bn(5–14), (b) [DPhe^{6}, Leu$^{13}\psi$Phe^{14}] Bn(6–14), ^{a} (c) [DPhe^{6},LeuNHEt^{13}, des-Met^{14}] Bn(6–14)	_	_	_	_	**Tyr**	**D-Phe**	Gln	Trp	Ala	Val	Gly	His	(a, b) **Leu-ψ**, (c) Leu-NHEt	(a, b) Phe-NH_2 (c) _	Breeman et al. (1999), Abd-Elgaliel et al. (2008)
18	[DTyr^{6},βAla^{11},Thi^{13}, Nle^{14}] Bn(6–14)	_	_	_	_	_	**D-Tyr**	Gln	Trp	Ala	Val	Ala	His	Tha	Met-NH_2	Zhang et al. (2004), Reubi et al. (2005), Maina et al. (2006), Dimitrakopoulou-Strauss et al. (2007)
19	Demobesin 1 [N4^{0}1, bzdig^{0},DPhe^{6},Leu-NHEt^{13},des-Met^{14}] Bn(6–13)	_	_	_	_	**N_4-bzdig**	**D-Phe**	Gln	Trp	Ala	Val	Gly	His	Leu-NHEt	_	Nock et al. (2003), Cescato et al. (2008), Schroeder et al. (2010)
20	RM1 [N_4^{0}DPhe^{6}, Sta^{13},Leu^{14}] Bn(6–14)	_	_	_	_	_	**N_4-DPhe**	Gln	Trp	Ala	Val	Gly	His	**Sta**	Leu-NH_2	Mansi et al. (2009), Abiraj et al. (2010)
21	[Lys^{6}]Bn(6–14)	_	_	_	_	_	**Lys**	Gln	Trp	Ala	Val	Gly	His	**Leu**	Met-NH_2	Achilefu et al. (2002)

(continued)

Table 2 (continued)

SN	Bombesin analog	Amino acid position relative to Bn sequence in bold														References
		1	2	3	4	5	6	7	8	9	10	11	12	13	14	
22	Bn(7–14)	–	–	–	–	–	–	Gln	Trp	Ala	Val	Gly	His	**Leu**	Met-NH_2	Van de Wiele et al. (2000), van de et al. (2001), Achilefu et al. (2002), Hu et al. (2002), La Bella et al. (2002), Hoffman et al. (2003), Smith et al. (2003a, b, c), Okarvi (2004), Rogers et al. (2004), Scopinaro et al. (2004), Wild et al. (2005), Alves et al. (2006), Yang et al. (2006), Zhang et al. (2006), Garcia et al. (2007a, b), Kunstler et al. (2007), Ma et al. (2007), Waser et al. (2007), Garrison et al. (2008), Lane et al. (2008), Gourni et al. (2009), Liu et al. (2009a, b), Mansi et al. (2009), Paterson et al. (2010), Retzloff et al. (2010), Schroeder et al. (2010)
23	(a) Demobesin 5 [$(N^4Bzdig)^0$] Bn(7–14), (b) Demobesin 6 [$(N^4Bzdig)^0$,Nle^{14}] Bn(7–14)	–	–	–	–	–	**N_4-Bzdig**	Gln	Trp	Ala	Val	Gly	His	**Leu**	(a) Met-NH_2, (b) Nle-NH_2	Moody et al. (2004), Nock et al. (2005)

(continued)

Table 2 (continued)

SN	Bombesin analog	Amino acid position relative to Bn sequence in bold														References
		1	2	3	4	5	6	7	8	9	10	11	12	13	14	
24	(a) [Cha^{13},Nle^{14}] Bn(7–14), (b) [Cha^{13}] Bn(7–14)	–	–	–	–	–	–	Gln	Trp	Ala	Val	Gly	His	**Cha**	(a) Nle-NH_2 (b) Met-NH_2	Garcia et al. (2007a,b), Brans et al. (2008), Maes et al. (2009)
25	[Nle^{14}]Bn(7–14)	–	–	–	–	–	–	Gln	Trp	Ala	Val	Gly	His	**Leu**	Nle-NH_2	Garcia et al. (2007a,b),
26	(a) [NMeGly^{11},Sta^{13}, Leu^{14}] Bn(7–14), (b) [FA01010^{13},Leu^{14}] Bn(7–14)	–	–	–	–	–	–	Gln	Trp	Ala	Val	NMe Gly	His	(a) **Sta**, (b) **FA01010**	Leu-NH_2	Hohne et al. (2008), Thomas et al. (2009)
27	[βAla^{11},Phe^{13},Nle^{14}] Bn(7–14)	–	–	–	–	–	–	Gln	Trp	Ala	Val	βAla	His	**Phe**	Nle-NH_2	de Visser et al. (2007)
28	[His(3Me)^{11},Sta^{13}, Leu^{14}]Bn (7–14)	–	–	–	–	–	–	Gln	Trp	Ala	Val	**His(3Me)**	His	**Sta**	Leu-NH_2	Hohne et al. (2008)
29	[des-Met^{14}] Bn(7–14)NH_2	–	–	–	–	–	–	Gln	Trp	Ala	Val	Gly	His	Leu-NH_2	–	Rogers et al. (1997)
30	[DTyr^6,des-Met^{14}] Bn(6–13)NHEt	–	–	–	–	–	D-Tyr	Gln	Trp	Ala	Val	Gly	His	Leu-NHEt	–	Breeman et al. (1999)
31	[Tyr^5,DPhe^6] Bn(5–13)NHEt	–	–	–	–	**Tyr**	**D-Phe**	Gln	Trp	Ala	Val	Gly	His	Leu-NHEt	–	Maina et al. (2006)
32	RC-3095 [D-Tpi^6, Leu^{13}, ψLeu^{14}] Bn(6–14)	–	–	–	–	–	D-Tpi	Gln	Trp	Ala	Val	Gly	His	**Leu**ψ^b	Leu-NH_2	Varvarigou et al. (2002)

(continued)

Table 2 (continued)

SN	Bombesin analog	Amino acid position relative to Bn sequence in bold														References
		1	2	3	4	5	6	7	8	9	10	11	12	13	14	
33	Pensin	–	–	–	–	–	**dPEG$_4$**	Gln	Trp	Ala	Val	Gly	His	**Leu**	Met-NH_2	Schroeder et al. (2010), Li et al. (2002)
34	AMBA	–	–	–	–	–	CH_2CO-Gly-4 amino benzyl	Gln	Trp	Ala	Val	Gly	His	**Leu**	Met-NH_2	Schroeder et al. (2010), Li et al. (2002), Schroeder et al. (2011)

(a) des-Met indicates deletion of the Bn 14th amino acid methionine. (b) ψ indicates a reduced peptide bond (–CH_2NH– instead of –CONH–)

On the other hand, for somatostatin receptors, receptor-mediated imaging has been shown to be safe and clinically useful and is now being widely used in clinical practice (Forrer et al. 2007; Van Essen et al. 2009). In the case of neuroendocrine tumors (carcinoids, pancreatic endocrine tumors), in most studies the majority (>80%) overexpress or ectopically express one or more of the five classes of G protein-coupled somatostatin receptors (sst1–5), usually the sst2 subtype (Krenning et al. 1993; Jensen 1997; Gibril and Jensen 2004; Forrer et al. 2007; Van Essen et al. 2009), in an analogous fashion to the tumors listed above, overexpressing one of the Bn receptor family. The use of ^{111}In-penetreotide for somatostatin receptor scintigraphy (SRS) is now a standard clinical method to image these tumors (Kwekkeboom et al. 2000; Gibril and Jensen 2004; Metz and Jensen 2008). Unfortunately, many of the common lethal tumors do not overexpress somatostatin receptors, as occurs in the neuroendocrine tumors. Therefore, if receptor-mediated imaging is going to be used for these tumors, some other family of receptors needs to be considered. The Bn family of receptors could fulfill this requirement for a number of these tumors (Zhou et al. 2004; Okarvi 2004, 2008; Gonzalez et al. 2008; Tweedle 2009; Schroeder et al. 2010).

BLPs also function as potent growth factors, sometimes in an autocrine fashion, for many common malignant tumors including those of lung, pancreas, head and neck, CNS (glioblastomas), kidney, prostate, breast, colon/rectum, ovary, and stomach (Preston et al. 1996; Moody et al. 2003; Yegen 2003; Jensen and Moody 2006). This raises the possibility that receptor antagonists of Bn receptors may have cytotoxic effects for a number of these tumors, and the possibility that targeting Bn receptors on these tumor cells may have additional cytotoxic effects by interrupting this autocrine stimulatory effect. There are no effective nonpeptide antagonists or agonists for GRPR or NMBR, which are primarily overexpressed by tumors. The pharmacology of these receptors has been well studied, especially in nonhuman cells. Both selective agonists and at least eleven chemical classes of antagonists, with varying degrees of selectivity, have been described (Battey et al. 1992; Jensen et al. 2008; Gonzalez et al. 2009). Therefore, pharmacologically, both agonists and antagonists exist that can be used for Bn receptor targeting strategies.

3.2 Gallium Radiometal

3.2.1 Radionuclide of Choice

To date, a wide variety of radionuclides (e.g., ^{99m}Tc, ^{188}Re, ^{90}Y, ^{111}In, ^{18}F, ^{64}Cu, ^{177}Lu, ^{149}Pm, and ^{68}Ga) have been used in the development of BB2-targeting peptides (Heppler Froidevaux Eberle et al. 2000; Hu et al. 2002; Hoffman et al. 2003; Smith et al. 2003a, c, d; Zhang et al. 2004, 2006, 2007; Garrison et al. 2007) (Table 2). The selection of the radionuclide for the GPR-R-targeted Bn analog is largely influenced by the desired function of the radiopharmaceutical. Diagnostic nuclear imaging agents that utilize radionuclides with gamma emission are suitable for single-photon emission computed tomography (SPECT), and those with positron emission can be used for positron emission tomography (PET). Radionuclides are chosen to deliver a maximum radiation dose to the cancerous tissue for targeted radiotherapy, at the same time attempting to ensure minimal damage to nontarget tissues (Volkert and Hoffman 1999).

An important aspect for wide use of ^{68}Ga in clinical PET is its chemical form and concentration after elution from the generator. There is concern about ^{68}Ge breakthrough and contamination of the generator column material. Gallium is a short-lived positron emitter and consists of two naturally occurring isotopes: ^{69}Ga (60.1% natural abundance) and ^{71}Ga (39.9% natural abundance). Three radioisotopes can be produced for labeling of radiopharmaceuticals. Two of these, ^{66}Ga ($t_{1/2} = 9.5$ h) and ^{68}Ga ($t_{1/2} = 68$ min), decay by β^+ emission and are therefore suitable for PET imaging; ^{67}Ga ($t_{1/2} = 8$ h) decays by γ emission and is used for SPECT imaging. Its production does not require a cyclotron since it is available as a generator nuclide. Different ^{68}Ge-carrier column materials have been proposed and used in the past, among them inorganic oxides such as Al_2O_3, TiO_2, or SnO_2. Recently, a TiO_2-based generator has become commercially available, being eluted with 0.1 mol/L HCl. Extraction of ^{68}Ga eluate from a ^{68}Ge/^{68}Ga generator has been reported (Meyer et al. 2005). Briefly, final concentration of 5.5 M HCl is used for extracting ^{68}Ga, which can be adsorbed on a strong anion exchanger as anionic chlorocomplexes of ^{68}Ga(III). Gallium adsorbed on resin is flushed with a stream of N_2 and then eluted with H_2O in small volumes.

This strategy separates ^{68}Ge, but it does not allow direct loading of ^{68}Ga(III) on the anion exchange resin from 0.1 N HCl, nor does it provide purification of Ga(III) from, for example, Zn(II) and Fe(III). The time needed to process the generator eluate, and to synthesize and purify the labeled product (e.g., ^{68}Ga-DOTA conjugated peptides), reduces the overall yields of the product. A final yield of 46 $\pm$ 5% for ^{68}Ga-labeled DOTA conjugated octreotide has been reported (Green and Welch 1989).

Several groups are using this generator and modifying it to allow safe management and to eliminate potential cationic impurities. The parent ^{68}Ge is accelerator-produced by the ^{69}Ga (p, 2n) reaction Lambrecht and Sajjad (1988) and decays with half-life of 270.8 days solely by orbital electron capture to ^{68}Ga. The latter disintegrates 89% by emission of positrons of 1.9 MeV maximum energy and 11% by electron capture to stable ^{68}Zn. The 270-day half-life of the parent ^{68}Ge allows use of the generator for a long period, potentially up to 1 year or even longer. The 68-min half-life of ^{68}Ga matches the pharmacokinetics of many peptides and other small molecules owing to rapid diffusion, localization at the target, and fast blood clearance. The only stable chemical form in aq. solution is the Ga(III) cation, which can hydrolyze and precipitate at pH 3–7 in the form of insoluble trihydroxide $Ga(OH)_3$ if the concentration exceeds nanomolar level. However, in the presence of stabilizing agents, precipitation can be avoided (Dymov and Savostin 1968; Green and Welch 1989). At physiological pH (7.4), the total solubility of Ga is high because of the almost exclusive formation of $[Ga(OH)_4]^-$ ions (Harris and Messori 2002). The other important contender in physiologic fluid for Ga^{3+} radiometals is transferrin. This Fe(III)-carrying protein binds Ga(III) with high affinity (log $K = 23.7$). Any application of a ^{68}Ga radiopharmaceutical needs to resist the exchange of Ga(III) from its chelate with transferrin and OH^- ions. The Ga(III) cation is classified as a hard acid metal. It forms stable complexes with many ligands containing oxygen and nitrogen as well as sulfur as donor atoms (Pearson 1963; Green and Welch 1989; Luyt and Katzenellenbogen 2002). The coordination chemistry of Ga(III) is defined by coordination number six and the octahedral coordination sphere.

3.3 Chelating Systems

The chelation system is responsible for the binding of the radiometal and preventing transchelation throughout the in vivo lifetime of the radiopharmaceutical. The selection of the chelation system is largely dependent on the chemical nature of the radionuclide; however, a variety of chelation systems (e.g., DOTA, TETA, and DTPA) have been shown to be effective in stabilizing a variety of radionuclides in vivo (Anderson and Welch 1999; Liu and Edwards 2001b; Garrison et al. 2007; Prasanphanich et al. 2007). The linking group provides a number of crucial roles in the bifunctional chelate design of BB2r-targeted Bn analogs; an evident role is to chemically connect the radiometal–chelation complex to the bombesin targeting vector. Selection of these groups takes into account prevention of interference by the radiometal–chelation complex with the binding of the bombesin targeting vector to the GPR-R.

Ga(III) can be coordinated by a bifunctional complexing agent covalently linked to a targeting vector, which in turn can bind to a target. The advantage of such a complex is that the bifunctional chelating agents can be labeled with various radiometals for certain diagnostic or therapeutic applications (Velikyan 2005). Acyclic bifunctional chelators, such as ethylenediaminetetraacetic acid (EDTA), diethylenetriaminepentaacetic acid (DTPA), desferrioxamine (DFO), *N,N′*-di(2-hydroxybenzyl)ethylenediamine-*N,N′*-diacetic acid (HBED), and their derivatives, has been used for labeling of macromolecules with ^{111}In, ^{67}Ga, ^{68}Ga, and ^{90}Y for tumor imaging and therapy (Fig. 3) (Wagner and Welch 1979; Hnatowich et al. 1981; Koizumi et al. 1987; Pochon et al. 1989; Mathias et al. 1990; Fichna and Janecka 2003). Most of these complexes show low stability in vivo and in vitro, which has been related to the tendency of such anionic complexes to undergo acid- or cation-promoted dissociation in vivo (Wagner and Welch 1979; Schuhmaker et al. 1986; Broan et al. 1991; Liu and Edwards 2001a).

The introduction of macrocyclic bifunctional chelating agents has led to more stable complexes (Craig et al. 1989; de Jong et al. 1997). Chelators such as 1,4,7-triazacyclononanetriacetic acid (NOTA), 1,4,7,10-triazacyclododecanetetraacetic acid (DOTA), 1,4,8,11-tetraazacyclotetradecan-1,4,8,11-tetraacetic acid (TETA) (Fig. 4) and their derivatives have been used for complexation with ^{64}Cu/^{67}Cu,

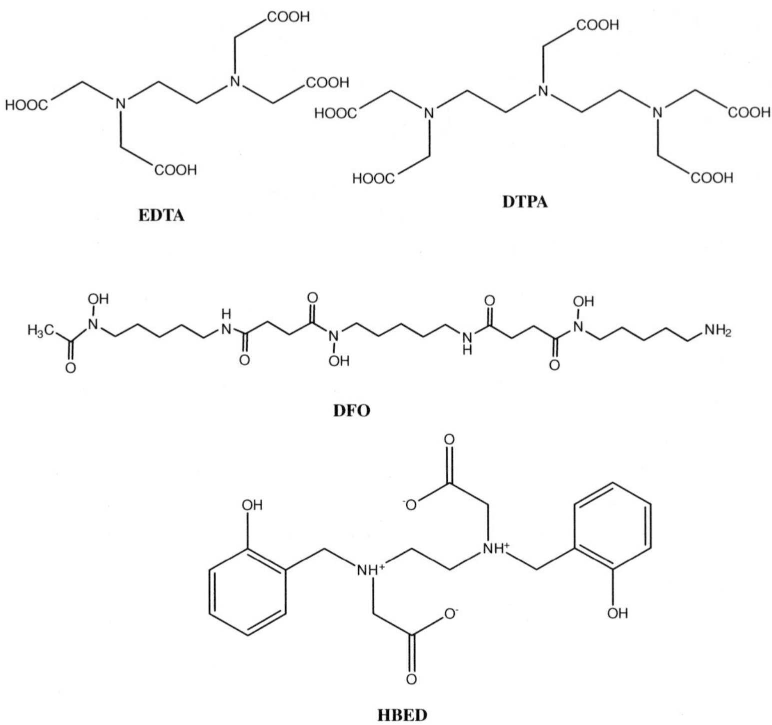

Fig. 3 Acyclic bifunctional chelator

$^{66}Ga/^{67}Ga/^{68}Ga$, $^{86}Y/^{90}Y$, ^{111}In, ^{177}Lu, and ^{225}Ac (Craig et al. 1989; Broan et al. 1991; Stimmel et al. 1995; Blower et al. 1996; Cutler et al. 2000; McDevitt et al. 2001; Chong et al. 2002; Eisenwiener et al. 2002; Fichna and Janecka 2003; Yoo et al. 2004; Uppal et al. 2011). DOTA and NOTA chelators can be attached to a carrier molecule via the carboxylate group or the functionalized skeleton carbon. The former methods allow a one-step coupling reaction to amines using carbodiimide chemistry (Lewis et al. 1994). Modification on the macrocyclic bifunctional chelators allow variation of the overall charge and hydrophilicity of the metal–chelate moiety, thus regulating the biodistribution pattern, excretion routes, and resistance to acid/cation-promoted dissociation over a wide pH range. The high stability of tetraazamacrocycle is provided by the extremely slow dissociation reactions. Typical dissociation values are 10^5–10^7 times lower than those of open-chain analogs.

A bifunctional chelator should meet the following criteria: (a) a chelator conjugated to the macromolecule should bind the radioisotope rapidly and sufficiently; and (b) the resulting complex should be kinetically stable to cation release over a pH range of 2–8 and in the presence of cations such as Ca(II), Zn(II), and Mg(II) which can be found in serum (Broan et al. 1991). Other factors to consider include redox properties, charge, and lipophilicity (Brunner et al. 1995; Reichert et al. 1999).

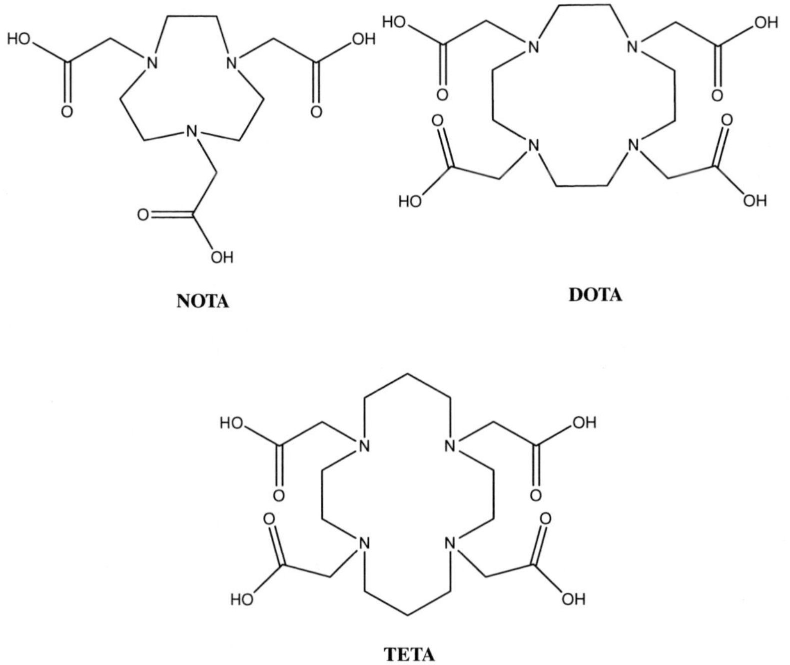

Fig. 4 Macrocyclic bifunctional chelator

Neutral complexes are less sensitive to acid/cation-promoted dissociation compared with anionic complexes. At very low pH, the neutral Ga(III)-NOTA complex has been shown to undergo acid-catalyzed dissociation only, whose occurrence is doubtful under physiological conditions. The log stability constant (log *K*) of Ga(III)-NOTA has been determined to 30.98, while the log *K* of the Ga(III) complex of DOTA has been determined to be 21.33 (Clarke and Martell 1991). X-ray crystallography study of the complex with Ga(III) revealed octahedral coordination of Ga(III) (Broan et al. 1991). A tetradentate tripodal (NOTA) S3N ligand was described, forming lipophilic tetrahedral Ga(III) complexes (Luyt and Katzenellenbogen 2002). The cavity of NOTA is defined by a facial triaza plane and an opposite facial plane consisting of three carboxylate oxygen atoms. The compactness of the triazanonane ring and the steric efficiency of the pendant acetate group lead to the formation of complexes with unusually high stability and selectivity for Ga(III). In the Ga(III) complex of DOTA-D-Phe-NH_2, DOTA adopts a *cis*-pseudooctahedral geometry with a folded macrocycle unit (Heppeler et al. 1999; Eisenwiener et al. 2002). Gallium radiopharmaceutical must be stable enough to avoid transchelation of Ga(III) to various iron-binding proteins, particularly transferrin. Transferrin has two binding sites, for which the gallium binding constant are 20.3 and 19.3 (Harris and Messori 2002). Therefore, a polydentate chelator, forming thermodynamically stable and kinetically inert complexes with six-coordinate Ga(III), is required. The kinetic stability of ^{67}Ga-DOTA-D-Phe1-Tyr3-octreotide (^{67}Ga-DOTATOC) under physiological conditions has been studied by measurement of the rate of radiometal exchange in blood serum, the half-life of which has been estimated to be 1,250 h (Eisenwiener et al. 2002). Moreover, Ga labeling of DOTA peptides ensures site-specific labeling and consequently higher in vivo stability compared, for example, with ^{99m}Tc, which can nonspecifically bind to peptides containing cysteine residues (Haubner et al. 2004). DOTA is a remarkable ligand for binding of gallium, and DOTA peptides can be rapidly and efficiently labeled with ^{68}Ga at high specific activities (Breeman et al. 2005; Velikyan et al. 2005), which implies that the mass of peptide to be administered can be very low (Breeman et al. 1995; Kung and Kung 2005). This is of great significance in the case of peptides with potential pharmacological side-effects, including substance P, CCK, and bombesin. Thus, Ga(III) is suitable for complexation with chelators, naked or conjugated with peptides or other macromolecules.

4 Special Focus on Gallium-Labeled Bombesin Analogs

The ^{68}Ga-labeled bombesin analogs have been reported in vitro and in vivo properties of various ^{68}Ga-Bn analogs conjugates and their results are summarized in Table 3 for imaging metastasized prostate, and gastrointestinal stromal tumors (Van de Wiele et al. 2000; Van de Dimitrakopoulou-Strauss et al. 2007; Van de Wiele et al. 2008). Many bombesin analog radiotracers have also been investigated for breast cancer imaging (Chen et al. 2004; Zhang et al. 2006). In the literature, various bombesin and analogs were labeled with different isotopes such as ^{99m}Tc, ^{111}In, ^{90}Y, ^{64}Cu, ^{177}Lu, ^{18}F or ^{68}Ga and investigated for GRPR-positive tumor-targeted imaging and therapy in both animal models and human trails (Chen et al. 2004; Zhang et al. 2004; Schuhmacher et al. 2005; Lantry et al. 2006; Yang et al. 2006; Zhang et al. 2006; Dimitrakopoulou-Strauss et al. 2007; Waser et al. 2007; Van de Wiele et al. 2008; Schweinsberg et al. 2008; Santos-Cuevas et al. 2008). A potent bombesin receptor antagonist (H-D-Phe-Gln-Trp-Ala-Val-Gly-His-Sta-Leu-NH_2) was obtained by replacing Leu-13 with a statyl residue (Llinares et al. 1999). Bombesin-based radiolabeled analogs have been described as targeting agents for prostate cancer in preclinical research (Zhang et al. 2004; Lin et al. 2005; Nock et al. 2005; Schuhmacher et al. 2005; Lantry et al. 2006; Parry et al. 2007) and clinical studies (Van de Wiele et al. 2000; Dimitrakopoulou-Strauss et al. 2007; Van de Wiele et al. 2008). A radiolabeled bombesin analog has been established for antagonistic properties potentially useful for imaging (SPECT, PET) and radionuclide therapy of GRPR-positive tumors (Mansi et al. 2009). PET studies with a ^{68}Ga-labeled bombesin analog were performed in 11 patients with prostate cancer (Hofmann et al. 2004). Accordingly, numerous bombesin analogs have been developed and labeled with Ga radiometals (Schuhmacher et al. 2005; Dimitrakopoulou-Strauss et al. 2006) to evaluate the

Table 3 ^{68}Ga-labeled bombesin analogs[218]

SN	Isotope	Linker	Bombesin analogs	Animal	Biodistribution	Imaging	Observation	Reference
1	^{68}Ga	DOTA-PEG_2 (PAN bombesin)	[D-Tyr6,-Ala^{11},Thi^{13},Nle^{14}] Bn(6–14) (BZH_3)	AR42 J tumor-bearing mice	Dose-dependent uptake of high-expressing GRPR tissues. Fast blood clearance	PET images 1 h after injection. Clear definition of tumor tissue and low uptake of nontarget tissues	With well-defined and low-background imaging, BZH_3 has prerequisites as a helpful compound in GRPR+ tumors	Reubi et al. (2005), Zhang et al. (2007)
2	^{68}Ga	DOTA-PEG_4	Bn(7–14)	PC-3 tumor-bearing mice	Rapid blood clearance. High uptake in tumor and pancreas. High retention in kidneys	PET and scintigraphy imaging show high uptake in tumor, pancreas, and kidneys	PEG4 spacer forms suitable compound for clinical studies	Zhang et al. (2007)
3	^{68}Ga	NOTA	RGD-BBN(7–14): cyclo (Arg-Gly-Asp-D-Tyr-Lys)-Glu-(Aca-Gln-Trp-Ala-Val-Gly-His-Leu-Met-NH_2)	(a) PC-3 tumor-bearing mice, (b) MDA-MB-435 tumor-bearing mice	High tumor and pancreas uptake	MicroPET images. Low uptake in PC-3 tumors	Dual receptor binding compound recognized to be useful in tumors where only one of the receptors is overexpressed	Liu et al. (2009a)
4	^{68}Ga	DOTA-AMBA	-Gly-4-aminobenzyl-Gln-Trp-Ala-Val-Gly-His-Leu-Met-NH_2	PC-3 tumors and VCaP tumor-bearing mice	High tumor uptake in colon and kidney	High uptake was seen in tumor tissue as well as in GRPR-positive pancreas tissue and in organs responsible for clearance (kidneys and bladder)	Bn analogs are superior to metabolism-based targeting using choline for scintigraphy of PC	Schroeder et al. (2011)
5	^{68}Ga	DOTA-(His)2-minigastrin (DOTA-MG0)	His–His-Glu-Ala-Tyr-Gly-Trp-Met-Asp-Phe-NH_2	AR42 J rat tumor cell line	High tumor uptake indicating CCK2/gastrin receptor-mediated uptake ($p = 0.0005$)	Besides tumor uptake, pronounced uptake was also seen in the kidneys	^{68}Ga-DOTA-MG0 is a promising tracer for PET imaging of CCK2/gastrin receptor–positive tumors in humans	Brom et al. (2011)

influence of ligand or chelator structure on the biokinetics of known radiopharmaceuticals.

In 2004, Shuhmacher et al. analyzed the Bn radiolabeled agonists $^{68/67}$Ga-DOTA-PEG2-[D-Tyr^{6},-Ala^{11},-Thi^{13},-Nle^{14}] Bn(6–14); $^{68/67}$Ga-BZH$_3$ in vitro and in vivo behavior and compared the results obtained with the same peptide radiolabeled with the radiolanthanide ^{177}Lu (Markwalder and Reubi 1999). In vitro studies were performed in the pancreatic tumor rat cell line AR42J, using the ^{67}Ga-BZH$_3$ conjugate. They reported hGRP receptor binding affinity of 0.46 nM for the new Bn analog (Table 3), which is three times higher than that for the ^{125}I-[Tyr^{4}]Bn radiocompound, used as standard control. ^{67}Ga-BZH$_3$ showed a high retention rate ($t_{1/2} = 13.5$ h, compared with 3 h for ^{125}I-[Tyr^{4}]Bn), probably due to the linker used for coupling. Biodistribution studies in tumor-bearing mice displayed a dose-dependent uptake for ^{67}Ga-BZH$_3$ in hGRP receptor-positive tissues (tumor and pancreas), with fast blood clearance. However, intestinal uptake was still high (Table 3). PET images were obtained using the ^{68}Ga-BZH$_3$ radioconjugate and indicated very sensitive localization of hGRP receptor-positive tumors in the mediastinal area. On the other hand, this $^{67/68}$Ga-radiolabeled compound could show some limitations in detection of metastatic prostate carcinoma, because of its high background signal in the abdomen (Schuhmacher et al. 2005).

In another study, the new Bn analog DOTA-PEG4-Bn(7–14) (DOTA-PESIN) (Table 3) was coupled with either ^{68}Ga or ^{177}Lu. In in vitro analysis in the human prostate cancer PC-3 cell line, they found a high hGRP receptor binding affinity for the ^{68}Ga-DOTA-PESIN conjugate (IC$_{50}$ 6.6 ± 3.0 nM). A longer time period (4 h) showed a higher ^{68}Ga-DOTA-PESIN uptake (Zhang et al. 2007). In vivo biodistribution and scintigraphy experiments using PC-3 cell xenografts showed fast tumor uptake and high level of tumor-to-liver ratio. Moreover, they found fast renal excretion and lower background for PET imaging (Zhang et al. 2007).

Use of $\alpha_v\beta_3$ integrin is justified by several studies that demonstrated its involvement in angiogenesis of most solid tumors (Friedlander et al. 1995; Brooks et al. 1994; Li et al. 2008). The efficiency of ^{99m}Tc-DOTA-$\alpha_V\beta_3$-tripeptide to target the receptor in vitro was assessed by receptor binding assays in tumor cell lines (U-87MG and BMG cell lines). The specific activity of the labeled peptide conjugate was found to be 1,890 MBq/mmol, which was high enough to saturate the receptors at nanomolar range. The ^{99m}Tc-labeled DOTA-$\alpha_V\beta_3$-tripeptide displayed selective affinity for human tumor cell line U-87MG (Varshney et al. 2011). Liu et al. (2009b) reported a heterodimeric peptide based on RGD Bn to investigate its dual receptor targeting properties for tumor $\alpha_v\beta_3$ integrin and gastrin-releasing peptide receptor. The multimeric radiocompound ^{68}Ga-NOTA-RGD-Bn (Table 3) was directed against both the $\alpha_v\beta_3$ integrin and hGRP receptors. The in vitro affinity for hGRP receptor was evaluated in the human prostate cancer cell line PC-3. Compared with native Bn and the compound with no linker (RGD-Bn), ^{68}Ga-NOTA-RGD-Bn showed comparable affinity with IC$_{50}$ values of 67.9 nM for RGD-Bn, 55.9 nM for NOTA-RGD-Bn, and 78.9 nM for Bn (Table 3). Cell uptake in PC-3 cells was higher for ^{68}Ga-NOTARGD-Bn than for ^{64}Cu- and ^{18}F-labeled Bn reported previously (Li et al. 2008; Liu et al. 2009c), but lower than that of ^{68}Ga-NOTA-Bn compound. MicroPET images, biodistribution studies, and immunofluorescence analysis in PC-3 tumor-bearing mice showed slightly higher tumor uptake of ^{68}Ga-NOTA-RGDBn than ^{68}Ga-NOTA-Bn (Table 3). The difference between in vitro and in vivo results was probably due to several factors including the presence of integrin receptors, which is much higher in the PC-3 tumor than in in vitro cells and the possibility that RGD was able to recognize the murine integrin $\alpha 3$, which is strongly expressed on tumor vasculature (as demonstrated by the immunofluorescence study). Moreover, the author hypothesized an in vivo synergistic interaction of the two motifs of the heterodimer compound that improved its binding affinity (Liu et al. 2009a).

^{68}Ga-labeled DOTA-MG0 is suited for PET, which could improve image quality. Targeting of cholecystokinin-2 (CCK2)/gastrin receptor-positive tumor cells with DOTA-MG0 labeled with ^{68}Ga in vitro was investigated using the AR42J rat tumor cell line and showed high receptor affinity. Biodistribution studies in BALB/c nude mice with a subcutaneous AR42J tumor revealed high tumor uptake of ^{68}Ga-DOTA-MG0 of 4.4 ± 1.3% ID/g at 1 h post injection. Coadministration of an excess unlabeled peptide blocked tumor uptake (0.7 ± 0.1% ID/g), indicating CCK2/gastrin receptor-mediated uptake ($p = 0.0005$). Subcutaneous and intraperitoneal tumors were clearly visualized by small-animal PET imaging with 5 MBq ^{68}Ga-DOTA-MG0. ^{68}Ga-labeled DOTA-MG0 specifically accumulates in CCK2/gastrin receptor-positive AR42J tumors with similar biodistribution apart from the kidneys. AR42J tumors were clearly visualized by microPET. Therefore, ^{68}Ga-DOTA-MG0 is a promising tracer for PET imaging of CCK2/gastrin receptor–positive tumors in humans. The results of the present study indicate that further clinical evaluation of GRPR-targeted nuclear imaging using Bn analogs is justified (Brom et al. 2011).

5 Conclusion

The discovery of the frequent overexpression and/or ectopic expression of various peptide/neurotransmitter receptors on many neoplasms has opened the potential for a new approach to both imaging these tumors and for targeted delivery. The introduction of ^{68}Ga-DOTA compounds has significantly improved the quality of neuroendocrine tumor imaging through improved PET resolution and higher affinity of the new generation of bombesin analogs. Bn analogs developed for labeling with radiometal may be of use for diagnostic imaging (PET and SPECT) and targeted radionuclide therapy. Through evaluation of binding affinity, internalization rate, efflux, and biodistribution in animals, PET imaging with ^{68}Ga has a major bearing on current and future clinical practice. Since the specificity of Bn analogs can be optimized to a very high degree, the synergistic effects of high image resolution and high target specificity may lead to widely available improvement in diagnostic efficacy.

References

Abd-Elgaliel WR, Gallazzi F, Garrison JC et al (2008) Design, synthesis, and biological evaluation of an antagonist bombesin analog as targeting vector. Bioconjug Chem 19:2040–2048

Abiraj K, Jaccard H, Kretzschmar M et al (2008) Novel DOTA-based prochelator for divalent peptide vectorization: synthesis of dimeric bombesin analogs for multimodality tumor imaging and therapy. Chem Commun (Camb) 28(28):3248–3250

Abiraj K, Mansi R, Tamma ML et al (2010) Tetraamine-derived bifunctional chelators for technetium-99m labeling: synthesis, bioconjugation and evaluation as targeted SPECT imaging probes for GRP-receptor-positive tumors. Chemistry 16:2115–2124

Achilefu S, Jimenez HN, Dorshow RB et al (2002) Synthesis, in vitro receptor binding, and in vivo evaluation of fluorescein and carbocyanine peptide-based optical contrast agents. J Med Chem 45:2003–2015

Akeson M, Sainz E, Mantey SA et al (1997) Identification of four amino acids in the gastrin-releasing peptide receptor that are required for high affinity agonist binding. J Biol Chem 272:17405–17409

Aloj L, Morelli G (2004) Design, synthesis and preclinical evaluation of radiolabeled peptides for diagnosis and therapy. Curr Pharm Des 10:3009–3031

Alves S, Correia JD, Santos I et al (2006) Pyrazolyl conjugates of bombesin: a new tridentate ligand framework for the stabilization of fac-[M(CO)3] + moiety. Nucl Med Biol 33:625–634

Anastasi A, Erspamer V, Bucci M (1971) Isolation and structure of bombesin and alytesin, two analogous active peptides from the skin of the European amphibians Bombina and Alytes. Experientia 27:166–167

Anderson CJ, Welch MJ (1999) Radiometal labeled agents (non-technetium) for diagnostic imaging. Chem Rev 99:2219–2234

Aprikian AG, Tremblay L, Han K et al (1997) Bombesin stimulates the motility of human prostate-carcinoma cells through tyrosine phosphorylation of focal adhesion kinase and of integrin-associated proteins. Int J Cancer 72:498–504

Avis IL, Kovacs TOG, Kasprzyk PG et al (1991) Preclinical evaluation of an anti-autocrine growth factor monoclonal antibody for treatment of patients with small cell lung cancer. J Natl Cancer Inst 83:1470–1476

Battey J, Wada E, Corjay M et al (1992) Molecular genetic analysis of two distinct receptors for mammalian bombesin-like peptides. J Natl Cancer Inst Monogr 13:141–144

Biddlecombe GB, Rogers BE, de Visser M et al (2007) Molecular imaging of gastrin-releasing peptide receptor-positive tumors in mice using 64Cu- and 86Y-DOTA-(Pro 1, Tyr 4)-bombesin(1–14). Bioconjug Chem 18:724–730

Blower PJ, Lewis JS, Zweit J (1996) Copper radionuclide and radiopharmaceuticals in nuclear medicine. Nucl Med Biol 23:957–980

Brans L, Maes V, Garcia-Garayoa E et al (2008) Glycation methods for bombesin analogs containing the (NalphaHis) Ac chelator for 99mTc(CO)3 radiolabeling. Chem Biol Drug Des 72:496–506

Breeman WA, Kwekkeboom DJ, Kooij PP et al (1995) Effect of dose and specific activity on tissue distribution of indium-111-pentetreotide in rats. J Nucl Med 36:623–627

Breeman WA, Hofland LJ, de Jong M et al (1999) Evaluation of radiolabeled bombesin analogs for receptortargeted scintigraphy and radiotherapy. Int J Cancer 81:658–665

Breeman WA, de Jong M, Erion JL et al (2002) Preclinical comparison of (111)In-labeled DTPA- or DOTA-bombesin analogs for receptor-targeted scintigraphy and radionuclide therapy. J Nucl Med 43:1650–1656

Breeman WA, de Jong M, de Blois E et al (2005) Radiolabeling DOTA-peptides with ^{68}Ga. Eur J Nucl Med Mol Imaging 32:478–485

Broan CJ, Cox JPL, Craig AS et al (1991) Structure and solution stability of indium and gallium complexes of 1,4,7-triazacyclononatriacetate and yttrium complexes of 1,4,7, 10-tetraazacyclododecanetetraacetate and related ligans: kinectically stable complexes for

use in imaging and radioimmunotherapy. X-ray molecular structure of the indium and gallium complexes of 1,4,7-triazacyclononane-1,4,7-triacetic acid. J Chem Soc Perkin Trans 2:87–99
Brom M, Joosten L, Laverman P et al (2011) Preclinical evaluation of ^{68}Ga-DOTA-minigastrin for the detection of cholecystokinin-2/gastrin receptor-positive tumors. Mol Imaging 10:144–152
Brooks PC, Clark RA, Cheresh DA (1994) Requirement of vascular integrin alpha v beta 3 for angiogenesis. Science 264:569–571
Brown M, Tache Y, Fisher D (1979) Central nervous system action of bombesin: mechanism to induce hyperglycemia. Endocrinology 105:660–665
Brunner UK, Renn O, Li M et al (1995) In principal of nuclear medicine, Philadelphia, pp 220–229
Bunnett N (1994) Gastrin-releasing peptide. In: Walsh JH, Dockray GJ (eds) Gut peptides: biochemistry, and physiology. Raven, New York, pp 423–445
Cai RZ, Reile H, Armatis P et al (1994) Potent bombesin antagonists with C terminal Leu-ψ(CH2-N)-Tac-NH2 or its derivatives. Proc Natl Acad Sci USA 91:12664–12668
Carlsson J, Forssell-Aronsson E, Hietala SO et al (2003) Tumor theraphy with radionuclides: assessment of progress and problems. Radiother Oncol 66:107–117
Cescato R, Maina T, Nock B et al (2008) Bombesin receptor antagonists may be preferable to agonists for tumor targeting. J Nucl Med 49:318–326
Chen X, Park R, Hou Y et al (2004) MicroPET and autoradiographic imaging of GRP receptor expression with 64Cu-DOTA-[Lys3]bombesin in human prostate adenocarcinoma xenografts. J Nucl Med 45:1390–1397
Chong HS, Garmestani K, Ma D et al (2002) Synthesis and biological evalution of novel macrocyclic ligands with pendent donor groups as potential yttrium chelators for radioimmunotheraphy with improved complex formation kinectics. J Med Chem 45:3458–3464
Christiansen J, Holst JJ, Kalaja E (1976) Inhibition of gastric acid in man by exogenous and endogenous pancreatic glucagon. Gastroenterology 70:688–692
Clarke ET, Martell AE (1991) Stabilities of the trivalent metal ion complexes of the tetracetate derivatives of 12-, 13-, and 14-membered tetraazamacrocycles. Inorg Chim Acta 190:37–46
Cornelio DB, Roesler R, Schwartsmann G (2007) Gastrin-releasing peptide receptor as a molecular target in experimental anticancer therapy. Ann Oncol 18:1457–1466
Craig AS, Parker D, Adams H et al (1989) Stability Ga-71 Nmr and crystal-structure of a Neutral Gallium (iii) complex of 1,4,7-Triazacyclononanetriacetate—a potential radiopharmaceutical. J Chem Soc-Chem Communications, pp 1793–1794
Cutler CS, Smith CJ, Ehrhardt GJ et al (2000) Current and potential therapeutic uses of lanthanide radioisotopes. Cancer Biother Radiopharm 15:531–545
Cuttitta F, Carney DN, Mulshine J et al (1985) Bombesin-like peptides can function as autocrine growth factors in human small-cell lung cancer. Nature 316:823–825
de Jong M, Bakker WH, Krenning EP et al (1997) Yttrium -90 and indium -111 labeling receptor binding and biodistribution of [DOTA0, d-Phe1, Tyr3]octreotide, a promising somastostatin analog for radionuclide theraphy. Eur J Nucl Med 24:368–371
de Visser M, Bernard HF, Erion JL et al (2007) Novel (111) In-labeled bombesin analogs analogs for molecular imaging of prostate tumors. Eur J Nucl Med Mol Imaging 34:1228–1238
Dimitrakopoulou-Strauss A, Hohenberger P, Eisenhut M et al (2006) J Nucl Med 47:102P
Dimitrakopoulou-Strauss A, Hohenberger P, Haberkorn U et al (2007) ^{68}Ga-labeled bombesin studies in patients with gastrointestinal stromal tumors: comparisonwith 18F-FDG. J Nucl Med 48:1245–1250
Durkan K, Lambrecht FY, Unak P et al (2007) Radiolabeling of bombesin-like peptide with 99 mTc: 99 mTc-litorin and biodistribution in rats. Bioconjug Chem 18:1516–1520
Dymov AM, Savostin AP (1968) Analytical chemistry of gallium. Ann Arbor: Ann Arbor Science, Moscow
Eary JF (2001) PET imaging for planning cancer theraphy. J Nucl Med 42:770–771
Eisenwiener KP, Prata MI, Buschmann I et al (2002) NODAGATOC, a new chelator-coupled somatostatin analog labeled with [$^{67/68}$Ga] and [111In] for SPECT, PET and targeted

therapeutic application of somatostatin receptor (hsst2) expressing tumors. Bioconjug Chem 13:530–541
Erspamer V (1988) Discovery, isolation and characterization of bombesin- like peptides. Ann N Y Acad Sci 547:3–9
Erspamer V, Erpamer GF, Inselvini M (1970) Some pharmacological actions of alytesin and bombesin. J Pharm Pharmacol 22:875–876
Faintuch BL, Teodoro R, Duatti A et al (2008) Radiolabeled bombesin analogs for prostate cancer diagnosis: preclinical studies. Nucl Med Biol 35:401–411
Fathi Z, Corjay MH, Shapira H et al (1993) BRS-3: a novel bombesin receptor subtype selectively expressed in testis, and lung carcinoma cells. J Biol Chem 268:5979–5984
Ferro-Flores G, Arteaga de Murphy C, Rodriguez-Cortes J et al (2006) Preparation and evaluation of 99 mTc-EDDA/HYNIC-[Lys 3]-bombesin for imaging gastrin-releasing peptide receptor-positive tumors. Nucl Med Commun 27:371–376
Fichna J, Janecka A (2003) Synthesis of target-specific radiolabed peptide for diagnostic imaging. Bioconjug Chem 14:3–17
Fischer JB, Schonbrunn A (1988) The bombesin receptor is coupled to a guanine nucleotide-binding protein which is insensitive to pertussis and cholera toxins. J Biol Chem 263:2808–2816
Forrer F, Valkema R, Kwekkeboom DJ et al (2007) Neuroendocrine tumors. Peptide receptor radionuclide therapy. Best Pract Res Clin Endocrinol Metab 21:111–129
Fragogeorgi EA, Zikos C, Gourni E et al (2009) Spacer site modifications for the improvement of the in vitro and in vivo binding properties of (99m)Tc-N(3)S-Xbombesin[2–14] derivatives. Bioconjug Chem 20:856–867
Friedlander M, Brooks PC, Shaffer RW et al (1995) Definition of two angiogenic pathways by distinct alpha v integrins. Science 270:1500–1502
Gambhir SS (2002) Molecular imaging of cancer with positron emission tomography. Nat Rev Cancer 2:683–693
Garcia GE, Ruegg D, Blauenstein P et al (2007a) Chemical and biological characterization of new Re(CO)3/[99 mTc](CO)3 bombesin analogs. Nucl Med Biol 34:17–28
Garcia GE, Schweinsberg C, Maes V et al (2007b) A new [99 mTc] bombesin analogs with improved biodistribution for targeting gastrin releasing-peptide receptorpositive tumors. Q J Nucl Med Mol Imaging 51:42–50
Garrison JC, Rold TL, Sieckman GL et al (2007) In vivo evaluation and small-animal PET/CT of a prostate cancer mouse model using 64Cu bombesin analogs: Side-by-side comparison of the CB-TE2A and DOTA chelation systems. J Nucl Med 48:1327–1337
Garrison JC, Rold TL, Sieckman GL et al (2008) Evaluation of the pharmacokinetic effects of various linking group using the 111In-DOTA-X-BBN (7–14)NH2 structural paradigm in a prostate cancer model. Bioconjug Chem 19:1803–1812
Ghatei MA, George SK, Major JH et al (1984) Bombesin-like immunoreactivity in the pancreas of man and other mammalian species. Experientia 40:884–886
Gibril F, Jensen RT (2004) Diagnostic uses of radiolabeled somatostatin-receptor analogs in gastroenteropancreatic endocrine tumors. Dig Liver Dis 36:S106–S120
Giraud AS, Dumesny C, Whitley JC et al (2010) Isolation, identification and biological activity of gastrin-releasing peptide 1–46 (GRP 1–46), the primary GRP gene-derived peptide product of the pregnant ovine endometrium. Peptides 31:284–290
Gonzalez N, Moody TW, Igarashi H et al (2008) Bombesin-related peptides and their receptors: recent advances in their role in physiology and disease states. Curr Opin Endocrinol Diabetes Obes 15:58–64
Gonzalez N, Mantey SA, Pradhan TK et al (2009) Characterization of putative GRP- and NMB-receptor antagonist's interaction with human receptors. Peptides 30:1473–1486
Gourni E, Paravatou M, Bouziotis P et al (2006) Evaluation of a series of new 99 mTc-labeled bombesin-like peptides for early cancer detection. Anticancer Res 26:435–438
Gourni E, Bouziotis P, Benaki D et al (2009) Structural assessment and biological evaluation of two N3S bombesin derivatives. J Med Chem 52:4234–4246

Green MA, Welch MJ (1989) Gallium radiopharmaceutical chemistry. Nucl Med Biol 16:435–448
Gugger M, Reubi JC (1999) Gastrin-releasing peptide receptors in non-neoplastic and neoplastic human breast. Am J Pathol 155:2067–2076
Hajri A, Koenig M, Balboni G et al (1996) Expression and characterization of gastrin-releasing peptide receptor in normal and cancerous pancreas. Pancreas 12:25–35
Halmos G, Schally AV (1997) Reduction in receptors for bombesin and epidermal growth factor in xenografts of human small-cell lung cancer after treatment with bombesin antagonist RC-3095. Proc Natl Acad Sci USA 94:956–960
Harris WR, Messori LA (2002) A comparative study of aluminium(III), gallium(III), indium(III), and thallium(III) binding to human serum tansferrin. Coord Chem Rev 228:237–262
Haubner R, Bruchertseifer F, Bock M et al (2004) Synthesis and biological evalution of a (99m) Tc-labeled Cyclic RGD peptide for imaging the alphabeta3 expression. Nuklearmedizin 43:26–32
Heasley LE (2001) Autocrine and paracrine signaling through neuropeptide receptors in human cancer. Oncogene 20:1563–1569
Hellmich MR, Ives KL, Udupi V et al (1999) Multiple protein kinase pathways are involved in gastrin-releasing peptide receptor-regulated secretion. J Biol Chem 274:23901–23909
Heppeler A, Froidevaux S, Macke HR et al (1999) Radiometal-labeled macrocyclic chelator-derivatised somastostatin analog with superb tumor-targeting properties and potential for receptor mediated internal radiotheraphy. Chem Eur J 5:1974–1981
Heppler A, Froidevaux S, Eberle AN et al (2000) Receptor imaging for tumor localisation and theraphy with radioisopes. Curr Med Chem 7:971–994
Hnatowich DJ, Friedman B, Clancy B et al (1981) Labeling of performed liposomes with Ga-67 and Tc-99 m by chelation. J Nucl Med 22:810–814
Ho CL, Chen LC, Lee WC et al (2009) Receptor-binding, biodistribution, dosimetry, and micro-SPECT/CT imaging of 111In-[DTPA(1), Lys(3), Tyr(4)]- bombesin analog in human prostate tumor-bearing mice. Cancer Biother Radiopharm 24:435–443
Hoffman TJ, Gali H, Smith CJ et al (2003) Novel series of 111In-labeled bombesin analogs as potential radiopharmaceuticals for specific targeting of gastrin-releasing peptide receptors expressed on human prostate cancer cells. J Nucl Med 44:823–831
Hofmann M, Maecke H, Borner R et al (2001) Biokinectics and imaging with the somatostatin receptor PET radioligand (68) Ga-DOTATOC: preliminary data. Eur J Nucl Med 28:1751–1757
Hofmann M, Machtens S, Stief C et al (2004) Feasibility of Ga-68-DOTABOM PET in prostate carcinoma patients [abstract]. J Nucl Med 45:449P
Hohne A, Mu L, Honer M et al (2008) Synthesis, 18F-labeling, and in vitro and in vivo studies of bombesin peptides modified with silicon-based building blocks. Bioconjug Chem 19:1871–1879
Hu F, Cutler CS, Hoffman T et al (2002) Pm-149 DOTA bombesin nalogs for potential radiotherapy—In vivo comparison with Sm-153 and Lu-177 labeled DO3A-amide-Ala-BBN(7–14)NH2. Nucl Med Biol 29:423–430
Jensen RT (1994) Receptors for bombesins. In: Johnson LR (ed) Physiology of the Gastrointestinal Tract. Raven, New York, pp 1387–1393
Jensen RT (1997) Peptide therapy. Recent advances in the use of somatostatin and other peptide receptor agonists and antagonists. In: Lewis JH, Dubois A (eds) Current clinical topics in gastrointestinal pharmacology. Blackwell Science, Malden, pp 144–223
Jensen RT, Coy DH (1991) Progress in the development of potent bombesin receptor antagonists. Trends Pharmacol Sci 12:13–19
Jensen RT, Moody TW (2006) Bombesin-related peptides and neurotensin: effects on cancer growth/proliferation and cellular signaling in cancer. In: Kastin AJ (ed) Handbook of biologically active peptides, 1st edn. Amsterdam, Elsevier, pp 429–434
Jensen RT, Battey JF, Spindel ER et al (2008) International Union of Pharmacology. LVIII. Mammalian Bombesin Receptors: Nomenclature, distribution, pharmacology, signalling and functions in normal and disease states. Pharmacol Rev 60:1–42

Kane MA, Toi-Scott M, Johnson GL et al (1996) Bombesin-like peptide receptors in human bronchial epithelial cells. Peptides 17:111–118

Kiehne K, Herzig KH, Folsch UR (2002) Differential activation of p43ERK2 and p125FAK by cholecystokinin and bombesin in the secretion and proliferation of the pancreatic amphicrine cell line AR42J. Pancreatology 2:46–53

Kim HJ, Evers BM, Guo Y et al (1996) Bombesin-mediated AP-1 activation in a human gastric cancer (SIIA). Surgery 120:130–136; discussion 136–137

Koh SW, Leyton J, Moody TW (1999) Bombesin activates MAP kinase in non-small cell lung cancer cells. Peptides 20:121–126

Koizumi M, Endo K, Kunimatsu M et al (1987) Preparation of 67 Ga-labeled antibodies using deferoxamine as a bifunctional chelate an improved method. J Immunological Methods 104:93–102

Koumarianou E, Mikolajczak R, Pawlak D et al (2009) Comparative study on DOTA-derivatized bombesin analog labeled with 90Y and 177Lu: in vitro and in vivo evaluation. Nucl Med Biol 36:591–603

Kowalski J, Henze M, Schumacher J et al (2003) Evalution of positron emission tomography imaging using [^{68}Ga]-DOTA-D-Phe(1)-Tyr(3)-Octreotide in comparison to [111In]-DTPAOC SPECT. First resuls in patients with neuroendocrine tumor. Mol Imaging Biol 5:42–48

Krenning EP, Kwekkeboom DJ, Bakker WH et al (1993) Somatostatin receptor scintigraphy with [111In-DTPA-D-Phe1]- and [123I-Tyr3]-octreotide: the Rotterdam experience with more than 1,000 patients. Eur J Nucl Med 20:716–731

Krenning EP, Kwekkeboom DJ, Valkema R et al (2004) Peptide receptor radionuclide therapy. Ann N Y Acad Sci 1014:234–245

Kroog GS, Jensen RT, Battey JF (1995) Mammalian bombesin receptors. Med Res Rev 15:389–417

Kung MP, Kung HF (2005) Mass effect of injected dose in small rodent imaging by SPECT and PET. Nucl Med Biol 32:673–678

Kunstler JU, Veerendra B, Figueroa SD et al (2007) Organometallic 99mTc(III) ‘4 + 1’ bombesin(7–14) conjugates: synthesis, radiolabeling, and in vitro/in vivo studies. Bioconjug Chem 18:1651–1661

Kwekkeboom D, Krenning EP, de Jong M (2000) Peptide receptor imaging and therapy. J Nucl Med 41:1704–1713

La Bella R, Garcia-Garayoa E, Langer M et al (2002) In vitro and in vivo evaluation of a 99 mTc(I)-labeled bombesin analog for imaging of gastrin releasing peptide receptor-positive tumors. Nucl Med Biol 29:553–560

Ladenheim EE, Taylor JE, Coy DH et al (1994) Blockade of feeding inhibition by neuromedin B using a selective receptor antagonist. Eur J Pharmacol 271:R7–R9

Lambrecht RM, Sajjad M (1988) Accelarator-derived radionuclide generators. Radiochim Acta 43:171–179

Lane SR, Veerendra B, Rold TL et al (2008) 99mTc(CO)3-DTMA bombesin conjugates having high affinity for the GRP receptor. Nucl Med Biol 35:263–272

Lantry LE, Cappelletti E, Maddalena ME et al (2006) 177Lu-AMBA: Synthesis and characterization of a selective 177Lu-labeled GRP-R agonist for systemic radiotherapy of prostate cancer. J Nucl Med 47:1144–1152

Laskin JJ, Sandler AB (2004) Epidermal growth factor receptor: a promising target insolid tumors. Cancer Treat Rev 30:1–17

Lebacq-Verheyden AM, Trepel J, Sausville EA et al (1990) Bombesin and gastrin-releasing peptide: neuropeptides, secretagogues, and growth factors. In: Sporn MB, Roberts AB (eds) Peptide growth factors and their receptors II. Springer, New York, pp 71–124

Lewis MR, Raubitschek A, Shively JE (1994) A facile, water soluble method for modification of proteins with DOTA. Use of elevated temperature and optimized pH to achieve high specific activity and high chelate stability in radiolabeled immunoconjugates. Bioconjug Chem 5:565–576

Li WP, Lewis JS, Kim J et al (2002) DOTA-D-Tyr1-octreotate: a somatostatin analog for labeling with metal and halogen radionuclides for cancer imaging and therapy. Bioconjug Chem 13:721–728
Li ZB, Wu Z, Chen K et al (2008) 18F-labeled BBN-RGD heterodimer for prostate cancer imaging. J Nucl Med 49:453–461
Liehr RM, Reidelberger RD, Rosewicz S et al (1992) Dose-related involvement of CCK in bombesin-induced pancreatic growth. Regul Pept 38:207–219
Lin TM, Warrick MW (1974) Action of acetylsalicyclic acid and glucagon on aicd secretion mucosal blood flow, bleeding, and net ionic effux in the fundic pouch of pentagastrin stimulated dogs. Arch Int Pharmacol Ther 210:279–287
Lin KS, Luu A, Baidoo KE et al (2005) A new high affinity technetium-99 m-bombesin analog with low abdominal accumulation. Bioconjug Chem 16:43–50
Liu S, Edwards DS (2001a) Synthesis and characterization of two (111)-In-labeled DTPA-peptide conjugates. Bioconjug Chem 12:630–634
Liu S, Edwards DS (2001b) Bifunctional chelators for therapeutic lanthanide radiopharmaceuticals. Bioconjug Chem 12:7–34
Liu Z, Niu G, Wang F et al (2009a) (68)Ga-labeled NOTARGD- BBN peptide for dual integrin and GRPR-targeted tumor imaging. Eur J Nucl Med Mol Imaging 36:1483–1494
Liu Z, Yan Y, Chin FT et al (2009b) Dual integrin and gastrin releasing peptide receptor targeted tumor imaging using 18F-labeled PEGylated RGD-bombesin heterodimer 18F-FBPEG3- Glu-RGD-BBN. J Med Chem 52:425–432
Liu Z, Li ZB, Cao Q et al (2009c) Small animal PET of tumors with (64)Cu-labeled RGD-bombesin heterodimer. J Nucl Med 50:1168–1177
Llinares M, Devin C, Chaloin O et al (1999) Syntheses and biological activities of potent bombesin receptor antagonists. J Pept Res 53:275–283
Lundqvist H, Tolmchev V (2002) Targeting peptides and positron emission tomography. Bioploymers 66:381–392
Luyt LG, Katzenellenbogen JA (2002) A trithiolate tripodal bifunctional ligan for the radiolabeling of peptides with gallium (III). Bioconjug Chem 13:1140–1145
Ma L, Yu P, Veerendra B et al (2007) In vitro and in vivo evaluation of Alexa Fluor 680- bombesin [7–14]NH2 peptide conjugate, a high-affinity fluorescent probe with high selectivity for the gastrin-releasing peptide receptor. Mol Imaging 6:171–180
Maecke HR, Hofmann M, Haberkorn U (2005) ^{68}Ga-labeled peptide in tumor imaging. J Nucl Med 46:172S–178S
Maes V, Brans L, Schweinsberg C et al (2009) Carbohydrated [99mTc(CO)3](NalphaHis) Ac-bombesin(7–14) analogs. Adv Exp Med Biol 611:409–410
Maina T, Nock B, Mather S (2006) Targeting prostate cancer with radiolabeled bombesins. Cancer Imaging 6:153–157
Mansi R, Wang X, Forrer F et al (2009) Evaluation of a therapeutic radionuclides tomography, positron emission tomography, and labeling with single-photon emission computed conjugated bombesin-based radioantagonist for the 1,4,7,10-tetraazacyclododecane-1,4,7,10-tetra-acetic acid. Clin Cancer Res 15:5240–5249
Mantey SA, Weber HC, Sainz E et al (1997) Discovery of a high affinity radioligand for the human orphan receptor, bombesin receptor subtype 3, which demonstrates that it has a unique pharmacology compared with other mammalian bombesin receptors. J Biol Chem 272:26062–26071
Markwalder R, Reubi JC (1999) Gastrin-releasing peptide receptors in the human prostate: relation to neoplastic transformation. Cancer Res 59:1152–1159
Mathias CJ, Sun YZ, Welch MJ et al (1990) N,N'-bis(2-hydroxybenzyl)-1-(4-bromoacetamidobenzyl)-1,2-ethylenediamine-N,N'-diacetic acid: a new bifunctional chelates for radiolabeling antibodies. Bioconjug Chem 1:204–211
Matsumoto K, Yamada K, Wada E et al (2003) Bombesin receptor subtype-3 modulates plasma insulin concentration. Peptides 24:83–90

McDevitt MR, Ma D, Lai LT et al (2001) Tumor theraphy with targeted atomic nanogenerators. Science 294:1537–1540

McDonald TJ, Jornvall H, Nilsson G et al (1979) Characterization of a gastrin releasing peptide from porcine non-antral gastric tissue. Biochem Biophys Res Commun 90:227–233

Metz DC, Jensen RT (2008) Gastrointestinal neuroendocrine tumors: pancreatic endocrine tumors. Gastroenterology 135:1469–1492

Meyer GJ, Gielow P, Borner AR et al (2005) Ga-67 and Ga-68 labeled DOTA-derivatised peptide-ligands. Nuklearmedizin 6:A192

Minamino N, Kangawa K, Matsuo H (1983) Neuromedin B: a novel bombesin-like peptide identified in porcine spinal cord. Biochem Biophys Res Commun 114:541–548

Minamino N, Kangawa K, Matsuo H (1984) Neuromedin C: a bombesinlike peptide identified in porcine spinal cord. Biochem Biophys Res Commun 119:14–20

Mollet A, Meier S, Grabler V et al (2003) Endogenous amylin contributes to the anorectic effects of cholecystokinin and bombesin. Peptides 24:91–98

Montet X, Weissleder R, Josephson L (2006) Imaging pancreatic cancer with a peptide nanoparticle conjugate targeted to normal pancreas. Bioconjug Chem 17:905–911

Moody TW, Crawley JN, Jensen RT (1982) Pharmacology and neurochemistry of bombesin-like peptides. Peptides 3:559–563

Moody TW, Chan D, Fahrenkrug J et al (2003) Neuropeptides as autocrine growth factors in cancer cells. Curr Pharm Des 9:495–509

Moody TW, Mantey SA, Pradhan TK et al (2004) Development of high affinity camptothecin-bombesin conjugates that have targeted cytotoxicity for bombesin receptor containing tumor cells. J Biol Chem 279:23580–23589

Moore JG (1973) Gastric acid suppression by inravenous glucose solutions. Gastroenterology 64:1106–1110

Moran TH, Moody W, Hostetler AM et al (1988) Distribution of bombesin binding sites in the rat gastrointestinal tract. Peptides 9:643–649

Mutic S, Malyapa RS, Grigsby PW et al (2003) PET-guided IMRT for cervical carcinoma with positive para-aortic lymph nodes-a-dose-escaltion treatment planning study. Int J Radiat Oncol Biol Phys 55:28–35

Nagalla SR, Gibson BW, Tang D et al (1992) Gastrinreleasing peptide (GRP) is not mammalian bombesin. Identification and molecular cloning of a true amphibian GRP distinct from amphibian bombesin in Bombina orientalis. J Biol Chem 267:6916–6922

Nanda PK, Lane SR, Retzloff LB et al (2010) Radiolabeled regulatory peptides for imaging and therapy. Curr Opin Endocrinol Diabetes Obes 17:69–76

Narayan S, Guo YS, Townsend CM et al (1990) Specific binding and growth effects of bombesin-related peptides on mouse colon cancer cells in vito. Cancer Res 50:6772–6778

Nemeroff CB, Osbahr AJ, Manberg PJ et al (1979) Alteration in nociception and body temperature after intracisternal administration of neurotensin, β-endorphin, other endogenous peptides, and morohine. Proc Natl Acad Sci USA 76:5368–5371

Nock B, Nikolopoulou A, Chiotellis E et al (2003) A novel potent bombesin analog for GRP receptor-targeted tumor imaging. Eur J Nucl Med Mol Imaging 30:247–258

Nock BA, Nikolopoulou A, Galanis A et al (2005) Potent bombesin-like peptides for GRP-receptor targeting of tumors with 99mTc: a preclinical study. J Med Chem 48:100–110

Okarvi SM (1999) Recent developments in 99mTc-labeled peptide-based radiopharmaceuticals: an overview. Nucl Med Commun 20:1093–1112

Okarvi SM (2004) Peptide-based radiopharmaceuticals: future tools for diagnostic imaging of cancers and other diseases. Med Res Rev 24:357–397

Okarvi SM (2008) Peptide-based radiopharmaceuticals and cytotoxic conjugates: potential tools against cancer. Cancer Treat Rev 34:13–26

Okarvi SM, Al-Jammaz I (2003) Synthesis, radiolabeling and biological characteristics of a bombesin peptide analog as a tumor imaging agent. Anticancer Res 23:2745–2750

Osumi Y, Aibara S, Sakae K et al (1977) Central noradrenergic inhibition of gastric mucosal blood flow and acid secretion in rats. Life Sci 20:1407–1416
Parry JJ, Andrews R, Rogers BE (2007) MicroPET imaging of breast cancer using radiolabeled bombesin analogs targeting the gastrin-releasing peptide receptor. Breast Cancer Res Treat 101:175–183
Paterson BM, Karas JA, Scanlon DB et al (2010) Synthesis, conjugation to bombesin (7–14)-NH2, and copper-64 radiolabeling. Inorg Chem 49:1884–1893
Pazos-Moura CC, Ortiga-Carvalho TM, Gaspar De Moura E (2003) The autocrine/paracrine regulation of thyrotropin secretion. Thyroid 13:167–175
Pearson RG (1963) Hard and soft acids and bases. J Am Chem Soc 85:3533–3539
Pochon S, Buchegger F, Pelegrin A et al (1989) A novel derivative of the chelon desferrioxamine for site-specific conjugation to antibodies. Int J Cancer 43:1188–1194
Pradhan TK, Katsuno T, Taylor JE et al (1998) Identification of a unique ligand which has high affinity for all four bombesin receptor subtypes. Eur J Pharmacol 343:275–287
Prasanphanich AF, Nanda PK, Rold TL et al (2007) [64Cu-NOTA-8-Aoc-BBN(7–14)NH2] targeting vector for positron-emission tomography imaging of gastrin-releasing peptide receptor-expressing tissues. Proc Natl Acad Sci USA 104:12462–12467
Preston SR, Miller GV, Primrose JN (1996) Bombesin-like peptides and cancer. Crit Rev Oncol Hematol 23:225–238
Reichert DE, Lewis JS, Andreson CJ (1999) Metal complexes as diagnostic tools. Coord Chem Rev 184:3–66
Retzloff LB, Heinzke L, Figureoa SD et al (2010) Evaluation of [99mTc-(CO)3-X-Y-bombesin(7–14)NH2] conjugates for targeting gastrin-releasing peptide receptors overexpressed on breast carcinoma. Anticancer Res 30:19–30
Reubi JC (1995) Neuropeptide receptors in health and disease: the molecular basis for in vivo imaging. J Nucl Med 36:1825–1835
Reubi JC (2003) Peptide receptors as molecular targets for cancer diagnosis and therapy. Endocr Rev 24:389–427
Reubi JC, Maecke HR (2008) Peptide-based probes for cancer imaging. J Nucl Med 49:1735–1738
Reubi JC, Wenger S, Schmuckli-Maurer J et al (2002) Bombesin receptor subtypes in human cancers: detection with the universal radioligand P 125PI-[DTy6, beta-AlaP11P, PheP 13 P, NleP14] bombesin(6–14). Clin Cancer Res 8:1139–1146
Reubi JC, Macke HR, Krenning EP (2005) Candidtae for peptide receptor radiotheraphy today and in the future. J Nucl Med 46:67S–75S
Rogers BE, Rosenfeld ME, Khazaeli MB et al (1997) Localization of iodine-125-mIP-Des-Met14-bombesin (7–13)NH2 in ovarian carcinoma induced to express the gastrin releasing peptide receptor by adenoviral vector-mediated gene transfer. J Nucl Med 38:1221–1229
Rogers BE, Manna DD, Safavy A (2004) In vitro and in vivo evaluation of a 64Cu-labeled polyethylene glycol-bombesin conjugate. Cancer Biother Radiopharm 19:25–34
Rozengurt E (1990) Bombesin stimulation of mitogenesis. Specific receptors, signal transduction and early events. Am Rev Respir Dis 142:S11–S15
Rozengurt E (1991) Neuropeptides as cellular growth factors: role of multiple signalling pathways. Eur J Clin Invest 21:123–134
Ryan RR, Weber HC, Hou W et al (1998) Ability of various bombesin receptor agonists and antagonists to alter intracellular signaling of the human orphan receptor BRS-3. J Biol Chem 273:13613–13624
Sancho V, Di Florio A, Terry W et al (2011) Bombesin receptor-mediated imaging and cytotoxicity: review and current status. Curr Drug Delivery 8:79–134
Santos-Cuevas CL, Ferro-Flores G, Arteaga de Murphy C et al (2008) Targeted imaging of gastrin-releasing peptide receptors with 99mTc-EDDA/HYNIC-[Lys3]-bombesin: biokinetics and dosimetry in women. Nucl Med Commun 29:741–747

Santos-Cuevas CL, Ferro-Flores G, Arteaga de Murphy C et al (2009) Design, preparation, in vitro and in vivo evaluation of (99m)Tc-N2S2-Tat(49–57)-bombesin: a target-specific hybrid radiopharmaceutical. Int J Pharm 375:75–83

Schroeder RP, Muller C, Reneman S et al (2010) A standardized study to compare prostate cancer targeting efficacy of five radiolabeled bombesin analogs. Eur J Nucl Med Mol Imaging 37:1386–1396

Schroeder RPJ, van Weerden WM, Krenning EP et al (2011) Gastrin-releasing peptide receptor-based targeting using bombesin analogs is superior to metabolism-based targeting using choline for in vivo imaging of human prostate cancer xenografts. Eur J Nucl Med Mol Imaging 38:1257–1266

Schuhmacher J, Zhang H, Doll J et al (2005) GRP receptor-targeted PET of a rat pancreas carcinoma xenograft in nude mice with a ^{68}Ga-labeled bombesin(6–14) analog. J Nucl Med 46:691–699

Schuhmaker J, Atys R, Hauser H et al (1986) Labeling of monoclonal antibodies with a 67 Ga phenolic aminocarboxylic acid chelate. Part I. Chemistry and labeling technique. Eur J Nucl Med 12:397–404

Schweinsberg C, Maes V, Brans L et al (2008) Novel glycated [99mTc(CO)3]-labeled bombesin analogs for improved targeting of gastrin-releasing peptide receptor-positive tumors. Bioconjug Chem 19:2432–2439

Scopinaro F, Varvarigou AD, Ussof W et al (2002) Technetium labeled bombesin-like peptide: preliminary report on breast cancer uptake in patients. Cancer Biother Radiopharm 17:327–335

Scopinaro F, De Vincentis G, Corazziari E et al (2004) Detection of colon cancer with 99mTc-labeled bombesin derivative (99mTc-leu13-BN1). Cancer Biother Radiopharm 19:245–252

Scopinaro F, Massari R, Varvarigou AD et al (2007) High resolution small animal single photon emission computed tomography: uptake of [99mTc]bombesin and [123I]ioflupane by rat brain. Q J Nucl Med Mol Imaging 51:204–210

Severi C, Coy DH, Jensen RT et al (1989) Pharmacological characterization of [13 Leu13ψ-CH2NH-Leu14]-bombesin as a specific bombesin receptor antagonist on isolated smooth muscle cells. J Pharmacol Exp Ther 251:713–717

Seybold VS, Parsons AM, Aanonsen LM et al (1990) Characterization and autoradiographic localization of gastrin releasing peptide receptors in the porcine gut. Peptides 11:779–787

Shipp MA, Tarr GE, Chen CY et al (1991) CD10/neutral endopeptidase 24.11 hydrolyzes bombesin-like peptides and regulates the growth of small cell carcinomas of the lung. Proc Natl Acad Sci USA 88:10662–10666

Signore A, Annovazzi A, Chianelli M et al (2001) Peptide radiopharmaceuticals for diagnosis and therapy. Eur J Nucl Med 28:1555–1565

Smith CJ, Gali H, Sieckman GL et al (2003a) Radiochemical investigations of 177Lu-DOTA-8-Aoc-BBN7- 14NH2: An in vitro/in vivo assessment of the targeting ability of this new radiopharmaceutical for PC-3 human prostate cancer cells. Nucl Med Biol 30:101–109

Smith CJ, Gali H, Sieckman GL et al (2003b) Radiochemical investigations of 99 mTc-N3S-X-BBN7-14NH2: An in vitro/in vivo structure-activity relationship study where X) 0-,3-,5-,8-, and 11-carbon tethering moieties. Bioconjug Chem 14:93–102

Smith CJ, Sieckman GL, Owen NK et al (2003c) T. J. Radio-Chemical investigations of gastrin-releasing peptide receptorspecific [(99m)Tc(X)(CO)3-Dpr-Ser-Ser–Ser-Gln-Trp-Ala-Val-Gly-His-Leu-Met-(NH2)] in PC-3, tumor-bearing, rodent models: syntheses, radiolabeling, and in vitro/in vivo studies where Dpr = 2,3-diaminopropionic acid and X = H_2O or $P(CH_2OH)_3$. Cancer Res 63:4082–4088

Smith CJ, Sieckman GL, Owen NK et al (2003d) Radiochemical investigation of [^{188}Re(H_2O)$(CO)_3$-diaminoproprionic acid-SSS-bombesin(7–14)NH2]: synthesis, radiolabeling and in vitro/in vivo GRP receptor targeting studies. Anticancer Res 23:63–70

Smith CJ, Volkert WA, Hoffman TJ (2003e) Gastrin releasing peptide (GRP) receptor targeted radiopharmaceuticals: a concise update. Nucl Med Biol 30:861–868

Smith CJ, Volkert WA, Hoffman TJ (2005) Radiolabeled peptide conjugates for targeting of the bombesin receptor superfamily subtypes. Nucl Med Biol 32:733–740

Spindel E (1986) Mammalian bombesin-like peptides. Trends Neurosci 9:130–133

Stimmel JB, Stockstill ME, Kull FC et al (1995) Yttrium-90 chelation properties of tetrazatetraacetic acid macrocycles, diethylenetriaminepentaacetic acid analogs, and a novel terpyridine acyclic chelator. Bioconjug Chem 6:219–225

Sunday ME, Kaplan LM, Motoyama E et al (1988) Gastrin-releasing peptide (mammalian bombesin) gene expression in health and disease. Lab Invest 59:5–24

Swope SL, Schonbrunn A (1988) The biphasic stimulation of insulin secretion by bombesin involves both cytosolic free calcium and protein kinase C. Biochem J 253:193–201

Tachf Y, Vale W, Rivier J et al (1980) Brain regulation of gastric secretion: influence of neuropeptides (bombesin/8-endorphin/central nervous system/gastric acid output). Proc Natl Acad Sci USA 77:5515–5519

Thomas R, Chen J, Roudier MM et al (2009) Vessella RL, Lantry LE, Nunn AD. In vitro binding evaluation of ^{177}Lu-AMBA, a novel ^{177}Lu-labeled GRP-R agonist for systemic radiotherapy in human tissues. Clin Exp Metastasis 26:105–119

Tofilon PJ, Saxman S, Coleman CN (2003) Molecular targets for radion theraphy: bringing preclinical data into clinical trials. Clin Cancer Res 9:3518–3520

Tweedle MF (2009) Peptide-targeted diagnostics and radiotherapeutics. Acc Chem Res 42:958–968

Upp JR, Poston GJ, Maclellan DG et al (1988) Mechanisms of the trophic actions of bombesin on the pancreas. Pancreas 3:193–198

Uppal JK, Hazari PP, Varshney R et al (2011) Design, synthesis and biological evaluation of choline based SPECT imaging agent: Ga(III)-DO3A-EA-choline. Org Bio Chem 9(1591):1599

Van de Wiele C, Dumont F, Vanden Broecke R et al (2000) Technetium-99 m RP527, a GRP analog for visualisation of GRP receptor-expressing malignancies: a feasibility study. Eur J Nucl Med 27:1694–1699

Van de Wiele C, Dumont F, Van Belle S et al (2001) Is there a role for agonist gastrin-releasing peptide-receptor radioligands in tumor imaging? Nucl Med Commun 22:5–15

Van de Wiele C, Phonteyne P, Pauwels P et al (2008) Gastrin-releasing peptide receptor imaging in human breast carcinoma versus immunohistochemistry. J Nucl Med 49:260–264

van de WC, Dumont F, Dierck RA et al (2001) Biodistribution and dosimetry of (99 m)Tc-RP527, a gastrin-releasing peptide (GRP) agonist for the visualization of GRP receptor-expressing malignancies. J Nucl Med 42:1722–1727

Van Essen M, Krenning EP, Kam BL et al (2009) Peptide-receptor radionuclide therapy for endocrine tumors. Nat Rev Endocrinol 5:382–393

Van Lommel A (2001) Pulmonary neuroendocrine cells (PNEC) and neuroepithelial bodies (NEB): chemoreceptors and regulators of lung development. Paediatr Respir Rev 2:171–176

Varshney R, Hazari PP, Uppal JK et al (2011) Solid phase synthesis, radiolabeling and biological evaluation of a 99mTc-labeled $\alpha V\beta 3$ tripeptide (RGD) conjugated to DOTA as a tumor imaging agent. Cancer Bio Therapy 11:1–9

Varvarigou AD, Scopinaro F, Leondiadis L et al (2002) Synthesis, chemical, radio-chemical and radiobiological evaluation of a new 99 mTc-labeled bombesin-like peptide. Cancer Biother Radiopharm 17:317–326

Varvarigou A, Bouziotis P, Zikos C et al (2004) Gastrin-releasing peptide (GRP) analog for cancer imaging. Cancer Biother Radiopharm 19:219–229

Velikyan I (2005) Syntesis, characterization and application of ^{68}Ga-labeled macromolecules. Digital comprehensive summaries of Uppsala dissertations from the Faculty of Science and Technology 73:1651–6214

Velikyan I, Sundberg AL, Lindhe O et al (2005) Preparation and evaluation of ^{68}Ga-DOTA-hEGF for visualization of EGFR expression in malignant tumors. J Nucl Med 46:1881–1888

Vigna SR, Giraud AS, Mantyh PS et al (1990) Characterization of bombesin receptors on canine antral gastrin cells. Peptides 11:259–264

Volkert WA, Hoffman TJ (1999) Therapeutic radiopharmaceuticals. Chem Rev 99:2269–2292
Von Schrenck T, Heinz-Erian P, Moran T et al (1989) Neuromedin B receptor in esophagus: evidence for subtypes of bombesin receptors. Am J Physiol 256:747–758
Wagner SJ, Welch MJ (1979) Gallium-68 labeling of albumin and albumin microspheres. J Nucl Med 20:428–433
Waser B, Eltschinger V, Linder K et al (2007) Selective in vitro targeting of GRP and NMB receptors in human tumors with the new bombesin tracer 177Lu-AMBA. Eur J Nucl Med Mol Imaging 34:95–100
Weiner RE, Thakur ML (2002) Radiolabeled peptides in the diagnosis and therapy of oncological diseases. Appl Radiat Isot 57:749–763
Whitley JC, Moore C, Giraud AS et al (1999) Molecular cloning, genomic organization and selective expression of bombesin receptor subtype 3 in the sheep hypothalamus and pituitary. J Mol Endocrinol 23:107–116
Wild D, Macke HR, Waser B et al (2005) ^{68}Ga-DOTANOC: a first compound for PET imaging with high affinity for somatostain receptor subtype 2 and 5. Eur J Nucl Med Mol Imaging 32:724
Yamaguchi I, Hiroi J, Kumada S (1977) Central and peripheral adrenergic mechanisms regulating gastric secretion in the rat. J Pharmacol Exp Ther 203:125–131
Yang YS, Zhang X, Xiong Z et al (2006) Comparative in vitro and in vivo evaluation of two 64Cu labeled bombesin analogs in a mouse model of human prostate adenocarcinoma. Nucl Med Biol 33:371–380
Yegen BC (2003) Bombesin-like peptides: candidates as diagnostic and therapeutic tools. Curr Pharm Des 9:1013–1022
Yoo J, Reichert DE, Welch MJ (2004) Comparative in vivo behaviour studies of cycle bases copper -64 complexes:regioselective synthesis, X-ray structure, radiochemistry, log P and biodistribution. J Med Chem 47:6625–6637
Zhang H, Chen J, Waldherr C et al (2004) Synthesis and evaluation of bombesin derivatives on the basis of pan-bombesin peptides labeled with indium-111, lutetium-177, and yttrium-90 for targeting bombesin receptor-expressing tumors. Cancer Res 64:6707–6715
Zhang X, Cai W, Cao F et al (2006) 18F-labeled bombesin analogs for targeting GRP receptor-expressing prostate cancer. J Nucl Med 47:492–501
Zhang HW, Schuhmacher J, Waser B et al (2007) DOTA-PESIN, a DOTA-conjugated bombesin derivative designed for the imaging and targeted radionuclide treatment of bombesin receptor-positive tumors. Eur J Nucl Med Mol Imaging 34:1198–1208
Zhou J, Chen J, Mokotoff M et al (2004) Targeting gastrinreleasing peptide receptors for cancer treatment. Anticancer Drugs 15:921–927

A Novel ^{68}Ga-Labeled Pteroic Acid-Based PET Tracer for Tumor Imaging via the Folate Receptor

Berit Kühle, Cristina Müller and Tobias L. Ross

Abstract

The folate receptor (FR) is a very attractive target in oncological imaging as it is overexpressed by a variety of cancer types, whereas the expression in healthy tissue is very limited. The synthesis of regioisomeric pure folic acid derivatives normally requires a regioselective approach and does not allow the use of native folic acid (FA). As the pharmacophore of FA is assumed to be pteroic acid, its use without the glutamic acid moiety may enable the possibility to considerably simplify the synthesis of a positron emission tomography (PET) tracer for FR imaging. In this work, DO3A-EA-Pte was successfully synthesized and labeled with ^{68}Ga. It is stable for up to 3 h in PBS and against transchelation by transferrin. It also displays a lipophilicity that allows the assumption that it will show favorable in vivo characteristics for FR imaging via PET.

Contents

B. Kühle (✉) · T. L. Ross
Johannes Gutenberg-University, Fritz-Strassmann-Weg 2,
55128 Mainz, Germany
e-mail: kuehle@uni-mainz.de

C. Müller
Center for Radiopharmaceutical Sciences of ETH, PSI and USZ,
Paul Scherrer Institute, 5232 Villigen-PSI, Switzerland

R. P. Baum and F. Rösch (eds.), *Theranostics, Gallium-68, and Other Radionuclides*,
Recent Results in Cancer Research 194, DOI: 10.1007/978-3-642-27994-2_13,

1 Introduction

Folic acid (FA) is a vitamin that plays a crucial role in cell division and proliferation of healthy cells (Leamon and Low 2001). Therefore, it is not surprising that a variety of malignant tissues (e.g., endometrial, ovarian, and lung cancer) (Toffoli et al. 1997; Ross et al. 1994) display high overexpression of the folate receptor (FR), which mediates uptake of FA via endocytosis (Kamen and Capdevila 1986). Healthy cells use the reduced folate carrier for FA uptake (Antony 1992), which makes FR such an interesting target for molecular imaging. Relevant FR expression in healthy tissues can only be found in the kidneys in the proximal tubule. Other expression sites (i.e., lung and choroid plexus) (Weitman et al. 1992) are also apical and cannot be reached by intravenous application of a drug.

Figure 1 shows the chemical structure of folic acid. Most approaches to conjugate FA for either drug targeting or development of imaging agents have used the glutamic acid moiety to connect FA to the respective molecule or probe (Mathias et al. 1998; Leamon et al. 2002; Ross et al. 2008). Starting from native FA, a mixture of regioisomers (α/γ-carboxy group) will be obtained, calling for laborious and complex separation procedures, thus regioselective retrosynthesis is necessary to obtain a defined monodisperse product. This synthetic challenge in combination with the widely accepted assumption that pteroic acid makes up for the pharmacophore of FA led us to a different approach in the development of FR-targeting structures based on pteroic acid only.

Whilst FA and its derivatives show excellent affinities to FR in the nanomolar range, solely pteroic acid shows a significant drop in affinity (Kamen and Capdevila 1986; Leamon et al. 2009). Interestingly, it has been shown that pteroic acid conjugated to moieties other than glutamic acid can show affinities in the low

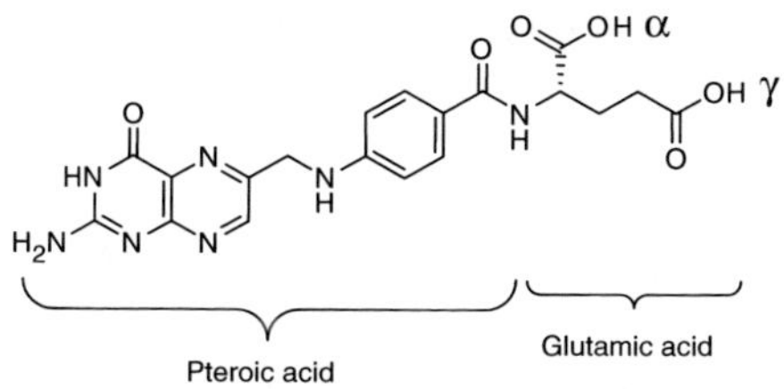

Fig. 1 Structure of folic acid

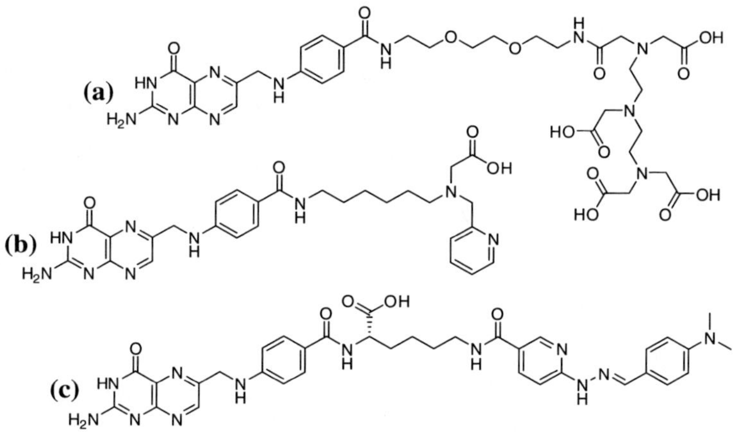

Fig. 2 Pteroic acid derivatives for labeling with ^{111}In (**a**) and ^{99m}Tc (**b**, **c**) (Ke et al. 2005; Guo et al. 2011; Müller et al. 2004)

nanomolar range again. Figure 2 shows three radiolabeled examples that were developed for SPECT imaging with ^{111}In and ^{99m}Tc and which exhibited promising results (Ke et al. 2005; Guo et al. 2011; Müller et al. 2004).

A range of ^{18}F-fluorinated FA derivatives show a tendency for improved in vivo behavior correlated to higher hydrophilicity of the substance (Ross et al. 2008). Therefore, polarity seems to be a critical property for the design of an ideal imaging agent for FR. To combine facilitated synthesis with the benefits of positron emission tomography (PET) as well as the good availability of a generator-based nuclide, we aim to develop ^{68}Ga-labeled pteroic acid-based agents. As the lack of glutamic acid decreases the hydrophilicity of the compound, it is unclear to date whether the introduction of the chelator (DOTA) would be sufficient to compensate the lost polarity. To investigate this systematically, a range of different spacers between the pteroic acid and the chelator are necessary—herein we report synthesis and preliminary in vitro evaluation of the first derivative, which is based on an ethyl spacer and will be used as reference for further compounds.

2 Results and Discussion

2.1 Synthesis

The synthetic route to the desired compound can be seen in Figs. 3 and 4. As FA is known to be sensitive to light and air and shows very poor solubility, we decided to introduce pteroic acid as late as possible into the molecule. The synthesis of an amine-bearing chelator **6** in five steps started with the Cbz protection of 2-aminoethanol and its subsequent bromination under Appel conditions. As the coupling to tris(*tert*-Bu)DO3A displayed severe problems regarding purification, compound **3** was connected to 1,4,7,10-tetraazacyclododecane (cyclene) according to Duimstra et al. (2005), yielding the monosubstituted derivative **4** exclusively, because no base was added to the reaction mixture. This was followed by introduction of *tert*-Bu-acetate side-chains to obtain a potent chelator for $^{68}Ga^{3+}$. The Cbz protecting group allows orthogonal deprotection by means of hydrogenation to yield tris(*tert*-Bu)DO3A-EA **6** as a protected chelator that can be coupled to target molecules that carry an acid function. Tris(*tert*-Bu)DO3A-EA **6** was successfully coupled to protected pteroic acid. Therefore, a novel peptide-coupling reagent, (1-cyano-2-ethoxy-2-oxoethylidenaminooxy)dimethylamino-morpholino-carbenium hexafluorophosphate (COMU), was used under typical conditions but the extractive standard workup had to be replaced by removal of the solvent and subsequent column chromatography of the residue. For deprotection we anticipated the need of two separate steps: one under acidic conditions to remove the *tert*-butyl ester groups from the chelator and a second one under basic conditions to remove the formyl- and dimethyl-aminomethylene groups at the pteroic acid. Interestingly, after incubation of compound **7** for 24 h in 1 M NaOH at 45°C, not only the formyl- and dimethylamino-methylene groups as expected, but also the *tert*-butyl esters, were already cleaved. The labeling precursor **8** could therefore be obtained in seven steps and overall yield of 8.3%.

2.2 Radiolabeling and In Vitro Studies

The eluate from a $^{68}Ge/^{68}Ga$ generator was purified via the cation exchange resin-based process (Zhernosekov et al. 2007) prior to use. A stock solution of the precursor in ethanol was prepared (0.5 mg/ml). Labeling was performed in 400 μl HEPES buffer (0.13 M) under conventional heating as well as under microwave support. Conventional heating was performed at 95°C, and different amounts of precursor (10, 20, 30 nmol, respectively) were investigated. The obtained results are shown in Fig. 5. Best results were obtained with 30 nmol after 10 min, yielding 75% radiochemical yield. Under microwave support the same results could be obtained, but only 10 nmol precursor was necessary and the reaction time could be considerably reduced to only 3 min.

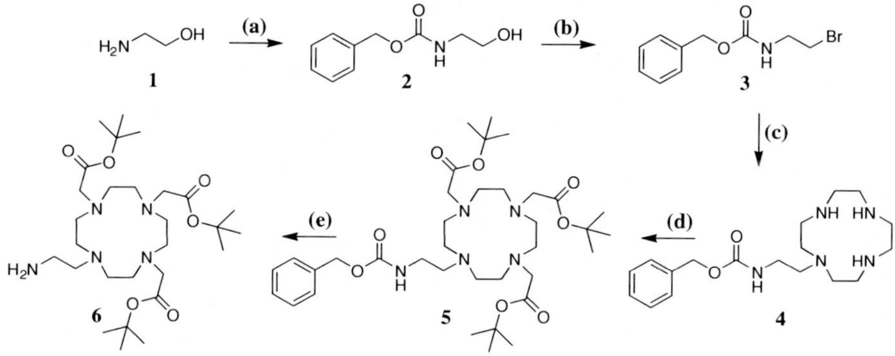

Fig. 3 Five-step synthesis of tris(*tert*-Bu)DO3A-EA. **a** H_2O, Na_2CO_3, Cbz-Cl, 0°C, 2 h; **b** THF, CBr_4, PPh_3, 0°C—rt, 2.5 h; **c** toluene, cyclene, reflux, overnight; **d** MeCN, α-bromo-*tert*-butyl acetate, Na_2CO_3, reflux, 24 h; **e** MeOH/TEA, H_2/Pd, rt, 6 h

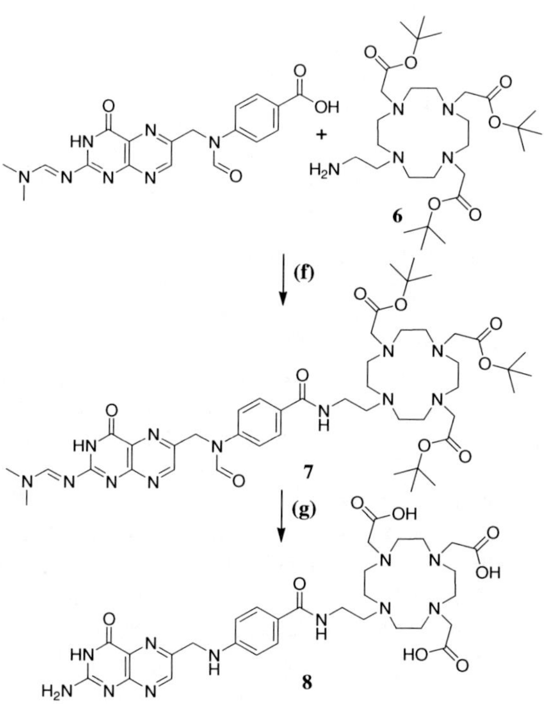

Fig. 4 Coupling and deprotection. **f** DMF, COMU, DIPEA, 0°C—rt, 3 h; **g** 1 M NaOH, 45°C, 24 h

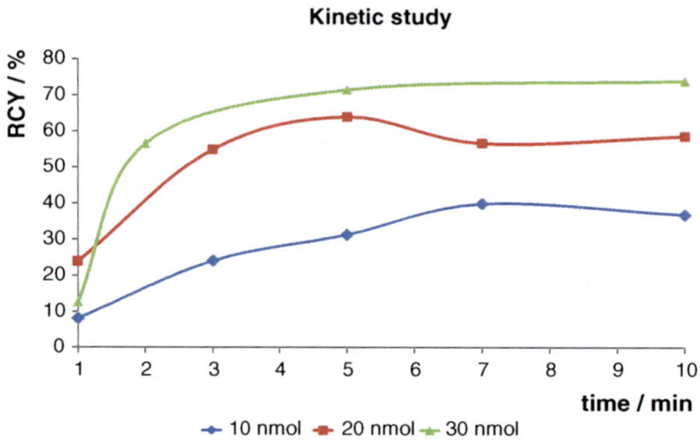

Fig. 5 Kinetic study. Labeling in HEPES (0.13 M) buffer at 95°C

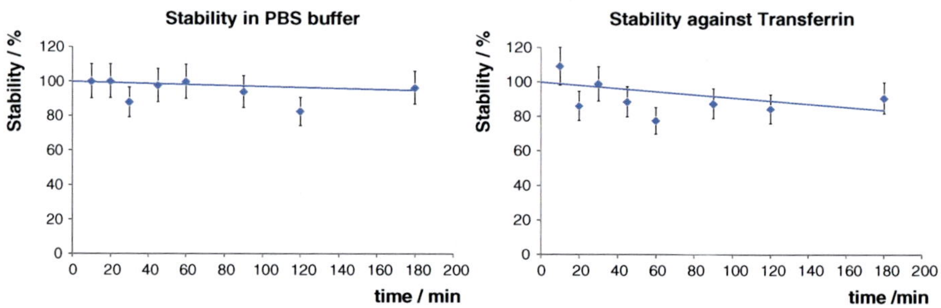

Fig. 6 Stability studies in PBS buffer and against transferrin at 37°C

For any in vivo application of a tracer, in vivo stability is essential. Therefore, we examined the complex's stability in PBS buffer as well as its behavior upon incubation with excessive transferrin. The results obtained were very promising, as in both cases no relevant degradation or transchelation could be detected for up to 3 h (Fig. 6).

Finally, the lipophilicity of the new tracer was determined by 1-octanol/PBS extraction. The organic phase was re-extracted twice, and the values of the first extraction were discarded. The obtained log*D* value of -0.1 ± 0.1 hints that the introduction of DOTA already adds reasonable values of polarity to the molecule, which is necessary for favorable in vivo behavior. It will be proven in in vivo experiments (μPET imaging) whether this is already enough or still needs to be improved.

3 Conclusion

To develop a pteroic acid-based PET tracer, synthesis of 2,2′,2″(10-(2-(4-((2-amino-4-oxo-3,4-dihydropteridin-6-yl)methylamino)benzamido)ethyl)-1,4,7,10-tetraazacyclododecane-1,4,7-triyl)triacetic acid **8** could successfully be achieved in seven steps. The conditions for labeling with ^{68}Ga have been investigated—good radiochemical yields can be achieved in 0.13 M HEPES buffer at 95°C for 10 min using 30 nmol of compound **8** or under microwave support with only 10 nmol precursor in only 3 min at 300 W. The ^{68}Ga complex is stable in PBS buffer as well as in the presence of excessive transferrin for at least 3 h. The log*D* value of -0.1 ± 0.1 for our novel tracer is in a range that allows favorable in vivo characteristics for PET imaging of FR to be assumed. After determining the affinity of our new ^{68}Ga radiotracer(s) to FR using human KB cells, they will be subject to further studies using in vivo μPET imaging.

4 Experimental

4.1 Benzyl-*N*-(2-hydroxyethyl)carbamate

To a cooled solution of 1.5 g (24.5 mmol) 2-aminoethanol in 15 ml water, 12.5 ml Na_2CO_3 (2 N) was added alternately with 3.5 ml benzylchloroformate (24.5 mmol) within 40 min. The mixture was allowed to stir for further 80 min at 0°C and was then extracted with ethyl acetate. After washing the organic phase with water, saturated $NaHCO_3$ solution, and brine, it was dried over Na_2SO_4. The solvent was evaporated to give the product as 3.45 g (17.7 mmol, 72%) of white crystals. ^{1}H-NMR (300 MHz, $CDCl_3$), δ [ppm] = 2.39 (1H, s, br, –O*H*), 3.32 (2H, m –NCH_2), 3.68 (2H, t, $J = 5.06$ Hz, –CH_2OH), 5.08 (2H, s, –CH_2–C6H5), 5.22 (1H, s, br, N*H*), 7.35–7.28 (5H, m, –CH_2–C_6H_5).

4.2 *N*-Benzyloxycarbonyl-2-bromoethylamine

A solution of 8.49 g (25.6 mmol) CBr_4 in 60 ml dry THF was added dropwise to a chilled solution of 6.71 g (25.6 mmol) PPh_3 in 50 ml THF and was allowed to stir for further 15 min. Then, a solution of 2.5 g (12.8 mmol) benzyl-*N*-(2-hydroxyethyl)carbamate in 100 ml dry THF was added, and after removal of the ice bath, the mixture was stirred at rt for 2 h. The precipitate was filtered and washed with ethyl acetate. The filtrate was washed with brine and dried with Na_2SO_4, and the solvent was evaporated in vacuo to yield the crude product. After column chromatography [SiO_2, petroleum ether/ethyl acetate (3:1)], 2.29 g (8.9 mmol, 70%) of the desired product was obtained as a white solid. ^{1}H-NMR (300 MHz, $CDCl_3$), δ [ppm] = 3.45 (2H, t, $J = 5.82$ Hz, –CH_2Br), 3.59 (2H, m, –NCH_2), 5.09 (2H, s, –CH_2–C_6H_5), 5.18 (1H, s, br, N*H*), 7.30–7.36 (5H, m, –C_6H_5). MS (FD) *m/z* (% rel. int.): 257.12 (100.00), 259.19 ($[M + H]^+$, 97.73); calculated: 258.12.

4.3 1-(*N*-Benzyloxycarbonyl-ethylamine)-1,4,7,10-tetraazacyclododecane

667 mg (3.87 mmol) 1,4,7,10-tetraazacyclododecane and 400 mg (1.55 mmol) *N*-benzyloxycarbonyl-2-bromoethylamine in 65 ml dry toluene were refluxed overnight. The reaction mixture was extracted twice with water; the aqueous phase was subsequently re-extracted with dichloromethane. The organic phase was dried over Na_2SO_4, and the solvent was removed under reduced pressure to obtain 500 mg (1.43 mmol, 92%) of a colourless oil. ^{1}H-NMR (300 MHz, $CDCl_3$), δ [ppm] = 2.34–2.78 (18H, m, br, cyclene + N–CH_2CH_2NHCbz), 3.23 (2H, m, N–CH_2CH_2 NHCbz), 5.03 (2H, s, C_6H_5–CH_2–OCONH–), 7.25–7.32 (5H, m, C_6H_5–). ^{13}C-NMR (75 MHz, $CDCl_3$), δ [ppm] = 166.22 (C=O), 128.52 (C_{ar}), 128.13 (C_{ar}), 127.35 (C_{ar}), 126.90 (C_{ar}), 87.72 (C_6H_5–CH_2–), 66.46 (Cbz–CH_2–), 55.11 (–CH_2–N_{ring}), 51.56 (–$C_{ring}H_2$–), 47.47 (–$C_{ring}H_2$–), 46.23 (–$C_{ring}H_2$–), 45.82 (–$C_{ring}H_2$–). MS (FD) *m/z* (% rel. int.): 350.42 ([M + H]$^+$, 100.00), 699.81 ([dimer + H]$^+$, 24.41); calculated: 349.48.

4.4 1-(*N*-Benzyloxycarbonyl-ethylamine)-4,7,10-tris(*tert*-butyl-acetate)-1,4,7,10-tetraaza-cyclododecane

51 mg (0.15 mmol) 1-(*N*-benzyloxycarbonyl-ethylamine)-1,4,7,10-tetraazacyclododecane, 155 mg (1.45 mmol) Na_2CO_3, and 142 mg (0.72 mmol) α-bromo-*tert*-butyl acetate were refluxed in 20 ml acetonitrile for 24 h. After filtration the solvent was removed in vacuo and the crude product was purified via column chromatography [SiO_2, dichloromethane/methanol (5:1)] to obtain 98 mg (0.14 mmol, 93%) of a light-yellow oil. ^{1}H-NMR (300 MHz, $CDCl_3$), δ [ppm] = 1.36 (27H, s, tris(C(CH_3)), 2.11–3.44 26H, m, br, ring + Cbz–NH–(CH_2)$_2$–), 4.94 (2H, s, C_6H_5–CH_2–OCONH–), 7.18–7.32 (5H, m, –C_6H_5). ^{13}C–NMR (75 MHz, $CDCl_3$), δ [ppm] = 172.73 (C=O (*tert*-Bu)), 166.22 (C=O (Cbz)), 128.39 (C_{ar}), 127.98 (C_{ar}), 127.90 (C_{ar}), 87.72 (C_6H_5–CH_2–), 82.86 (–CH_2–COO–*tert*–Bu), 82.27 (–CH_2–COO–*tert*–Bu), 66.56 (Cbz–NH–CH_2–), 56.47 (–CH_2–N_{ring}), 55.68 (–$C_{ring}H_2$–), 54.05 (–$C_{ring}H_2$–), 50.37 (–$C_{ring}H_2$–), 27.94 (–C(CH_3)$_3$), 27.84 (–C(CH_3)$_3$). MS (FD) *m/z* (% rel. int.): 692.95 ([M + H]$^+$, 16.68), 714.96 ([M + Na]$^+$, 100.00); calculated: 691.92.

4.5 1-(Aminoethyl)-4,7,10-tris(*tert*-butyl-acetate)-1,4,7,10-tetraazacyclododecane

20 mg (0.03 mmol) 1-(*N*-benzyloxycarbonyl-ethylamine)-4,7,10-tris(*tert*-butyl-acetate)-1,4,7,10-tetraazacyclododecane was dissolved in 5 ml dry methanol/triethylamine (3:1), and 1 mg Pd/C (10%) was added. Hydrogen was passed through the solution for 6 h, then the solvent was removed and the residue purified by column chromatography [SiO_2, dichloromethane/methanol (5:1)] to obtain 12 mg

(0.022 mmol, 73%) as a colorless oil. ^{1}H-NMR (300 MHz, $CDCl_3$), δ [ppm] = 1.41 (27H, s, tris-($C(CH_3)_3$)), 2.03–3.33 (26H, m, br, ring + $-(CH_2)_2-NH_2$ + tris($-CH_2-COOC(CH_3)_3$)). MS (FD) *m/z* (% rel. int.): 558.79 ($[M + H]^+$, 100.00); calculated: 557.78.

4.6 *tert*-Butyl 2,2′,2″-(10-(2-(4-(*N*-((2-((dimethylamino) methyleneamino)-4-oxo-3,4-dihydropteridin-6-yl) methyl)formamido)benzamido)ethyl)-1,4,7,10-tetraazacyclododecane-1,4,7-triyl)triacetate

20 mg (0.055 mmol) protected pteroic acid was dissolved in 3 mL DMF and cooled to 0°C. Then, 13.9 μl (0.083 mmol) diisopropylethylamine, 24 mg (0.055 mmol) COMU (dissolved in 3 ml DMF), and 31 mg (0.055 mmol) 1-(aminoethyl)-4,7,10-tris(*tert*-butyl-acetate)-1,4,7,10-tetraazacyclododecane (dissolved in 3 ml DMF) were added successively. Ice-cooling was removed after 5 min, and the mixture was stirred for 2.5 h at rt. The solvent was removed under reduced pressure and the residue purified via column chromatography [SiO_2, dichloromethane/methanol (20:1 → 5:1)] to obtain 10.9 mg (0.012 mmol, 21%) as a yellow oil. ^{1}H-NMR (300 MHz, MeOH-d_4), δ [ppm] = 1.31–1.56 (39H, m, tris(*tert*-Bu) + tris(CH_2COO–*tert*–Bu) + $-N(CH_3)_2$), 2.25–3.71 (20H, m, cyclene + spacer), 5.36 (2H, s, pteridine–CH_2–N–), 7.52 (2H, d, J = 8.46 Hz, phenyl), 7.92 (2H, d, J = 8.46 Hz, phenyl), 8.77 (1H, s, pteridine-*H*), 8,80 (1H, s $(CH_3)_2$ N–*CH*=N–), 8.84 (1H, s, br, formyl-*H*). ^{13}C–NMR (75 MHz, MeOH-d_4), δ [ppm] = 28.35, 28.38, 35.58, 37.55, 39.46, 39.99, 41.76, 56.54, 56.91, 57.62, 83.17, 83.23, 123.80, 130.27, 133.81, 144.76, 150.30, 150.52, 155.44, 156.65, 156.86, 160.93, 164.45, 169.50, 174.47, 174.59. MS (ESI) *m/z* (% rel. int.): 957.55 ($[M + Na]^+$, 100.00), 958.58 (56.70), 959.59 (6.19); calculated: 935.15.

4.7 2,2′,2″(10-(2-(4-((2-Amino-4-oxo-3,4-dihydropteridin-6-yl) methylamino)benzamido)ethyl)-1,4,7,10-tetraazacyclododecane-1,4,7-triyl)triacetic acid

3 mg (3.2 μmol) of 1-(*N2-N,N*-dimethylaminomethylene-10-formyl-pteroic acid-ethylamide)-4,7,10-tris(*tert*-butylacetate)-1,4,7,10-tetraazacyclododecane was heated to 45°C in 3 ml 1 M NaOH for 24 h. Afterwards, the product could be precipitated with 3 M HCl. The suspension was centrifuged for 5 min at 10,000 rpm, the supernatant was discarded, and the pellet was washed with 30 μl water. The centrifugation process was repeated, and the pellet was dried in vacuo to obtain 2.3 mg (3.19 μmol, 99% → calculated as hydrochloride) of yellow solid. ^{1}H-NMR (400 MHz, DMSO-d_6), δ [ppm] = 2.79–3.49 (m, br, spacer + chelator), 4.49 (2H, s, pteridine–CH_2–N–), 6.63 (2H, d, J = 8.80 Hz, phenyl), 7.65 (2H, d, J = 8.80 Hz, phenyl), 8.65 (1H, s, pteridine-*H*). MS (ESI) *m/z* (% rel. int.): 684.36 ($[M]^+$, 100.00); calculated: 683.72 (mass spectrum was obtained under addition of formic acid).

4.8 Radiolabeling

10, 20 or 30 nmol (from stock solution of 0.5 mg/ml ethanol) of precursor **8** was added to 400 μl HEPES buffer [277 mg 4-(2-hydroxyethyl)piperazine-1-ethane-sulfonic acid sodium salt in 8 ml 0.1 M HCl]. The generator eluate was post-processed using a cation exchange resin as described in the literature (Zhernosekov et al. 2007). Purified eluate (400 μl) was added to the reaction mixture and either heated for ten minutes at 95°C or processed with microwave heating. The microwave settings were 300 W, 120°C maximum temperature, constant cooling, 1 min ramp followed by 2 min hold. Radiochemical yields were determined by radioTLC [silica gel, sodium citrate buffer (0.1 M, pH 4.0)] and analyzed with an Instant Imager (Canberra Packard).

4.9 Stability Studies

Four vials of 1 ml PBS buffer were tempered at 37°C before addition of the radiotracer. For the transferrin study, a solution of 3 mg/ml PBS was prepared and equally distributed and tempered at 37°C. As control, free ^{68}Ga from the generator eluate was added to an extra vial containing PBS/PBS + transferrin. Samples were taken at 10, 20, 30, 45, 60, 90, 120, and 180 min and analyzed by the above-mentioned TLC system.

4.10 Lipophilicity Assay

For the determination of the log*D* value the radiotracer was extracted with 1-octanol and PBS buffer ($n = 4$). For each extraction, 700 μl of each phase was used, and the vials were shaken at 1,500 rpm on a heating thermoMixer (MHR13, Ditabis, Germany) and centrifuged afterwards for 2 min at 12,000 rpm to resep-arate the phases. Three microliters of each phase was spotted on absorptive paper, and the activity was quantified with the Instant Imager, while 400 μl of the 1-octanol phase was used for further re-extraction under the same conditions. This was repeated twice, and only the values obtained from the last two extractions were included in the calculation.

Acknowledgments We gratefully thank Merck and Cie, Schaffhausen, Switzerland for providing us with the protected pteroic acid.

References

Antony AC (1992) The biological chemistry of folate receptors. Blood 79:2807–2820

Duimstra JA, Femia FJ, Meade TJ (2005) A gadolinium chelate for detection of β-glucuronidase: a self-immolative approach. J Am Chem Soc 127:12847–12855

Guo H, Xie F, Zhu M et al (2011) The synthesis of pteroyl-lys conjugates and its application as technetium-99m labeled radiotracer for folate receptor-positive tumor targeting. Bioorg Med Chem Lett 21:2025–2029

Kamen BA, Capdevila A (1986) Receptor-mediated folate accumulation is regulated by the cellular folate content. Proc Natl Acad Sci USA 83:5983–5987

Ke C-Y, Mathias CJ, Green MA (2005) Targeting the tumor-associated folate receptor with an ^{111}In–DTPA conjugate of pteroic acid. J Am Chem Soc 127:7421–7426

Leamon CP, Low PS (2001) Folate-mediated targeting: from diagnostics to drug and gene delivery. Drug Discov Today 6:44–51

Leamon CP, Parker MA, Vlahov IR et al (2002) Synthesis and biological evaluation of EC20: a new folate-derived, ^{99m}Tc-based radiopharmaceutical. Bioconjugate Chem 13:1200–1210

Leamon C, You F, Santhapuram H et al (2009) Properties influencing the relative binding affinity of pteroate derivatives and drug conjugates thereof to the folate receptor. Pharm Res 26:1315–1323

Mathias CJ, Wang S, Waters DJ et al (1998) Indium-111-DTPA-folate as a potential folate receptor-targeted radiopharmaceutical. J Nucl Med 39:1579–1585

Müller C, Dumas C, Hoffmann U et al (2004) Organometallic ^{99m}Tc-technetium(I)- and Re-rhenium(I)-folate derivatives for potential use in nuclear medicine. J Organomet Chem 689:4712–4721

Ross JF, Chaudhuri PK, Ratnam M (1994) Differential regulation of folate receptor isoforms in normal and malignant tissues in vivo and in established cell lines. Physiologic and clinical implications. Cancer 73:2432–2443

Ross TL, Honer M, Lam PYH et al (2008) Fluorine-18 click radiosynthesis and preclinical evaluation of a new 18F-labeled folic acid derivative. Bioconjugate Chem 19:2462–2470

Toffoli G, Cernigoi C, Russo A et al (1997) Overexpression of folate binding protein in ovarian cancers. Int J Cancer 74:193–198

Weitman SD, Weinberg AG, Coney LR et al (1992) Cellular localization of the folate receptor: potential role in drug toxicity and folate homeostasis. Cancer Res 52:6708–6711

Zhernosekov KP, Filosofov DV, Baum RP et al (2007) Processing of generator-produced ^{68}Ga for medical application. J Nucl Med 48:1741–1748

Measurement of Protein Synthesis: In Vitro Comparison of ^{68}Ga-DOTA-Puromycin, [^{3}H]Tyrosine, and 2-Fluoro-[^{3}H]tyrosine

Sebastian Eigner, Denis R. Beckford Vera, Marco Fellner, Natalia S. Loktionova, Markus Piel, Frantisek Melichar, Frank Rösch, Tobias L. Roß, Ondrej Lebeda and Katerina Eigner Henke

Abstract

Aim: Puromycin has played an important role in our understanding of the eukaryotic ribosome and protein synthesis. It has been known for more than 40 years that this antibiotic is a universal protein synthesis inhibitor that acts as a structural analog of an aminoacyl-transfer RNA (aa-tRNA) in eukaryotic ribosomes. Due to the role of enzymes and their synthesis in situations of need (DNA damage, e.g., after chemo- or radiation therapy), determination of protein synthesis is important for control of antitumor therapy, to enhance long-term survival of tumor patients, and to minimize side-effects of therapy. Multiple attempts to reach this goal have been made through the last decades, mostly using radiolabeled amino acids, with limited or unsatisfactory success. The aim of this study is to estimate the possibility of determining protein synthesis ratios by using ^{68}Ga-DOTA-puromycin (^{68}Ga-DOTA-Pur), [^{3}H]tyrosine, and 2-fluoro-[^{3}H]tyrosine and to estimate the possibility of different pathways due to the fluorination of tyrosine. *Methods*: DOTA-puromycin was synthesized using a puromycin-tethered controlled-pore glass (CPG) support by the usual protocol for automated DNA and RNA synthesis following our design. ^{68}Ga was obtained from a ^{68}Ge/^{68}Ga generator as described previously by Zhernosekov et al. (J Nucl Med 48:1741–1748, 2007). The purified eluate was used for labeling of DOTA-puromycin at 95°C for 20 min. [^{3}H]Tyrosine

S. Eigner (✉) · D. R. Beckford Vera · F. Melichar · O. Lebeda · K. E. Henke
Department of Radiopharmaceuticals, Nuclear Physics Institute,
Academic of Sciences of the Czech Republic, Rez, Czech Republic
e-mail: eigner@ujf.cas.cz

M. Fellner · N. S. Loktionova · M. Piel · F. Rösch · T. L. Roß
Institute for Nuclear Chemistry, Johannes Gutenberg-University Mainz,
Mainz, Germany

R. P. Baum and F. Rösch (eds.), *Theranostics, Gallium-68, and Other Radionuclides*,
Recent Results in Cancer Research 194, DOI: 10.1007/978-3-642-27994-2_14,

and 2-fluoro-[^{3}H]tyrosine of the highest purity available were purchased from Moravek (Bera, USA) or Amersham Biosciences (Hammersmith, UK). In vitro uptake and protein incorporation as well as in vitro inhibition experiments using cycloheximide to inhibit protein synthesis were carried out for all three substances in DU145 prostate carcinoma cells (ATCC, USA). ^{68}Ga-DOTA-Pur was additionally used for μPET imaging of Walker carcinomas and AT1 tumors in rats. Dynamic scans were performed for 45 min after IV application (tail vein) of 20–25 MBq ^{68}Ga-DOTA-Pur. *Results*: No significant differences in the behavior of [^{3}H]tyrosine and 2-fluoro-[^{3}H]tyrosine were observed. Uptake of both tyrosine derivatives was decreased by inhibition of protein synthesis, but only to a level of 45–55% of initial uptake, indicating no direct link between tyrosine uptake and protein synthesis. In contrast, ^{68}Ga-DOTA-Pur uptake was directly linked to ribosomal activity and, therefore, to protein synthesis. ^{68}Ga-DOTA-Pur μPET imaging in rats revealed high tumor-to-background ratios and clearly defined regions of interest in the investigated tumors. *Summary*: Whereas the metabolic pathway of ^{68}Ga-DOTA-Pur is directly connected with the process of protein synthesis and shows high tumor uptake during μPET imaging, neither [^{3}H]tyrosine nor 2-fluoro-[^{3}H]tyrosine can be considered useful for determination of protein synthesis. *Research Support*: This work has been supported by the Ministry of Education, Youth, and Sports of the Czech Republic and The Grant Agency of the Czech Republic.

Contents

1 Introduction

Due to the role of DNA damage-repair enzymes and their synthesis in situations of need (DNA damage, e.g., after chemo- or radiation therapy), determination of protein synthesis is important for control of antitumor therapy, to enhance long-term survival of tumor patients, and to minimize side-effects of therapy. Multiple attempts to reach this goal have been made through the last decades, mostly using radiolabeled amino acids.

Many amino acids have been radiolabeled to study their potential imaging characteristics. These radiolabeled amino acids differ in ease of synthesis, biodistribution, and formation of metabolites in vivo. To date, the most frequently used amino acid tracers are [^{11}C-methyl]-L-methionine (MET) for PET and 3-[^{123}I]iodo-α-methyl-L-tyrosine (IMT) for SPECT (Jager et al. 2001). Due to the short physical half-life of the ^{11}C label (20.38 min), MET PET remains restricted to a few PET centers with a cyclotron on site and could not be established in routine clinical practice despite convincing clinical results. IMT SPECT offers more widespread application (Langen et al. 2002), but the spatial resolution of SPECT is considerably lower than that of PET and does not allow for quantification. Therefore, a number of attempts have been undertaken to label amino acids with ^{18}F (109.7 min half-life), but the yield of the radiosynthesis of these ^{18}F-labeled amino acids was rather ineffective (Coenen 1993; Laverman et al. 2002). *O*-(2-[^{18}F]fluoroethyl)-L-tyrosine (FET) (Fig. 1) is one of the first ^{18}F-labeled amino acids that can be produced in large amounts for clinical purposes and is applicable for PET studies in a satellite concept similar to the widely used FDG (Wester et al. 1999; Hamacher and Coenen 2002).

Despite all efforts, the success of utilizing radiolabeled amino acids to measure protein synthesis in vivo is still limited or unsatisfactory. The difficulties in utilizing radiolabeled amino acids for in vivo determination of protein synthesis are due to the wide variety of possible metabolic pathways of amino acids (Haubner 2010).

Puromycin has played an important role in our understanding of the eukaryotic ribosome and protein synthesis. It has been known for more than 40 years that this antibiotic is a universal protein synthesis inhibitor that acts as a structural analog of an aminoacyl-tRNA (aa-tRNA) (Yarmolinsky and Haba 1959) in eukaryotic ribosomes (Fig. 2). Nathans (1964) demonstrated that the eukaryotic ribosome mistakenly inserts puromycin in place of aa-tRNA, resulting in truncated proteins containing the drug at their C-termini. In a later examination of this mechanism, Miyamoto-Sato et al. (2000) concluded that puromycin inhibits translation solely through C-terminal labeling of peptides and not through additional pathways. This classic model for puromycin action admits only a single mode of action, i.e., covalent attachment to the nascent peptide chain (Starck and Roberts 2002).

Puromycin–deoxycytidine conjugates (puromycin–dC conjugates) labeled with biotin have been utilized by molecular biologists to determine in vivo protein synthesis during the last years (Miyamoto-Sato et al. 2000; Starck and Roberts 2002;

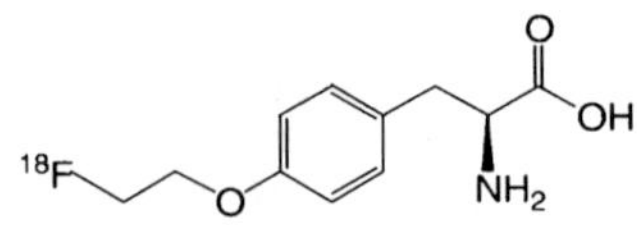

Fig. 1 (2-[^{18}F]fluoroethyl)-L-tyrosine

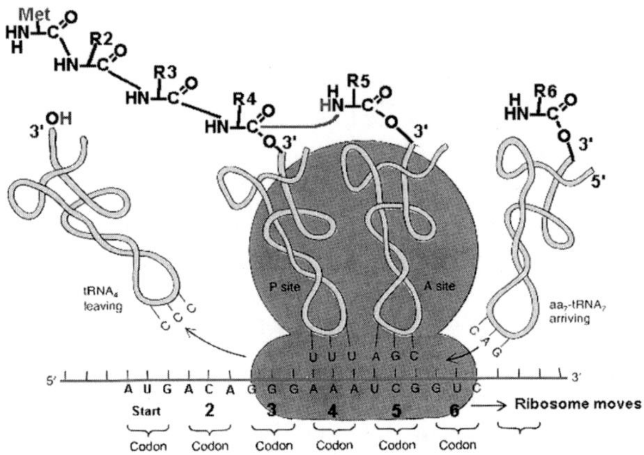

Fig. 2 Active ribosomal complex; modified from Griffiths et al. (1996)

Nemoto et al. 1999). Their metabolism has been proven to be only involved in protein synthesis mimicking aa-tRNA. We decided to replace biotin, which is used as fluorescent dye for detection, with the chelator 1,4,7,10-tetraazacyclododecane-1,4,7,10-tetraacetic acid (DOTA) (Fig. 3). Both molecules, biotin and DOTA, are inserted to the puromycin precursors as activated *N*-hydroxysuccinimide (NHS) esters. In this context, positron-emitting radio metals such as ^{68}Ga can be used for labeling.

Consequently, the purpose of this study is to investigate whether ^{68}Ga-labeled puromycin-based DOTA conjugates can be utilized for imaging of protein synthesis in vivo and to demonstrate the differences between natural amino acids and their fluorinated analogs in metabolic pathways involved in protein synthesis utilizing [^{3}H]tyrosine (representing natural amino acids) and 2-fluoro-[^{3}H]tyrosine as its fluorinated analog.

2 Methods

2.1 Equipment and Reagents

DOTA-Pur (Fig. 1) was purchased from Purimex (Grebenstein, Germany). [^{3}H]tyrosine and 2-fluoro-[^{3}H]tyrosine of the highest purity available were purchased from Moravek (Bera, USA) or Amersham Biosciences (Hammersmith,

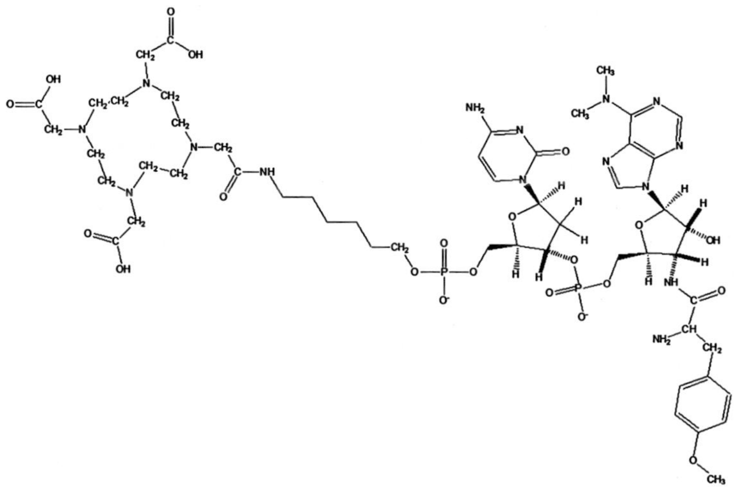

Fig. 3 DOTA-NHC$_6$-dC-puromycin: DOTA-NHC$_6$-deoxycytidine-puromycin was produced at Purimex (Grebenstein, Germany), analogous to the biotin derivatives developed by Starck and Roberts (2002) (puromycin-2P)

UK). Chelex 100 in sodium form and human serum albumin (HSA) were purchased from Sigma (Steinheim, Germany). All other reagents were purchased from Merck (Darmstadt, Germany) or Fluka (Steinheim, Germany) with the highest purity available. Ultrapure water (Aquatec Water Systems, Inc., CA, USA) was used for all procedures. To avoid metal contamination, all solutions used in conjugation and radiolabeling reactions were passed through a Chelex 100 column (1 × 10 cm). All glassware was washed with 2 M HCl and ultrapure water.

2.2 ^{68}Ga Production

^{68}Ga was produced from a commercially available 1 110-MBq ^{68}Ge-^{68}Ga generator based on a TiO_2 phase adsorbing $^{68}Ge^{4+}$ (Cyclotron Co. Ltd., Russia). Generator-eluted ^{68}Ga is preconcentrated and purified using miniaturized column with organic cation exchanger. The method used for separation of ^{68}Ga from ^{68}Ge is the most effective method to eliminate ^{68}Ge breakthrough and the generator column material contaminants from the product, and was developed by Zhernosekov et al. (2007) and published previously.

2.3 Synthesis of DOTA-NHC$_6$-dC-Puromycin (DOTA-Pur)

DOTA-Pur was synthesized using a puromycin-tethered CPG support by the usual protocol for automated DNA and RNA synthesis [phosphoramidite method (Starck and Roberts 2002)] following our design by Purimex (Grebenstein, Germany).

2.4 ^{68}Ga-Labeling of DOTA-Pur

DOTA-Pur (50 μl) in H_2O (1.11 nmol/μl) was added to 30 MBq ^{68}Ga in 100 μl 0.2 M HCl and incubated in a heating block at 90°C for 20 min while shaking. The reaction mixture was purified on a reversed-phase C-18 cartridge (Strata-X 33 μm Polymeric Sorbent, 60 mg/mL; Phenomenex, Inc., USA). After transfer to the cartridge, the product was washed with 2 mL H_2O. ^{68}Ga-DOTA-Pur was eluted from the resin in 300 μl ethanol. The ethanol was then evaporated and the product dissolved in 0.9% saline to a final volume activity of 30 MBq/ml.

2.5 In Vitro Studies

All described in vitro studies were carried out in DU145 (HTB-81™, human prostate carcinoma) and BJ (CRL-2522™, human foreskin fibroblasts) cells. Cells were purchased between 2 and 4 months before conducting the experiments. Cells are commercially available at LGC/ATCC, Lomianki, Poland.

2.6 In Vitro Uptake and Protein Incorporation

DU145 cells were routinely cultivated in standardized supplemented full media [RPMI1640 + 10% fetal calf serum (FCS) +1% penicillin/streptomycin (PAA, Czech Republic)] at 37°C in a humidified atmosphere containing 5% CO_2. Cell preparation for the experiments was carried out 48 h beforehand, seeding 2×10^5 living cells per well in 6-well plates (Becton, Dickinson and Company, USA) using 2 mL normal media. Therefore, cells were harvested by trypsinization, and the number of living cells was determined utilizing a CASY TT cell analyzing system (Innovatis, Reutlingen, Germany). During the experiments, the number of living cells was counted for each measurement using CASY TT. All data were normalized to 1×10^6 living cells.

Total cellular uptake was measured after incubation of the cells with 84 pmol of tracer (^{68}Ga-DOTA-Pur, [^{3}H]tyrosine, or 2-fluoro-[^{3}H]tyrosine) per well for 2 h. Incubation was stopped by discarding the treatment media and washing the cells twice with ice-cold PBS. In the next step, cells were dissolved in 500 μl lysis buffer [10% NaOH + 5% sodium dodecyl sulfate (SDS)], and the total sample activity was measured in a fully automated gamma counter (2,470 Wizard; Perkin Elmer, USA). For measuring protein incorporation, proteins were then precipitated and isolated by addition of trichloroacetic acid (TCA) to final concentration $\geq$10%. After centrifugation, the supernatant was removed and the precipitate washed twice with TCA solution. Activity contained in the acid solution and protein pellet were determined in the automated gamma counter. Results were calculated using GraphPad Prism software (GraphPad Software, Inc., CA, USA).

2.7 Inhibition of ^{68}Ga-DOTA-Pur, [^{3}H]Tyrosine, and 2-Fluoro-[^{3}H]tyrosine Incorporation into Proteins

Experiments using 3-[2-(3,5-dimethyl-2-oxocyclohexyl)-2-hydroxyethyl] glutarimide (cycloheximide) (Fluka, Steinheim, Germany) as noncompetitive inhibitor of protein synthesis were carried out in 6-well plates (Becton, Dickinson and Company, USA) with 2 × 10^5 cells/well inhibitor. Cycloheximide exerts its effect by interfering with the translocation step in protein synthesis (movement of two tRNA molecules and mRNA in relation to the ribosome), thus blocking translational elongation.

DU145 and BJ cells were treated simultaneously with 84 pmol/well tracer (^{68}Ga-DOTA-Pur, [^{3}H]tyrosine, or 2-fluoro-[^{3}H]tyrosine) and inhibitor (cycloheximide) concentrations between 10 pmol/well and 20 nmol/well. Cells were incubated for 1 h, and total cellular uptake and protein incorporation were measured as described above. Results were calculated as response in percent of noncompeting uptake and plotted semilogarithmically against inhibitor concentration using GraphPad Prism software (GraphPad Software, Inc., CA, USA).

2.7.1 ^{68}Ga-DOTA-Pur μPET Imaging in Tumor-Bearing Rats

All used cell lines and animals were provided by the Institute of Physiology, Johannes Gutenberg-University Mainz, Germany. Rat cell lines AT1 (subline of Dunning R3327 rat prostate carcinoma) and Walker carcinoma 256 (subcutaneous solid tumor) were used in all experiments. AT1 cells were grown in RPMI medium supplemented with 10% FCS and Walker cells in DMEM (Gibco No. 430–1,600; Gibco, Darmstadt, Germany) containing 5% FCS, 2.5 μg/mL amphoterin B, 50 μg/mL kanamycin, 100 μg/mL streptomycin, and 100 U/mL penicillin at 37°C under a humidified 5% CO_2 atmosphere. Medium was changed routinely every 2 days, and passages were done once a week.

For tumor implantation with AT1 cells and Walker cells, male Copenhagen rats (Charles River Wiga, Sulzfeld, Germany; body weight 150–200 g) and male CD(SG)IGS rats (Charles River Wiga, Sulzfeld, Germany; body weight 150–200 g) were used, respectively. Animals were housed in the animal care facility of the Johannes Gutenberg-University Mainz and allowed access to food and water ad libitum before the investigation. All experiments had previously been approved by the regional Animal Ethics Committee and were conducted in accordance with the German Law for Animal Protection and the UK Coordinating Committee on Cancer Research (UKCCCR) Guidelines. Solid carcinomas of both cell lines were heterotopically induced by injection of the cells (0.4 ml, 10^4 cells/μL) subcutaneously into the dorsum of the hind foot. Tumors grew was flat, solid spherical. Volumes were determined by measuring the three orthogonal diameters (*d*) of the tumors and using an ellipsoid approximation with the formula: $V = (\pi/6) \times d_1 \times d_2 \times d_3$. Animals were used for μPET studies when the tumors reached volumes between 1.0 and 2.0 mL, approximately 10–14 days after tumor cell inoculation.

μPET imaging was performed on a μPET Focus 120 small animal PET (Siemens/ Concorde, Knoxville, TN, USA). During PET measurements, anesthetized (3% isoflurane in oxygen) animals (230–270 g body weight) were placed tail first supine in the field of view. To keep the body temperature of the animals stable, an infrared light source was placed near the animals. ^{68}Ga-DOTA-puromycin (20–25 MBq) in 0.7–0.9 ml 0.9% NaCl solution was administered as a bolus via a previously inserted catheter in the tail vein while the animals were already placed inside the μPET.

Time–activity curves (TAC) were obtained with varying time frames (1–5 min) for a total measuring interval of 45 min. The PET list-mode data were histogrammed into 12 frames and reconstructed using interlaced ordered subset expectation-maximization (OSEM 2d) algorithm. Volumes of interest (VOIs) were defined for tumor and reference tissue (testis). Tissue concentration in testis was nearly constant for all animals at a low level, indicating low tracer uptake. Ratios of tumor to reference tissue were calculated from TAC. Optical reconstruction and estimation of TACs was performed using PMOD (PMOD Technologies Ltd., Zürich, Switzerland).

2.8 Statistical Analysis

Quantitative data are expressed as mean ± SD. Means were compared using Student's *t*-test; *p* values less than 0.05 were considered statistically significant.

3 Results

3.1 Synthesis of DOTA-NHC$_6$-dC-Puromycin

Using originally 4,000 nmol immobilized puromycin for fully automated synthesis of DOTA-NHC$_6$-dC-puromycin, an average amount of 333 nmol HPLC-purified, desalted, and lyophilized precursor was obtained.

3.2 ^{68}Ga-Labeling of DOTA-Pur

Overall recovery after purification on reversed-phase C-18 cartridges was 65.0 ± 6.0%. Specific activity of ^{68}Ga-DOTA-Pur was 1.5 ± 0.1 GBq/μmol.

3.3 In Vitro Uptake and Protein Incorporation

3.3.1 ^{68}Ga-DOTA-Pur

Uptake in the tumor cells (DU145) after 2 h was 2.0 ± 0.1% of the applied dose per 1×10^6 cells; in normal skin fibroblasts (BJ) it was 0.2 ± 0.1% of the applied dose per 1×10^6 cells. Tumor-to-normal cell ratio was approximately 10:1.

Protein incorporation after 2 h in tumor and normal cell line was ≥93% of the uptake and was 2.0 ± 0.1% of applied dose per 1 × 10^6 cells for tumor cells and 0.2 ± 0.1% per 1 × 10^6 cells for normal cells.

3.3.2 [^{3}H]Tyrosine

Uptake in tumor cells (DU145) after 2 h was 7.7 ± 0.9% of the applied dose per 1 × 10^6 cells; in normal skin fibroblasts (BJ) it was 2.0 ± 0.2% of the applied dose per 1 × 10^6 cells. Tumor-to-normal cell ratio was approximately 4:1. Protein incorporation after 2 h in the tumor cell line was ≥73% of the uptake and 5.1 ± 0.5% of applied dose per 1 × 10^6 cells. Protein incorporation for normal cells was ≥57% of the uptake and 1.2 ± 0.2% of applied dose per 1 × 10^6 cells.

3.3.3 2-Fluoro-[^{3}H]tyrosine

Uptake in the tumor cells (DU145) after 2 h was 4.5 ± 0.5% of the applied dose per 1 × 10^6 cells; in normal skin fibroblasts (BJ) it was 1.4 ± 0.5% of the applied dose per 1 × 10^6 cells. Tumor-to-normal cell ratio was approximately 3:1. Protein incorporation after 2 h in the tumor cell line was ≥73% of the uptake and 3.3 ± 0.7% of applied dose per 1 × 10^6 cells. Protein incorporation for normal cells was ≥33% of the uptake and 0.4 ± 0.2% of applied dose per 1 × 10^6 cells.

3.4 Inhibition of Protein Synthesis

3.4.1 ^{68}Ga-DOTA-Pur

Inhibition of protein synthesis utilizing cycloheximide for noncompetitive inhibition reduced cellular uptake of ^{68}Ga-DOTA-Pur to ≤15.7 ± 0.2% of the administered dose for inhibitor concentrations ≥200 pmol, while protein incorporation was reduced to ≤6.2 ± 0.5% of the administered dose. Inhibitor concentrations exceeding 2 nmol resulted in nearly complete blockage of uptake and incorporation (Fig. 4).

3.4.2 [^{3}H]Tyrosine

Inhibition of protein synthesis utilizing cycloheximide for noncompetitive inhibition reduced cellular uptake of [^{3}H]tyrosine to ≤57.2 ± 5.5% of the administered dose for inhibitor concentrations ≥200 pmol, while protein incorporation was reduced to ≤20.1 ± 3.5% administered dose. Inhibitor concentrations exceeding 2 nmol resulted in nearly complete blockage of incorporation while the uptake values remained nearly unaffected (Fig. 5).

3.4.3 2-Fluoro-[^{3}H]tyrosine

Inhibition of protein synthesis utilizing cycloheximide for noncompetitive inhibition reduced cellular uptake of 2-fluoro-[^{3}H]tyrosine to ≤59.2 ± 1.1% of the

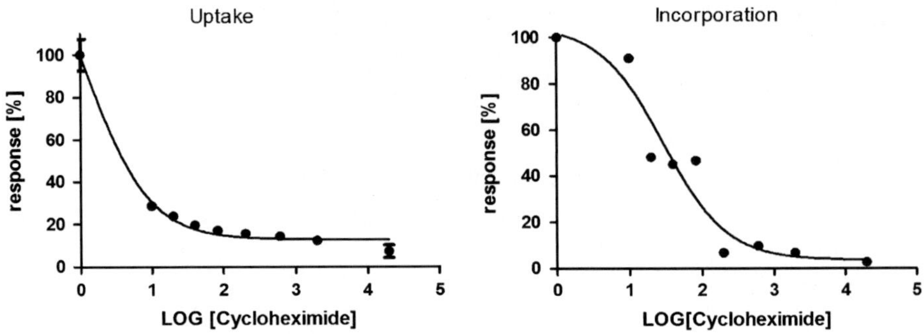

Fig. 4 Noncompetitive inhibition of ^{68}Ga-DOTA-Pur uptake (*left*) and incorporation (*right*) using increasing concentrations from 10 to 20 nmol/well of cycloheximide to inhibit protein synthesis. Reduction of cellular uptake to normal cell level for inhibitor concentrations $\geq$200 nmol/well and blockage of uptake and incorporation for inhibitor concentration exceeding 2 nmol

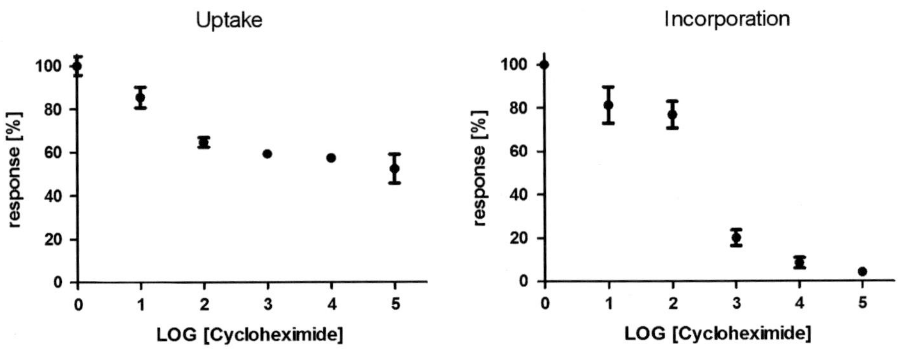

Fig. 5 Inhibition of protein synthesis utilizing cycloheximide for noncompetitive inhibition reduced the cellular uptake of [^{3}H]tyrosine to $\leq$57.2 $\pm$ 5.5% administered dose for inhibitor concentrations $\geq$200 pmol while protein incorporation was reduced to $\leq$20.1 $\pm$ 3.5% administered dose. Inhibitor concentrations exceeding 2 nmol resulted in nearly complete blockage of incorporation while the uptake values remained nearly unaffected

administered dose for inhibitor concentrations $\geq$200 pmol, while protein incorporation was reduced to $\leq$9.5 $\pm$ 0.6% of the administered dose. Inhibitor concentrations exceeding 2 nmol resulted in nearly complete blockage of incorporation, while the uptake values remained nearly unaffected (Fig. 6).

3.5 µPET Imaging in Tumor-Bearing Rats

To test feasibility of DOTA-Pur for imaging of protein synthesis in tumors, ^{68}Ga-DOTA-Pur was injected intravenously into Walker carcinoma and AT1

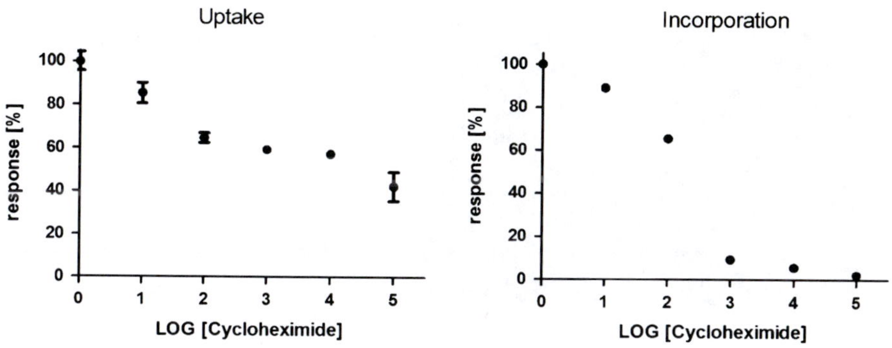

Fig. 6 Inhibition of protein synthesis utilizing cycloheximide for noncompetitive inhibition reduced cellular uptake of 2-fluoro-[^{3}H]tyrosine to ≤59.2 ± 1.1% administered dose for inhibitor concentrations ≥200 pmol while protein incorporation was reduced to ≤9.5 ± 0.6% administered dose. Inhibitor concentrations exceeding 2 nmol resulted in nearly complete blockage of incorporation while the uptake values remained nearly unaffected

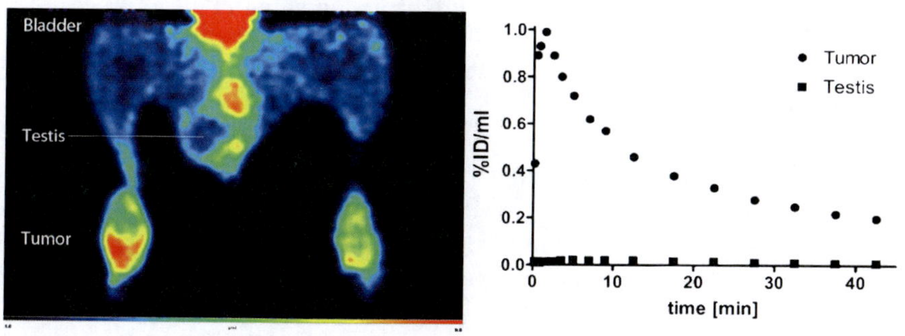

Fig. 7 Summarized μPET image (*left*), coronal slice, colors expressed as SUV (0–9) (3–20 min, dynamic scan) of Walker carcinomas on hind feet of CD rats and 0–45 min TACs of tumor and testis (reference). Obtained TAC (*right*) shows rapid uptake and slow washout caused retention of ^{68}Ga-DOTA-Pur as aa-tRNA-analogon within eukaryotic ribosomal A-site

tumor-bearing rats and μPET scans were performed from 0 to 45 min p.i. Summarized image of Walker carcinoma from 3 to 20 min and tumor as well as reference tissue TACs from 0 to 45 min p.i. obtained from dynamic scans are shown in Fig. 7. Summarized image of AT1 tumors from 3 to 20 min and tumor as well as reference tissue TACs from 0 to 60 min p.i. obtained from dynamic scans are shown in Fig. 8. Both tumors are clearly visualized with high tumor-to-background contrast (≥40:1). Highest tumor uptake was measured between 3 and 6 min p.i.

Most of the AT1 tumors showed necrotic tissue inside the tumor when removed for ex vivo biodistribution. The necrotic regions of the tumors were clearly visible inside the tumor outlines. Prominent activity was located in the kidneys and

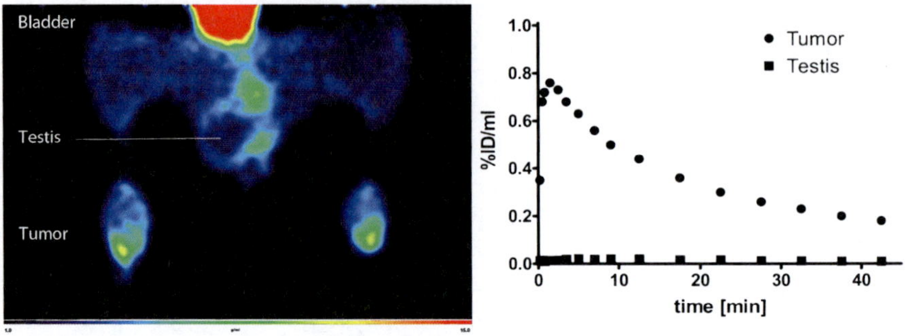

Fig. 8 Summarized µPET-image, coronal slice, colors expressed as SUV (0–15) (3–20 min, dynamic scan) of AT1 tumors on hind feet of Copenhagen rats and 0–45 min TAC of tumor and testis (reference); obtained TAC shows rapid uptake and slow washout caused by retention of ^{68}Ga-DOTA-Pur as aa-tRNA-analogon within eukaryotic ribosomal A-site

urinary bladder, the major excretion pathway of DOTA-Pur. Tumor-to-testis and tumor-to-muscle ratios were sufficiently high for imaging at all times.

4 Discussion

Synthesis of proteins is a fundamental process for all cellular functions. Because of the uncontrolled and accelerated growth of cancer, the process of protein synthesis in tumors is increased. As a consequence, the demand for proteins, the building blocks of cellular structures and enzymes, is increased. It is, therefore, expected that radiolabeled amino acid tracers will also accumulate in tumors. Nearly all amino acids and slightly modified variants have been radiolabeled, but only a few satisfy the requirements (reliable production, stability in vivo, adequate tumor uptake, etc.) to a degree sufficient for clinical use. In brain tumor imaging, use of radiolabeled amino acids is quite well established. In most other tumors, the data are not sufficient to permit definite conclusions (Haubner 2010; Jager et al. 2005).

Amino acid tracers were initially developed with the intention to measure protein synthesis rates. However, the rate of amino acid transport rather than the protein synthesis rate seems to be the major determinant of tracer uptake in tumor imaging studies. This study showed that fluorination of tyrosine caused a significant change in its biological behavior, when tested under idealized conditions in cell culture. Even without the presence of interfering parameters, such as effecting plasma proteins or defluorination, uptakes measured on natural and fluorinated analogs were significantly different. The second major setback for use of amino acids for measurement of protein synthesis is explained and illustrated by the data obtained from the protein synthesis inhibition experiments: For both amino acids, the uptake is not dependent on the amount of amino acid used for protein synthesis.

The most important biochemical property of an analog tracer to be tested for assessment of protein synthesis in vivo is its acceptance by aa-tRNA synthetase and its subsequent incorporation into peptide chains by ligase enzyme systems. The generally applied method of isolating proteins from tissue homogenates by TCA precipitation is rather crude. It does not particularly discriminate between real incorporation into the peptide chain and possible binding as false substrate to one or several enzymes with which it would be coprecipitated by TCA (Hamacher and Coenen 2002). Since it has been demonstrated by Nathans (Haubner 2010) and Smith (Yarmolinsky and Haba 1959) that there is only one possible pathway for puromycin and puromycin conjugates inside cells, this method can be applied to determine exactly the protein-bound fractions of ^{68}Ga-DOTA-Pur. For the used amino acids, we performed coprecipitations with added surplus of amino acids to determine if the used compounds are coprecipitated or not. In both cases, coprecipitation could not be observed.

As the protein-bound fraction of ^{68}Ga-DOTA-Pur after 2 h is $\geq$93% of the cellular uptake, direct dependency of the uptake on the protein incorporation ratio is essential. Inhibition of protein synthesis experiments performed on eukaryotic tumor cells showed significant reduction of cellular uptake to the level of normal cells used as reference. Therefore, the visible accumulation of activity in tumors correlates with the amount of active ribosomes and, therefore, with protein synthesis in the region of interest.

^{68}Ga exhibits several attractive properties as a PET nuclide such as excellent availability (from ^{68}Ge/^{68}Ga generators), 89% decay via positron emission with maximum energy of 1.92 MeV, and negligible accompanying gamma radiation. The short half-life of ^{68}Ga (68 min) permits application of ^{68}Ga activities suitable for imaging while keeping the radiation burden to the patient at acceptable level. Since we can synthesize ready-to-use injection solution of ^{68}Ga-DOTA-Pur after 62 min, the half-life of ^{68}Ga does not cause significant technical hindrance of its clinical use.

The labeling efficiency of DOTA-Pur and the overall recovery was between 55% and 65%, which still presents an opportunity for improvement but is comparable to labeling yields for DOTA derivatives of peptides labeled with ^{68}Ga (Meyer et al. 2004).

TACs revealed that, after 1 h, more than 95% of the injected activity has been excreted via the renal system. Since protein synthesis is a rather slow process, it will be necessary to prolong the half-life in blood for further improvement of tumor accumulation of DOTA-Pur, which results in increase of compound's concentration inside the tumor over time. Starck and Roberts (2002) showed that puromycin oligonucleotides reveal steric restrictions for ribosome entry and multiple modes of translation inhibition. Therefore, changes in the structure of the conjugate might result in decrease of the biological activity of the modified molecule. Even if the half-life in blood could be prolonged by modifications, it might result in decreased ribosomal acceptance and thus reduced accumulation of the puromycin conjugate in tumor tissue.

Due to the cytotoxicity of puromycin administered in ≥ 1 mmol concentrations (resulting in nonfunctional protein fragments), increasing the dose to achieve an increased amount of protein incorporation is not an option.

Since ribosomal activity can only be found during protein synthesis, determination of ribosomal activity is a direct equivalent for protein synthesis. The more active ribosomes that are present, the higher the retention of ^{68}Ga-DOTA-Pur in the cell, as shown in the blocking experiments utilizing cycloheximide.

Optical imaging of fluorophores such as biotin in tissue is limited due to a tissue penetration of maximum range 0.5–2.0 cm. Hence, their use for diagnostics in human beings is not feasible. In contrast, the penetration depth and attenuation of 511-keV photons allow for use of the radiolabeled DOTA-puromycin conjugate as a suitable tool for PET imaging with all its advantages (high resolution and precise quantification), being thus superior to any optical-photon-based imaging agent.

Taking all these facts into account, the most suitable possibility for increasing the half-life in blood might be use of infusion pumps for administration of a steady dose over time instead of application in a bolus injection.

5 Conclusions

As shown in this study, utilizing fluorinated amino acids for in vivo determination of protein synthesis in general will not be feasible.

On the other hand, ^{68}Ga-DOTA-Pur is promising to become useful in imaging of protein synthesis for both therapy control and target identification for therapy, due to both its favorable metabolic pathway and the favorable physical properties of ^{68}Ga.

References

Coenen HH (1993) Biochemistry and evaluation of fluoroamino acids. In: Mazoyer BM, Heiss WD, Comar D (eds) PET studies on aminoacid metabolism and protein synthesis. Kluwer Academic, Dordrecht, pp 109–129

Griffiths AJF et al (1996) An introduction to genetic analysis, 6th edn. Freeman, New York

Hamacher K, Coenen HH (2002) Efficient routine production of the 18F-labelled amino acid O-2-18F fluoroethyl-L-tyrosine. Appl Radiat Isot 57(6):853–856

Haubner R (2010) PET radiopharmaceuticals in radiation treatment planning - synthesis and biological characteristics. Radiother Oncol 96(3):280–287

Jager PL, Vaalburg W, Pruim J, Vries EGEd, Langen K-J, Piers DA (2001) Radiolabeled amino acids: basic aspects and clinical applications in oncology. J Nucl Med 42:14

Jager PL, de Korte MA, Lub-de Hooge MN, van Waarde A, Koopmans KP, Perik PJ, de Vries EG (2005) Molecular imaging: what can be used today. Cancer Imaging, 5 Spec No A: S27–32

Langen KJ, Pauleit D, Coenen HH (2002) 3-[(123)I]Iodo-alpha-methyl-L-tyrosine: uptake mechanisms and clinical applications. Nucl Med Biol 29(6):625–631

Laverman P, Boerman OC, Corstens FH, Oyen WJ (2002) Fluorinated amino acids for tumour imaging with positron emission tomography. Eur J Nucl Med Mol Imaging 29(5):681–690

Meyer GJ, Macke H, Schuhmacher J, Knapp WH, Hofmann M (2004) 68 Ga-labelled DOTA-derivatised peptide ligands. Eur J Nucl Med Mol Imaging 31(8):1097–1104

Miyamoto-Sato E, Nemoto N, Kobayashi K, Yanagawa H (2000) Specific bonding of puromycin to full-length protein at the C-terminus. Nucleic Acids Res 28(5):1176–1182

Nathans D (1964) Puromycin inhibition of protein synthesis: incorporation of puromycin into peptide chains. Proc Natl Acad Sci USA 51:585–592

Nemoto N, Miyamoto-Sato E, Yanagawa H (1999) Fluorescence labeling of the C-terminus of proteins with a puromycin analogue in cell-free translation systems. FEBS Lett 462(1–2): 43–46

Starck SR, Roberts RW (2002) Puromycin oligonucleotides reveal steric restrictions for ribosome entry and multiple modes of translation inhibition. RNA 8:15

Wester HJ, Herz M, Weber W, Heiss P, Senekowitsch-Schmidtke R, Schwaiger M, Stocklin G (1999) Synthesis and radiopharmacology of O-(2-[18F]fluoroethyl)-L-tyrosine for tumor imaging. J Nucl Med 40(1):205–212

Yarmolinsky MB, Haba GL (1959) Inhibition by puromycin of amino acid incorporation into protein. Proc Natl Acad Sci USA 45(12):1721–1729

Zhernosekov KP, Filosofov DV, Baum RP, Aschoff P, Bihl H, Razbash AA, Jahn M, Jennewein M, Rosch F (2007) Processing of generator-produced 68Ga for medical application. J Nucl Med 48(10):1741–1748

Hypoxia Imaging Agents Labeled with Positron Emitters

Lathika Hoigebazar and Jae Min Jeong

Abstract

Imaging hypoxia using positron emission tomography (PET) is of great importance for therapy of cancer. [^{18}F]Fluoromisonidazole (FMISO) was the first PET agent for hypoxia imaging, and various radiolabeled nitroimidazole derivatives such as [^{18}F]fluoroerythronitroimidazole (FETNIM), [^{18}F]1-α-D-(2-deoxy-2-fluoroarabinofuranosyl)-2-nitroimidazole (FAZA), [^{18}F]2-(2-nitro-1*H*-imidazol-1-yl)-*N*-(2,2,3,3,3-pentafluoropropyl) acetamide (EF-5), and [^{18}F]fluoroetanidazole (FETA) have been developed successively. To overcome the high cost of cyclotron installation, ^{68}Ga-labeled nitroimidazole derivatives also have been developed. Another important hypoxia imaging agent is ^{64}Cu-diacetyl-bis(N^4-methylthiosemicarbazone) (^{64}Cu-ATSM), which can distribute in cancer tissue rapidly due to high lipophilicity. However, its application is limited due to high cost of radionuclide production. Although various hypoxia imaging agents have been reported and tested, hypoxia PET images still have to be improved, because of the low blood flow in hypoxic tissues and resulting low uptake of the agents.

Contents

L. Hoigebazar · J. M. Jeong (✉)
Department of Nuclear Medicine, Seoul National University College of Medicine,
101 Daehangno Jongno-gu, 110-744 Seoul, Korea
e-mail: radiopharmaceutical@gmail.com

R. P. Baum and F. Rösch (eds.), *Theranostics, Gallium-68, and Other Radionuclides*,
Recent Results in Cancer Research 194, DOI: 10.1007/978-3-642-27994-2_15,

1 Introduction

Hypoxia is an important cause of cancer resistance to radiation and chemotherapies. Thus, imaging of hypoxia has been an important issue in nuclear medicine. The cause of hypoxia in cancer and various hypoxia imaging agents labeled with positron emitters produced either from cyclotron or generator are discussed in this chapter.

2 Hypoxia

Decreased blood supply to cells can lead to reduction of oxygen delivery, which makes cells hypoxic while remaining viable. Such hypoxia occurs due to interruption of vascular supply such as stroke or myocardial infarction, or due to poorly organized tumor vasculature as in tumor outgrowing its vascular supply. Hypoxia in tumor tissues is a characteristic feature of solid tumors. Tumor cells close to the blood vessels are normoxic and rapidly growing, but cells far from vessels are anoxic and necrotic. Cells in the central areas of tumors are hypoxic and less susceptible to radiation.

Hypoxia is an important factor influencing the prognosis of many diseases such as stroke and cancers. Increase in tumor aggressiveness, failure of local control, and metastatic potential of solid tumors are believed to be highly associated with presence of hypoxia within the cancer (Antunes et al. 2007).

Thus, there are three distinct types of tumor hypoxia (Vaupel and Harrison 2004): (1) Acute (perfusion-related) hypoxia results from inadequate blood flow in tumors, which is generally the consequence of recognized structural and functional abnormalities of the tumor neovasculature; this kind of acute hypoxia is often transient, and may lead to ischemic hypoxia. (2) Chronic (diffusion-related) hypoxia is caused by increased oxygen diffusion distances, related to tumor expansion and affecting cells greater than 70 μm from the nearest capillary, depending on where tumor cells lie in relation to the arterial or venous end of a capillary. (3) Anemic hypoxia relates to reduced O_2 transport capacity of blood which is tumor associated.

3 Why Is Detection of Tumor Hypoxia Important?

Hypoxic tumor imaging is useful for planning radiation therapy as well as bioreductive drug therapy of tumors. The former is because tumor resistance against radiation therapy is correlated in part with the development of hypoxic regions (Ballinger 2001), and the latter is because bioreductive drugs can be activated in hypoxic tumors (Nunn et al. 1995). Hypoxic regions develop as a tumor grows beyond the ability of its blood supply to deliver oxygen, exacerbated by vascular spasm or compression caused by increased interstitial fluid pressure. However, hypoxia is heterogeneous, and the extent of hypoxia is variable.

Hypoxia is an important adverse prognostic factor for tumor progression and is a major cause of failure of radiation therapy (Brown 1999) due to the lack of oxygen, a potent radiosensitizer. Furthermore, hypoxia is a predictive factor for increased tumor aggressiveness, manifested as a higher rate of recurrence and metastasis (Brizel et al. 1996; Graeber et al. 1996; Hockel et al. 1996). Determining the extent of tumor hypoxia is important for treatment planning of cancer or myocardial ischemia (Padhani 2005). When tumor grows beyond 2 mm, tumor neovascularization should occur (He et al. 2008). However, these new tumor vessels formed are functionally and structurally abnormal and less efficient compared with normal tissues, which have a well-organized vasculature (Overgaard 1994). Despite the potential importance of oxygen levels in tissue, difficulty in making this measurement in vivo has limited its role in clinical decision-making. In case of short-term hypoxia, the metabolism can recover to normal, but if hypoxia persists, irreversible cell damage and death may occur. So, a hypoxia marker would be very useful in oncology. Although the existence of tumor hypoxia was suggested more than 50 years ago (Thomlinson and Gray 1955), its real importance in cancer has been known only for 15 years (He et al. 2008). However, measurement of hypoxia extent within normal and tumor tissues is difficult (Lord et al. 1993). Earlier tumor hypoxia measurements have been made using diverse technologies including biological, chemical, and physical methods (Stone et al. 1993).

Tissue hypoxia cannot be predicted from biopsy or conventional imaging methods. Thus, either direct or indirect measurements might help to identify the presence of hypoxic tissues. There are limitations to direct measurements because they are invasive and may be subject to sampling error, cannot reach all tissue sites, and are often undertaken at time of surgery. Thus, development of noninvasive imaging methods for assessing tumor hypoxia has attracted substantial interest. The most widely used method is positron emission tomography (PET) (Lawrentschuk et al. 2005). Several hypoxic tracers suitable for PET have been reported.

2-Nitroimidazole, which is thought to be reduced and to accumulate in sites of hypoxia, has been labeled with ^{18}F, ^{123}I, and ^{99m}Tc and used for imaging purposes with both SPECT (Parliament et al. 1992; Rumsey et al. 1995) and PET (Nunn et al. 1995). Among these, [^{18}F]fluoromisonidazole (FMISO) and ^{123}I-iodoazomycin arabinoside (IAZA) have been most commonly used. Other than nitroimidazole derivatives, nonnitro bioreductive complexes, such as ^{60}Cu-, ^{62}Cu-, and ^{64}Cu-thiosemicarbazone ATSM and ^{99m}Tc-butylene amineoxime (BnAO or HL91), have been developed. Although ^{99m}Tc-BnAO does not contain a nitroimidazole group and its mechanism of localization in hypoxic site is not understood, it might be analogous to that proposed for Cu-ATSM in which the redox state of the metal is involved in its selective retention under hypoxic conditions. In preclinical studies, [^{123}I]IAZA and ^{60}Cu-ATSM have shown correlation with response to radiotherapy (Ballinger 2001).

4 Nature of an Ideal Hypoxia Imaging Agent for Hypoxia Imaging

The tracer should easily cross the blood capillary membrane, preferably without using membrane transporter systems, which otherwise might complicate the interpretation of tracer study results. Thus, rapid membrane permeation and localization to the target viable hypoxic tissue with high specificity is essential.

Low redox potential is important for selective retention in hypoxic tissue. For higher specificity, it should be preferably reduced by enzymes with abnormally high electron concentration in hypoxic cells.

For clinical application, it should have favorable dosing and safety profiles in human. Thus, favorable rate of excretion is required.

These parameters also influence the target-to-background ratio that ultimately determines the ability to detect tissue hypoxia. Although none of the presently available hypoxia tracers completely meet all these preconditions, some currently available nitroimidazoles and a few nonnitroimidazole derivatives satisfy several of these prerequisites.

5 Nitroimidazole as Hypoxic Agent

Several invasive procedures to detect and measure hypoxia in tumors have been developed, but none of these are in routine clinical use because of technical complexity, inconvenience, and inability to obtain repeated measures. A group of oxygen-sensitive compounds known as 2-nitroimidazoles, originally developed as antibacterial agents, have now been adapted as hypoxia imaging agents after radiolabeling (Ballinger 2001; Hossmann 2003).

PET is a promising approach for visualizing hypoxia (Lewis et al. 1999). Use of PET with radiolabeled molecules which undergo chemical reduction in the absence of oxygen has led to a number of promising agents. Several bioreductive substances, especially nitroimidazole derivatives, have been advocated for imaging hypoxic tissue (Kumar et al. 2010). Nitroimidazole derivatives are known to undergo different intracellular metabolism depending on the availability of oxygen in the tissue (Fig. 1). In particular, 2-nitroimidazole can be reduced to form reactive chemical species that can bind irreversibly to cell components in the absence of sufficient oxygen, a property exploited for their antibacterial action, and thus development of radiolabeled nitroimidazole derivatives for imaging of hypoxia remains an active field of research to improve cancer therapy results. When a nitroimidazole enters hypoxic cells, the molecule undergoes an enzymatic

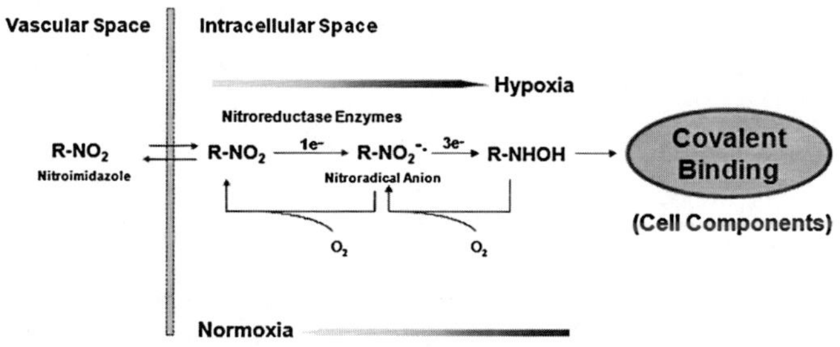

Fig. 1 Schematic representation of the proposed mechanism underlying binding of nitroimidazole tracers in hypoxic cell. Reprinted with permission from Stroke 2008, 39, 1629–1637. Copyright (2008) American Stroke Association

single-electron reduction depending on the availability of oxygen, which forms a radical anion (Fig. 2). The process is initiated by an enzyme-mediated single-electron reduction to form a free radical.

In normal oxygen level, the free radical anion is rapidly reversed to its original compound (Fig. 2). The rate of oxidation is dependent on the intracellular concentration of oxygen. In hypoxic tissue, the reduced compound is not able to be reoxidized and is further reduced, resulting in association of the reduced nitroimidazole with various intracellular components. The association is not irreversible, since these agents clear from hypoxic tissue over time. So, under hypoxic conditions, bioreductive metabolism leads to further stepwise reduction to amine ($6e^-$) derivatives (Fig. 2), and binds to cell components, thus the associated radiolabel is selectively retained in hypoxic cells. The cellular components that covalently bind the free radical-type nitroimidazoles have not been clearly identified, but might be intracellular macromolecules such as proteins or DNA (Nunn et al. 1995). Labeled nitroimidazole derivatives are therefore potential radiopharmaceuticals for imaging hypoxic areas. So, development of radiolabeled derivatives of nitroimidazole for hypoxia imaging is important for improving clinical outcome.

Naturally occurring nitroaromatic compounds are not common, but most classes of organisms including bacteria, protozoa, fungi, plants, and mammals can metabolize them using nitroreductase. It is difficult to say which particular enzyme is responsible for reduction of the nitro group in mammalian cells, but several enzymes are capable of this. Various nitroreductase enzymes are associated with the cytoplasm, microsomes, and mitochondria (McManus et al. 1982; Walton and Workman 1987).

Particularly for nitroimidazole derivatives, as discussed above, the amount of tracer delivered to the target via the blood–brain barrier (BBB) and faster washout from normoxic tissues with the high rate of trapping in hypoxic tissue is very important, as this determines the duration of the experiment sufficient to reach adequate contrast between normoxic and hypoxic tissue, as well as the presence of the intracellular macromolecular components necessary for binding (Nunn et al. 1995).

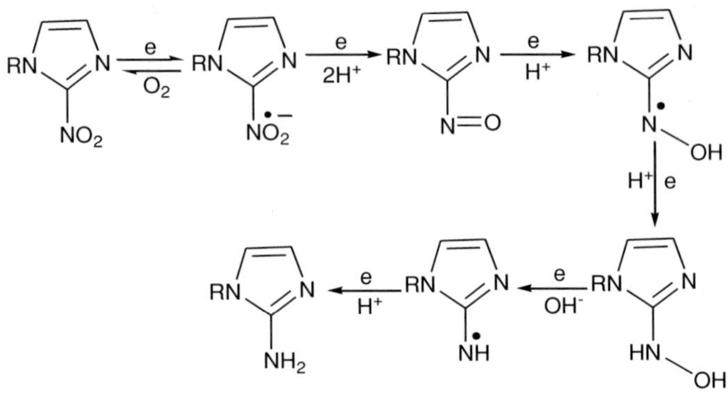

Fig. 2 Proposed mechanism for nitroimidazole reduction

[^{18}F]FMISO is the first and most widely studied nitroimidazole agent for in vivo PET imaging (Lee and Scott 2007; Martin et al. 1989; Rajendran et al. 2006). It has been evaluated extensively for detection of tumor hypoxia preclinically using different animal models. The first clinical study to image tumor hypoxia using [^{18}F]FMISO was performed by Rasey et al. (1996), who used [^{18}F]FMISO to quantify the hypoxic fraction in patients with lung, head and neck, and prostate cancers. Both animal and clinical studies using [^{18}F]FMISO showed feasibility of this tracer as a hypoxia imaging agent (Kubota et al. 1999). However, [^{18}F]FMISO has failed to obtain wider acceptance for routine clinical application because it is rather lipophilic, which may contribute to the finding that hypoxia-specific accumulation is rather slow. The need to wait several hours to permit clearance of the agent from the normoxic background tissue (contrast between lesion and background typically <2:1 at about 90 min after injection) is a serious fault of ^{18}F-labeled agents having a relatively short half-life (110 min). In addition, due to the relatively low uptake of [^{18}F]FMISO in hypoxic tissues, its clinical application has seen limited success. Therefore, considerable efforts have been made to develop more feasible compounds for clinical use, i.e., nitroimidazoles with either increased specific tumor uptake or faster clearance. Clinical experience with nitroimidazole agents other than [^{18}F]FMISO is limited. However, one such candidate used for clinically is ^{18}F-labeled fluoroerythronitroimidazole ([^{18}F]FETNIM) (Yang et al. 1995; Gronroos et al. 2004), which is more hydrophilic than [^{18}F]FMISO and shows rapid elimination from nontarget tissues via excretion through the urinary pathway. The log *P* value of [^{18}F]FETNIM was reported to be 0.17.

[^{18}F]FETNIM used in patients with head and neck cancer showed higher and heterogeneously distributed uptake in tumors than in adjacent neck muscle. Also, the tumor-to-blood ratio with [^{18}F]FETNIM at 4 h after injection was significantly higher than with [^{18}F]FMISO. Although it showed lower background than [^{18}F]FMSIO at 90 min post injection, it was found to be largely perfusion dependent (Lehtio et al. 2001). Halogenated nitroimidazoles, such as

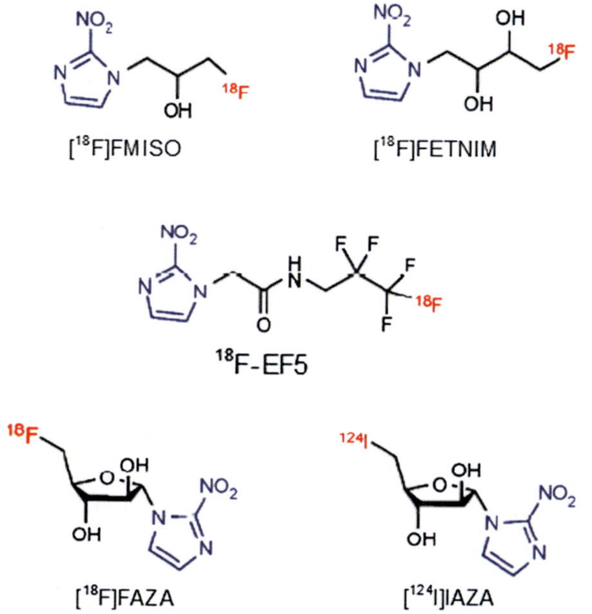

Fig. 3 Known nitroimidazole agents for hypoxia imaging

1-α-D-(2-deoxy-2-[^{18}F]fluoroarabinofuranosyl)-2-nitroimidazole ([^{18}F]FAZA) (Grosu et al. 2007; Piert et al. 2005; Postema et al. 2009; Souvatzoglou et al. 2007), 1-(5-[^{123}I]iodo-5-deoxy-β-D-arabinofuranosyl)-2-nitroimidazole (iodoazomycin arabinoside) ([^{124}I]IAZA) (Reischl et al. 2007), 2-(2-nitro-1*H*-imidazol-1-yl)-*N*-(2,2,3,3,3-[^{18}F]pentafluoropropyl) acetamide ([^{18}F]EF-5) (Dolbier et al. 2001; Komar et al. 2008; Yapp et al. 2007), and fluoroetanidazole ([^{18}F]FETA) (Rasey et al. 1999), are other known hypoxia imaging agents (Fig. 3) developed to improve imaging performance by improving the target-to-nontarget ratio by increasing excretion rates. [^{18}F]FAZA, developed to undergo more rapid clearance from blood and nontarget tissues than [^{18}F]FMISO, was introduced to image tumor hypoxia with PET (Sorger et al. 2003). Because of its improved imaging properties, [^{18}F]FAZA is recommended for further preclinical and clinical study for imaging tumor hypoxia. Compared with [^{18}F]FMISO, [^{18}F]FAZA displays a lower octanol:water partition coefficient (log $P = 1.1$) (Kumar et al. 1999), which indicates the potential for both rapid diffusion through tissue and faster renal excretion for [^{18}F]FAZA (Kumar et al. 1999). Also, the significantly lower tumor-to-blood ratio resulting from [^{18}F]FAZA is related to either renal or hepatobiliary excretion, leading to a lower radiation burden and more favorable imaging result than with [^{18}F]FMISO (Sorger et al. 2003). Another agent is [^{18}F]fluoroetanidazole ([^{18}F]FETA), which is a well-known 2-nitroimidazole analog with *P* value of 0.16 (Barthel et al. 2004) and also showed significantly lower levels of retention in the liver and lung than those of [^{18}F]FMISO (Rasey et al. 1999).

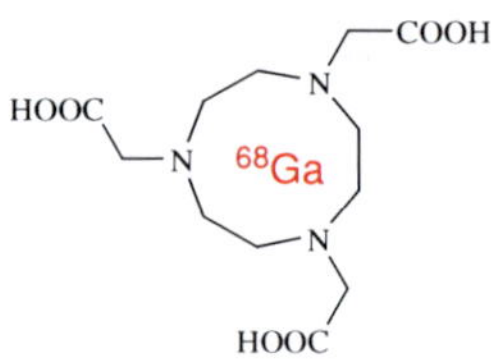

^{68}Ga-NOTA

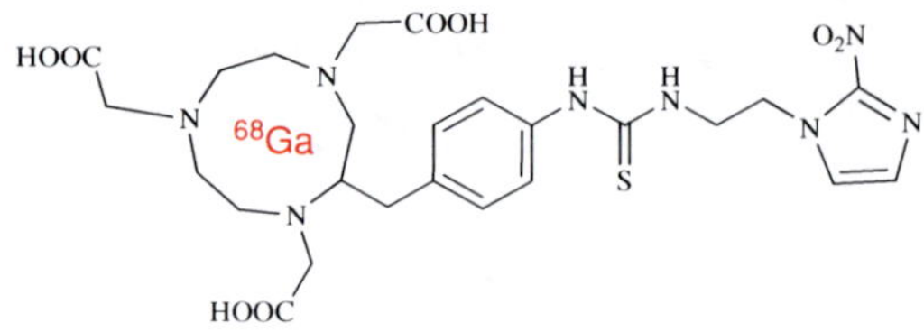

^{68}Ga-SCN-NOTA-nitroimidazole

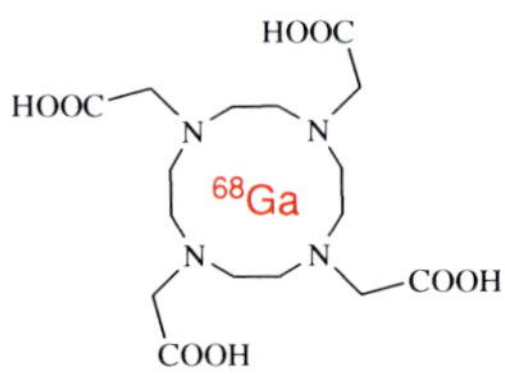

^{68}Ga-DOTA

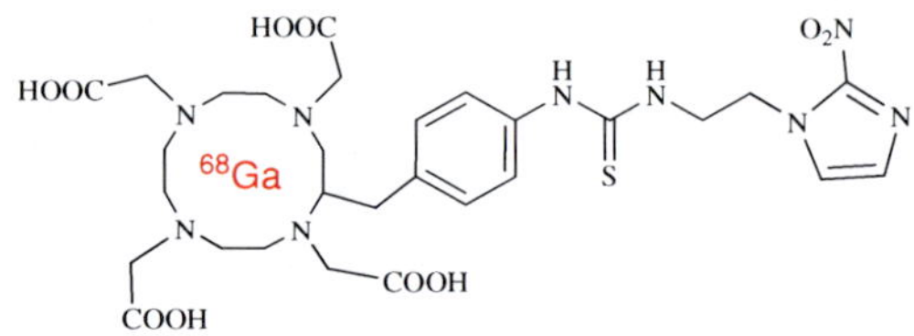

^{68}Ga-SCN-DOTA-nitroimidazole

Fig. 4 Structures of ^{68}Ga-labeled nitroimidazole derivatives

However, being more hydrophilic compounds, diffusion of PET tracers into tumoral tissues might be limited (Hoigebazar et al. 2011). So, a new class of more lipophilic derivatives, 2-(2-nitroimidazol-1-yl)-*N*-(3,3,3-trifluoropropyl)-acetamide (EF3) and EF5, were developed. Preliminary animal experiments involving these fluorinated derivatives showed more homogeneous distribution in normal tissues along with clearance through the kidneys and accumulation in hypoxic tumors (Busch et al. 2000; Koch 2002).

However, production of these radiotracers is limited on cyclotron systems, which are expensive as well as difficult to handle. Other than cyclotron-produced radioisotopes, an alternative method to label biomolecules is use of ^{68}Ga, which can be obtained from a commercially available radionuclide generator system (Antunes et al. 2007; Breeman and Verbruggen 2007; Green and Welch 1989; Hnatowich 1977; Jeong et al. 2008; Shetty et al. 2010a, b). ^{68}Ga is an economical alternative to cyclotron-produced radionuclides. Compounds characterized by high hydrophilicity were thought to be better for imaging hypoxia because of rapid blood clearance and high target-to-nontarget ratio. Recently, ^{68}Ga-labeled nitroimidazole analogs were developed (Hoigebazar et al. 2010, 2011) for PET hypoxia imaging (Fig. 4). These derivatives showed elevated uptakes in hypoxic condition compared with normoxic condition in in vitro study. Also, good tumor uptake at 30 and 60 min and high tumor-to-muscle ratios were demonstrated by biodistribution and PET studies (Fig. 5).

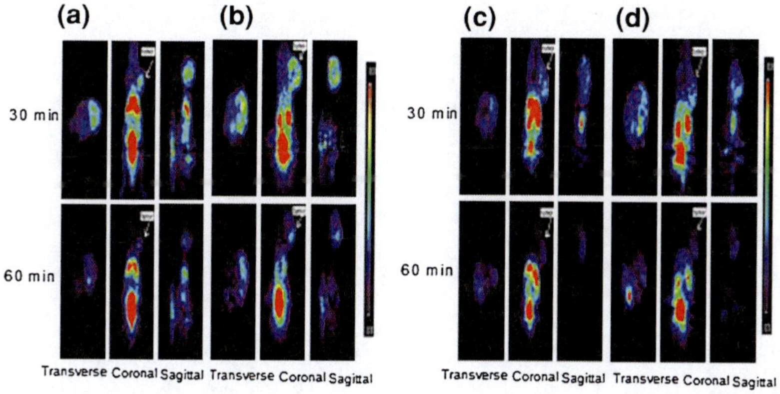

Fig. 5 Small-animal PET images of mice bearing a CT-26 xenograft on the right shoulder: **a** ^{68}Ga-NOTA-nitroimidazole (26.64 MBq/0.15 mL), **b** ^{68}Ga-DOTA-nitroimidazole (24.05 MBq/0.15 mL), **c** ^{68}Ga-SCN-NOTA-nitroimidazole (34.04 MBq/0.15 mL), and **d** ^{68}Ga-SCN-DOTA-nitroimidazole (39.26 MBq/0.15 mL) injected through tail vein at 30 and 60 min post administration. Reprinted with permission from Hoigebazar et al. (2010). Copyright (2011) American Chemical Society. Reprinted with permission from Hoigebazar et al. (2011). Copyright (2011) Elsevier

6 Copper(II)-Diacetyl-bis(*N*^{4}-methylthiosemicarbazone) (Cu-ATSM) as Hypoxic Agent

Other than nitroimidazole agents, ^{64}Cu-ATSM has been developed for hypoxia PET (Fujibayashi et al. 1997). ^{64}Cu-ATSM is an agent that shows rapid delineation of tumor hypoxia (<1 h) with high tumor-to-blood ratios $\gg$2.0. It has been shown to be selective for hypoxic cancers and ischemic myocardial tissue. Hypoxia selectivity of ^{64}Cu-ATSM was reported first in an isolated rat heart ischemia model (Fujibayashi et al. 1997).

In the chemistry of copper, there are two principle oxidation states, I and II, whose biochemistry and metabolism are known in human as they are omnipresent. Use of copper-labeled radiopharmaceuticals for PET is attractive because of the increasing availability of four positron-emitting radionuclides of copper: ^{60}Cu ($t_{1/2} = 0.40$ h, $\beta^+ = 93\%$, EC = 7%), ^{61}Cu ($t_{1/2} = 3.32$ h, $\beta^+ = 62\%$, EC = 38%), ^{62}Cu ($t_{1/2} = 0.16$ h, $\beta^+ = 98\%$, EC = 2%), and ^{64}Cu ($t_{1/2} = 12.7$ h, $\beta^+ = 17.4\%$, EC = 43%) (Blower et al. 1996). ^{62}Cu can be produced by a generator (^{62}Zn/^{62}Cu generator) system (Fukumura et al. 2006; Haynes et al. 2000), whereas ^{60}Cu, ^{61}Cu, and ^{64}Cu are produced by cyclotron (McCarthy et al. 1997, 1999) using reliable and reproducible target methods. Among copper isotopes, ^{64}Cu is most commonly used, as it is well suited for PET studies with half-life of 12.7 h and β^+ maximum energy of 0.66 MeV. This long half-life allows distribution of the nuclide from regional production centers to imaging centers that do not have an in-house cyclotron. ^{64}Cu also decays by electron capture (43%)

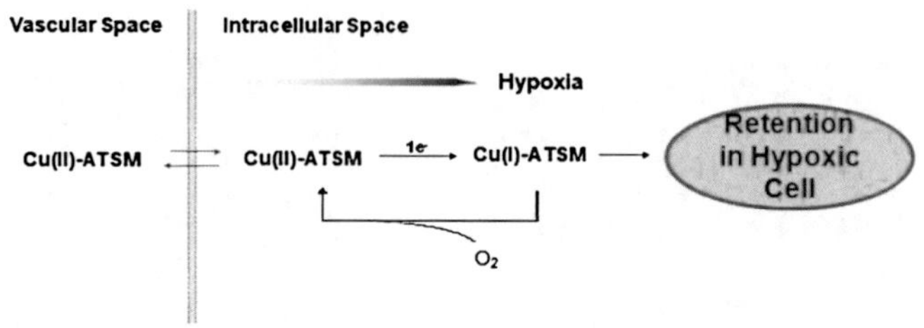

Fig. 6 Schematic representation of the proposed mechanism for Cu-ATSM in hypoxic cell

and β^- (43%) and therefore has been studied as both a diagnostic and therapeutic radionuclide (Blower et al. 1996).

A comparative biodistribution study was carried out in BALB/c mice bearing EMT6 tumors after intravenous injection of ^{64}Cu-ATSM and copper-pyruvaldehyde-bis(N^4-methylthiosemicarbazone) (^{64}Cu-PTSM) (Lewis et al. 1999). The data showed optimal tumor uptake of both agents at 10 min post injection, suggesting a rapid trapping mechanism for these agents in solid tumors. Ex vivo autoradiography of tumor slices after co-injection of ^{64}Cu-ATSM and ^{60}Cu-PTSM into the same animal was also studied. The result obtained showed uniform spreading of ^{60}Cu-PTSM throughout the EMT6 tumor, but heterogeneous uptake of ^{64}Cu-ATSM suggested trapping of this agent in hypoxic region of the tumors.

A proposed mechanism of Cu-ATSM retention was first reported by Fujibayashi et al. According to their research, Cu(II)-ATSM reduction only occurred in hypoxic cells and it was then irreversibly trapped (Fujibayashi et al. 1997) (Fig. 6). Later, a mechanistic study of Cu-ATSM in tumor cells was performed and found that Cu-ATSM was reduced mainly in microsome/cytosol fraction rather than in mitochondria (Obata et al. 2001). The reduction process in the microsome/cytosol (heat-sensitive) was enhanced by adding exogenous NADPH, indicating enzymatic reduction of Cu-ATSM in tumor cells. Additionally, it was found that the bioreductive enzymes, NADH-cytochrome b5 reductase and NADPH-cytochrome P450 reductase in the microsomes, play a major role in the reductive retention of Cu-ATSM in tumors, and this enzymatic reduction was enhanced by induction of hypoxia. Further studies of Dearling et al. (2002) and Maurer et al. (2002) suggested that Cu(II)-ATSM undergoes reduction in both normoxic and hypoxic cells, resulting in unstable Cu(I)-ATSM. This unstable species would be reoxidized to Cu(II)-ATSM in normoxic cells and diffuse back out of the cells. However, in case of hypoxic cells, it would completely dissociate and be irreversibly trapped inside the cells.

The crystal structure of Cu(II)-ATSM could be determined, but isolation of Cu(I) was not possible (Cowley et al. 2002). However, the novel dimeric species $[Cu_2(ATSMH_2)_2]^{2+}$ could be purified as a $[PF_6]^-$ salt. The X-ray crystal structure of this agent showed a dimeric structure with each of the ATSM ligands acting as a bidentate N–S donor to each Cu(I) ion to generate a novel helical structure which is unprecedented for bis(thiosemicarbazone) complexes. Cu-ATSM has several advantages over other radiopharmaceuticals used for hypoxia PET, including a simple synthesis method, faster clearance from normoxic tissue allowing a short waiting time for imaging, and a simpler method for quantification. ^{64}Cu-ATSM (Lewis et al. 1999; Vavere and Lewis 2007) and ^{60}Cu-ATSM (Lewis et al. 2008) show fast clearance rate from normoxic tissue and allow a shorter waiting time for imaging. Although Cu-ATSM is not perfect and may not be applicable for all cancer types, it holds exceptional potential as a hypoxia PET agent.

7 Retention of Radiolabeled Compounds in EMT6 Cells

Lewis et al. performed a washout study using Cu-ATSM in which the radioactivities from normoxic and hypoxic cells were observed. Samples were taken at 1, 5, 15, 30, 45, and 60 min after addition of radiotracer. Over 42% of ^{64}Cu-ATSM was washed out from normoxic cells after 1 h, but in hypoxic cells this value was only 27%, suggesting selective retention of the complex in a more reducing cellular environment (Lewis et al. 1999). The hypoxic retention of ^{64}Cu-ATSM was proved to be a reversible phenomenon dependent only pO_2 but not due to irreversible cellular damage such as membrane disruption (Fujibayashi et al. 1997). ^{64}Cu-ATSM is a small lipophilic molecule having neutral square planar structure with high membrane permeability and low redox potential for selective retention within hypoxic tissue (Green 1987; Taniuchi et al. 1997). BALB/c mice were injected subcutaneously into each flank with EMT6 cells from cell culture. After 10 days, ^{64}Cu-ATSM (0.2 MBq) was injected through the tail vein and biodistribution studies were carried out. The uptake of ^{64}Cu-ATSM into the EMT6 tumor showed optimal uptake after 10 min.

Direct comparison of cellular uptake of ^{64}Cu-ATSM and [^{18}F]FMISO in vitro was done by Lewis et al. They found selective uptake of both tracers in hypoxic cells. However, the peak cellular uptake of [^{18}F]FMISO was approximately 15% that of ^{64}Cu-ATSM and occurred after a much longer incubation time (2 h versus 15 min) (Lewis et al. 1999, 2001). This reflects the greater membrane permeability of ^{64}Cu-ATSM than of [^{18}F]FMISO. Also, these studies were confirmed in an in vivo rodent tumor model, in which uptake of ^{64}Cu-ATSM was shown to be dependent upon tissue pO_2, with greater retention of this tracer in hypoxic tissues. These preclinical studies suggested that ^{60}Cu-ATSM could be used clinically to identify hypoxic components of human tumors by PET. However, production of ^{60}Cu and ^{64}Cu requires a special solid target processing system and expensive target material, and hence, its use is likely to be limited.

8 Conclusions

Since detection of hypoxia is very important for therapy, developing hypoxia imaging agents has become an inevitable part of research. Many nitroimidazole and nonnitroimidazole derivatives have been developed for detecting hypoxia, among which a few are already used for clinical studies. Although [^{18}F]FMISO is the first agent used to detect hypoxia, many derivatives are competing with [^{18}F]FMISO, to give better results and become potential agents for imaging of hypoxia tissue. Despite the fact that these derivatives are not perfect hypoxic agents, they definitely hold exceptional potential as hypoxic PET agents.

References

Antunes P, Ginj M, Zhang H, Waser B, Baum RP, Reubi JC, Maecke H (2007) Are radiogallium-labelled DOTA-conjugated somatostatin analogues superior to those labelled with other radiometals? Eur J Nucl Med Mol Imaging 34:982–993

Ballinger JR (2001) Imaging hypoxia in tumors. Semin Nucl Med 31:321–329

Barthel HWH, Collingridge DR, Brown G, Osman S, Luthra SK (2004) In vivo evaluation of [18F]fluoroetanidazole as a new marker for imaging tumour hypoxia with positron emission tomography. Br J Cancer 90:2232–2242

Blower PJ, Lewis JS, Zweit J (1996) Copper radionuclides and radiopharmaceuticals in nuclear medicine. Nucl Med Biol 23:957–980

Breeman WA, Verbruggen AM (2007) The 68Ge/68Ga generator has high potential, but when can we use 68Ga-labelled tracers in clinical routine? Eur J Nucl Med Mol Imaging 34:978–981

Brizel DM, Scully SP, Harrelson JM, Layfield LJ, Bean JM, Prosnitz LR, Dewhirst MW (1996) Tumor oxygenation predicts for the likelihood of distant metastases in human soft tissue sarcoma. Cancer Res 56:941–943

Brown JM (1999) The hypoxic cell: a target for selective cancer therapy—eighteenth Bruce F. Cain memorial award lecture. Cancer Res 59:5863–5870

Busch TM, Hahn SM, Evans SM, Koch CJ (2000) Depletion of tumor oxygenation during photodynamic therapy: detection by the hypoxia marker EF3 [2-(2-nitroimidazol-1[H]-yl)-N-(3,3,3-trifluoropropyl)acetamide]. Cancer Res 60:2636–2642

Cowley AR, Dilworth JR, Donnelly PS, Labisbal E, Sousa A (2002) An unusual dimeric structure of a Cu(I) bis(thiosemicarbazone) complex: implications for the mechanism of hypoxic selectivity of the Cu(II) derivatives. J Am Chem Soc 124:5270–5271

Dearling JL, Lewis JS, Mullen GE, Welch MJ, Blower PJ (2002) Copper bis(thiosemicarbazone) complexes as hypoxia imaging agents: structure-activity relationships. J Biol Inorg Chem 7:249–259

Dolbier WR Jr, Li AR, Koch CJ, Shiue CY, Kachur AV (2001) [18F]-EF5, a marker for PET detection of hypoxia: synthesis of precursor and a new fluorination procedure. Appl Radiat Isot 54:73–80

Fujibayashi Y, Taniuchi H, Yonekura Y, Ohtani H, Konishi J, Yokoyama A (1997) Copper-62-ATSM: a new hypoxia imaging agent with high membrane permeability and low redox potential. J Nucl Med 38:1155–1160

Fukumura T, Okada K, Suzuki H, Nakao R, Mukai K, Szelecsenyi F, Kovacs Z, Suzuki K (2006) An improved 62Zn/62Cu generator based on a cation exchanger and its fully remote-controlled preparation for clinical use. Nucl Med Biol 33:821–827

Graeber TG, Osmanian C, Jacks T, Housman DE, Koch CJ, Lowe SW, Giaccia AJ (1996) Hypoxia-mediated selection of cells with diminished apoptotic potential in solid tumours. Nature 379:88–91

Green MA (1987) A potential copper radiopharmaceutical for imaging the heart and brain: copper-labeled pyruvaldehyde bis(N4-methylthiosemicarbazone). Int J Radiat Appl Instrum B 14:59–61

Green MA, Welch MJ (1989) Gallium radiopharmaceutical chemistry. Nucl Med Biol 16:435

Gronroos T, Bentzen L, Marjamaki P, Murata R, Horsman MR, Keiding S, Eskola O, Haaparanta M, Minn H, Solin O (2004) Comparison of the biodistribution of two hypoxia markers [18F]FETNIM and [18F]FMISO in an experimental mammary carcinoma. Eur J Nucl Med Mol Imaging 31:513–520

Grosu AL, Souvatzoglou M, Roper B, Dobritz M, Wiedenmann N, Jacob V, Wester HJ, Reischl G, Machulla HJ, Schwaiger M, Molls M, Piert M (2007) Hypoxia imaging with FAZA-PET and theoretical considerations with regard to dose painting for individualization of radiotherapy in patients with head and neck cancer. Int J Radiat Oncol Biol Phys 69:541–551

Haynes NG, Lacy JL, Nayak N, Martin CS, Dai D, Mathias CJ, Green MA (2000) Performance of a 62Zn/62Cu generator in clinical trials of PET perfusion agent 62Cu-PTSM. J Nucl Med 41:309–314

He FQ, Deng XL, Wen BX, Liu YP, Sun XR, Xing LG, Minami A, Huang YH, Chen Q, Zanzonico PB, Ling CC, Li GC (2008) Noninvasive molecular imaging of hypoxia in human xenografts: comparing hypoxia-induced gene expression with endogenous and exogenous hypoxia markers. Cancer Res 68:8597–8606

Hnatowich DJ (1977) A review of radiopharmaceutical development with short-lived generator-produced radionuclides other than 99mTc. Int J Appl Radiat Isot 28:169–181

Hockel M, Schlenger K, Aral B, Mitze M, Schaffer U, Vaupel P (1996) Association between tumor hypoxia and malignant progression in advanced cancer of the uterine cervix. Cancer Res 56:4509–4515

Hoigebazar L, Jeong JM, Choi SY, Choi JY, Shetty D, Lee YS, Lee DS, Chung JK, Lee MC, Chung YK (2010) Synthesis and characterization of nitroimidazole derivatives for Ga-68-labeling and testing in tumor xenografted mice. J Med Chem 53:6378–6385

Hoigebazar L, Jeong JM, Hong MK, Kim YJ, Lee JY, Shetty D, Lee YS, Lee DS, Chung JK, Lee MC (2011) Synthesis of (68)Ga-labeled DOTA-nitroimidazole derivatives and their feasibilities as hypoxia imaging PET tracers. Bioorg Med Chem 19:2176–2181

Hossmann KA (2003) Non-invasive imaging methods for the characterization of the pathophysiology of brain ischemia. Acta Neurochir Suppl 86:21–27

Jeong JM, Hong MK, Chang YS, Lee YS, Kim YJ, Cheon GJ, Lee DS, Chung JK, Lee MC (2008) Preparation of a promising angiogenesis PET imaging agent: 68Ga-labeled c(RGDyK)-isothiocyanatobenzyl-1,4,7-triazacyclononane-1,4,7-triacetic acid and feasibility studies in mice. J Nucl Med 49:830–836

Koch CJ (2002) Measurement of absolute oxygen levels in cells and tissues using oxygen sensors and 2-nitroimidazole EF5. Redox Cell Biol Genet, Part A 352:3–31

Komar G, Seppanen M, Eskola O, Lindholm P, Gronroos TJ, Forsback S, Sipila H, Evans SM, Solin O, Minn H (2008) 18F-EF5: a new PET tracer for imaging hypoxia in head and neck cancer. J Nucl Med 49:1944–1951

Kubota K, Tada M, Yamada S, Hori K, Saito S, Iwata R, Sato K, Fukuda H, Ido T (1999) Comparison of the distribution of fluorine-18 fluoromisonidazole, deoxyglucose and methionine in tumour tissue. Eur J Nucl Med 26:750–757

Kumar P, Naimi E, McEwan AJ, Wiebe LI (2010) Synthesis, radiofluorination, and hypoxia-selective studies of FRAZ: a configurational and positional analogue of the clinical hypoxia marker, [18F]-FAZA. Bioorg Med Chem 18:2255–2264

Kumar PSD, Xia H, McEwan AJB, Machulla H-J, Wiebe LI (1999) Fluoroazomycin arabinoside (FAZA): synthesis, 2H and 3H-labelling and preliminary biological evaluation of a novel 2-nitroimidazole marker of tissue hypoxia. J Labelled Compds Radiopharm 42:3–16

Lawrentschuk N, Poon AMT, Foo SS, Putra LGJ, Murone C, Davis ID, Bolton DM, Scott AM (2005) Assessing regional hypoxia in human renal tumours using 18F-fluoromisonidazole positron emission tomography. BJU Int 96:540–546

Lee ST, Scott AM (2007) Hypoxia positron emission tomography imaging with 18f-fluoromisonidazole. Semin Nucl Med 37:451–461

Lehtio K, Oikonen V, Gronroos T, Eskola O, Kalliokoski K, Bergman J, Solin O, Grenman R, Nuutila P, Minn H (2001) Imaging of blood flow and hypoxia in head and neck cancer: initial evaluation with [O-15]H2O and [F-18]fluoroerythronitroimidazole PET. J Nucl Med 42:1643–1652

Lewis JS, Laforest R, Dehdashti F, Grigsby PW, Welch MJ, Siegel BA (2008) An imaging comparison of 64Cu-ATSM and 60Cu-ATSM in cancer of the uterine cervix. J Nucl Med 49:1177–1182

Lewis JS, McCarthy DW, McCarthy TJ, Fujibayashi Y, Welch MJ (1999) Evaluation of 64Cu-ATSM in vitro and in vivo in a hypoxic tumor model. J Nucl Med 40:177–183

Lewis JS, Sharp TL, Laforest R, Fujibayashi Y, Welch MJ (2001) Tumor uptake of copper-diacetyl-bis(N(4)-methylthiosemicarbazone): effect of changes in tissue oxygenation. J Nucl Med 42:655–661

Lord EM, Harwell L, Koch CJ (1993) Detection of hypoxic cells by monoclonal antibody recognizing 2-nitroimidazole adducts. Cancer Res 53:5721–5726

Martin GV, Caldwell JH, Rasey JS, Grunbaum Z, Cerqueira M, Krohn KA (1989) Enhanced binding of the hypoxic cell marker [3H]fluoromisonidazole in ischemic myocardium. J Nucl Med 30:194–201

Maurer RI, Blower PJ, Dilworth JR, Reynolds CA, Zheng Y, Mullen GE (2002) Studies on the mechanism of hypoxic selectivity in copper bis(thiosemicarbazone) radiopharmaceuticals. J Med Chem 45:1420–1431

McCarthy DW, Bass LA, Cutler PD, Shefer RE, Klinkowstein RE, Herrero P, Lewis JS, Cutler CS, Anderson CJ, Welch MJ (1999) High purity production and potential applications of copper-60 and copper-61. Nucl Med Biol 26:351–358

McCarthy DW, Shefer RE, Klinkowstein RE, Bass LA, Margeneau WH, Cutler CS, Anderson CJ, Welch MJ (1997) Efficient production of high specific activity 64Cu using a biomedical cyclotron. Nucl Med Biol 24:35–43

McManus ME, Lang MA, Stuart K, Strong J (1982) Activation of misonidazole by rat liver microsomes and purified NADPH-cytochrome c reductase. Biochem Pharmacol 31:547–552

Nunn A, Linder K, Strauss HW (1995) Nitroimidazoles and imaging hypoxia. Eur J Nucl Med 22:265–280

Obata A, Yoshimi E, Waki A, Lewis JS, Oyama N, Welch MJ, Saji H, Yonekura Y, Fujibayashi Y (2001) Retention mechanism of hypoxia selective nuclear imaging/radiotherapeutic agent cu-diacetyl-bis(N4-methylthiosemicarbazone) (Cu-ATSM) in tumor cells. Ann Nucl Med 15:499–504

Overgaard J (1994) Clinical evaluation of nitroimidazoles as modifiers of hypoxia in solid tumors. Oncol Res 6:509–518

Padhani AR (2005) Where are we with imaging oxygenation in human tumours? Cancer Imaging 5:128–130

Parliament MB, Chapman JD, Urtasun RC, McEwan AJ, Golberg L, Mercer JR, Mannan RH, Wiebe LI (1992) Non-invasive assessment of human tumour hypoxia with 123I-iodoazomycin arabinoside: preliminary report of a clinical study. Br J Cancer 65:90–95

Piert M, Machulla HJ, Picchio M, Reischl G, Ziegler S, Kumar P, Wester HJ, Beck R, McEwan AJB, Wiebe LI, Schwaiger M (2005) Hypoxia-specific tumor imaging with F-18-fluoroazomycin arabinoside. J Nucl Med 46:106–113

Postema EJ, McEwan AJ, Riauka TA, Kumar P, Richmond DA, Abrams DN, Wiebe LI (2009) Initial results of hypoxia imaging using 1-alpha-D: -(5-deoxy-5-[18F]-fluoroarabinofuranosyl)-2-nitroimidazole (18F-FAZA). Eur J Nucl Med Mol Imaging 36:1565–1573

Rajendran JG, Schwartz DL, O'Sullivan J, Peterson LM, Ng P, Scharnhorst J, Grierson JR, Krohn KA (2006) Tumor hypoxia imaging with [F-18] fluoromisonidazole positron emission tomography in head and neck cancer. Clin Cancer Res 12:5435–5441

Rasey JS, Hofstrand PD, Chin LK, Tewson TJ (1999) Characterization of [F-18]fluoroetanidazole, a new radiopharmaceutical for detecting tumor hypoxia. J Nucl Med 40:1072–1079

Rasey JS, Koh WJ, Evans ML, Peterson LM, Lewellen TK, Graham MM, Krohn KA (1996) Quantifying regional hypoxia in human tumors with positron emission tomography of [18F]fluoromisonidazole: a pretherapy study of 37 patients. Int J Radiat Oncol Biol Phys 36:417–428

Reischl G, Dorow DS, Cullinane C, Katsifis A, Roselt P, Binns D, Hicks RJ (2007) Imaging of tumor hypoxia with [I-124] IAZA in comparison with [F-18] FMISO and [F-18]FAZA—first small animal PET results. J Pharm Pharm Sci 10:203–211

Rumsey WL, Patel B, Linder KE (1995) Effect of graded hypoxia on retention of technetium-99m-nitroheterocycle in perfused rat heart. J Nucl Med 36:632–636

Shetty D, Jeong JM, Ju CH, Kim YJ, Lee JY, Lee YS, Lee DS, Chung JK, Lee MC (2010a) Synthesis and evaluation of macrocyclic amino acid derivatives for tumor imaging by gallium-68 positron emission tomography. Bioorg Med Chem 18:7338–7347

Shetty D, Jeong JM, Ju CH, Lee YS, Jeong SY, Choi JY, Yang BY, Lee DS, Chung JK, Lee MC (2010b) Synthesis of novel 68Ga-labeled amino acid derivatives for positron emission tomography of cancer cells. Nucl Med Biol 37:893–902

Sorger D, Patt M, Kumar P, Wiebe LI, Barthel H, Seese A, Dannenberg C, Tannapfel A, Kluge R, Sabri O (2003) [18F]Fluoroazomycinarabinofuranoside (18FAZA) and [18F]Fluoromisonidazole (18FMISO): a comparative study of their selective uptake in hypoxic cells and PET imaging in experimental rat tumors. Nucl Med Biol 30:317–326

Souvatzoglou M, Grosu AL, Roper B, Krause BJ, Beck R, Reischl G, Picchio M, Machulla HJ, Wester HJ, Piert M (2007) Tumour hypoxia imaging with [18F]FAZA PET in head and neck cancer patients: a pilot study. Eur J Nucl Med Mol Imaging 34:1566–1575

Stone HB, Brown JM, Phillips TL, Sutherland RM (1993) Oxygen in human tumors: correlations between methods of measurement and response to therapy. Summary of a workshop held at the National Cancer Institute, Bethesda, Maryland, 19–20 Nov 1992. Radiat Res 136: 422–434

Taniuchi H, Fujibayashi Y, Yonekura Y, Konishi J, Yokoyama A (1997) Hyperfixation of copper-62-PTSM in rat brain after transient global ischemia. J Nucl Med 38:1130–1134

Thomlinson RH, Gray LH (1955) The histological structure of some human lung cancers and the possible implications for radiotherapy. Br J Cancer 9:539–549

Vaupel P, Harrison L (2004) Tumor hypoxia: causative factors, compensatory mechanisms, and cellular response. Oncologist 9(Suppl 5):4–9

Vavere AL, Lewis JS (2007) Cu-ATSM: a radiopharmaceutical for the PET imaging of hypoxia. Dalton Trans 43:4893–4902

Walton MI, Workman P (1987) Nitroimidazole bioreductive metabolism. Quantitation and characterisation of mouse tissue benznidazole nitroreductases in vivo and in vitro. Biochem Pharmacol 36:887–896

Yang DJ, Wallace S, Cherif A, Li C, Gretzer MB, Kim EE, Podoloff DA (1995) Development of F-18-labeled fluoroerythronitroimidazole as a PET agent for imaging tumor hypoxia. Radiology 194:795−800

Yapp DT, Woo J, Kartono A, Sy J, Oliver T, Skov KA, Koch CJ, Adomat H, Dragowska WH, Fazli L, Ruth T, Adam MJ, Green D, Gleave M (2007) Non-invasive evaluation of tumour hypoxia in the shionogi tumour model for prostate cancer with 18F-EF5 and positron emission tomography. BJU Int 99:1154–1160

^{177}Lu/^{90}Y Intermediate-Affinity Monoclonal Antibodies Targeting EGFR and HER2/c-neu: Preparation and Preclinical Evaluation

Denis R. Beckford Vera, Sebastian Eigner, Katerina Eigner Henke, Rene Leyva Montaña, Frantisek Melichar and Milos Beran

Abstract

The epidermal growth factor receptor (EGFR) is a rational target of anticancer therapies due to its overexpression in a variety of malignant epithelial tumors. Nevertheless, this antigen is also present in normal tissues. Consequently, monoclonal antibodies which selectively bind to EGFR-overexpressing tumors will be choice drug candidates for development of radioimmunoconjugates (RIC). Nimotuzumab (h-R3) and trastuzumab are monoclonal antibodies (mAbs) which would preferentially target tissues with EGFR and HER2 overexpression, respectively. In this chapter, we describe preparation and evaluation of the targeting properties of RIC formed by ^{177}Lu/^{90}Y and monoclonal antibodies which selectively target EGFR- and HER2/c-neu-overexpressing tissues. mAbs were labeled with n.c.a. ^{177}Lu/^{90}Y using bifunctional chelating agents. RIC binding properties and toxicity were evaluated in vitro using cell lines with varying antigen expression. In vivo tumor targeting properties of RIC were evaluated in mice bearing colorectal (SNU-C2B) and A431 tumor xenografts. RICs were prepared with specific activities up to 2 GBq/mg without significant loss in biological activity. ^{90}Y-h-R3/trastuzumab increased cell growth inhibition compared with unmodified mAbs or $^{90}YCl_3$ alone in cell lines with overexpression of the target antigen. ^{177}Lu-h-R3 showed significantly higher uptake in A431

D. R. Beckford Vera (✉) · S. Eigner · K. E. Henke · F. Melichar · M. Beran
Department of Radiopharmaceuticals, Nuclear Physics Institute,
Academy of Sciences of the Czech Republic, 250 68 Rez,
Prague, Czech Republic
e-mail: denis.beckford@gmail.com

R. L. Montaña
Department of Radiopharmacy, Center of Isotopes, Guanabacoa,
Ciudad de La Habana, Cuba

R. P. Baum and F. Rösch (eds.), *Theranostics, Gallium-68, and Other Radionuclides*, Recent Results in Cancer Research 194, DOI: 10.1007/978-3-642-27994-2_16,

(22.8 ± 3.1% ID/g) than in SNU-C2B (8.8 ± 4.1% ID/g) xenografts at 72 h post injection, indicating strong association between tumor uptake and EGFR expression levels.

Contents

1 Introduction

Investigation of target-specific radiopharmaceuticals based on monoclonal antibodies (mAbs), their fragments, and peptides for therapy and molecular imaging is increasing due to the availability of new radioisotopes and biomolecules with improved characteristics. As evidence, in the last decade two radioimmunoconjugates (Zevalin and Bexxar) have been approved by the US Food and Drug Administration (FDA) for radioimmunotherapy of refractory non-Hodgkin's lymphoma, which is a great achievement for this therapeutic modality. Unfortunately, the success of RIT in hematologic disease has not been translated to solid tumors yet. Nevertheless, treatment of minimal residual disease, locoregional application, and pretargeted RIT have shown some advances. In addition, several radioimmunoconjugates are under preclinical investigation, and some of them which have shown promising results are already under clinical development (Eckelman 2011).

The epidermal growth factor receptor (EGFR) is a rational target of anticancer therapies due to its overexpression in a variety of malignant epithelial tumors and its correlation with poor prognosis (Rocha-Lima et al. 2007). Among the EGFR family members, FGFR1 (EGFR) and EGFR2 (HER2/neu) are the targeting agents which have shown the most encouraging results in drug development. One of the most widely studied approaches to inhibit EGFR oncogenic expression is use of monoclonal antibodies which bind the extracellular domain of this receptor, inhibiting dimerization and autophosporylation (Kamath and Buolamwini 2006). While EGFRs are overexpressed in tumors, they are ever present in normal tissues. Recently, studies have suggested that, for EGFR associate antigens tumors, monoclonal antibodies with intermediate affinity will favor uptake in EGFR-overexpressing tissues followed by reduction of toxicity in normal tissues (Garrido et al. 2011; Talavera et al. 2009; Li et al. 2005).

Trastuzumab (Herceptin; Genentech Inc., San Francisco, CA, USA) was the first mAb approved by the FDA for treatment of HER2-positive breast cancer. Later, cetuximab (Erbitux) was approved for treatment of metastatic colorectal cancer and squamous cell carcinoma. Relatively new mAbs against EGFRs such as panitumumab, matuzumab, MDX-447, nimotuzumab, and mAb806 are currently under preclinical and clinical evaluation (Rocha-Lima et al. 2007; Reichert 2011).

Nimotuzumab (h-R3; Thera-CIM, BIOMAb-EGFR, Oncosciences) is an IgG1 with intermediate affinity and high specificity to the external domain of the EGFR (Morales-Morales et al. 1999; Mateo et al. 1997; Vallis et al. 2002; Boland and Bebb 2009; Rojo et al. 2010). This drug is approved for marketing in some countries for treatment of squamous cell carcinoma of the head and neck and for glioma for pediatric and adult patients (Reichert 2011). Nimotuzumab is under phase III clinical trials in patients with glioblastoma multiforme and patients with advanced nasopharyngeal cancer (Reichert 2011). ^{99m}Tc-h-R3 has been used for radioimmunoscintigraphy of nodal metastatic disease, but poor correlation between EGFR expression and positive tumor imaging was observed (Vallis et al. 2002; Boswell and Brechbiel 2007). However, encouraging results have been obtained in RIT (phase I clinical trial) of recurrent high-grade glioma after intracavitary administration of h-R3 labeled with ^{188}Re (Boswell and Brechbiel 2007; Casaco et al. 2008).

Residualizing radionuclides, such as ^{90}Y and ^{177}Lu, are potentially more suitable for RIT (Brouwers et al. 2004). ^{90}Y is of particular interest for radiotherapy due to its high-energy pure β-particle emission (Liu 2008; Liu and Edwards 2001a). ^{90}Y is a generator-produced radionuclide, resulting from the decay of ^{90}Sr. ^{90}Y has half-life of 2.7 days, which is short enough to achieve a critical dose rate and at the same time long enough to allow the radiopharmaceutical to be manufactured and delivered for clinical use (Liu 2008; Liu and Edwards 2001a). ^{90}Y forms a very stable complex with 1,4,7,10-tetraazacyclododecane-1,4,7,10-tetraacetate acid (DOTA) derivatives in vivo, hence it is well suited for receptor-based therapeutic radiopharmaceuticals (Liu 2008; Liu and Edwards 2001a; Liu et al. 2002; DeNardo et al. 2003). ^{90}Y is the radionuclide in one of the two FDA-approved radioimmunotherapeutic products for indolent non-Hodgkin's lymphoma. ^{177}Lu ($t_{1/2} = 6.7$ days, $E_\gamma = 0.208$ MeV, $\beta^- = 0.497$ MeV, max range of tissue penetration = 2.0 mm) is being strongly considered for RIT, since it combines the advantages of both ^{90}Y and ^{131}I and the ability to form stable complexes with macrocyclic and acyclic ligands (Liu 2008;

Liu and Edwards 2001a; Ehrhardt et al. 1998; Mausner and Srivastava 1993). Its half-life is appropriate for successful delivery of therapeutic doses to the tumor by radioimmunoconjugates such as monoclonal antibodies. In addition, ^{177}Lu emits two low-energy γ lines with energy of 113 and 208 keV that are suitable for imaging and assessment of delivered doses.

In this chapter, we describe the radiochemistry and preclinical evaluation for successful preparation of radioimmunoconjugates formed by ^{90}Y/^{177}Lu and monoclonal antibodies with intermediate affinity to EGFR (nimotuzumab) and HER2/neu (trastuzumab). Part of the following results has been recently published (Vera et al. 2011; Beckford Vera et al. 2011).

2 Materials and Methods

2.1 Conjugation of Monoclonal Antibodies

Modification of nimotuzumab and trastuzumab with DOTA-NHS, p-SCN-Bn-DOTA, and p-SCN-Bn-DTPA (Macrocyclics, Dallas, TX, USA) was performed as previously described (Vera et al. 2011; Beckford Vera et al. 2011; Xiques et al. 2009). Monoclonal antibodies were mixed with 10-, 20-, 50-, 100-, and 150-fold molar excess of the selected bifunctional chelating agent, and the reaction mixture was incubated overnight at 4°C. The immunoconjugates were purified by ultrafiltration on Vivaspin 6 until the absorbance in the ultrafiltrate at 280 nm was nearly zero. Protein concentration was determined by Bradford assay. Conjugates were stored at 4°C for further use. Immunoconjugates were characterized by SE-HPLC to verify conjugate integrity. About 20 μL of conjugates was injected onto TSK-Gel SW 3,000 (7.5 × 300 mm, 10 μm; TosoHass) column using NaCl 0.9%/NaN_3 0.05% as mobile phase. The flow rate was maintained at 1 mL/min, and the elution was monitored by UV at 280 nm. The average number of chelates linked to an antibody molecule was determined using ^{90}Y by a radioactive method previously described (Lewis et al. 2001). Briefly, 49 μg (10 μL) of the conjugates was added to 30–50 μL NH_4OAc 0.5 mol/L, pH 7.0; afterward, 10–30 μL (3.33×10^{-4} mol/L) of standardized YCl_3 spiked with ^{90}Y solution was added. Immunoconjugates were also analyzed by sodium dodecyl sulfate polyacrylamide gel electrophoresis (SDS–PAGE) under reducing and nonreducing conditions as described previously (Laemmli 1970) using NuPAGE® minigels 4–12% Bis–Tris (10 mm × 10 wells). The electrophoresis was run in an Amersham Biosciences electrophoretic system using NuPAGE® running buffer. Proteins in the gel were visualized by staining and destaining the gel with Coomassie Blue R-250 (BioRad, CA, USA) solutions.

2.2 Flow Cytometric Analysis

Reactivity of DOTA-h-R3 conjugates, with increasing molar excess of DOTA-NHS, to H-125 human lung adenocarcinoma cell line was determined by flow cytometry analysis. Cells were harvested and adjusted to 10^6 cells/mL in RPMI 1640 supplemented with 10.0% fetal bovine serum (FBS; Gibco Laboratories) and penicillin–streptomycin–neomycin antibiotics. Two hundred microliters of cell suspension was added to Lp3 tubes and centrifuged at 3,000 rpm for 5 min. Cells were washed twice with PBD solution pH 7.4, resuspended in 20 μL of saturating amounts of antibody concentration 3.0 μg/mL, and incubated at 4°C for 30 min. The cells were washed twice again with PBS solution and resuspended in 100 μL of 1:20 dilution of the goat anti-human IgG conjugated with fluorescein isothiocyanate (FITC; Dako, Denmark) and incubated at 4°C for 30 min. After washing, cells were resuspended in 500 μL PBS solution and analyzed for immunofluorescence with a fluorescence-activated cell scan (FACS; Ortho Diagnostic Systems, Johnson and Johnson). The immunoreactivity of the DOTA-h-R3 conjugates was expressed as the percentage of positive cells obtained after subtraction of the value given by incubating the cells with isotypic matching nonspecific anti-HLA antibody and with h-R3 alone.

2.3 Radiolabeling

^{177}Lu non-carrier added (n.c.a in 0.05 mol/L HCl), produced indirectly via the $^{176}Yb(n,\gamma)^{177}Yb \rightarrow (\beta^-) \rightarrow {}^{177}Lu$ reaction, was generously donated by Isotope Technologies Garching (ITG, Garching GmbH). Radiolabeling was performed as previously described. Briefly, aliquots of $^{177}LuCl_3$ were mixed with 0.5 mol/L NH_4OAc buffer at pH 7.0, followed by the conjugates. $^{90}YCl_3$ (555 MBq in 22 μL 0.05 M HCl) was purchased from PerkinElmer. Aliquots of $^{90}YCl_3$ (25–518 MBq, 1–12 μL) were added to 20–50 μL 0.5 mol/L NH_4OAc buffer at pH 7.0, followed by 20–50 μL (0.05–0.250 mg) of conjugates. In some cases 5 μL ascorbic acid solution 100 mg/mL was added. Afterward, the reaction mixture was incubated at 42°C for 30 or 60 min.

2.4 Quality Control

For stopping the reaction and binding of any free radiometal, 1/10 of the total radiolabeling reaction volume of DTPA 0.01 mol/L pH 6.0 was added and the mixture was incubated for 15 min at room temperature. Radiometal labeling efficiency and radiochemical purity were determined by thin-layer chromatography performed on SG-ITLC plates (Pall Corporation, USA), using 10% (w/v) ammonium acetate:methanol (1:1) as mobile phase. SE-HPLC was also employed using TSK-Gel SW 3,000 (7.5 × 300 mm, 10 μm; TosoHass) column, with isocratic mobile phase of NaCl 0.9%/NaN_3 0.05% and flow rate of 1.0 mL/min. When needed, radiolabeled conjugates were purified from unbound radiometal by size-exclusion chromatography on PD-10 column eluted with phosphate-buffered saline at 0.01 mol/L.

2.5 Cell Culture

The following human cell lines were used in the in vitro experiments: squamous carcinoma A431 and SCC25, colorectal carcinoma SNU-C2B, glioblastoma-astrocytoma U373 MG, prostate carcinoma DU145, and mama carcinomas HCC-1419 and SK-BR-3. In addition, the human skin fibroblast cell line BJ was used as control. A431, SK-BR-3, and SCC25 cell lines were cultured in DMEM high-glucose medium. U373 MG, SNU-C2B, DU145, and BJ cell lines were cultured in RPMI 1640. All media were supplemented with 10% fetal calf serum and penicillin/streptomycin (penicillin 100 IU/mL, streptomycin 100 μg/mL). During cell culture and cell experiments (unless otherwise stated), cells were grown at 37°C in incubators with humidified air, equilibrated with 5% CO_2.

2.6 Binding Saturation and Competitive Assays

For saturation binding and competitive experiments, A431, SNU-C2B, HCC-1419, and SK-BR-3 cells were cultured at $\sim 2 \times 10^5$ cells/well on 12-well plates (BD Falcon™; Becton–Dickinson, UK) in 1 mL medium for 24 h prior to the studies. Cells were treated with solutions of different concentrations (100 μL/well, 2.7–120.0 nmol/L) of radiolabeled conjugates for the saturation binding assay. For the competitive binding assay, cells were incubated with 100 μL/well (50 ng, ~75,000 cpm/well) of radio-immunoconjugates in cell culture medium and increasing concentrations of unmodified mAbs. After incubating the cells for 3 h at 4°C or 37°C, the medium was discarded and cells were washed with ice-cold phosphate buffer solution (PBS). Cells were lysed using 0.5 mL 0.5 M NaOH containing 5% SDS, and radioactivity was measured in an automatic γ- or β-counter. The nonspecific background binding was studied by adding a 100 times excess of native nimotuzumab or trastuzumab to some wells. Triplicate cell dishes were used for each measuring point. For cell counting, a representative parallel sample from the experiments was trypsinized for about 15 min, and the cells were counted using a fully automated cell analysis system (CASY TT; Roche Innovatis AG, Germany). The mean was used as the cell number for all wells. Dissociation constants (K_d), half-maximal inhibitory concentration (IC_{50}), and maximal binding sites (B_{max}) were estimated from nonlinear fitted curves using GraphPad Prism software (GraphPad Software, Inc., CA, USA). The immunoreactivity fraction of the radio-immunoconjugates was determined using the method described by Konishi et al. (2004) based on competitive binding assay using fixed cell concentration.

2.7 Cytotoxicity Study

For cytotoxic study, A431, SNU-C2B, SCC25, HCC-1419, U373 MG, PC-3, and SK-BR-3 cells were cultured at $\sim 2 \times 10^5$ cells/well on 12-well plates for 48 h. Cells were treated with ^{90}Y-DOTA-Bn-h-R3/Herc with different DOTA-Bn/mAb molar ratios Theraloc®, Herceptin™, and $^{90}YCl_3$ for 10 days, and cell proliferation was then assessed. At corresponding time point, cells were trypsinized, and living cells were counted using CASY TT. The increase in cell number was compared with control samples.

2.8 In Vivo Studies

As previously reported (Vera et al. 2011; Beckford Vera et al. 2011), animal experiments were performed according to the Animals Ethics Committees of the Faculty of Pharmacy (Charles University, Hradec Kralove, Czech Republic) or Institute of Nuclear Research (Husinec-Rez, Czech Republic).

2.9 Influence of Increasing Amount of BFC per mAb

Specific pathogen-free male Wistar rats (3 months old, 165–210 g; Bio Test s.r.o., Konárovice, Czech Republic) were used for biodistribution studies in healthy animals. Each rat was intravenously injected with 0.2 mL ^{177}Lu-DOTA-Bn-h-R3. Three preparations with different DOTA/h-R3 ratios (9, 13, and 15) were tested. The animals were anesthetized, bled, sacrificed, and dissected at 5 min, 1, 24, 48, and 72 h after injection, and organs of interest were collected, rinsed of residual blood, and weighed. Sample activity was measured in an automatic γ-counter (Wizard 3). Tissue activity was calculated in percent of injected dose per gram of tissue (% ID/g) as average of three animals.

2.10 Influence of the Nature of the Chelate on the In Vivo Behavior of the Radioimmunoconjugate

^{177}Lu-DOTA-Bn-h-R3 or ^{177}Lu-DTPA-Bn-h-R3 conjugate ($\sim$10 μg in 0.1 mL normal saline solution, 150–250 kBq) was intravenously injected via tail vein into healthy mice weighing 20–26 g. At 24, 72, and 168 h after injection the mice were anesthetized, euthanized by cervical dislocation, and dissected. Organs of interest were collected, rinsed of residual blood, and weighed. Sample activity was measured in an automatic γ-counter. Tissue activity was calculated in percent of injected dose per gram of tissue (% ID/g) as an average of three or four animals. The influence of the number of chelates per antibody molecule and the nature of the ligand on the in vivo behavior of the conjugates was studied.

2.11 Biodistribution of ^{177}Lu-Nimotuzumab in Mice Bearing SNU-C2B Xenograft

The in vivo studies of ^{177}Lu-DOTA-Bn-h-R3 in tumor model were conducted in female SNU-C2B xenograft-bearing athymic mice. The mice were injected subcutaneously with SNU-C2B tumor cells ($\sim$6–8 million cells per tumor in 100 μL cell culture medium). The tumors were allowed to grow for 2 weeks before the experiments were performed. Mice were tail vein injected with approximately 100 kBq (50 μL, 10 μg) ^{177}Lu-DOTA-Bn-h-R3. Preparation with 50-fold excess of p-SCN-Bn-DOTA to modify nimotuzumab was used. Groups of three animals were anesthetized, bled, sacrificed, and dissected at 3, 24, 48, 72, and 144 h after injection. In addition to the tumors, blood, liver, kidney, muscle, stomach, and skin were collected, weighed, and measured in a γ-counter. The tails were also measured for radioactive content to determine the accuracy of the injections. The percentage of injected dose per gram tissue was determined.

2.12 Biodistribution of ^{177}Lu-Nimotuzumab in Mice Bearing A431 Xenograft

Mice bearing A431 human epithelial carcinoma xenografts were injected intravenously via tail vein with approximately 100–280 kBq (100 μL, 10 μg) ^{177}Lu-DOTA-Bn-h-R3. Groups of three to four animals were anesthetized, euthanized by cervical dislocation, and dissected at 24, 72, 96, 168, 216, and 264 h after injection. In addition, ^{177}Lu-DOTA-Bn-h-R3 conjugate was applied directly into the volume of the tumor tissue for a second group of mice, to study the in vivo behavior of locoregionally applied radioimmunoconjugate. Groups of four animals were anesthetized, euthanized by cervical dislocation, and dissected at 24, 72, and 96 h after injection. At the selected time points for each experiment, blood was collected by cardiac puncture and tumors and main organs were collected, weighed, and measured in an automatic γ-counter. The percent of injected dose per gram of tissue was determined using standards representing the injected dose per animal, and tumor-to-nontumor (T/nT) tissue ratios were also calculated.

2.13 Statistical Analysis

Statistical analysis was performed to compare the results from radiolabeling, in vitro studies, and the differences in tissue uptake among the conjugates using Student's t-test ($p < 0.05$) or analysis of variance (one- or two-way ANOVA test) using the software package GraphPad Prism. The ANOVA test was followed by Bonferroni's multiple-comparison test ($p < 0.05$). The same approach was used to determine the differences between intravenous and locoregional application.

3 Results and Discussion

3.1 Antibody Modification and Radiochemistry

Antitumor antibody therapy has tended to use monoclonal antibodies with the highest affinities. Nevertheless, due to the feature of EGFR, which is overexpressed in tumors but also present in normal tissues, mAbs with very high affinity

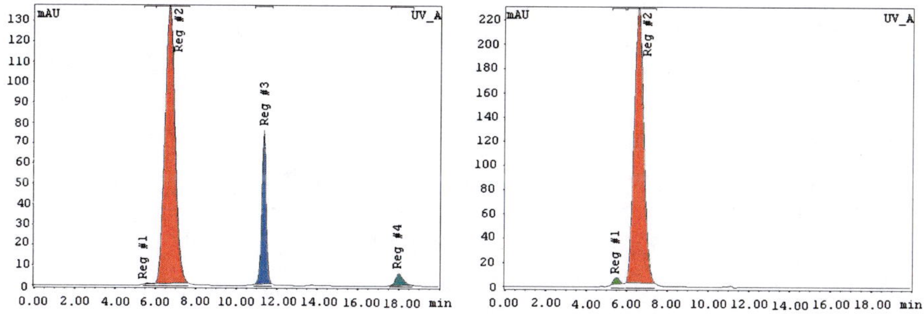

Fig. 1 HPLC profiles of DOTA-mAbs conjugations. (*Right*) reaction mixture. (*Left*) purified conjugate

may negatively affect the biodistribution (Rudnick and Adams 2009). Recent study suggested that nimotuzumab would preferentially target tissues with EGFR overexpression because this antibody relies on bivalent binding for stable attachment to cellular surface (Garrido et al. 2011). Trastuzumab selectively exerts antitumor effects in experimental animals and patients with HER2-amplified breast tumors but not in tumors with normal HER2 expression (Nahta and Esteva 2006; Jasnis and Fiszman 2011). However, the clinical efficacy of trastuzumab is limited, since a significant number of patients with HER2-overexpressing tumors will be initially or eventually resistant to trastuzumab (Jasnis and Fiszman 2011; Vogel et al. 2002). An overall response rate (complete + partial responses) ranging from 15 to 30% has been obtained when used as single agent; however, higher response rates (50–80%) have been reported when used in combination with standard chemotherapy for metastatic disease (Romond et al. 2005). The previous findings led us to choose nimotuzumab and trastuzumab as a $^{90}Y/^{177}Lu$ carrier for anti-EGFR RIT.

Conjugates with high purity and low-grade aggregation were obtained (Fig. 1). The concentration of conjugates ranged from 4.6 to 6.0 mg/mL as determined by Bradford assay. Conjugation reaction gave final chelate-to-mAb ratios of 4, 9, 12, and 15 for 20:1, 50:1, 100:1, and 150:1 chelate-to-mAb molar ratios, respectively. The nature of the ligand did not affect the efficiency of conjugation. The results of flow cytometric analysis suggested that modification of h-R3 through the amino groups, at least until 15 DOTA groups per h-R3, might occur outside of the complementary determining regions which are responsible for the interaction with the antigen (Fig. 2).

Several groups have reported radiolabeling of mAbs with ^{90}Y and ^{177}Lu using acyclic and cyclic ligands (Kukis et al. 1998; Motta-Hennessy et al. 1991; Blend et al. 2003; Griffiths et al. 2003; Coliva et al. 2005; Mohsin et al. 2007; Papi et al. 2010). ^{90}Y and ^{177}Lu were selected due to their appropriate half-lives for labeling mAbs, well-known chelation chemistry, residualization after internalizing mAbs, and reasonable availability (Liu 2008; Nayak and Brechbiel 2009). Since ^{90}Y and ^{177}Lu are used for endoradiotherapeutic purposes, this study was undertaken

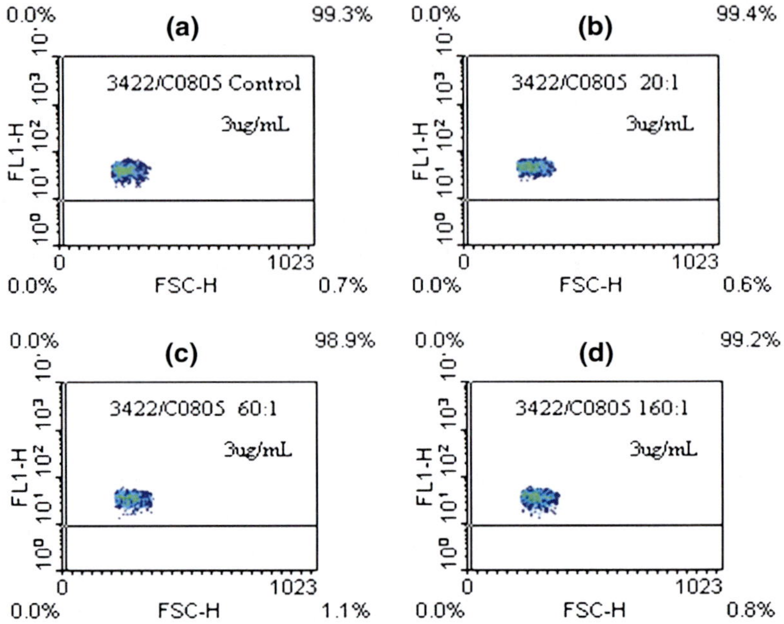

Fig. 2 Flow cytometric analysis. **a** Unmodified nimotuzumab, **b** (DOTA-Bz-SCN)4-5-h-R3, **c** (DOTA-Bz-SCN)8-9-h-R3, **d** (DOTA-Bz-SCN)14-15-h-R3

to obtain radioimmunoconjugates with high specific activities. Radioimmunoconjugates with high chemical and radiochemical purity (>98%) and specific activity up to 2 GBq/mg (Fig. 3) were obtained. The quality of the radionuclide and the volume of radiolabeling mixture influenced the radiolabeling efficiency (Vera et al. 2011). The radiolabeling yields were higher and more reproducible for radioimmunoconjugates formed with p-SCN-Bn-DOTA. Our results are similar to or higher than those previously reported (Xiques et al. 2009; Blend et al. 2003; Coliva et al. 2005; Mohsin et al. 2007; Papi et al. 2010; Liu et al. 2010; Beckford Vera et al. 2007; Lee et al. 2005; Zacchetti et al. 2009). The radiolabeling yields and specific activities achieved are suitable for radiopharmaceutical preparation. It seems to be that the radioactive concentration, not only in the radionuclide preparation but also in the final reaction mixture, plays an important role in the labeling of mAbs with radiometals.

3.2 In Vitro Studies

Radioimmunoconjugates without significant loss of biological activity were obtained. The binding of the radioimmunoconjugate to the cell lines was receptor specific as estimated by the ability to compete with native unmodified mAbs

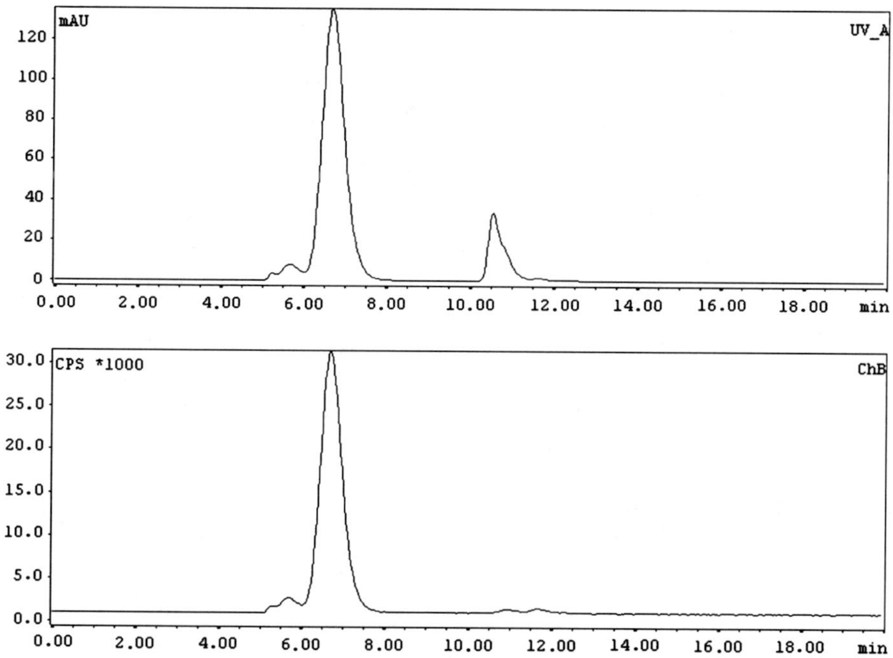

Fig. 3 Typical radioHPLC profile of the $^{177}Lu/^{90}Y$-DOTA-(nimotuzumab/trastuzumab). (*Upper panel*) UV profile in which the main peak (*left*) and the second peak (*right*) correspond to the radioimmunoconjugate DTPA added for quality control, respectively. (*Lower panel*) Radioactive profile; almost all the activity is associated with the mAb

(Vera et al. 2011; Beckford Vera et al. 2011). The immunoreactivity fraction of labeled mAbs was higher than 90%. The results showed that the conjugation and radiolabeling did not significantly affect the immunoreactivity, specificity, and affinity of the conjugate.

The results from the cell proliferation assay with ^{90}Y-mAbs conjugates, unmodified mAbs, and ^{90}Y showed that ^{90}Y-mAbs conjugates increased cell growth proliferation compared with unmodified mAbs and ^{90}Y (Fig. 4). The cell proliferation study showed that ^{90}Y-DOTA-Bn-h-R3 conjugates, such as nimotuzumab, selectively bound to cells with moderate to high EGFR expression due to the necessity for bivalent binding in order to have stable attachment to the cell surface (Garrido et al. 2011). The increased cell proliferation inhibition of ^{90}Y-DOTA-Bn conjugates over unmodified mAbs or ^{90}Y alone in treated cells might be explained due to the crossfire effect of the ^{90}Y radiation and its residualization.

In a previous study (Costantini et al. 2007), trastuzumab labeled with ^{111}In showed 1.2-fold higher toxicity in cultured SKBR3 cells than unlabeled trastuzumab, whereas in a recent study (Rasaneh and Rajabi 2010), trastuzumab labeled with ^{177}Lu showed 4.5-fold higher toxicity in cultured SKBR3 cells than unlabeled

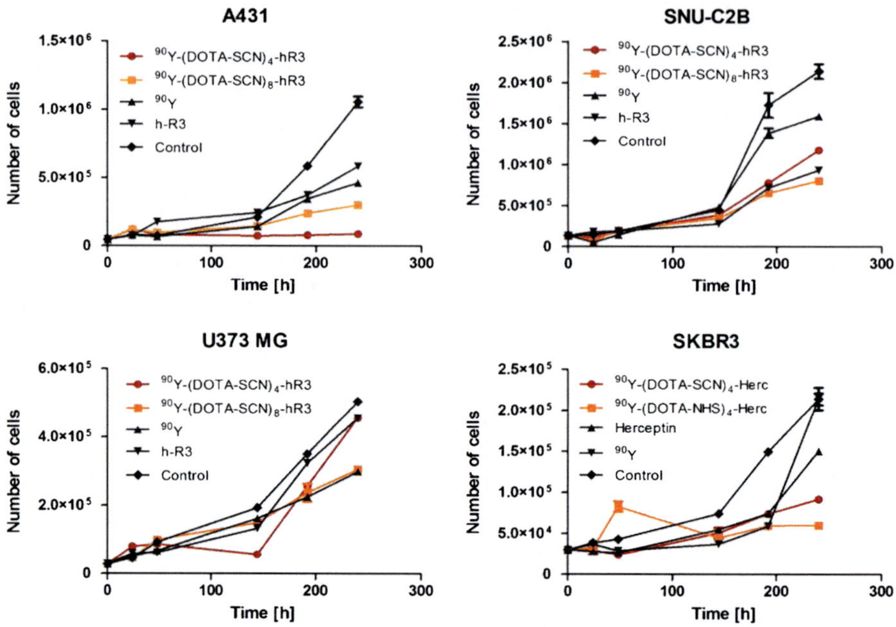

Fig. 4 Cell growth inhibition assay

trastuzumab. In this study, it was observed that ^{90}Y-(DOTA-NHS)$_{8\text{-}9}$-Herceptin and ^{90}Y-(DOTA-Bn)$_{8\text{-}9}$-Herceptin showed 3.0- and 1.7-fold higher toxicity, respectively, than unlabeled trastuzumab.

Consequently, targeted RIT with ^{90}Y-(h-R3 or trastuzumab) could be a promising approach to increase the apoptotic effect of h-R3 and trastuzumab in cells with intermediate to high EGFR expression. Due to the energy and maximal tissue penetration of the beta particles emitted by ^{90}Y and the results of the cytotoxicity studies, ^{90}Y-h-R3/Herc might be suitable for treatment of large-diameter solid tumors.

3.3 In Vivo Studies

Uptake of the ^{177}Lu-DOTA-Bn-h-R3 conjugate in healthy animals behaves similarly to mAbs labeled with radiolanthanides through macrocyclic ligands (Mohsin et al. 2006, 2007). It is well known that monoclonal antibodies are cleared through the reticuloendothelial organs, so spleen and liver uptakes should be commonly observed (Mohsin et al. 2006, 2007). The study revealed that the number of chelators bound to the monoclonal antibody influenced blood clearance and liver uptake. Liver uptake was significantly higher for the ^{177}Lu-DOTA-Bn-h-R3 conjugate with the higher DOTA/h-R3 ratio ($p < 0.01$). These results are in agreement with those reported by Knogler et al. (2006). The uptakes in liver, spleen, and bones observed in our study were lower than those reported by Mohsin et al. (2007) for conjugates modified with 4–5 groups of p-SCN-Bn-DOTA or p-SCN-Bn-DTPA. The release of the radiometal from the conjugate and its metabolism produces nonspecific accumulation of the radioactivity in different tissues and gives us an idea of the stability of the conjugate. Tumor-to-blood ratio calculations are useful for this estimation. The liver-to-blood ratio slightly increased over time for ^{177}Lu-(DTPA-Bn)$_{4\text{-}5}$-h-R3 and ^{177}Lu-(DOTA-Bn)$_{8\text{-}9}$-h-R3 but for ^{177}Lu-(DOTA-Bn)$_{4\text{-}5}$-h-R3, indicating its relatively higher stability compared with the first two mentioned conjugates. The bone-to-blood ratio did not increase with time for all radioimmunoconjugates, suggesting high stability of the metal–ligand complexes.

DOTA derivatives were chosen over DTPA derivatives for labeling the mAbs with ^{90}Y and ^{177}Lu based on the cumulative published data where it is stated that macrocyclic ligands form highly stable complexes with yttrium for in vivo applications (Kukis et al. 1998; Liu et al. 2003; Liu and Edwards 2001b). However, even when those ligands are commercially available, they have the disadvantage of the several parameters which can affect the radiolabeling (Liu 2008). The results of the biodistribution study of ^{177}Lu-DOTA-Bn-h-R3 in mice with SNU-C2B tumor xenograft, previously reported (Vera et al. 2011), showed significant uptake in blood, liver, kidneys, tumor, and skin connected to tumor. The maximum and average uptake of radioimmunoconjugate for SNU-C2B tumor was 10.0 $\pm$ 1.9% ID/g. In this study (Vera et al. 2011), tumor uptake of ^{177}Lu-DOTA-Bn-h-R3 was higher than reported by Alejo Morales-Morales et al. (1999), Velikyan et al. (2005), and Lee et al. (2009), and similar to that reported by Milenic et al. (2002).

Biodistribution studies of ^{177}Lu-(DOTA-Bn)$_n$-h-R3 ($n = 4$–5) were conducted in A431 human epidermal carcinoma xenografts in BALB/c nude mice. Tumor uptake reached a maximum value of 22.4 $\pm$ 3.1% ID/g at 72 h. From 72 to 216 h the average tumor uptake was 18.3 $\pm$ 0.3% ID/g. Bone uptake was low, with maximum value of 2.7 $\pm$ 1.1% ID/g at 24 h and an average of 1.6 $\pm$ 0.5% ID/g from 72 to 264 h. Tumor-to-nontumor tissue ratios reached maximum values of 2.6, 2.4, 6.1, 6.6, 23.5, and 17.5 for blood, liver, spleen, kidneys, muscle, and bone, respectively. When ^{177}Lu-(DOTA-Bn)$_n$-h-R3 ($n = 4$–5) conjugate was applied locoregionally to A431 xenografts in BALB/c nude mice, tumor uptake was significantly higher at 24 and 72 h than observed for intravenous application ($p < 0.001$). Tumor uptake peaked at 32.7 $\pm$ 2.9% ID/g at 72 h. Locoregionally application of the ^{177}Lu-DOTA-Bn-h-R3 conjugate showed T/nT ratios 4.6, 9.8, 10.5, 9.8, and 11.7 times higher for blood, liver, spleen, lungs, and kidneys, respectively, than those calculated for IV application. At 72 h, the T/nT ratios mentioned above were two times higher for locoregional (LR) than IV application. In this study, the tumor uptake values and tumor-to-nontumor ratios are higher than those previously reported for h-R3 and the parental murine mAb labeled with ^{99m}Tc and ^{90}Y (Almqvist et al. 2006; Tabrizi et al. 2006; Morales et al. 2000).

Dosimetric calculations showed that the ^{177}Lu-DOTA-h-R3 radioimmunoconjugate will deliver the highest dose to the tumor. The smaller the tumor, the higher the dose deposited. The results obtained are in agreement with those previously reported for similar ^{177}Lu conjugates (Brouwers et al. 2004; Zacchetti et al. 2009). The results from extrapolation of animal data to humans in this study showed doses to normal organs lower than those reported by Iznaga-Escobar et al. (1998) for ^{99m}Tc-h-R3. It is necessary to mention that, in the extrapolation of the animal data obtained in this study to humans, cross-reactivity of nimotuzumab is not taken into account. In this respect locoregional anti-EGFR RIT might be a more promising option.

4 Conclusion

Radioimmunoconjugates with high radiolabeling yield, radiochemical purity, and specific activity were obtained without significant loss in biological activity. Cytotoxicity studies showed the potential of the radioimmunoconjugates over unmodified monoclonal antibodies to inhibit cell proliferation in cell lines with intermediate to high EGFR/HER2 expression. ^{177}Lu-DOTA-h-R3 may have potential for further evaluation as a radiopharmaceutical for RIT of EGFR-over-expressing tumors.

Acknowledgments We gratefully acknowledge Isotope Technologies Garching GmbH (ITG), Munich, Germany for providing the ^{177}Lu n.c.a. The authors would like to thank Dr. Normando Iznaga and Dr. Angel Casacó (Center of Molecular Immunology) for their outstanding support in the flow cytometric study.

References

Almqvist Y, Steffen AC, Tolmachev V, Divgi CR, Sundin A (2006) In vitro and in vivo characterization of ^{177}Lu-huA33: a radioimmunoconjugate against colorectal cancer. Nucl Med Biol 33(8):991–998

Beckford Vera DR, Eigner S, Beran M, Henke KE, Laznickova A, Laznicek M et al (2011) Preclinical evaluation of (177)lu-nimotuzumab: a potential tool for radioimmunotherapy of epidermal growth factor receptor-overexpressing tumors. Cancer Biother Radiopharm 26(3): 287–297

Beckford Vera DR, Eigner S, Henke KE, Lebeda O, Melichar F, Beran M (2011) Preparation and preclinical evaluation of ^{177}Lu-nimotuzumab targeting epidermal growth factor receptor overexpressing tumors. Nucl Med Biol 39(1):3–13

Beckford Vera DR, Xiques Castillo A, Leyva Montaña R, Pérez Malo M, Gonzalez Casanova E, Zamora Barrabi M (2007) New radioimmunoconjugate 90Y-DOTA-h-R3. Synthesis and radiolabeling. Nucleus 41:3–8

Blend MJ, Stastny JJ, Swanson SM, Brechbiel MW (2003) Labeling anti-HER2/neu monoclonal antibodies with ^{111}In and ^{90}Y using a bifunctional DTPA chelating agent. Cancer Biother Radiopharm 18(3):355–363

Boland WK, Bebb G (2009) Nimotuzumab: a novel anti-EGFR monoclonal antibody that retains anti-EGFR activity while minimizing skin toxicity. Expert Opin Biol Ther 9(9):1199–1206

Boswell CA, Brechbiel MW (2007) Development of radioimmunotherapeutic and diagnostic antibodies: an inside-out view. Nucl Med Biol 34(7):757–778

Brouwers AH, van Eerd JE, Frielink C, Oosterwijk E, Oyen WJ, Corstens FH et al (2004) Optimization of radioimmunotherapy of renal cell carcinoma: labeling of monoclonal antibody cG250 with ^{131}I, ^{90}Y, ^{177}Lu, or ^{186}Re. J Nucl Med 45(2):327–337

Casaco A, Lopez G, Garcia I, Rodriguez JA, Fernandez R, Figueredo J et al (2008) Phase I single-dose study of intracavitary-administered Nimotuzumab labeled with 188 Re in adult recurrent high-grade glioma. Cancer Biol Ther 7(3):333–339

Coliva A, Zacchetti A, Luison E, Tomassetti A, Bongarzone I, Seregni E et al (2005) ^{90}Y Labeling of monoclonal antibody MOv18 and preclinical validation for radioimmunotherapy of human ovarian carcinomas. Cancer Immunol Immunother 54(12):1200–1213

Costantini DL, Chan C, Cai Z, Vallis KA, Reilly RM (2007) (111)In-labeled trastuzumab (Herceptin) modified with nuclear localization sequences (NLS): an Auger electron-emitting radiotherapeutic agent for HER2/neu-amplified breast cancer. J Nucl Med 48(8):1357–1368

DeNardo SJ, DeNardo GL, Yuan A, Richman CM, O'Donnell RT, Lara PN et al (2003) Enhanced therapeutic index of radioimmunotherapy (RIT) in prostate cancer patients: comparison of radiation dosimetry for 1,4,7,10-tetraazacyclododecane-N, N', N", N"'-tetraacetic acid (DOTA)-peptide versus 2IT-DOTA monoclonal antibody linkage for RIT. Clin Cancer Res 9(10 Pt 2):3938S–3944S

Eckelman W (2011) Review of new clinical applications of radiometal labeled radiopharmaceuticals. Nucl Med Biol 38(5):613–616

Ehrhardt GJ, Ketring AR, Ayers LM (1998) Reactor-produced radionuclides at the University of Missouri Research Reactor. Appl Radiat Isot 49(4):295–297

Garrido G, Tikhomirov IA, Rabasa A, Yang E, Gracia E, Iznaga N et al (2011) Bivalent binding by intermediate affinity of nimotuzumab: a contribution to explain antibody clinical profile. Cancer Biol Ther 11(4):373–382

Griffiths GL, Govindan SV, Sharkey RM, Fisher DR, Goldenberg DM (2003) ^{90}Y-DOTA-hLL2: an agent for radioimmunotherapy of non-Hodgkin's lymphoma. J Nucl Med 44(1):77–84

Iznaga Escobar N, Morales AM, Duconge J, Torres IC, Fernandez E, Gomez JA (1998) Pharmacokinetics, biodistribution and dosimetry of ^{99m}Tc-labeled anti-human epidermal growth factor receptor humanized monoclonal antibody R3 in rats. Nucl Med Biol 25(1):17–23

Jasnis MA, Fiszman GL (2011) Molecular Mechanisms of Trastuzumab Resistance in HER2 Overexpressing Breast Cancer. Int J Breast Cancer 2011:11

Kamath S, Buolamwini JK (2006) Targeting EGFR and HER-2 receptor tyrosine kinases for cancer drug discovery and development. Med Res Rev 26(5):569–594

Knogler K, Grunberg J, Novak-Hofer I, Zimmermann K, Schubiger PA (2006) Evaluation of ^{177}Lu-DOTA-labeled aglycosylated monoclonal anti-L1-CAM antibody chCE7: influence of the number of chelators on the in vitro and in vivo properties. Nucl Med Biol 33(7):883–889

Konishi S, Hamacher K, Vallabhajosula S, Kothari P, Bastidas D, Bander N et al (2004) Determination of immunoreactive fraction of radiolabeled monoclonal antibodies: what is an appropriate method? Cancer Biother Radiopharm 19(6):706–715

Kukis DL, DeNardo SJ, DeNardo GL, O'Donnell RT, Meares CF (1998) Optimized conditions for chelation of yttrium-90-DOTA immunoconjugates. J Nucl Med 39(12):2105–2110

Laemmli UK (1970) Cleavage of structural proteins during the assembly of the head of bacteriophage T4. Nature 227(5259):680–685

Lee FT, Mountain AJ, Kelly MP, Hall C, Rigopoulos A, Johns TG et al (2005) Enhanced efficacy of radioimmunotherapy with ^{90}Y-CHX-A"-DTPA-hu3S193 by inhibition of epidermal growth factor receptor (EGFR) signaling with EGFR tyrosine kinase inhibitor AG1478. Clin Cancer Res 11(19 Pt 2):7080s–7086s

Lee S-Y, Hong Y-D, Felipe PM, Pyun M-S, Choi S-J (2009) Radiolabeling of monoclonal anti-CD105 with ^{177}Lu for potential use in radioimmunotherapy. Appl Radiat Isot 67(7–8):1366–1369

Lewis MR, Kao JY, Anderson AL, Shively JE, Raubitschek A (2001) An improved method for conjugating monoclonal antibodies with N-hydroxysulfosuccinimidyl DOTA. Bioconjug Chem 12(2):320–324

Li S, Schmitz KR, Jeffrey PD, Wiltzius JJ, Kussie P, Ferguson KM (2005) Structural basis for inhibition of the epidermal growth factor receptor by cetuximab. Cancer Cell 7(4):301–311
Liu S (2008) Bifunctional coupling agents for radiolabeling of biomolecules and target-specific delivery of metallic radionuclides. Adv Drug Deliv Rev 60(12):1347–1370
Liu S, Edwards DS (2001a) Bifunctional chelators for therapeutic lanthanide radiopharmaceuticals. Bioconjug Chem 12(1):7–34
Liu S, Edwards DS (2001b) Stabilization of (90)Y-labeled DOTA-biomolecule conjugates using gentisic acid and ascorbic acid. Bioconjug Chem 12(4):554–558
Liu S, Pietryka J, Ellars CE, Edwards DS (2002) Comparison of yttrium and indium complexes of DOTA-BA and DOTA-MBA: models for (90)Y- and (111)In-labeled DOTA-biomolecule conjugates. Bioconjug Chem 13(4):902–913
Liu S, Ellars CE, Edwards DS (2003) Ascorbic acid: useful as a buffer agent and radiolytic stabilizer for metalloradiopharmaceuticals. Bioconjug Chem 14(5):1052–1056
Liu Z, Liu Y, Jia B, Zhao H, Jin X, Li F et al (2010) Epidermal growth factor receptor-targeted radioimmunotherapy of human head and neck cancer xenografts using ^{90}Y-labeled fully human antibody panitumumab. Mol Cancer Ther 9(8):2297–2308
Mateo C, Moreno E, Amour K, Lombardero J, Harris W, Perez R (1997) Humanization of a mouse monoclonal antibody that blocks the epidermal growth factor receptor: recovery of antagonistic activity. Immunotechnology 3(1):71–81
Mausner LF, Srivastava SC (1993) Selection of radionuclides for radioimmunotherapy. Med Phys 20(2 Pt 2):503–509
Milenic DE, Garmestani K, Chappell LL, Dadachova E, Yordanov A, Ma D et al (2002) In vivo comparison of macrocyclic and acyclic ligands for radiolabeling of monoclonal antibodies with ^{177}Lu for radioimmunotherapeutic applications. Nucl Med Biol 29(4):431–442
Mohsin H, Jia F, Sivaguru G, Hudson MJ, Shelton TD, Hoffman TJ et al (2006) Radiolanthanide-labeled monoclonal antibody CC49 for radioimmunotherapy of cancer: biological comparison of DOTA conjugates and 149Pm, 166Ho, and ^{177}Lu. Bioconjug Chem 17(2):485–492
Mohsin H, Fitzsimmons J, Shelton T, Hoffman TJ, Cutler CS, Lewis MR et al (2007) Preparation and biological evaluation of ^{111}In-, ^{177}Lu- and ^{90}Y-labeled DOTA analogues conjugated to B72.3. Nucl Med Biol 34(5):493–502
Morales AA, Duconge J, Alvarez-Ruiz D, Becquer-Viart ML, Nunez-Gandolff G, Fernandez E et al (2000) Humanized versus murine anti-human epidermal growth factor receptor monoclonal antibodies for immunoscintigraphic studies. Nucl Med Biol 27(2):199–206
Morales-Morales A, Duconge J, Caballero-Torres I, Nunez-Gandolff G, Fernandez E, Iznaga-Escobar N (1999) Biodistribution of ^{99m}Tc-labeled anti-human epidermal growth factor receptor (EGF-R) humanized monoclonal antibody h-R3 in a xenograft model of human lung adenocarcinoma. Nucl Med Biol 26(3):275–279
Motta-Hennessy C, Sharkey RM, Goldenberg DM (1991) Labeling of monoclonal antibody conjugates with ^{90}Y. Int J Rad Appl Instrum A 42(5):421–426
Nahta R, Esteva FJ (2006) HER2 therapy: molecular mechanisms of trastuzumab resistance. Breast Cancer Res 8(6):215
Nayak TK, Brechbiel MW (2009) Radioimmunoimaging with longer-lived positron-emitting radionuclides: potentials and challenges. Bioconjug Chem 20(5):825–841
Papi S, Martano L, Garaboldi L, Rossi A, Cremonesi M, Grana CM et al (2010) Radiolabeling optimization and reduced staff radiation exposure for high-dose ^{90}Y-ibritumomab tiuxetan (HD-Zevalin). Nucl Med Biol 37(1):85–93
Rasaneh S, Rajabi H (2010) Hossein Babaei M, Johari Daha F. Toxicity of trastuzumab labeled ^{177}Lu on MCF7 and SKBr3 cell lines. Appl Radiat Isot 68(10):1964–1966
Reichert JM (2011) Antibody-based therapeutics to watch in 2011. MAbs 3(1):76–99
Rocha-Lima CM, Soares HP, Raez LE, Singal R (2007) EGFR targeting of solid tumors. Cancer Control 14(3):295–304
Rojo F, Gracias E, Villena N, Cruz T, Corominas JM, Corradino I et al (2010) Pharmacodynamic trial of nimotuzumab in unresectable squamous cell carcinoma of the head and neck: a SENDO foundation study. Clin Cancer Res 16(8):2474–2482

Romond EH, Perez EA, Bryant J, Suman VJ, Geyer CE Jr, Davidson NE et al (2005) Trastuzumab plus adjuvant chemotherapy for operable HER2-positive breast cancer. N Engl J Med 353(16):1673–1684

Rudnick SI, Adams GP (2009) Affinity and avidity in antibody-based tumor targeting. Cancer Biother Radiopharm 24(2):155–161

Tabrizi M, Tseng C, Roskos L (2006) Elimination mechanisms of therapeutic monoclonal antibodies. Drug Discov Today 11(1–2):81–88

Talavera A, Friemann R, Gomez-Puerta S, Martinez-Fleites C, Garrido G, Rabasa A et al (2009) Nimotuzumab, an antitumor antibody that targets the epidermal growth factor receptor, blocks ligand binding while permitting the active receptor conformation. Cancer Res 69(14):5851–5859

Vallis KA, Reilly RM, Chen P, Oza A, Hendler A, Cameron R et al (2002) A phase I study of ^{99m}Tc-hR3 (DiaCIM), a humanized immunoconjugate directed towards the epidermal growth factor receptor. Nucl Med Commun 23(12):1155–1164

Velikyan I, Sundberg AL, Lindhe O, Hoglund AU, Eriksson O, Werner E et al (2005) Preparation and evaluation of (68)Ga-DOTA-hEGF for visualization of EGFR expression in malignant tumors. J Nucl Med 46(11):1881–1888

Vogel CL, Cobleigh MA, Tripathy D, Gutheil JC, Harris LN, Fehrenbacher L et al (2002) Efficacy and safety of trastuzumab as a single agent in first-line treatment of HER2-overexpressing metastatic breast cancer. J Clin Oncol 20(3):719–726

Xiques CA, Olive KI, Gonzalez EC, Beckford D, Montaña RL, Alvarez AM, Alvarez EO (2009) An adapted purification procedure to improve the quality of ^{90}Y for clinical use. Radiochim Acta 97(97):739–746

Zacchetti A, Coliva A, Luison E, Seregni E, Bombardieri E, Giussani A et al (2009) (177)Lu- labeled MOv18 as compared to (131)I- or (90)Y-labeled MOv18 has the better therapeutic effect in eradication of alpha folate receptor-expressing tumor xenografts. Nucl Med Biol 36(7):759–770

Part III
Molecular Imaging Using ^{68}Ga labeled Tracers

Divergent Role of ^{68}Ga-Labeled Somatostatin Analogs in the Workup of Patients with NETs: AIIMS Experience

Niraj Naswa and C. S. Bal

Abstract

Neuroendocrine tumors (NETs) encompass a wide range of rare and heterogeneous neoplasms arising from the neural crest. Diagnosis of NETs is conventionally done by a combination of common clinical symptoms and biochemical evidence of hormonal excess, which these tumors are known to secrete. After a diagnosis of NET is established, a search for its localization is carried out using common morphologic imaging methods such as ultrasonography, computed tomography (CT), and magnetic resonance imaging (MRI). The main problem with structural imaging is, however, its inability to distinguish between endocrine and exocrine lesions. Functional imaging of NETs started with use of iodine-131-meta-iodobenzylguanidine (^{131}I-MIBG) and has come a long way since. From accurate demonstration of functioning tumors to detection of small and occult lesions, functional imaging has penetrated almost every aspect of NET management. Procedures such as $^{131/123}$I-MIBG, ^{111}In-Octreoscan and others are rapidly giving way to use of PET/CT based on the superior resolution of the system and the availability of target-specific positron-emitting radiotracers. The availability of ^{68}Ga from generator-based radionuclide systems, namely ^{68}Ge/^{68}Ga generators, opened up a new era of molecular imaging for NETs. A multitude of somatostatin analogs can be easily radioliganded with ^{68}Ga using heterocyclic macromolecular bifunctional chelating systems for targeted diagnosis of somatostatin receptor-expressing tumors, used most effectively to date for detection of NETs. This chapter focuses on our experience at the All India Institute of Medical Sciences, New Delhi regarding the divergent roles of ^{68}Ga-labeled somatostatin analogs in the workup of patients with NETs.

N. Naswa · C. S. Bal (✉)
Department of Nuclear Medicine, AIIMS, Ansari Nagar,
New Delhi 110029, India
e-mail: CSBal@hotmail.com

R. P. Baum and F. Rösch (eds.), *Theranostics, Gallium-68, and Other Radionuclides*,
Recent Results in Cancer Research 194, DOI: 10.1007/978-3-642-27994-2_17,

Contents

1 Introduction

Neuroendocrine tumors (NETs) constitute a heterogeneous group of neoplasms that have been postulated to originate from a common precursor cell population (Rindi et al. 2001). The system includes endocrine glands, such as the pituitary, the parathyroid, and the [neuroendocrine (NE)] adrenals, as well as endocrine islets within glandular tissue (thyroid or pancreas) and cells dispersed between exocrine cells, such as endocrine cells of the digestive and respiratory tracts, and the diffuse endocrine system (Solcia et al. 1999, 2000; Rindi et al. 2000). Because these cells share a number of antigens with nerve elements, the term "neuroendocrine" is also used to denote such cell types (Rindi et al. 2000).

NETs originating from the gastrointestinal (GI) tract, along with similar tumors originating from the lungs and thymus, have traditionally been defined as "carcinoid tumors" (Oberg 2002). Some NETs may occasionally show very aggressive behavior and become highly malignant (poorly differentiated NETs) and retain many multipotent differentiation capacities (Solcia et al. 2000). Such features include the ability to produce and secrete a variety of metabolically active substances (amines and peptides) and cause distinct clinical syndromes (Lamberts et al. 2001).

In addition, NETs possess neuroamine uptake mechanisms and/or specific receptors at the cell membrane, such as somatostatin (SSTRs) receptors, which can be of great value in identifying and localizing these tumors as well as being useful in their therapy (Kaltsas et al. 2001). NETs may occur either sporadically or as part of familial syndromes; the latter are associated with particular genetic defects, a number of which have recently been delineated at molecular level (Calender 2000).

2 Epidemiology

NETs are very rare tumors (fewer than 2 cases per 100,000). They account for only 0.5% of all malignancies. Female preponderance has been observed under the age of 50 years in appendiceal location. Main primary sites are gastrointestinal tract (62–67%) and lung (22–27%). In the last decades, the incidence has been rising. This might be due to greater awareness, improved diagnostic tools, or a change in definition. Presentation with metastatic disease accounts for 12–22% cases. In metastatic disease, survival has increased since 1992, when treatment with octreotide became largely available in The Netherlands (Taal and Visser 2004). The 5-year survival is mainly associated with stage: 93% in local disease, 74% in regional disease, and 19% in metastatic disease.

3 Our Study

^{68}Ga-Somatostatin receptor (SR) PET/CT using 1,4,7,10-tetraazacyclododecane-1,4,7,10-tetraacetic acid (DOTATOC)-Phe^{1}-Tyr^{3}-octreotide or DOTANOC (DOTA)-NaI^{3}-octreotide started at our center from October 2006, and so far 700 patients with various types of neuroendocrine tumors have been imaged for different indications. For a better overview, the role of ^{68}Ga somatostatin receptor (SR) PET/CT has been divided into sections in this chapter to discuss the role of the tracer in each NET, in order of frequency performed at our center. Figure 1 illustrates the relative frequencies of the different NETs imaged at our center. For simplicity of discussion in the text, the results of ^{68}Ga-DOTANOC PET/CT have been highlighted.

4 Gastroenteropancreatic Neuroendocrine Tumors (GEP-NETs)

Perhaps of all the NETs, tumors arising from the gastrointestinal tract are the most common. GEP-NETs have been traditionally classified into two main groups:

1. Carcinoids
2. Endocrine pancreatic tumors (EPTs).

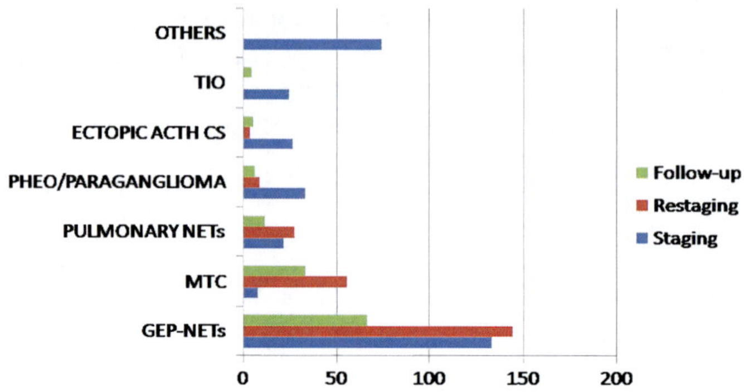

Fig. 1 Bar diagram showing the approximate frequencies of different neuroendocrine tumors referred for ^{68}Ga-SR PET/CT imaging at our center. The most common indication for referral has been gastroenteropancreatic tumors (GEP-NETs)

The diverse and amorphous nature of GEP-NETs has led to a confused, overlapping, and changing terminology. In general, aggressiveness (malignancy), secretion (of hormones), and anaplasia (dissimilarity between tumor cells and normal cells) tend to go together, but there are many exceptions, which have contributed to the confusion in terminology. A proper understanding of the classification is thus important.

5 Classification

In 2000, the WHO introduced a classification system for NETs, which was updated in 2004 and most recently in 2010, differentiating between the terms NET and neuroendocrine carcinoma (NEC) (Kloppel et al. 2004). Important parameters in this classification include angioinvasion, proliferation index (Ki-67, MIB-1), and mitoses. Current classification of these tumors includes three categories and is presented in Table 1.

Although the WHO classification provides substantial information on tumor biology, complete prognostic assessment using these parameters is not enough. The most common NETs are the gastroenteropancreatic tumors (GEP-NETs), representing a heterogeneous group with different clinical behavior and prognosis. Hence, proper stratification is required to separate these tumors into different entities so that a group-selective treatment plan can be adopted. This prompted the European Neuroendocrine Tumor Society (ENETS) to issue guidelines on GEP-NETs (Rindi et al. 2006, 2007). A tumor–node–metastases (TNM) classification was later found to be clinically relevant by Fisher et al. (2008). In addition, a tumor grading system based on the mitotic count per square millimeter of tumor and the Ki-67 index has been proposed by ENETS (G1, G2, and G3) (Table 1).

Table 1 WHO classification of neuroendocrine tumors. Also shown in the extreme right column is the grading system proposed by the European Neuroendocrine Tumor Society (ENETS)

Type	Size (cm)	Ki-67 index (%)	Tumor grade (proposed later by ENETS)
Well-differentiated NETs	<2	<2	G1
Well-differentiated NECs	>2	>2, angioinvasion	G2
Poorly differentiated NECs	>2	>20	G3

6 Functional Imaging of GEP-NETs

Primary neuroendocrine tumors (NETs) are often small and grow slowly. This often makes their identification and localization difficult. The introduction in 1994 of routine clinical use of single-photon emission computed tomography (SPECT) with metalloradiopharmaceutical ^{111}In-diethylene-triamine-pentaacetic acid (DTPA)-octreotide (Octreoscan) spurred the development of somatostatin analogs labeled with therapeutic and PET radiometals. However, the acyclic bifunctional chelator (BFC) DTPA conjugated via one of the carboxyl group with the targeting vector molecule turned out to be unsuitable for use with radiometals other than In(III) because of its in vivo instability (Harrison et al. 1991). Consequently, a DOTA-substituted octreotide DOTA-D-Phe^1-Tyr^3-octreotide (DOTATOC) was synthesized (Heppeler et al. 1999). One of the most widely used macrocyclic frameworks to design BFCs is 1,4,7,10-tetraazacyclododecane (Mäcke and Good 2003). 1,4,7,10-tetraazacyclododecane-1,4,7,10-tetraacetic acid (DOTA) is an octacoordinating ligand based on tetraazacyclododecane, in which each nitrogen atom bears an acetic substituent. Macrocyclic chelators provide exceptional inertness as well as high thermodynamic stability of the complexes. A disadvantage is the requirement for harsh labeling conditions (high temperature) to achieve high labeling yield because of the low kinetics of complex formation.

7 Studies with SRS (Somatostatin Receptor Scintigraphy)

^{111}In-Pentetreotide (Octreoscan) has proven to be an important diagnostic tool for GEP-NETs (Lamberts et al. 1990, 1991; Krausz et al. 1998; Schillaci et al. 1997, 2000; Krenning et al. 1993). It has been reported to be more sensitive than conventional imaging modalities (CIM) by some authors (Krenning et al. 1993). Somatostatin receptor scintigraphy (SRS) with ^{111}In-DTPA-octreotide however suffers from the drawbacks of the limited resolution of SPECT technology as well as unfavorable biodistribution in liver and spleen, obscuring small lesions.

8 Studies with ^{68}Ga-Labeled Octreotide Analogs

Several different DOTA peptides (DOTATOC, DOTANOC, and DOTATATE) have been used in this clinical setting for either NET diagnosis or peptide-based radioreceptor therapy (PRRT). The utility of ^{68}Ga-SR PET/CT in this regard ranges from diagnosis of disease extent and as a preliminary procedure to evaluate SSTR expression before the start of PRRT or cold somatostatin analog (SSA) treatment. Several studies in the past have established the efficacy of ^{68}Ga PET/CT imaging in NETs with varying results (Srirajaskanthan et al. 2010; Ambrosini et al. 2010; Maecke et al. 2005; Gabriel et al. 2007).

At our center, the most important application of this radiotracer has undoubtedly been evaluation of patients with GEP-NETs. This is a well-established and regular procedure and penetrates into many aspects of GEP-NET management which include: (a) staging patients with already diagnosed NETs, (b) detection of sites of recurrence in patients with treated NETs (restaging), (c) diagnosis of patients suspected of having NET based on clinical features or biochemical evidence of hormone excess, (d) selection of potential candidates for cold SSA or PRRT, and (e) monitoring response to therapy in such patients.

9 ^{68}Ga-DOTATOC/NOC Synthesis

^{68}Ga-DOTANOC synthesis was carried out by the Radiopharmacy Unit of the Nuclear Medicine Department, All India Institute of Medical Sciences (AIIMS), following procedures previously detailed by Zhernosekov et al. (2007) and briefly summarized here. A 30–50 mCi ^{68}Ge/^{68}Ga generator (Cyclotron Co. Ltd.; Obninsk, Russia) was eluted using 0.1 M HCl. The eluent was loaded on a miniaturized column of organic cation exchanger resin for preconcentration and prepurification (using 80% acetone/0.15 M HCl). The processed ^{68}Ga (half-life, 68.3 min; β^+ 88%; $E^{\beta+}$ maximum, 1.9 MeV) was directly eluted with 97.7% acetone/0.05 M HCl into the reaction vial containing 30–50 μg DOTANOC/TOC. Synthesis was carried out at approximately 126°C for 10–15 min. This was followed by removal of labeled peptide from unlabeled peptide using reversed-phase C-18 column, using 400 μL ethanol. This was further diluted with normal saline and passed through 0.22-μm filter to obtain sterile preparation for injection. Labeling yield >95% was achieved within 10–15 min.

10 ^{68}Ga-DOTA-Peptide Imaging Protocol

^{68}Ga-DOTANOC PET/CT was performed on a dedicated PET/CT unit (Biograph 2, Siemens Healthcare). Somatostatin analog therapy was stopped prior to PET/CT: short-acting analogs for 3 days before PET/CT and long-acting analogs for 4–6 weeks. Fasting was not mandatory. A dose of 132–222 MBq (4–6 mCi) of

^{68}Ga-DOTANOC was injected intravenously (IV). After a 45- to 60-min uptake period, patients underwent PET/CT. No IV contrast agent was used. In the PET/CT system, the CT acquisition was performed with slice thickness of 4 mm and pitch of 1 on a helical dual-slice CT unit. Images were acquired using a matrix of 512 × 512 pixels and pixel size of 1 mm. After the CT acquisition, the table was moved toward the field of view (FOV) of PET, and PET acquisition of the same axial range was started with the patient in the same position. The PET components of the PET/CT system are based on a full-ring lutetium oxyorthosilicate PET system. Three-dimensional PET acquisition was performed from the base of the skull, including the pituitary fossa, to the mid thighs. Additional spot views were obtained when necessary. PET data were acquired using a matrix of 128 × 128 pixels and slice thickness of 1.5 mm. CT-based attenuation correction of the emission images was used. PET images were reconstructed by iterative method using ordered subset expectation maximization (two iterations and eight subsets). After completion of PET acquisition, the reconstructed attenuation-corrected PET images, CT images, and fused images of matching pairs of PET and CT images were available for review in the axial, coronal, and sagittal planes, as well as in maximum-intensity projections and in 3D cine mode.

11 Normal Biodistribution of ^{68}Ga-Labeled Somatostatin Peptides

^{68}Ga-DOTANOC is a tracer for somatostatin receptor-based PET imaging. It has predominant affinity for somatostatin receptors 2, 3, and 5 (SSTR2, 3, 5) (Kaemmerer et al. 2011). Hence it is physiologically distributed in organs which normally express high levels of SSTRs. It is important to be aware of the physiologic distribution of this tracer before attempting to interpret the pathologic sites of uptake. The highest uptake of ^{68}Ga-DOTANOC is seen in the spleen, which is often considered the reference organ on ^{68}Ga-DOTANOC PET/CT imaging (Fig. 2). Uptake in the pituitary and adrenal glands is also physiologic and constant. Mild uptake is seen in the liver and the thyroid gland, although uptake in the thyroid gland is quite variable. Mild, variable uptake has also been reported in the pancreas, especially the uncinate process (Castellucci et al. 2011). Physiologic excretion through the kidneys and the urinary bladder makes these organs evident on the PET/CT scan.

12 Sporadic GEP-NETs

The average sensitivity and specificity of ^{68}Ga-DOTANOC PET/CT imaging for GEP-NET evaluation have been 78.2 and 92.5%, respectively, for detection of primary tumor (Fig. 3). These values are rather similar to those previously described in previous studies with this agent (Gabriel et al. 2007). Most disappointing has been however detection of biochemically confirmed diagnosis of insulinoma, with a detection rate of only 18%. This limitation of SRS-based

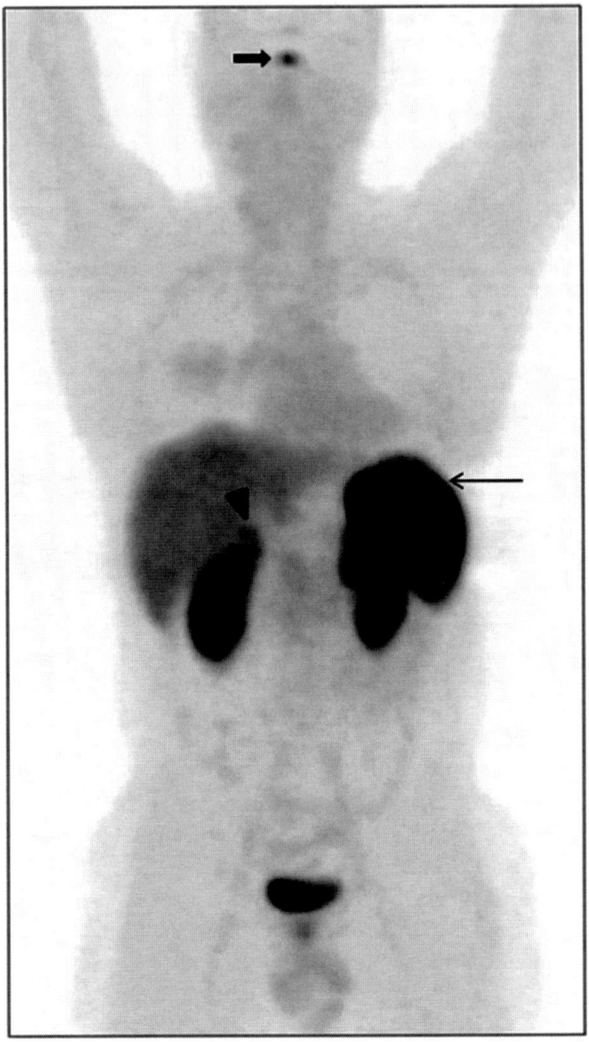

Fig. 2 ^{68}Ga-DOTANOC whole-body maximum-intensity projection (MIP) image showing the biodistribution of the radiotracer. Spleen shows the highest uptake on PET imaging and can be considered as the reference organ (*arrow*). Physiological uptake is seen in the pituitary (*bold arrow*) and adrenal glands (*arrowhead*). Mild uptake is seen in the liver, while excretion of the tracer through the urinary tract renders visualization of kidneys and urinary bladder evident

imaging has been previously acknowledged (Zimmer et al. 1996). Uptake analysis has shown that pancreatic tumors have higher uptake than other primary sites. This might be because of the fact that pancreatic NETs are usually well differentiated with higher expression of SSTR2A receptor (Prasad et al. 2010; Campana et al. 2010) (Fig. 4). One of the important concerns in this aspect has been the occasional high degree of uptake in the pancreatic head, which can give rise to false positives leading to unnecessary surgical procedures. Recent reviews routinely mention this finding of increased uptake in the head of pancreas as physiological (Ruf et al. 2011). However, this problem has not been a concern of late with increased experience in reporting such studies and was therefore a part of the

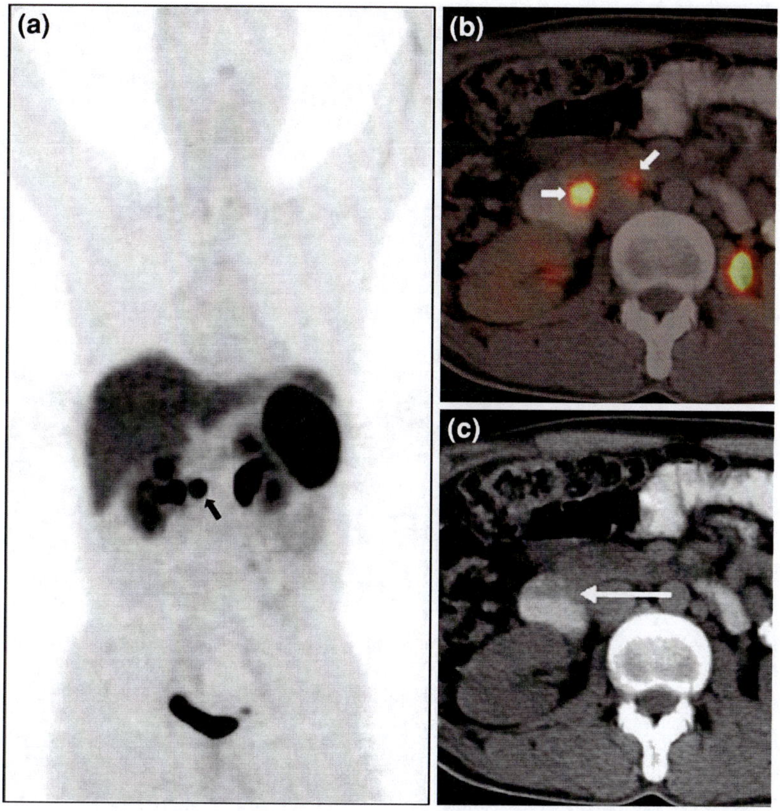

Fig. 3 A 38-year-old male with clinical features suggestive of gastrinoma and elevated serum gastrin level (1,400 pg/ml) who presented with no apparent abnormality on conventional contrast-enhanced CT (CECT) and a suspicious lesion in the duodenum on upper-GI endoscopy underwent ^{68}Ga-DOTANOC PET imaging for confirmation of diagnosis and localization of a possible source. Whole-body PET MIP image shows a focal area of increased tracer uptake in the abdomen (**a**, *bold arrow*). Axial PET/CT image (**b**) shows two focal areas of uptake in the region of duodenum (*bold arrows*), later found to be the primary tumor in second part of duodenum, and a small regional lymph node confirmed to be well-differentiated NET on histopathological analysis. ^{68}Ga-DOTANOC PET/CT not only helped in confirming the diagnosis but also revealed the involved regional node, removal of which reduces the chances of recurrence in this case. Axial unenhanced CT shows no apparent abnormality in the duodenum (**c**, *arrow*)

preliminary hardships. The average sensitivity and specificity of ^{68}Ga-DOTANOC PET/CT for detecting metastatic disease are 97.4% and 100%, respectively. The high rate of positivity obtained with in vivo ^{68}Ga-DOTANOC PET/CT is not surprising since high-affinity somatostatin binding sites have been found in vitro on most GEP endocrine tumors (Ruf et al. 2011; Reubi et al. 1991). The majority of these tumors contain high numbers of SSTRs, homogeneously distributed throughout the tumor and expressed at both primary and metastatic sites (Reubi et al. 1991) (Fig. 5).

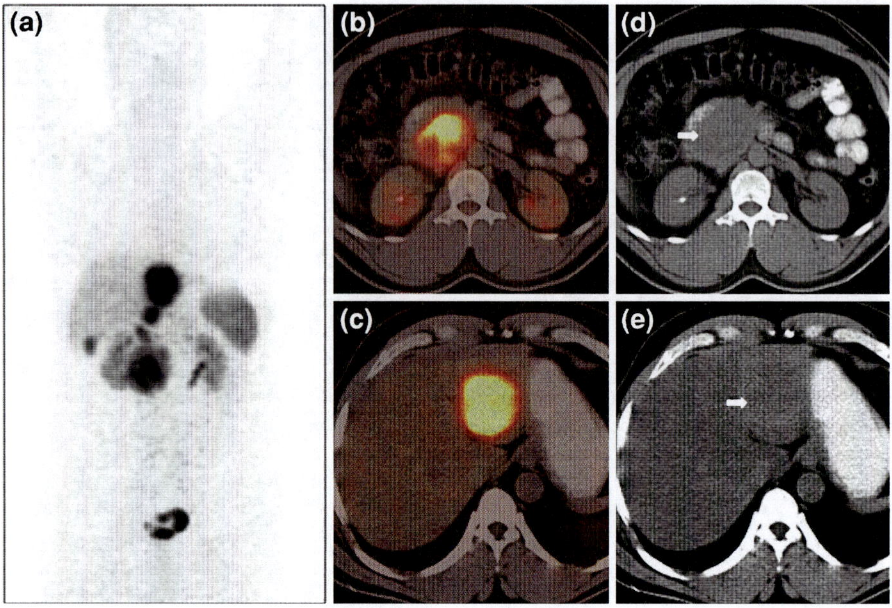

Fig. 4 A 50-year-old male with well-differentiated neuroendocrine carcinoma of pancreas with liver metastases underwent staging ^{68}Ga-DOTANOC PET/CT imaging. Whole-body PET MIP image shows intense tracer uptake in the abdomen at multiple locations (**a**). Axial PET/CT images show increase tracer uptake in the pancreatic head (**b**) and liver (**c**). Corresponding unenhanced CT images show a homogeneous soft tissue mass involving the head of pancreas (**d**, *bold arrow*) and liver lesion on a fatty liver background (**e**, *bold arrow*). The patient is under treatment with ^{177}Lu-DOTATATE PRRT therapy and shows stable disease on follow-up imaging

This has been the best modality to detect metastases in lymph nodes and bones (Putzer et al. 2009), including at our center, leading to comprehensive whole-body assessment and subsequent therapy planning. Liver is the most common site of metastases of GEP-NETs. Although no significant difference is seen in the evaluation of liver lesions when compared with CT or MRI, it is important from a prognostic point of view. Patients with documented liver metastases routinely undergo ^{68}Ga-DOTANOC and ^{18}F-FDG (fluorodeoxyglucose) PET/CT at our center, if possible. This often helps in selecting the best possible treatment for such patients, as a combination of these two imaging modalities is known to help classify these tumors into appropriate differentiation categories with an acceptable degree of accuracy. Well-differentiated tumors are mostly treated with octreotide-based regimes, while less-differentiated neoplasms are known to respond to combined chemotherapy using etoposide and cisplatin (Reubi et al. 1991; Moertel et al. 1991; Hainsworth et al. 2006).

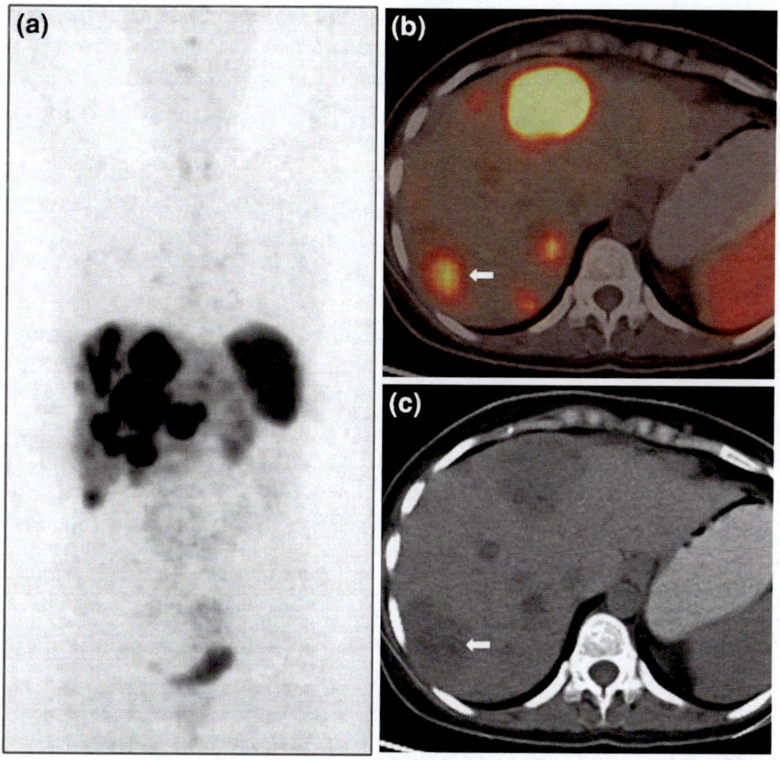

Fig. 5 A 35-year-old female with carcinoid tumor of colon (post surgery) and multiple liver metastases underwent restaging ^{68}Ga-DOTANOC PET/CT imaging to explore the possibility of octreotide therapy. ^{68}Ga-DOTANOC whole-body maximum-intensity projection (MIP) image revealed intense tracer avidity in the liver lesions (**a**) shown on PET/CT (**b**) and unenhanced CT images (**c**). Patient underwent therapy with long-acting octreotide analog (Sandostatin) and is stable 6 months post therapy on follow-up PET imaging

13 Metastatic GEP-NETs with Occult/Uncertain Primary Tumor

Neuroendocrine tumors account for about 2–4% of carcinoma of unknown primary site (CUP) and are often mentioned separately because this entity belongs to a treatable subset (Hainsworth et al. 2006). Identification of the primary site is of prime importance as many aspects of tumor management are dependent on it, ranging from disease prognosis, treatment outcomes, to survival rates. Although detection of the primary tumor in patients with metastatic NET may not change the disease stage, its detection and removal can prevent the patient from having significant local symptoms; e.g., small bowel NETs are notorious for causing desmoplastic reaction and adjacent fibrosis which can cause obstructive features. SRS using ^{111}In-DTPA-octreotide has also been explored to detect occult primary sites in patients with metastatic GEP-NETs with a detection rate of 39% (Savelli et al. 2004). The role of PET/CT using ^{68}Ga-labeled somatostatin analogs to localize the primary tumor in patients with CUP-NET was first assessed by Prasad et al. (2010). They demonstrated that ^{68}Ga-DOTANOC PET/CT was able to localize the primary tumor in 59% of the patients enrolled, with an overall change in management in 10% of cases. A study from our center has found similar results, although the number of patients was less compared with their study (Naswa et al. 2012). A detection rate of 60% has been observed in our series, with midgut being the most common site of primary tumor localization (Fig. 6). In patients where no primary could be localized, several hypotheses can be put forward as explanations. First, there may be receptor downregulation which hinders tracer binding and detection. The size of the tumor might be too small to be detected by the resolution of the imaging system. Finally, dedifferentiation of tumor cells is another possibility, causing failure to detect on ^{68}Ga-DOTANOC PET/CT, giving way to ^{18}F-FDG-PET/CT imaging in this regard. However, the role of ^{18}F-FDG-PET/CT still remains to be explored in this subset of patients, as the low metabolic rate and indolent nature of NETs might cause too many false-negative results (Adams et al. 1998). Even in patients in whom no primary tumor is localized, additional sites of metastatic disease are observed when compared with conventional imaging, the most common being lymph nodes and bone. Although detection of such additional metastatic lesions do change management in these patients, they are certainly important from a prognostic point of view.

14 Gastroenteropancreatic Neuroendocrine Tumors in Patients with Hereditary Syndromes

The most common hereditary cancer syndrome associated with GEP-NETs is the multiple endocrine neoplasia (MEN1) syndrome. GEP tumors associated with MEN1 syndrome are usually functional and commonly include gastrinomas (60%) and insulinomas (10%), although carcinoid tumors are also known to occur (Thakker 2000). Most of these tumors belong to the category of well-differentiated neuroendocrine tumors and are known to express SSTR on tumor cell surface (Kaltsas et al. 2004). Functional imaging with ^{111}In-DTPA-octreotide is a proven method to image neuroendocrine gastroenteropancreatic tumors, but currently lacks full evaluation in MEN1 syndrome, including its usefulness for early diagnosis of tumors (Shi et al. 1998). However, it is considered to be the procedure of choice for screening endocrine tumor metastases in MEN1 patients (Langer et al. 2004). High degree of uptake on SRS imaging (both SPECT and PET) has been previously mentioned by Ezziddin et al. (2006) and Campana et al. (2010) in their studies. However, they could not find any significant difference in tracer uptake of functioning and nonfunctioning NETs. A higher degree of ^{68}Ga-DOTANOC uptake, however, has been shown to have a better long-term outcome than tumors with low maximum standardized uptake value (SUV_{max}) values even in patients with advanced stage of the disease (Campana et al. 2010). Indeed in our series of seven such patients, the median SUV_{max} of the detected

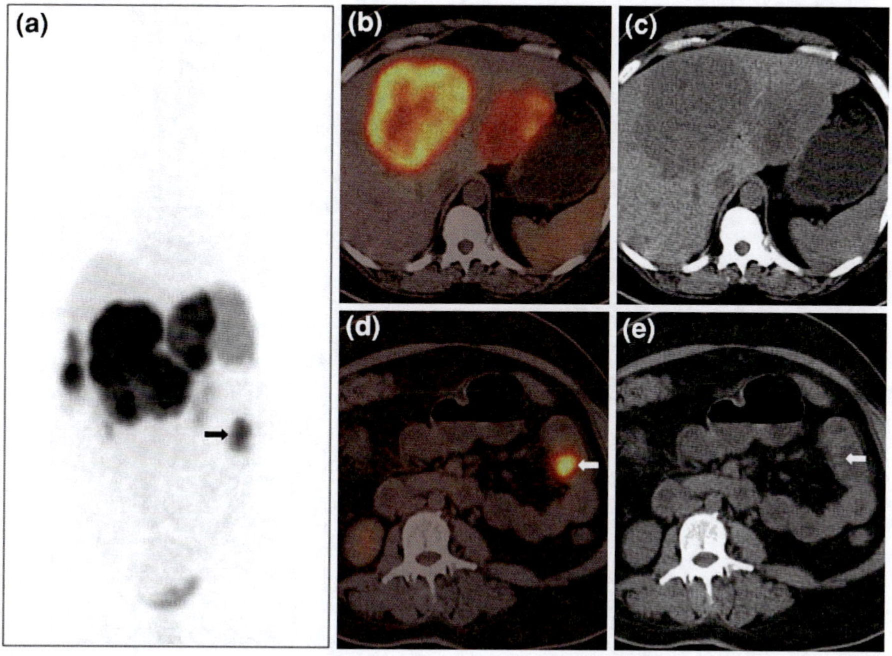

Fig. 6 A 46-year-old female with NET metastases to liver and a suspected primary tumor in the small bowel underwent ^{68}Ga-DOTANOC PET/CT imaging. Whole-body PET MIP image shows multiple areas of increased tracer uptake in the liver suggestive of liver secondaries and an area of abnormal uptake in the left side of abdomen (**a**, *bold arrow*). Axial PET/CT image (**b**) reveals increased tracer uptake in the liver, while corresponding CT image (**c**) shows the large hypodense lesions with a necrotic center. A focal area of uptake is seen in a jejunal loop on PET/CT (**d**), while no definite abnormality is seen on the CT section (**e**, *bold arrow*)

lesions was 36.1, with all of them showing stable disease after median follow-up of 2 years, clinically and radiologically (Fig. 7).

SUV_{max} is a semiquantitative parameter of tumor uptake and has now been proven to be an important and independent prognostic factor in the natural history of patients with neuroendocrine tumors. Campana et al. (2010) prospectively investigated the prognostic value of ^{68}Ga-DOTANOC SUV_{max} in 47 NET patients and found that SUV_{max} was significantly higher in patients with well-differentiated NETs. Among primary tumor sites, pancreas had higher uptake than other tumor sites. Patients with higher tumor SUV_{max} values showed a stable pattern of disease or partial remission on follow-up, with a cutoff value of 17.9–19.3 being the best prognostic indicator of favorable prognosis. Tumors with lower SUV_{max} progressed more often. Results from our center are in agreement with this observation. The average SUV_{max} values of different tumors and sites are shown in Table 2. However, among the primary tumors, histological subtypes do not influence the uptake of ^{68}Ga-DOTANOC. No significant difference is observed in the SUV_{max} of carcinoid with gastrinoma and NET not otherwise specified (NOS) (Naswa et al. 2011).

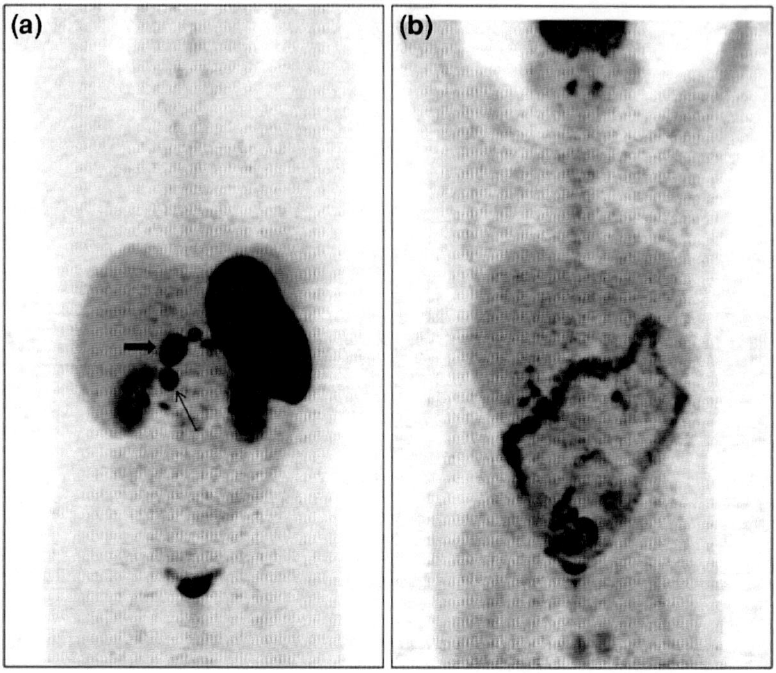

Fig. 7 A 32-year-old male with MEN1 syndrome had presence of a pyloric tumor with regional lymph node involvement. ^{68}Ga-DOTANOC whole-body MIP image shows abnormal areas of uptake in the abdomen (**a**, *bold arrow*-primary tumor, *arrow*-regional lymph node). ^{18}F-FDG PET MIP image (**b**) shows normal distribution of tracer with no abnormal uptake within the abdomen. Histopathology (HP) analysis of the primary tumor revealed features of a well-differentiated NET with Ki-67 index <1%

15 Correlation of Tumor Uptake with Cellular Differentiation

Uptake of somatostatin analogs has been shown to be dependent on a number of variables (Ezziddin et al. 2006). Perhaps the most important amongst these is the degree of cellular differentiation. The system recently proposed for gastroenteropancreatic NETs by the ENETS and also now recommended by the WHO uses either mitotic rate or Ki-67 labeling index (Rindi et al. 2007) (Table 1). Ki-67 is a nuclear antigen expressed in proliferating cells (G1, S, G2, and M phases) but not in resting cells (G0 phase). Cell proliferative activity is an important indicator of the growth and behavior of various human malignant tumors, because tumors with higher Ki-67 expression are associated with poorer prognosis (Lee 1996). Kimura et al. have shown that Ki-67 is an excellent indicator to assess progression of neuroendocrine tumors. Tumors with high Ki-67 values (>50 labeled nuclei/field) progress rapidly with the worst outcome; tumors with moderately high Ki-67

Table 2 Results of semiquantitative analysis on ^{68}Ga DOTANOC PET/CT

Site	SUV_{max}, median (range)
Primary (all)	13 (1–125)
Carcinoid	13 (3.3–125)
Gastrinoma	11 (4.5–58.2)
Insulinoma	29.3 (23.5–48.3)
NET (NOS)	11.3 (1–69)
Metastasis (all)	14.5 (1.3–145)
Liver	16.8 (4.3–145)
Lymph node	9.6 (2.3–50)
Bone	5.5 (1.3–53)

values (20–50 labeled nuclei) progress slowly but with poor outcome; and tumors with very low Ki-67 values (<10 labeled nuclei) have no metastases and good prognosis (Kimura et al. 1994). Belhocine et al. in their study on 17 patients with carcinoid tumors, correlated findings on somatostatin receptor scintigraphy (SRS) with the histological characteristics of the lesion. They found low expression of Ki-67 (<10%) in all well-differentiated carcinoid tumors, although no clear relationship could be found between proliferative activity and SRS results (Belhocine et al. 2002). In another study, Adams et al. showed the linear relationship between higher proliferative rate and FDG uptake. They concluded that PET imaging of gastroenteropancreatic tumors reveals increased glucose metabolism only in less-differentiated GEP tumors with high proliferative activity and that additional ^{18}F-FDG PET should be performed only if somatostatin receptor scintigraphy is negative (Adams et al. 1998). A comparison of ^{68}Ga-DOTANOC and ^{18}F-FDG studies done at our center in 26 patients has shown that well-differentiated GEP-NETs with low Ki-67 index have higher tumor uptake, while uptake on ^{18}F-FDG PET is higher in poorly differentiated tumors. However, a level of statistical significance could not be reached in this comparison. This holds true for both primary and metastatic sites. Also tumors with higher SUV_{max} values tend to follow a stable pattern of disease over time, while tumors with lower uptake and low SUV values progress over time. Hence, tumor SUV_{max} values on PET/CT can be considered an in vivo proxy of the prognostic value which Ki-67 holds.

16 Correlation of Tumor Uptake with SSTR Subtypes

The effects of somatostatin and its analogs are mediated via specific cell membrane-bound high-affinity receptors located on target cells. Five subtypes of SSTRs, SSTRs 1–5, have been cloned, and they belong to a distinct group within the superfamily of G-protein-coupled receptors with seven transmembrane regions (Reisine et al. 1995). Of practical importance is the division of the five receptor subtypes into two groups, where SSTRs 2, 3, and 5 differ from SSTRs 1 and 4 regarding amino acid homology and pharmacological profile. Short somatostatin analogs bind to the first group of receptor subtypes. Octreotide has highest affinity to SSTR 2 and lower affinity to SSTRs 3 and 5. ^{68}Ga-DOTANOC seems to be the most promising peptide for broad SSTR subtype affinity (binding to SSTR2, SSTR3, and SSTR5) (Wild et al. 2003). In a study by Miederer et al. in 18 patients, ^{68}Ga-DOTATOC PET/CT scans were quantified by SUV calculations and correlated to a cell membrane-based SSTR2-immunohistochemistry (IHC) score (0–3). They found that negative IHC scores were consistent with SUV values below 10, and all scores of 2 and 3 specimens corresponded with high SUV values (above 15). This validates the use of SSTR2 IHC in patients missing a preoperative PET scan to indicate ^{68}Ga-DOTA PET/CT as a method for restaging and follow-up in individual patients (Miederer et al. 2009). IHC correlation of SSTR subtypes with tumor uptake is however not available at our center.

17 Impact on Management

It is evident from the discussion above that ^{68}Ga-DOTANOC is clearly superior to any other currently available imaging modality in detection of gastroenteropancreatic neuroendocrine tumors. The main question in this regard, however, is whether detection of a greater number of lesions transforms into an overall survival advantage and creates a change in the management proposed. Ambrosini et al. were first to demonstrate that ^{68}Ga-DOTANOC PET/CT either affected stage or caused a therapy modification in more than half the patient population studied ($n = 90$; 55.5%), confirming the clinical role of ^{68}Ga-DOTANOC PET in management of NETs (Ambrosini et al. 2010). A study of 109 gastroenteropancreatic tumors at our center showed an overall influence in almost half of the patients (48%) regarding management decisions (change in 19%, support in 29%) (Naswa et al. 2011). The main advantage of PET in this regard is its impact on management decisions, rather than a change in stage. Important in this regard is either the inclusion or exclusion of surgical procedures. Also, in vivo demonstration of SSTR expression offers the physician a chance to treat these tumors with octreotide analogs, both cold SSA analogs and peptide-based radionuclide therapy (PRRT). Treatment with both these agents has shown to reduce signs and symptoms of hormone hypersecretion, to produce an overall improvement in quality of life, and to slow tumor growth, thus conferring a survival advantage to the patient (Bodei et al. 2009). It is also important in this regard to understand that a negative finding (no tracer uptake) on ^{68}Ga-DOTANOC PET in a demonstrated morphologic abnormality is as important as its ability to detect true-positive lesions. Targeted therapy would not be an effective therapy for such patients but rather than a switch to chemotherapy will provide a better option; hence, ^{68}Ga-DOTANOC PET becomes a mandatory procedure in patients with GEP-NETs to select the appropriate treatment strategy (Moertel et al. 1991).

18 Role of FDG-PET/CT

The workhorse of PET imaging, ^{18}F-FDG, exploits the increased glycolytic activity of tumor cells, which appears lacking in most NETs (Hawkins 1995; Kayani et al. 2008). This appears to be the predominant reason for the limited sensitivity of ^{18}F-FDG in this category of tumor and has been repeatedly mentioned in the literature (Adams et al. 1998). The importance of ^{18}F-FDG-PET imaging in GEP-NETs is, however, to target a different issue: detection of tumor cells with increased metabolic activity, which has an impact on prognosis and management (Strauss and Ponti 1991). A total tumor population characterization using a combination of ^{18}F-FDG and ^{68}Ga-labeled octreotide analog therefore seems a plausible approach (Fig. 8). This can map the entire extent of tumor cell differentiation in the same patient (Kayani et al. 2008), detect occult primary tumors as well as metastatic sites (which can change management), select the appropriate mode of treatment based on predominant cellular differentiation (somatostatin therapy for well-differentiated and conventional chemotherapy for less well-differentiated tumors), and select potential candidates for undergoing peptide-based radionuclide therapy in GEP-NETs when they are surgically unresectable. Hence, ^{18}F-FDG PET/CT must be considered complementary to ^{68}Ga-DOTANOC PET imaging, rather than contrasting (Binderup et al. 2010).

19 Pulmonary Neuroendocrine Tumors

The recent WHO classification of pulmonary neuroendocrine tumors classifies these neoplasms in order of increasing malignant potential into typical and atypical carcinoids, and large cell and small cell neuroendocrine tumors (Brambilla et al. 2001). Patients with pulmonary neuroendocrine tumor often present with recurrent pneumonia, cough, hemoptysis, or chest pain. Most pulmonary carcinoids are typical carcinoids with metastases in only 15% and a high 5-year survival rate of over 90% (Morandi et al. 2006). They are 3–4 times more common than atypical carcinoids, which tend to occur in older patients, are usually larger, and more often arise peripherally. They metastasize in about 30–50% of cases with a 5-year survival rate of 40–60% (Srirajaskanthan et al. 2008). Pulmonary carcinoids, especially the typical variety, are considered indolent with a very low metabolic rate and express a very high density of somatostatin receptors at the cell surface. Various studies in the past have explored somatostatin receptor-based PET/CT with ^{68}Ga-labeled somatostatin analogs in pulmonary neuroendocrine tumors, often in conjunction with ^{18}F-FDG PET, and most of them have reached a rather common opinion that typical bronchial carcinoids show a high degree of ^{68}Ga-DOTA-octreotide uptake while high-grade atypical bronchial carcinoids tend to show less uptake (Figs. 9, 10). They are, however, intensely FDG avid (Kayani et al. 2009). A combination of the two functional imaging procedures can be used for presurgical planning in primary bronchial carcinoids and for restaging

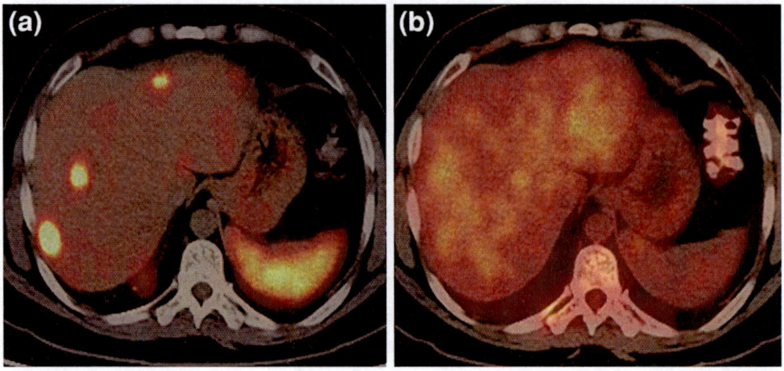

Fig. 8 A 35-year-old male with well-differentiated NET (gastrinoma) underwent restaging PET/CT. Increased tracer uptake is seen in the multiple liver metastases on ^{68}Ga-DOTANOC PET/CT axial image (**a**) with no avidity to FDG on ^{18}F-FDG PET/CT imaging (**b**)

recurrent pulmonary neuroendocrine tumors. Similar results and experiences have been reported from our center in the past (Jindal et al. 2011).

20 Medullary Carcinoma Thyroid

Medullary thyroid carcinoma (MTC) is a rare neuroendocrine tumor arising from the C-cells of the thyroid gland. Although classified under thyroidal malignancies, its biological behavior, management, and prognosis differ from the differentiated thyroid malignancies (papillary and follicular carcinomas). MTC may occur in sporadic (75%) or familial (25%) forms that include multiple endocrine neoplasia types IIA and IIB and isolated familial MTC (Marsh et al. 1995; Leboulleux et al. 2004). Lymph nodes are the most common site of metastases throughout the clinical course, with incidence of 71–80% during initial staging (Dralle et al. 1992), followed by bones, liver, and lungs, while incidence for distant metastases at initial presentation ranges from 10% to 15% (Bergholm et al. 1989). Surgery remains the primary mode of treatment, total thyroidectomy including neck dissection being the standard surgical procedure (Scollo et al. 2003). Post surgery, elevated basal serum calcitonin and carcinoembryonic antigen (CEA) levels suggest persisting tumor tissue (Elisei et al. 2004), and testing of the levels of these plasma markers is therefore the most frequently applied method in long-term follow-up. Conventional nuclear medicine studies with ^{99m}Tc(V) dimercaptosuccinic acid (DMSA), ^{99m}Tc-sestamibi, and ^{131}I-metaiodobenzylguanidine (MIBG) have variable and often limited sensitivity (Ugur et al. 1996; Gao et al. 2004). The advent of ^{18}F-FDG PET added another imaging tool for detection of recurrent MTC. ^{18}F-FDG has been successfully used in the follow-up of patients with differentiated thyroid cancer (Dietlein et al. 1997); however, for imaging MTC, the literature presents a wide spectrum of results, with

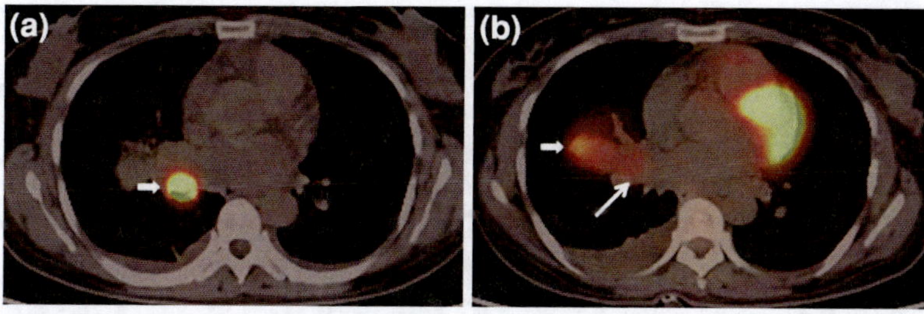

Fig. 9 A 40-year-old female presented with cough and hemoptysis. CT imaging revealed a nodular tumor occluding a portion of right bronchus intermedius, suspicious of a carcinoid tumor. Dual PET/CT imaging was undertaken to characterize the tumor. ^{68}Ga-DOTANOC PET/CT image (**a**) shows intense radiotracer uptake in the tumor, while ^{18}F-FDG-PET/CT showed no avidity for the same (**b**, *arrow*). However, the collapsed pulmonary segment shows increased FDG uptake (**b**, *bold arrow*). Histopathological assessment of the primary tumor after surgery revealed features compatible with a typical pulmonary carcinoid, while features of obstructive pneumonitis were seen in the collapsed lung segment

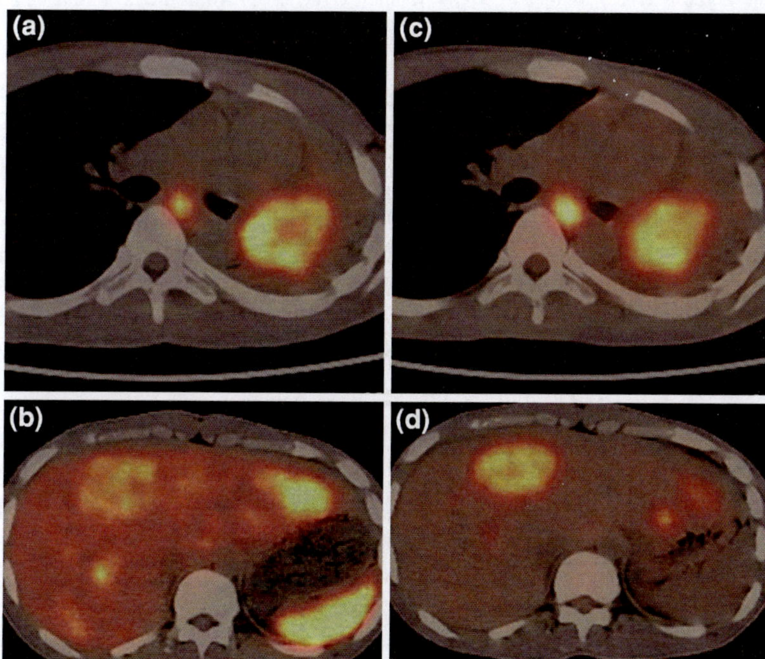

Fig. 10 A 20-year-old male with atypical carcinoid tumor of left lung shows increased tracer uptake on both ^{68}Ga-DOTANOC (**a**, **b**) and ^{18}F-FDG PET/CT imaging (**c**, **d**) in both primary lung tumor and liver metastases. Intensity of uptake in liver lesions is greater on FDG imaging (**b**, **d**)

most studies being limited by small sample sizes and a paucity of direct calcitonin correlations (Brandt et al. 2000; Diehl et al. 2001). Another modality used for imaging recurrent MTC has been somatostatin receptor scintigraphy (SRS) using

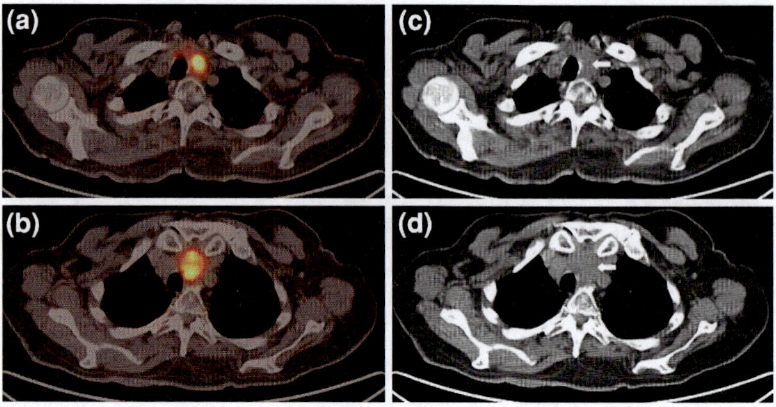

Fig. 11 A 65-year-old male with history of treated medullary carcinoma thyroid (MTC) presented with elevated serum calcitonin level of 3,195 pg/mL on follow-up. Neck ultrasound demonstrated a recurrence suspicion in the thyroid bed. ^{68}Ga-DOTANOC PET/CT was done for restaging. Axial PET/CT images (**a**, **b**) show intense tracer uptake in the neck and mediastinum suggestive of recurrence. Corresponding unenhanced axial CT sections show soft tissue masses in the left thyroid bed (**c**, *bold arrow*) and a superior mediastinal lymph node (**d**, *arrow*)

^{111}In-pentetreotide, which targets somatostatin receptors (SSTRs) expressed on tumor cell surface (Lamberts et al. 1991), including that of MTC (Zatelli et al. 2006).

MTC cells are also known to express SSTRs owing to their neuroendocrine origin and behavior. ^{68}Ga-DOTANOC PET/CT has so far demonstrated a detection rate of 80.7% for localization of biochemically recurrent MTC at our center, which is in general lower than for identification of other NETs (Ambrosini et al. 2010; Campana et al. 2010). The most common site of disease recurrence is in the form of nodal metastases in the neck and the mediastinum (Fig. 11). However, the main advantage stems from its ability to detect occult sites of metastasis especially in the bones. No direct correlations are observed between serum calcitonin levels and presence of metastatic disease, although the probability of disease detection is higher when the calcitonin level is >500 pg/mL. ^{18}F-FDG PET/CT is also routinely performed at our center in MTC patients, and a brief comparison of the two tracers is presented here. Our results demonstrate sensitivity of 63.4%, which is low compared with the available literature. The overall low sensitivity of ^{18}F-FDG PET/CT is probably explained by the nature and biological behavior of the tumor. MTC belongs to the group of well-differentiated neuroendocrine tumors with a low level of glucose metabolism, and its uptake and localization on ^{18}F-FDG PET are therefore expected to be low, a finding confirmed by Musholt et al. (1997) in their study. ^{68}Ga-DOTANOC PET/CT appears marginally superior to ^{18}F-FDG PET/CT in detecting disease recurrence. This difference is, however, not statistically significant ($p = 0.063$). A 75% concordance has been observed between the two imaging agents, with discordance mainly in lymph node groups, some of which appeared avid on ^{68}Ga-DOTANOC PET/CT and some on ^{18}F-FDG PET/CT. This might imply that some of the lymph nodes within such groups have started dedifferentiating (hence being FDG avid) and portend poorer prognosis. Distant metastases are detectable on both modalities. Liver metastases are especially avid to FDG and more frequently negative on ^{68}Ga-DOTANOC PET.

Only one study so far has systematically compared ^{18}F-FDG with SRS-based PET/CT using the tracer ^{68}Ga-DOTATATE in 18 recurrent MTC patients (Brendon et al. 2010). The calculated sensitivity was higher for ^{18}F-FDG (77.8%) than for ^{68}Ga-DOTATATE (72.2%), but the overall difference was not statistically significant. Results from our center are not very different from theirs, but the rate of lesion detection has so far been higher with ^{68}Ga-DOTANOC PET/CT than with ^{18}F-FDG PET/CT, with no significant difference in the overall diagnostic accuracy of the two modalities ($p = 0.063$) (Naswa et al. 2012). This small difference between the two studies might be because of the different receptor affinity profile of DOTATATE and DOTANOC. ^{68}Ga-DOTANOC has a broader affinity profile for SSTR subtypes SSTR2, SSTR3, and SSTR5, while ^{68}Ga-DOTATATE is more active at SSTR2 and SSTR3 (Reubi et al. 2000).

21 Pheochromocytoma and Paraganglioma

Pheochromocytomas are catecholamine-producing tumors derived from the sympathetic nervous system (Gifford et al. 1994; Werbel and Ober 1995). About 90% of these neoplasms occur as solitary benign tumors of the adrenal gland (Manger and Gifford 1995), and the rest can be localized in extra-adrenal sites (Neumann et al. 1993). About 10–20% of the tumors are malignant (Neumann et al. 1993). In addition to sporadic forms, pheochromocytomas are a feature of disorders with an autosomal dominant pattern of inheritance [e.g., multiple endocrine neoplasia type 2 in about one-fourth of unselected cases (Neumann et al. 1993)]. They are the cause of hypertension in less than 1% of the hypertensive population, but may be fatal if untreated or improperly treated. Thus, precise localization of pheochromocytomas is critical to management (Moreira and Pow-Sang 2002; Bravo 1994). Paragangliomas, or glomus tumors, like pheochromocytomas, arise from extra-adrenal chromaffin tissue and frequently cause symptoms by overproduction of catecholamines (Capella et al. 1988). About 9% of paragangliomas are familial (Grufferman et al. 1980). Multicentricity of paragangliomas is present in about 10% of unselected series, but may be as high as 32% in familial cases (Kliewer et al. 1989). Malignant behavior occurs in about 10% of patients (Lack et al. 1979).

The diagnosis of pheochromocytoma/paragangliomas is established biochemically by measuring the level of urinary and plasma catecholamines and their metabolites (24-h total metanephrine and/or catecholamine) (Kudva et al. 2003). However, imaging is important for tumor localization and excluding the possibility of multifocal lesions before surgery (Neumann et al. 1999). Computed tomography (CT) or magnetic resonance imaging (MRI) provide excellent morphologic details and have high sensitivity in the depiction of pheochromocytoma, but they often fail in the discrimination between pheochromocytoma and other causes of adrenal gland enlargement (Quint et al. 1987), and occasional false positives can lead to unnecessary surgery (Connor et al. 1988). Scintigraphy with ^{123}I-metaiodobenzylguanidine (MIBG) is currently the functional imaging method of choice for localization of adrenal or extra-adrenal pheochromocytomas and provides high sensitivity and specificity. However, it presents some disadvantages such as limited spatial resolution (making it difficult to detect tumors smaller than 1.5–2.0 cm in diameter, or when large tumors have extensive necrosis and/or hemorrhage), lack of tracer uptake in some tumors, and interference with certain medications, all of which lead to false-negative results (Khafagi et al. 1989). ^{111}In-Pentetreotide has been shown to be superior to MIBG in patients with malignant, metastatic, and extra-adrenal lesions. However, the overall sensitivity of this method is less than 30% (Van der Harst et al. 2000).

There has been little experience with PET imaging of pheochromocytomas. Two different studies, by Taieb et al. and Shuklin et al. opined that most pheochromocytomas accumulate FDG, especially the malignant variety, and this can be more useful for defining the distribution of those pheochromocytomas that fail to concentrate MIBG. Another useful remark by this study was to refrain from concluding that absence of FDG uptake excludes pheochromocytoma (Taíeb et al. 2009; Shuklin et al. 1999). Other PET-based radionuclides such as ^{11}C-hydroxyephedrine and ^{18}F-fluorodihydroxyphenylalanine (FDOPA) have also been evaluated in such tumors, with both providing a high level of accuracy in these group of tumors (Trampal et al. 2004; Hoegerle et al. 2002). Systematic studies with SR PET/CT in the detection of pheochromocytomas and paragangliomas has, however, not been described so far. Only one small series by Win et al. compared the PET tracer ^{68}Ga-DOTATATE with ^{123}I-MIBG in five patients with pheochromocytoma (Win et al. 2007). In that series, ^{68}Ga-DOTATATE PET showed more lesions, with higher uptake and better resolution, compared with ^{123}I-MIBG.

A series of 35 consecutive patients with known/suspected chromaffin cell tumors were analyzed at our center using ^{68}Ga-DOTANOC PET/CT. High diagnostic accuracy of 97.1% on per-patient and 98% on lesion-wise analysis was observed (Fig. 12). Negative results were seen mainly in patients with normal conventional imaging results, marginally elevated serum catecholamine level, and no significant tracer uptake on ^{131}I-MIBG scintigraphy. Alternative diagnoses were suggested in these patients later on follow-up (renal artery stenoses, essential hypertension). These situations are not uncommon in clinical practice. A large survey revealed that 4.2% of incidentalomas were pheochromocytomas, but only 43% of these patients were hypertensive, despite urinary catecholamine elevations in 86% (Mantero et al. 2000). ^{68}Ga-DOTANOC PET/CT was therefore considered as true negative in such patients, stressing the importance of this imaging technique in ruling out such tumors, apart from diagnosis and localization at the same time (Fig. 13). No significant relationship was, however, observed between the degree of tracer uptake (SUV_{max}) and lesion size and or between adrenal and extra-adrenal lesions (Naswa et al. 2012). Direct correlation of tumor SSTR status and succinate dehydrogenase (SDH) gene mutations which are common in such

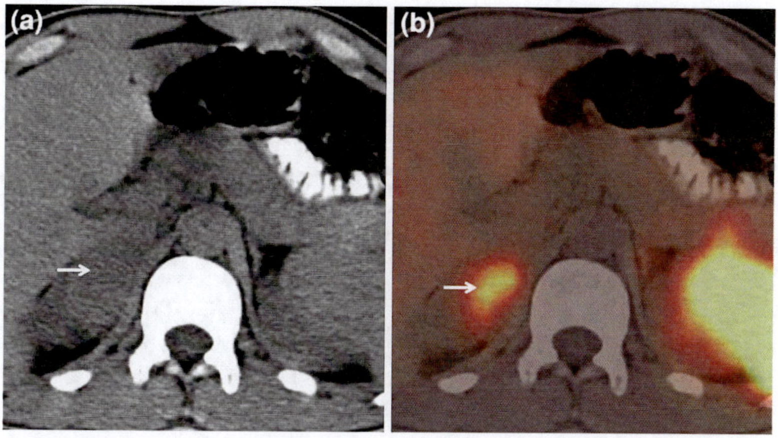

Fig. 12 A 32-year-old male with clinical suspicion of pheochromocytoma and biochemically confirmed diagnosis underwent PET/CT imaging in view of strong family history to rule out possibility of multifocal lesions before surgery. ^{68}Ga-DOTANOC PET imaging revealed increased tracer uptake corresponding to the right adrenal gland. Axial unenhanced CT shows the right adrenal lesions (**a**, *arrow*). Axial PET/CT image shows intense tracer uptake in the adrenal mass (**b**, *arrow*)

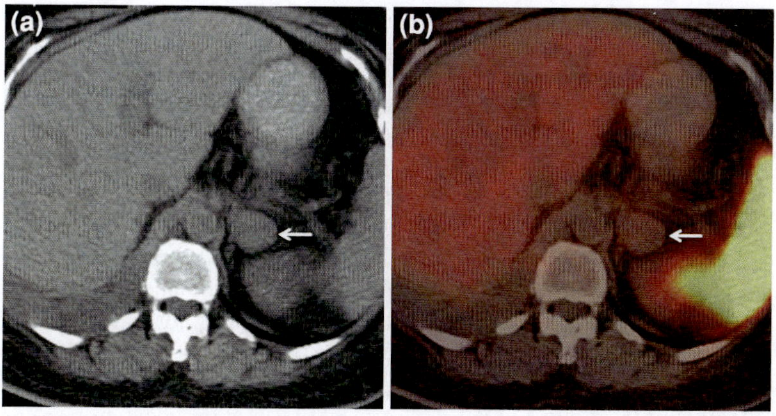

Fig. 13 A 44-year-old male with hypertension and marginally elevated serum catecholamines was found to have a left adrenal nodule on CECT imaging with a possible diagnosis of pheochromocytoma. ^{68}Ga-DOTANOC PET/CT was done to support the diagnosis. Unenhanced CT portion of the study shows the left adrenal nodule (**a**, 1.7 × 1.8 cm; 34 HU). Axial ^{68}Ga-DOTANOC PET/CT image shows no apparent increase in uptake in the left adrenal nodule (**b**, *arrow*), and a diagnosis of pheochromocytoma was questioned. The patient subsequently underwent surgery, and HP revealed features of a lipid-poor adenoma, thus highlighting the importance of negative SR PET/CT imaging

tumors especially the malignant and extra-adrenal ones, with tumor biomarkers could not be done as these were not available; hence, prognostic assessment of such tumors was not possible.

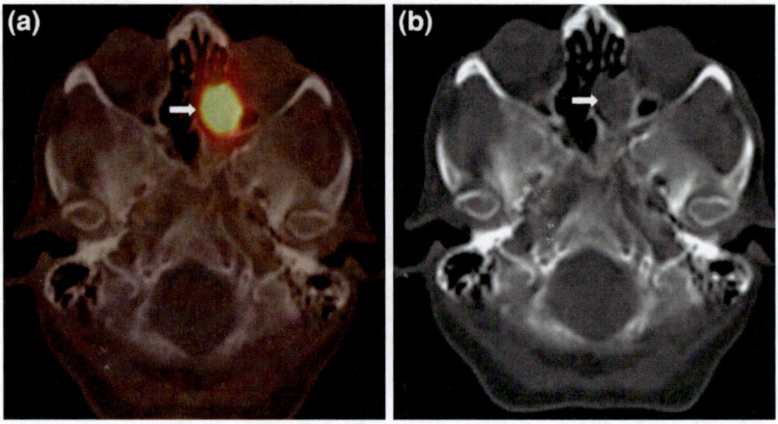

Fig. 14 A 55-year-old female with clinical diagnosis of tumor-induced osteomalacia and no obvious cause after extensive workup underwent ^{68}Ga-DOTANOC PET/CT imaging for search of a possible etiology. Intense tracer uptake was noticed in the region of left ethmoid sinus (**a**, *bold arrow*). Corresponding CT image (**b**) shows the soft tissue mass in the left ethmoid group of sinuses. The patient underwent excision of the lesion, and biopsy revealed features of a mesenchymal phosphaturic tumor (hemangiopericytoma). The patient is clinically well on follow-up with near-normal level of serum phosphate

22 Ectopic ACTH-Producing Tumors

Ectopic (Adrenocorticotropic hormone) ACTH-producing tumors occur in approximately 10% of cases of patients with Cushing's syndrome. Although a biochemical diagnosis of Cushing's syndrome is easily achieved, localization of the tumor is more difficult (Ilias et al. 2005; Tsagarakis et al. 2003). The majority of these tumors are of neuroendocrine origin and consequently may show high expression of somatostatin receptors. A bronchial carcinoid tumor is the type of ectopic ACTH-producing lesion responsible in most cases (Weiss et al. 1994). To investigate the exact location of such tumors, multiple imaging modalities are required, and at present no single modality can pinpoint the location of a suspected lesion (Grossman et al. 2006). The diagnostic utility of ^{111}In or ^{99m}Tc-labeled octreotide acetate scintigraphy in patients with suspected lesions has been debated. Some believe that it is not helpful, whereas others have reported radionuclide imaging to be a useful diagnostic tool (Isidori et al. 2006). An analysis of studies examining the usefulness of SRS in the ectopic ACTH syndrome demonstrated diagnostic sensitivities ranging from 33% to 80% for tumor localization (Tsagarakis et al. 2003; Tabarin et al. 1999). In addition, two previous studies aimed at localization of the ectopic source (Tabarin et al. 1999; Torpy et al. 1999) have shown that, in case of negative baseline ^{111}In-pentetreotide scan, future repeated scintigraphy would prove useless. However, the advantages of this technique cannot be ignored either. It provides whole-body information, which is a major

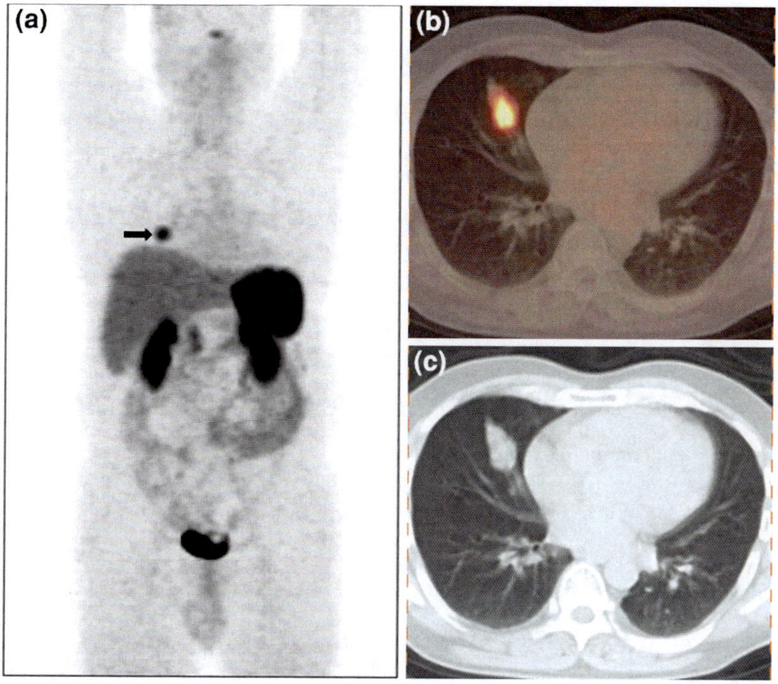

Fig. 15 A patient with Cushing's syndrome and possibility of ectopic ACTH source as cause underwent PET/CT imaging for localization. Focal area of increased uptake is noted in the right lung region on ^{68}Ga-DOTANOC MIP image (**a**, *bold arrow*). A fibronodular lesion in the right lung field is seen, showing increased uptake on the axial PET/CT and CT image (**b**, **c**)

advantage over conventional radiology. Particularly, detection of brain or skeletal metastases, as described in one of the patients in the study by Torpy et al. can significantly alter the therapeutic approach in these patients (Torpy et al. 1999). This technique also provides additional functional information; a positive scintigram points to the presence of functional receptors for octapeptide somatostatin analogs (Phlipponneau et al. 1994). Treatment of these scan-positive patients with octapeptide somatostatin analogs may then result in correction of hypercortisolism and thus improve metabolic control and tissue healing before performing curative surgery. However, the specificity of ^{111}In-pentetreotide scintigraphy is low, which can lead to unnecessary interventions. The role of ^{68}Ga-labeled somatostatin analogs has not been addressed in a systematic manner for detection of these lesions. Results from our center have also not been too encouraging. Only four patients so far have shown localization (lungs in three patients, pancreas in one). Systematic future studies are required to better address this issue (Fig. 14).

Apart from these common and unusual situations where ^{68}Ga-DOTANOC PET has been found useful, certain other clinical scenarios exist where this tracer can be of immense utility such as meningiomas and tumor induced osteomalacia (TIO), (Fig. 15).

23 Conclusions

^{68}Ga somatostatin receptor imaging is a novel concept of PET imaging to detect neuroendocrine tumors. It penetrates into many aspects of tumor management and can be considered as the first-line imaging investigation for evaluation of such lesions, especially GEP-NETs.

References

Adams S, Baum R, Rink T, Schumm-Dräger PM, Usadel KH, Hör G (1998) Limited value of fluorine-18 fluorodeoxyglucose positron emission tomography for the imaging of neuroendocrine tumors. Eur J Nucl Med 25:79–83

Ambrosini V, Campana D, Bodei L et al (2010) ^{68}Ga-DOTANOC PET/CT clinical impact in patients with neuroendocrine tumors. J Nucl Med 51:669–673

Belhocine T, Foidart J, Rigo P, Najjar F, Thiry A, Quatresooz P, Hustinx R (2002) Fluorodeoxyglucose positron emission tomography and somatostatin receptor scintigraphy for diagnosing and staging carcinoid tumors: correlations with the pathological indexes p53 and Ki-67. Nucl Med Commun 23:727–734

Bergholm U, Adami HO, Bergstrom R et al (1989) Clinical characteristics in sporadic and familial medullary thyroid carcinoma: a nationwide study of 249 patients in Sweden from 1959 through 1981. Cancer 63:1196–1204

Binderup T, Knigge U, Loft A, Mortensen J, Pfeifer A, Federspie B et al (2010) Functional imaging of neuroendocrine tumors: A head-to-head comparison of somatostatin receptor scintigraphy, ^{123}I-MIBG Scintigraphy, and ^{18}F-FDG PET. J Nucl Med 51:704–712

Bodei L, Ferone D, Grana CM et al (2009) Peptide receptor therapies in neuroendocrine tumors. J Endocrinol Invest 32:360–369

Brambilla E, Travis WD, Colby TV, Corrin B, Shimosato Y (2001) The new World Health Organization classification of lung tumors. Eur Respir J 18:1059–1068

Brandt MK, Muller SP, Gorges R, Saller B, Bockisch A (2000) The value of fluorine-18 fluorodeoxyglucose PET in patients with medullary thyroid cancer. Eur J Nucl Med 27:490–496

Bravo EL (1994) Evolving concepts in the pathophysiology, diagnosis and treatment of pheochromocytoma. Endocr Rev 15:356–368

Brendon GC, Nikolaos DP, Prakash V, Kayani I, Caplin M, Mahmood S et al (2010) Comparison of ^{68}Ga-DOTATATE and ^{18}F-fluorodeoxyglucose PET/CT in the detection of recurrent medullary thyroid carcinoma. Eur J Nucl Med Mol Imaging 37:49–57

Calender A (2000) Molecular genetics of neuroendocrine tumors. Digestion 62(Suppl 1):3–18

Campana D, Ambrosini V, Pezzilli R, Fanti S, Labate AMM, Santini D et al (2010) Standardized uptake values of ^{68}Ga-DOTANOC PET: a promising prognostic tool in neuroendocrine tumors. J Nucl Med 51:353–359

Capella C, Riva C, Cornaggia M et al (1988) Histopathology, cytology and cytochemistry of pheochromocytomas and paragangliomas including chemodectomas. Path Res Pract 183: 176–187

Castellucci P, Ucha JP, Fuccio C, Rubello D, Ambrosini V, Montini GC et al (2011) Incidence of increased ^{68}Ga-DOTANOC uptake in the pancreatic head in a large series of extrapancreatic NET patients studied with sequential PET/CT. J Nucl Med 52:886–890

Connor CS, Hermreck AS, Thomas JH (1988) Pitfalls in the diagnosis of pheochromocytoma. Am Surg 54:634–636

Diehl M, Risse JH, Brandt-Mainz K et al (2001) Fluorine-18 fluorodeoxyglucose positron emission tomography in medullary thyroid cancer: results of a multicentre study. Eur J Nucl Med 28:1671–1676

Dietlein M, Scheidhauer K, Voth E, Theissen P, Schicha H (1997) Fluorine-18 fluorodeoxyglucose positron emission tomography and iodine-^{131} whole-body scintigraphy in the follow-up of differentiated thyroid cancer. Eur J Nucl Med 24:1342–1348

Dralle H, Damm I, Scheumann GF, Kotzerke J, Kupsch E (1992) Frequency and significance of cervicomediastinal lymph node metastases in medullary thyroid carcinoma: results of a compartment-oriented microdissection method. Henry Ford Hosp Med J 40:264–267

Elisei R, Bottici V, Luchetti F, Di Coscio G, Romei C, Grasso L et al (2004) Impact of routine measurement of serum calcitonin on the diagnosis and outcome of medullary thyroid cancer: experience in 10,864 patients with nodular thyroid disorders. J Clin Endocrinol Metab 89:163–168

Ezziddin S, Logvinski T, Yong-Hing C, Ahmadzadehfar H, Fischer HP, Palmedo H et al (2006) Factors predicting tracer uptake in somatostatin receptor and MIBG scintigraphy of metastatic gastroenteropancreatic neuroendocrine tumors. J Nucl Med 47:223–233

Fischer L, Kleeff J, Esposito I et al (2008) Clinical outcome and long-term survival in 118 consecutive patients with neuroendocrine tumors of the pancreas. Br J Surg 95(5):627–635

Gabriel M, Decristoforo C, Kendler D et al (2007) ^{68}Ga-DOTA-Tyr 3 -octreotide PET in neuroendocrine tumors: comparison with somatostatin receptor scintigraphy and CT. J Nucl Med 48:508–518

Gao Z, Biersack H, Ezziddin S, Logvinski T, An R (2004) The role of combined imaging in metastatic medullary thyroid carcinoma: ^{111}In-DTPA-octreotide and ^{131}I/^{123}I-MIBG as predictors for radionuclide therapy. J Cancer Res Clin Oncol 130:649–656

Gifford RW Jr, Manger WM, Bravo EL (1994) Pheochromocytoma. Endocrinol Metab Clin North Am 23:387–404

Grossman AB, Kelly P, Rockall A, Bhattacharya S, McNicol A, Barwick T (2006) Cushing's syndrome caused by an occult source: difficulties in diagnosis and management. Nat Clin Pract Endocrinol Metab 2:642–647

Grufferman S, Gillman MW, Pasternak LR et al (1980) Familial carotid body tumors: case report and epidemiologic review. Cancer 46:2116–2122

Hainsworth JD, Spigel DR, Litchy S, Greco FA (2006) Phase II trial of paclitaxel, carboplatin, and etoposide in advanced poorly differentiated neuro-endocrine carcinoma: a minnie pearl cancer research network study. J Clin Oncol 24:3548–3554

Harrison A, Walker CA, Parker D, Jankowski KJ, Cox JPL, Craig AS et al (1991) The in vivo release of 90Y from cyclic and acyclic ligand-antibody conjugates. Int J Radiat Appl Instrum B 18(5):469–476

Hawkins RA (1995) Pancreatic tumors: imaging with PET. Radiology 195:320

Heppeler A, Froidevaux S, Mäcke HR, Jermann E, Behe M, Powell P (1999) Radiometal-labelled macrocyclic chelator-derivatised somatostatin analogue with superb tumour-targeting properties and potential for receptor-mediated internal radiotherapy. Chem Eur J 5:1974–1981

Hoegerle S, Nitzsche E, Altehoefer C et al (2002) Pheochromocytomas: detection with ^{18}F DOPA whole-body PET—initial results. Radiology 222:507–512

Ilias I, Torpy DJ, Pacak K, Mullen N, Wesley RA, Nieman LK (2005) Cushing's syndrome due to ectopic corticotropin secretion: twenty years' experience at the National Institutes of Health. J Clin Endocrinol Metab 90:4955–4962

Isidori AM, Kaltsas GA, Pozza C, Frajese V, Newell-Price J, Reznek RH, Jenkins PJ, Monson JP, Grossman AB, Besser GM (2006) The ectopic adrenocorticotropin syndrome: clinical features, diagnosis, management, and long-term follow-up. J Clin Endocrinol Metab 91:371–377

Jindal T, Kumar A, Venkitaraman B, Meena M, Kumar R, Malhotra A, Dutta R (2011) Evaluation of the role of [^{18}F]FDG-PET/CT and [^{68}Ga]DOTATOC-PET/CT in differentiating typical and atypical pulmonary carcinoids. Cancer Imaging Jun 15(11):70–75

Kaemmerer D, Peter L, Lupp A, Schulz S, Sänger J, Prasad V et al (2011) Molecular imaging with (^{68}) Ga-SSTR PET/CT and correlation to immunohistochemistry of somatostatin receptors in neuroendocrine tumors. Eur J Nucl Med Mol Imaging 38:1659–1668

Kaltsas GA, Mukherjee JJ, Grossman AB (2001) The value of radiolabelled MIBG and octreotide in the diagnosis and management of neuroendocrine tumors. Ann Oncol 12(Suppl 2):S47–S50

Kaltsas G, Rockall A, Papadogias D, Reznek R, Grossman AB (2004) Recent advances in radiological and radionuclide imaging and therapy of neuroendocrine tumors. Eur J Endocrinol 151:15–27

Kayani I, Bomanji JB, Groves A et al (2008) Functional imaging of neuroendocrine tumors with combined PET/CT using ^{68}Ga-DOTATATE (DOTA-DPhe1, Tyr3-octreotate) and ^{18}F-FDG. Cancer 112:2447–2455

Kayani I, Conry BG, Groves AM, Win T, Dickson J, Caplin M et al (2009) A comparison of ^{68}Ga-DOTATATE and ^{18}F-FDG PET/CT in pulmonary neuroendocrine tumors. J Nucl Med 50:1927–1932

Khafagi FA, Shapiro B, Fig LM et al (1989) Labetalol reduces ^{131}I MIBG uptake by pheochromocytoma and normal tissues. J Nucl Med 30:481–489

Kimura N, Miura W, Noshiro T, Miura Y, Ookuma Y, Nagura H (1994) Ki-67 is an indicator of progression of neuroendocrine tumors. Endocr Pathol 5:223–228

Kliewer KE, Wen DR, Cancilla PA et al (1989) Paragangliomas: assessment of prognosis by histologic, immunohistochemical, and ultrastructural techniques. Hum Pathol 20:29–39

Kloppel G, Perren A, Heitz PU (2004) The gastroenteropancreatic neuroendocrine cell system and its tumors: the WHO classification. Ann N Y Acad Sci 1014:13–27

Krausz Y, Bar-Ziv J, de Jong R et al (1998) Somatostatin receptor scintigraphy in the management of gastro enteropancreatic tumors. Am J Gastroenterol 93:66–70

Krenning EP, Kwekkeboom DJ, Bakker WH et al (1993) Somatostatin receptor scintigraphy with [^{111} In-DTPA-D Phe1]- and [^{123} I-Tyr3]-octreotide: the Rotterdam experience with more than 1000 patients. Eur J Nucl Med 20:716–731

Kudva YC, Sawka AM, Young WF Jr (2003) Clinical review 164: the laboratory diagnosis of adrenal pheochromocytoma—the Mayo Clinic experience. J Clin Endocrinol Metab 88:4533–4539

Lack EE, Cubilla AL, Woodruff JM (1979) Paragangliomas of the head and neck region. A pathologic study of tumors from 71 patients. Hum Pathol 10:191–218

Lamberts SWJ, Hofland LJ, van Koetsueld PM et al (1990) Parallel in vivo and in vitro detection of functional somatostatin receptors in human endocrine pancreatic tumors: consequences with regard to diagnosis, localization and therapy. J Clin Endocrinol Metab 71:566–574

Lamberts SWJ, Krenning EP, Reubi JC (1991) The role of somatostatin and its analogs in the diagnosis and treatment of tumors. Endocr Rev 12:450–482

Lamberts SW, Hofland LJ, Nobels FR (2001) Neuroendocrine tumor markers. Front Neuroendocrinol 22:309–339

Langer P, Kann PH, Fendrich V, Richter G, Diehl S, Rothmund M et al (2004) Prospective evaluation of imaging procedures for the detection of pancreaticoduodenal endocrine tumors in patients with multiple endocrine neoplasia type 1. World J Surg 28:1317–1322

Leboulleux S, Baudin E, Travagli JP, Schlumberger M (2004) Medullary thyroid carcinoma. Clin Endocrinol (Oxf) 61:299–310

Lee CS (1996) Differences in cell proliferation and prognostic significance of proliferating cell nuclear antigen and Ki-67 antigen immunoreactivity in in situ and invasive carcinomas of the extrahepatic biliary tract. Cancer 78:1881–1887

Mäcke HR, Good S (2003) Radiometals (non-Tc, non-Re) and bifunctional labeling chemistry. In: Vértes A, Nagy S, Klencsár Z (eds) Handbook of nuclear chemistry. Amsterdam, 4: 279–314

Maecke HR, Hofmann M, Haberkorn U (2005) ^{68}Ga-labeled peptides in tumor imaging. J Nucl Med 46(suppl 1):172S–178S

Manger WM, Gifford RW (1995) Pheochromocytoma: a clinical overview. In: Laragh JH, Brenner BM (eds) Hypertension: pathophysiology, diagnosis and management. Raven, New York, pp 225–244

Mantero F, Massimo T, Arnoldi G et al (2000) A survey on adrenal incidentaloma in Italy. J Clin Endocrinol Metab 85:637–644

Marsh DJ, Learoyd DL, Robinson BG (1995) Medullary thyroid carcinoma: recent advances and management update. Thyroid 5:407–424

Miederer M, Seidl S, Buck A, Scheidhauer K, Wester HJ, Schwaiger M, Perren A (2009) Correlation of immunohistopathological expression of somatostatin receptor 2 with standardised uptake values in ^{68}Ga-DOTATOC PET/CT. Eur J Nucl Med Mol Imaging 36(1):48–52

Moertel CG, Kvols LK, O'Connell MJ, Rubin J (1991) Treatment of neuroendocrine carcinomas with combined etoposide and cisplatin: evidence of major therapeutic activity in the anaplastic variants of these neoplasms. Cancer 68:227–232

Morandi U, Casali C, Rossi G (2006) Bronchial typical carcinoid tumors. Semin Thorac Cardiovasc Surg 18:191–198

Moreira SG Jr, Pow-Sang JM (2002) Evaluation and management of adrenal masses. Cancer Control 9:326–334

Musholt TJ, Musholt PB, Dehdashti F, Moley JF (1997) Evaluation of fluorodeoxyglucose-positron emission tomographic scanning and its association with glucose transporter expression in medullary thyroid carcinoma and pheochromocytoma: a clinical and molecular study. Surgery 122:1049–1060

Naswa N, Sharma P, Kumar A, Nazar AH, Kumar R, Chumber S, Bal C (2011) Gallium-68-DOTA-NOC PET/CT of patients with gastroenteropancreatic neuroendocrine tumors: A prospective single-center study. AJR 197:1–8

Naswa N, Sharma P, Sudhir Suman KC, Lata S, Kumar R, Malhotra A, C Bal (2012) Prospective evaluation of ^{68}Ga-DOTA-NOC PET-CT in patients with Recurrent Medullary Thyroid Carcinoma (MTC): comparison with 18F-FDG PET-CT. Nucl Med Commun (in Press)

Naswa N, Sharma P, Nazar AH, Agarwal KK, Kumar R, Ammini AC (2012) Prospective evaluation of ^{68}Ga-DOTA-NOC PET-CT in phaeochromocytoma and paraganglioma: preliminary results from a single centre study. Eur Radiol 22:710–719. DOI 10.1007/s00330-011-2289-x

Naswa N, Sharma P, Kumar A, Soundararajan R, Kumar R, Malhotra A, Ammini AC, Bal C (2012) ^{68}Ga-DOTANOC PET/CT in patients with carcinoma of unknown primary of neuroendocrine origin. Clin Nucl Med 37(3):245–251

Neumann HPH, Berger DP, Sigmund G et al (1993) Pheochromocytomas, multiple endocrine neoplasia type 2, and von Hippel- Lindau disease. N Engl J Med 329:1531–1538

Neumann HPH, Bender BU, Reincke M et al (1999) Adrenal sparing surgery for pheochromocytoma. Br J Surg 84:94–97

Oberg K (2002) Carcinoid tumors: molecular genetics, tumor biology, and update of diagnosis and treatment. Curr Opin Oncol 14:38–45

Prasad V, Ambrosini V, Hommann M, Hoersch D, Fanti S, Baum RP (2010) Detection of unknown primary neuroendocrine tumors (CUP-NET) using ^{68}Ga-DOTANOC receptor PET/CT. Eur J Nucl Med Mol Imaging 37(1):67–77

Phlipponneau M, Nocaudie M, Epelbaum J et al (1994) Somatostatin analogs for the localization and preoperative treatment of an adrenocorticotropin-secreting bronchial carcinoid tumor. J Clin Endocrinol Metab 78:20–24

Putzer D, Gabriel M, Henninger B, Kendler D, Uprimny D, Dobrozemsky G (2009) Bone metastases in patients with neuroendocrine tumor: ^{68}Ga-DOTA-Tyr3-octreotide PET in comparison to CT and bone scintigraphy. J Nucl Med 50:1214–1221

Quint LE, Glazer GM, Francis IR et al (1987) Pheochromocytoma and paraganglioma: comparison of MRI imaging with CT and ^{131}I MIBG scintigraphy. Radiology 165:89–93

Reisine T, Bell GI (1995) Molecular biology of somatostatin receptors. Endocr Rev 16:427–442

Reubi JC, Kvols L, Krenning E, Lamberts SWJ (1991) In vitro and in vivo detection of somatostatin receptors in human malignant tissues. Acta Oncol 30:463–468

Reubi JC, Schar JC, Waser B, Wenger S, Heppeler A, Schmitt JS et al (2000) Affinity profiles for human somatostatin receptor subtypes SST1-SST5 of somatostatin radiotracers selected for scintigraphic and radiotherapeutic use. Eur J Nucl Med 27:273–282

Rindi G, Villanacci V, Ubiali A (2000) Biological and molecular aspects of gastroenteropancreatic neuroendocrine tumors. Digestion 62(Suppl 1):19–26

Rindi G, Villanacci V, Ubiali A, Scarpa A et al (2001) Endocrine tumors of the digestive tract and pancreas: histogenesis, diagnosis, and molecular basis. Expert Rev Mol Diagn 1:323–333

Rindi G, Kloppel G, Alhman H et al (2006) TNM staging of foregut (neuro) endocrine tumors: a consensus proposal including a grading system. Virchows Arch 449(4):395–401

Rindi G, Kloppel G, Couvelard A et al (2007) TNM staging of midgut and hindgut (neuro) endocrine tumors: a consensus proposal including a grading system. Virchows Arch 451(4):757–762

Ruf J, Schiefer J, Furth C et al (2011) ^{68}Ga-DOTATOC PET/CT of neuroendocrine tumors: spotlight on the CT phases of a triple-phase protocol. J Nucl Med 52:697–704

Savelli G, Lucignani G, Seregni E, Marchianò A, Serafini G, Aliberti G et al (2004) Feasibility of somatostatin receptor scintigraphy in the detection of occult primary gastro-entero-pancreatic (GEP) neuroendocrine tumors. Nucl Med Commun 25:445–449

Schillaci O, Annibale B, Scopinaro F, delle Fave GF, Colella AC (1997) Somatostatin receptor scintigraphy of malignant somatostatinoma with indium-111-pentetreotide. J Nucl Med 38:886–887

Schillaci O, Massa R, Scopinaro F (2000) Indium-^{111}-pentetreotide scintigraphy in the detection of insulinomas: importance of SPECT imaging. J Nucl Med 41:459–462

Scollo C, Baudin E, Travagli JP, Caillou B, Bellon N, Leboulleux S et al (2003) Rationale for central and bilateral lymph node dissection in sporadic and hereditary medullary thyroid cancer. J Clin Endocrinol Metab 88:2070–2075

Shi W, Johnston CF, Buchanan KD, Ferguson WR, Laird JD, Crothers JG, Maclirath EM (1998) Localization of neuroendocrine tumors with [^{111}In] DTPA-octreotide scintigraphy (Octreoscan): a comparative study with CT and MR imaging. QJM 91:295–301

Shuklin BL, Thompson NW, Shapiro B et al (1999) Pheochromocytomas: imaging with 2-[fluorine-18] fluoro-2-deoxy-D-glucose PET. Radiology 212:35–41

Solcia E, Rindi G, Paolotti D, La Rosa S, Capella C, Fiocca R (1999) Clinicopathological profile as a basis for classification of the endocrine tumors of the gastroenteropancreatic tract. Ann Oncol 10(Suppl 2):S9–S15

Solcia E, Kloppel G, Sobin LH (2000) Histological typing of endocrine tumors, 2nd edn. World Health Organization, Heidelberg

Srirajaskanthan R, Toumpanakis C, Karpathakis A et al (2008) Surgical management and palliative treatment in bronchial neuroendocrine tumors: a clinical study of 45 patients. Lung Cancer 65:68–73

Srirajaskanthan R, Kayani I, Quigley AM, Soh J, Caplin ME, Bomanji J (2010) The role of ^{68}Ga-DOTATATE PET in patients with neuroendocrine tumors and negative or equivocal findings on ^{111} In-DTPA-octreotide scintigraphy. J Nucl Med 51:875–882

Strauss LG, Ponti PS (1991) The application of PET in clinical oncology. J Nucl Med 32:623–648

Taal BG, Visser O (2004) Epidemiology of neuroendocrine tumors. Neuroendocrinology 80(Suppl 1):3–7

Tabarin A, Valli N, Chanson P et al (1999) Usefulness of somatostatin receptor scintigraphy in patients with occult ectopic ACTH syndrome. J Clin Endocrinol Metab 84:1193–1202

Taíeb D, Sebag F, Barlier A et al (2009) ^{18}F-FDG avidity of pheochromocytomas and paragangliomas: A new molecular imaging signature? J Nucl Med 50:711–717

Thakker RV (2000) Multiple endocrine neoplasia type 1. In: De Groot LJ, Jameson JL (eds) Endocrinology, 4th edn. Saunders, Philadelphia, pp 2503–2517

Torpy DJ, Chen DD, Mullen N et al (1999) Lack of utility of ^{111}In-pentetreotide scintigraphy in localizing ectopic ACTH producing tumors: follow-up of 18 patients. J Clin Endocrinol Metab 84:1186–1192

Trampal C, Engler H, Juhlin C et al (2004) Pheochromocytomas: detection with ^{11}C Hydroxyephedrine PET. Radiology 230:423–428

Tsagarakis S, Christoforaki M, Giannopoulou H, Rondogianni F, Housianakou I, Malagari C, Rontogianni D, Bellenis I, Thalassinos N (2003) A reappraisal of the utility of somatostatin receptor scintigraphy in patients with ectopic adrenocorticotropin Cushing's syndrome. J Clin Endocrinol Metab 88:4754–4758

Ugur O, Kostakğlu L, Gü ler N, Caner B, Uysal U, Elahi N, Haliloğ lu M, Yü ksel D, Aras T, Bayhan H, Bekdik C (1996) Comparison of 99mTc(V)-DMSA, 201Tl and 99mTc-MIBI imaging in the follow-up of patients with medullary carcinoma of the thyroid. Eur J Nucl Med 23:1367–1371

Van der Harst E, De Herder WW, Bruining HA et al (2000) ^{123}[I] Metaiodobenzylguanidine and ^{111}[In] octreotide uptake in benign and malignant pheochromocytomas. J Clin Endocrinol Metab 86:685–693

Weiss M, Yellin A, Husza'r M, Eisenstein Z, Bar-Ziv J, Krausz Y (1994) Localization of adrenocorticotropic hormone-secreting bronchial carcinoid tumor by somatostatin-receptor scintigraphy. Ann Intern Med 121:198–199

Werbel SS, Ober KP (1995) Pheochromocytoma: update on diagnosis, localization, and management. Med Clin North Am 79:131–153

Wild D, Schmitt JS, Ginj M et al (2003) DOTANOC, a high-affinity ligand of somatostatin receptor subtypes 2, 3 and 5 for labelling with various radiometals. Eur J Nucl Med Mol Imaging 30:1338–1347

Win Z, Al-Nahhas A, Towey D et al (2007) ^{68}Ga-DOTATATE PET in neuroectodermal tumours: first experience. Nucl Med Commun 28(359):363

Zatelli MC, Piccin D, Tagliati F, Bottoni A, Luchin A, Vignali C et al (2006) Selective activation of somatostatin receptor subtypes differentially modulates secretion and viability in human medullary thyroid carcinoma primary cultures: potential clinical perspectives. J Clin Endocrinol Metab 91:2218–2224

Zhernosekov KP, Filosofov DV, Baum RP, Aschoff P, Bihl H, Razbash AA et al (2007) Processing of generator-produced ^{68}Ga for medical application. J Nucl Med 48:1741–1748

Zimmer T, Stolzel U, Bader M, Koppenhagen K, Hamm B, Buhr H et al (1996) Endoscopic ultrasonography and somatostatin receptor scintigraphy in the pre-operative localisation of insulinomas and gastrinomas. Gut 39:562–568

Differential Uptake of ^{68}Ga-DOTATOC and ^{68}Ga-DOTATATE in PET/CT of Gastroenteropancreatic Neuroendocrine Tumors

Thorsten D. Poeppel, Ina Binse, Stephan Petersenn, Harald Lahner, Matthias Schott, Gerald Antoch, Wolfgang Brandau, Andreas Bockisch and Christian Boy

Abstract

Purpose: Abundant expression of somatostatin receptors (sst) is a characteristic of neuroendocrine tumors (NET). Thus, radiolabeled somatostatin analogs have emerged as important tools for both in vivo diagnosis and therapy of NET. The two compounds most often used in functional imaging with positron emission tomography (PET) are ^{68}Ga-DOTATATE and ^{68}Ga-DOTATOC. Both analogs share a quite similar sst binding profile. However, the in vitro affinity of ^{68}Ga-DOTATATE in binding the sst subtype 2 (sst2) is approximately tenfold higher than that of ^{68}Ga-DOTATOC. This difference may affect their efficiency in detection of NET lesions, as sst2 is the predominant receptor subtype on gastroenteropancreatic NET. We thus compared the diagnostic value of PET/CT with both radiolabeled somatostatin analogs (^{68}Ga-DOTATATE and ^{68}Ga-DOTATOC) in the same patients with gastroenteropancreatic NET. *Patients and Methods*: Twenty-seven patients with metastatic gastroenteropancreatic NET underwent ^{68}Ga-DOTATOC and ^{68}Ga-DOTATATE PET/CT as part of the

T. D. Poeppel (✉) · I. Binse · W. Brandau · A. Bockisch · C. Boy
Department of Nuclear Medicine, University Hospital Essen,
Hufelandstr. 55, D-45122, Essen, Germany
e-mail: thorsten.poeppel@uni-due.de

S. Petersenn · H. Lahner
Department of Endocrinology, University Essen, Essen, Germany

M. Schott
Department of Endocrinology, University Dusseldorf, Dusseldorf, Germany

G. Antoch
Department of Diagnostic and Interventional Radiology, University Dusseldorf,
Dusseldorf, Germany

R. P. Baum and F. Rösch (eds.), *Theranostics, Gallium-68, and Other Radionuclides*, Recent Results in Cancer Research 194, DOI: 10.1007/978-3-642-27994-2_18,

workup before prospective peptide receptor radionuclide therapy (PRRT). The performance of both imaging methods was analyzed and compared for detection of individual lesions per patient and for eight defined body regions. A region was regarded as positive if at least one lesion was detected in that region. In addition, radiopeptide uptake in terms of the maximal standardized uptake value (SUV_{max}) was compared for concordant lesions and renal parenchyma. *Results*: Fifty-one regions were found positive with both ^{68}Ga-DOTATATE and ^{68}Ga-DOTATOC. Overall, however, significantly fewer lesions were detected with ^{68}Ga-DOTATATE in comparison with ^{68}Ga-DOTATOC (174 versus 179, $p < 0.05$). Mean ^{68}Ga-DOTATATE SUV_{max} across all lesions was significantly lower compared with ^{68}Ga-DOTATOC (16.9 ± 6.8 versus 22.1 ± 12.0, $p < 0.01$). Mean SUV_{max} for renal parenchyma was not significantly different between ^{68}Ga-DOTATATE and ^{68}Ga-DOTATOC (12.6 ± 2.6 versus 12.6 ± 2.7). *Conclusions*: ^{68}Ga-DOTATOC and ^{68}Ga-DOTATATE possess similar diagnostic accuracy for detection of gastroenteropancreatic NET lesions (with a potential advantage of ^{68}Ga-DOTATOC) despite their evident difference in affinity for sst2. Quite unexpectedly, maximal uptake of ^{68}Ga-DOTATOC tended to be higher than its ^{68}Ga-DOTATATE counterpart. However, tumor uptake shows high inter- and intraindividual variance with unpredictable preference of one radiopeptide. Thus, our data encourage the application of different sst ligands to enable personalized imaging and therapy of gastroenteropancreatic NET with optimal targeting of tumor receptors.

Keywords
^{68}Ga-DOTATOC PET/CT · ^{68}Ga-DOTATATE PET/CT · NET

Contents

1 Introduction

Abundant expression of somatostatin receptors (sst) is a characteristic of neuroendocrine tumors (NET). To date, five somatostatin receptor subtypes have been cloned and characterized to bind somatostatin with nanomolar affinity (sst1–sst5) (Hoyer et al. 1995; Reubi et al. 2000). NET typically express several sst subtypes in a pattern related to tumor type, origin, and grade of differentiation (Reubi and Waser 2003; Reubi et al. 2001). In most gastroenteropancreatic NET, sst2 binding sites predominate on the majority of tumors (Reubi and Waser 2003; Reubi et al. 2001). Structural differences between sst subtypes allow for receptor targeting with subtype-specific radiolabeled somatostatin analogs (Boy et al. 2011). Several of these are used for peptide receptor radionuclide therapy (PRRT) and scintigraphic or positron emission tomographic (PET) imaging of NET. In particular, sst scintigraphy and PET have become key diagnostic techniques as NET are often difficult to identify with morphological imaging (lesions are frequently small-sized and present in variable anatomical locations). Moreover, recent research demonstrated the superiority of sst PET over scintigraphy and CT (Buchmann et al. 2007; Gabriel et al. 2007).

The efficiency of a given somatostatin analog in detection of NET lesions or PRRT depends on its specific binding profile. Particularly, its affinity to sst2 is essential. Two compounds most frequently used for sst PET and PRRT are DOTA-D-Phe1-Tyr3-octreotide (DOTATOC) and DOTA-D-Phe1-Tyr3-octreotate (DOTATATE). Reubi et al. determined the binding profiles of these and several other radiolabeled somatostatin analogs. There were significant differences in subtype-specific affinity after minor structural changes in the radioligand molecule, the introduction of a radiometal, or the use of different radiometals and chelators (Reubi et al. 2000). However, data regarding the analog with the highest uptake in NET show discrepancies between in vitro and animal data on the one side (Reubi et al. 2000; de Jong et al. 1998; Storch et al. 2005) and human data on the other (Forrer et al. 2004): Reubi and colleagues determined the affinity of ^{68}Ga-DOTATATE in binding sst2 (0.2 ± 0.04 nM) to be approximately tenfold higher than that of ^{68}Ga-DOTATOC (2.5 ± 0.5 nM) (Reubi et al. 2000). De Jong et al. (1998) compared ^{111}In-DTPA-Tyr3-octreotide and ^{111}In-DTPA-Tyr3-octreotate (and others) in rats bearing sst-expressing tumors: octreotate exhibited the highest uptake from all compounds tested. Storch et al. (2005) reported similar results of a comparison including ^{111}In-DTPA-Tyr0-octreotide and ^{111}In-DOTA-Tyr3-octreotate (also animal data). However, Forrer et al. (2004) could not find relevant differences in tumor uptake of ^{111}In-DOTATOC versus ^{111}In-DOTATATE in a direct comparison in patients with metastasized NET. Moreover, Poeppel et al. (2011) found the uptake of ^{68}Ga-DOTATOC to be higher than that of ^{68}Ga-DOTATATE in patients with different types of NET.

The controversy regarding the optimal radiopeptide extends into the therapeutic setting as both compounds are used in PRRT. Since nephrotoxicity is a major concern in PRRT, the dose-limiting factor is often the radiation absorbed dose to the kidneys (Rolleman et al. 2010). The dose is determined by the radiometal and the uptake/retention of the radiopeptide (Rolleman et al. 2010; Bodei et al. 2008; Valkema et al. 2005). Hence, the tumor-to-kidney ratio of a radiopeptide is crucial, as the efficacy of PRRT relies on the tumor dose, which is limited by the maximum dose that can be safely administered to the kidney. While Forrer et al. (2004) reported a higher tumor-to-kidney ratio for ^{90}Y-DOTATOC than ^{90}Y-DOTATATE, Esser et al. (2006) reported results in favor of ^{177}Lu-DOTATATE versus ^{177}Lu-DOTATOC.

Currently, there is no direct comparison of ^{68}Ga-DOTATATE and ^{68}Ga-DOTATOC available regarding tumor uptake and ability to detect gastroenteropancreatic NET. Thus, it is unclear which radiopeptide is preferable for imaging and therapy of those NET patients.

Therefore, the aim of this study is to compare the tumor uptake of ^{68}Ga-DOTATOC versus ^{68}Ga-DOTATATE and their diagnostic value in PET/CT in the same patients with gastroenteropancreatic NET.

2 Patients and Methods

2.1 Patients

Twenty-seven patients (21 males, 6 females, average age 62 ± 10 years, range 46–81 years) were imaged as part of the workup before prospective PRRT. As the two peptides DOTATOC and DOTATATE are readily available in our department, imaging is routinely performed with both ^{68}Ga-DOTATOC and ^{68}Ga-DOTATATE to determine optimal uptake for treatment with either ^{90}Y-DOTATOC or ^{90}Y-DOTATATE. All patients suffered from histologically verified gastroenteropancreatic NET and had prior imaging evidence of primary or residual or recurrent disease (primary tumor, metastases, or both). All aspects of patient care and treatment were performed at the discretion of the treating clinicians and according to routine procedures of the department, which are in accordance with the guidelines of the European Neuroendocrine Tumor Society (Plockinger et al. 2004). The imaging workup was performed in accordance with guidelines issued by the university hospital institutional review board. Written informed consent was obtained from all patients. A somatostatin analog therapy was discontinued at least 4 weeks prior to the imaging procedures.

2.2 Radiopharmaceutical Preparation

In-house synthesis of ^{68}Ga-peptides was performed according to the method described by Zhernosekov et al. (2007). ^{68}Ga was obtained from a ^{68}Ge/^{68}Ga radionuclide generator (Eckert & Ziegler, Germany). Peptides were obtained from Bachem (Switzerland). Overall preparation time was about 60 min with radiochemical yield of 60–70%. Quality control carried out with two thin-layer chromatography systems revealed radiochemical purity of >98%.

2.3 ^{68}Ga-DOTATOC and ^{68}Ga-DOTATATE Imaging

All patients underwent ^{68}Ga-DOTATOC/^{68}Ga-DOTATATE imaging with an average time interval between the two examinations of less than 14 days. Three patients received the ^{68}Ga-DOTATATE scan initially, whereas all others received the ^{68}Ga-DOTATOC scan first.

Imaging was performed using two (ECAT) EXACT HR + PET scanners: one stand-alone system (CTI/Siemens), the other the PET component of an integrated PET/CT scanner (Biograph Emotion Duo, Siemens). Both PET systems had been cross-calibrated. Imaging was performed as previously described (Boy et al. 2011; Antoch et al. 2002, 2004). In short, attenuation-corrected whole-body (skull base to upper thighs) scans were acquired in three-dimensional mode (4 min emission time per bed position, 3 min transmission time on the stand-alone PET, Fourier rebinning attenuation-weighted ordered-subset expectation-maximization reconstruction algorithm, smoothing with 5-mm Gaussian kernel). In PET/CT, the CT was performed first in a limited breath-hold technique [CT acquisition parameters for full (low) dose protocol: 130 (15) mAs, 130 (110) kV, slice width 5 mm, rotation time 0.8 s, table speed 8 mm per rotation]. Iodinated contrast material was given intravenously by using an automated injector. The small bowel was distended by administration of a water-equivalent oral contrast agent (Antoch et al. 2004). To minimize radiation exposure and to avoid repeated use of contrast agents, each patient received only one full-dose contrast-enhanced CT scan. Thus, 25 patients received both examinations on the PET/CT (first scan in full-dose, second scan in low-dose technique in 21 patients; both scans in low-dose technique in 4 patients) and 2 patients (with recent external whole-body contrast-enhanced CT) were evaluated on the stand-alone scanner.

2.4 Image Evaluation

Images were initially interpreted visually by two experienced nuclear medicine physicians blinded to the results of the other imaging examinations by counting the number of lesions with pathologically increased radiopeptide uptake in eight regions: "head/neck," "mediastinum," "lung," "liver," "pancreas," "abdomen/pelvis" (excluding liver and pancreas), "bone," and "lymph nodes" (whole body, i.e., composite of several regions). Only lesions with a morphologic correlate on the CT of the full-dose PET/CT or on follow-up examinations were considered. Thus, only 20 of the patients with a full-dose PET/CT were analyzed in this manner. If more than five lesions were visualized within one region, the number of lesions was truncated at five for that region to avoid bias (Binderup et al. 2010; Therasse et al. 2000). In a second semiquantitative approach, maximal standardized uptake values (SUV_{max}) were determined in all patients on a lesion-by-lesion basis by one of the initial readers. SUV measurements were carried out side-by-side on corresponding lesions on fused image data sets. Spherical volumes of interest (VOI) were drawn closely encircling a lesion, and the SUV_{max} was obtained. If more than five lesions were visualized within one organ, only the first five lesions in craniocaudal direction were considered, with the exception of the liver where the lesions were traced in caudocranial direction to avoid attenuation artifacts. Spherical reference VOIs were drawn in unaffected liver tissue, the erector spinae muscles, and the gluteal muscles on the left or right side (as appropriate). The native SUV_{max} of the lesions were normalized to the SUV_{max} of the liver reference region and to the average SUV_{max} of the muscle reference regions. A further spherical VOI was placed in the renal cortex avoiding the pelvis and calyces in the left or right kidney (as appropriate).

2.5 Statistical Analysis

Analysis was performed at three levels. The first level addressed the aforementioned eight regions. A region was regarded as positive if at least one lesion was detected therein. The second level analyzed the individual count of lesions per region that were detected in an imaging session. At the third level, the SUV_{max} of corresponding lesions (overall and in five subgroups: hepatic metastases, lymphatic metastases, bone metastases, pulmonary metastases, and primary tumor) was compared.

Nonparametric methods were used. Positive regions were compared using McNemar's test for paired observations of dichotomous traits. The number of lesions per region from the regional analysis and the SUV_{max} of corresponding lesions from the lesional analysis were compared using Wilcoxon signed-rank test for paired observations. Scanning parameters were tested for possible differences with Mann–Whitney U test for independent samples. Potential correlations were tested with Kruskal–Wallis ANOVA or Spearman's rank correlation coefficient as appropriate. Significance level was 0.05, two-sided. Bonferroni correction was applied as appropriate. Analyses were performed with STATISTICA version 8 (StatSoft, Inc.).

3 Results

Scan parameters and patient characteristics are presented in Tables 1 and 2, respectively. There was no significant difference between both imaging procedures regarding the scanning parameters (uptake time, injected activity, specific activity, injected peptide mass).

3.1 Regional and Lesional Analyses

Fifty-one regions (excluding the composite region "lymph nodes") were found positive with both ^{68}Ga-DOTATATE and ^{68}Ga-DOTATOC (Table 3). There was no discrepant region. On average three positive regions were found per patient with each of the imaging procedures. There was no significant difference between the two imaging procedures regarding the number of detected regions per patient

Table 1 Patient characteristics

Pat. no.	Age (years)	Sex	Primary NET site	Previous treatments	Ki-67	SUV_{max} ^{68}Ga-DOTATATE	SUV_{max} ^{68}Ga-DOTATOC
1	49	Male	Foregut (gastric)	Surgery, SIRT, PRRT	30	11.1	13.8
2	77	Female	Midgut	Surgery, chemotherapy	5	25.5	29.2
3	70	Male	Midgut	Chemotherapy	<1	17.8	26.2
4	62	Female	Midgut (appendiceal)	Surgery, chemotherapy, PRRT	5	8.5	12.3
5	72	Male	Midgut (cecal)	Surgery	<1	24.1	30.0
6	72	Male	Midgut (duodenal)	Surgery	N.a.	7.4	10.7
7	65	Male	Midgut (ileal)	Surgery, somatostatin analogs	<2	13.8	18.4
8	79	Male	Midgut (ileal)	Surgery, chemotherapy, interferon alpha, PRRT	N.a.	18.2	21.1
9	58	Male	Midgut (ileal)	Surgery, somatostatin analogs	5	19.1	12.3
10	61	Male	Midgut (ileal)	Surgery	1	10.3	14.5
11	57	Male	Midgut (ileal)	Somatostatin analogs, PRRT	1	15.6	30.2
12	46	Male	Midgut (ileal)	Surgery, somatostatin analogs	<2	15.6	32.4
13	69	Female	Midgut (ileal)	Surgery, SIRT	40	28.0	12.9
14	54	Male	Midgut (ileal)	Surgery, somatostatin analogs, PRRT, chemoembolization	<1	17.0	12.1
15	70	Male	Midgut (ileocecal)	Surgery, somatostatin analogs, PRRT	<1	11.2	15.5
16	81	Male	Midgut (ileocecal)	Surgery, somatostatin analogs	<2	10.3	10.1
17	71	Male	Midgut (jejunal)	Surgery, somatostatin analogs	10	28.2	22.2

(continued)

Table 1 (continued)

Pat. no.	Age (years)	Sex	Primary NET site	Previous treatments	Ki-67	SUV_{max} ^{68}Ga-DOTATATE	SUV_{max} ^{68}Ga-DOTATOC
18	66	Male	Midgut (jejunal)	None	<1	9.9	12.0
19	48	Female	Pancreas	Surgery, somatostatin analogs	<2	6.8	6.9
20	59	Male	Pancreas	None	30	20.0	28.1
21	46	Male	Pancreas	Surgery (metastases), chemotherapy, PRRT	3	27.0	33.8
22	56	Female	Pancreas	Surgery, chemotherapy, SIRT, TACE, PRRT	10	18.9	20.0
23	55	Female	Pancreas	PRRT	5	20.0	25.5
24	67	Male	Pancreas	Surgery	5	16.4	21.5
25	66	Male	Pancreas	Surgery	5	12.8	18.1
26	53	Male	Pancreatic gastrinoma	Surgery	<1	13.8	46.6
27	50	Male	Pancreatic insulinoma	Somatostatin analogs	N.a.	30.2	60.5

CUP cancer of unknown primary, *NET* neuroendocrine tumor, *N.a.* not available, *PRRT* peptide receptor radionuclide therapy, *SIRT* selective internal radiation therapy, *TACE* transarterial chemoembolization

Table 2 Scan parameters

Scan parameter	^{68}Ga-DOTATATE			^{68}Ga-DOTATOC		
	Mean	SD	Range	Mean	SD	Range
Uptake time (min)	56	32	24–161	68	32	29–162
Activity per dose (MBq)	102	13	60–123	88	16	52–111
Specific activity (MBq/nmol)	48.9	24.1	16.0–95.6	41	20.6	10.9–81
Peptide per dose (μg)	6	3	2–13	6	3	2–12

Table 3 Regional analyses: positive regions per patient

Pat. no. (n = 20)	Regions positive*	
	^{68}Ga-DOTATATE	^{68}Ga-DOTATOC
1	2	2
3	3	3
4	4	4
5	1	1
6	1	1
9	2	2
10	2	2
11	2	2
12	2	2
14	1	1
15	2	2
17	2	2
18	4	4
19	2	2
21	4	4
22	1	1
23	5	5
24	6	6
25	3	3
26	2	2
Sum	*51*	*51*
Mean	3	3

* Excluding the composite region "lymph nodes"

Table 4 Regional analyses: lesions per region

Region	Number of patients	
	^{68}Ga-DOTATATE	^{68}Ga-DOTATOC
Head/neck	1	1
Mediastinum	6	6
Lung	1	1
Liver	17	17
Pancreas	5	5
Abdomen/pelvis	14	14
Bone	7	7
Lymph nodes*	15	15

* Composite region

or the number of patients with at least one lesion within one of the eight regions (including the composite region "lymph nodes") (Table 4).

Within the defined regions (excluding the composite region "lymph nodes") 174 lesions were detected with ^{68}Ga-DOTATATE versus 179 lesions with ^{68}Ga-DOTATOC (versus Table 5). The difference was significant ($p = 0.043$). The five lesions that were detected additionally with ^{68}Ga-DOTATOC were found in five patients and were distributed among the following regions: "liver" (two patients), "pancreas," "abdomen/pelvis," and "bone." On average 8.7 lesions were found per patient with ^{68}Ga-DOTATATE versus 9.0 lesions with ^{68}Ga-DOTATOC. There was no significant difference between the two imaging procedures in lesion detection with respect to tumor grading or tumor origin (foregut, midgut, pancreas).

3.2 SUV Analyses

Mean ^{68}Ga-DOTATATE SUV_{max} across all lesions was 16.9 ± 6.8, versus 22.1 ± 12.0 with ^{68}Ga-DOTATOC (Table 6). The difference was significant ($p = 0.007$) and retained its significance for the normalized values ($p < 0.05$). The difference retained its significance across the subgroups hepatic metastases (24 patients, $p = 0.003$) and lymphatic metastases (16 patients, $p = 0.002$). No significance test was applied to the subgroups bone metastases (10 patients), primary tumor (8 patients), and pulmonary metastases (1 patient) owing to the small sample size.

The mean difference between ^{68}Ga-DOTATATE and ^{68}Ga-DOTATOC SUV_{max} across all lesions was 7.6 ± 8.0 (range 0.1–32.8). There was no significant relation between the differences of SUV_{max} measurements between ^{68}Ga-DOTATATE and ^{68}Ga-DOTATOC and tumor grading or tumor origin (foregut, midgut, pancreas).

Even though 22 out of 27 patients exhibited on average higher ^{68}Ga-DOTATOC SUV_{max} than ^{68}Ga-DOTATATE SUV_{max}, the tumor uptake varied considerably both within and between patients: 13 patients displayed only lesions with

Table 5 Regional analyses: lesions per patient

Pat. no. (n = 20)	Lesions per patient*	
	^{68}Ga-DOTATATE	^{68}Ga-DOTATOC
1	10	10
3	9	9
4	15	16
5	5	5
6	1	1
9	6	6
10	7	7
11	7	7
12	6	7
14	5	5
15	6	7
17	8	8
18	15	15
19	10	10
21	8	8
22	5	5
23	18	18
24	19	19
25	11	12
26	3	4
Sum	*174*	*179*
Mean	*8.7*	*9.0*

* Excluding the composite region "lymph nodes"

higher uptake of ^{68}Ga-DOTATOC than ^{68}Ga-DOTATATE (Fig. 1), 11 patients displayed a mixture of lesions with either higher uptake of ^{68}Ga-DOTATATE or (predominantly) of ^{68}Ga-DOTATOC, and 3 patients displayed only lesions with higher uptake of ^{68}Ga-DOTATATE than ^{68}Ga-DOTATOC (Fig. 2).

There was no significant difference between measurements of SUV_{max} in patients with or without prior somatostatin analog therapy.

Mean ^{68}Ga-DOTATATE SUV_{max} for renal parenchyma was 12.6 ± 2.6 versus 12.6 ± 2.7 with ^{68}Ga-DOTATOC (Table 6). The difference was not significant for both the native and the normalized values. Tumor-to-kidney ratio was 1.5 ± 0.8 for ^{68}Ga-DOTATATE versus 1.8 ± 1.2 for ^{68}Ga-DOTATOC. The difference was significant ($p = 0.005$). The correlation coefficient of mean SUV_{max} ^{68}Ga-DOTATATE and ^{68}Ga-DOTATOC for renal parenchyma was 0.50.

Table 6 Tumor uptake: SUV_{max}

Group (no. of patients)	^{68}Ga-DOTATATE			^{68}Ga-DOTATOC		
	Mean SUV_{max}			Mean SUV_{max}		
	Native	Normalized (liver)	Normalized (muscle)	Native	Normalized (liver)	Normalized (muscle)
All ($n = 27$)	16.9	2.2	8.8	22.1	2.3	10.5
Hepatic metastases ($n = 24$)	20.2	2.6	10.2	24.4	2.6	11.9
Bone metastases ($n = 10$)	12.1	1.6	6.6	15.6	1.9	8.8
Lymphatic metastases ($n = 16$)	17.4	2.1	9.3	23.8	2.5	11.1
Pulmonary metastases ($n = 1$)	4.4	0.5	1.9	4.7	0.4	2.3
Primary tumor ($n = 8$)	19.6	2.7	12.7	37.4	3.0	16.7

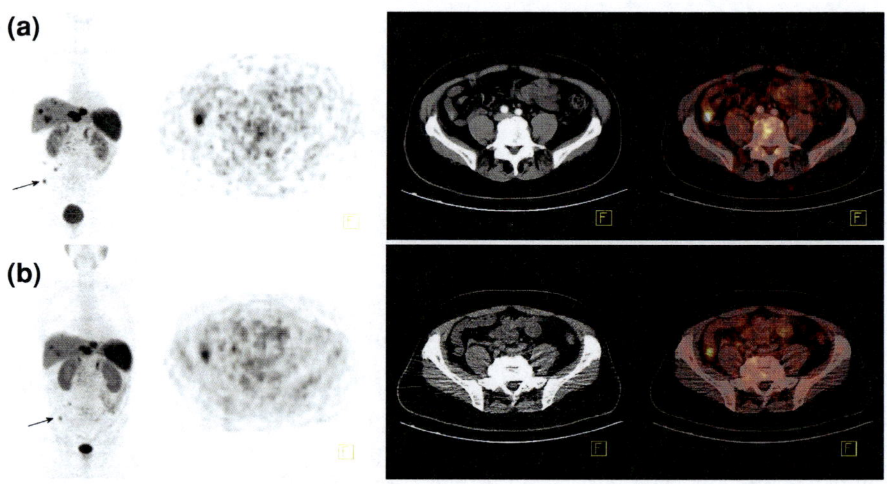

Fig. 1 Example of lesions with exclusively higher uptake of ^{68}Ga-DOTATOC than ^{68}Ga-DOTATATE (patient no. 11). **a** From *left* to *right*: ^{68}Ga-DOTATOC-PET maximum-intensity projection, ^{68}Ga-DOTATOC PET, CT, PET/CT fusion. **b** From *left* to *right*: ^{68}Ga-DOTATATE PET maximum-intensity projection, ^{68}Ga-DOTATATE PET, CT, PET/CT fusion. *Arrow* Ileal carcinoid (SUV_{max} ^{68}Ga-DOTATOC: 21.0; SUV_{max} ^{68}Ga-DOTATATE: 8.2)

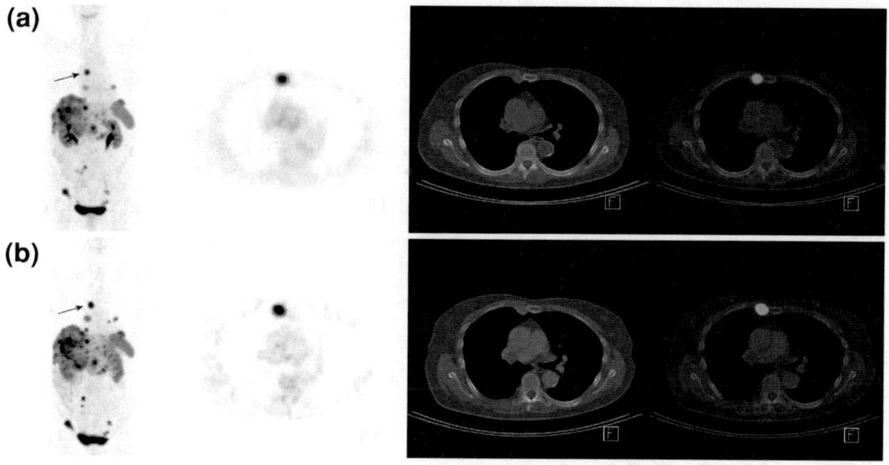

Fig. 2 Example of lesions with exclusively higher uptake of ^{68}Ga-DOTATATE than ^{68}Ga-DOTATOC (patient no. 13). **a** From *left* to *right*: ^{68}Ga-DOTATOC-PET maximum-intensity projection, ^{68}Ga-DOTATOC PET, CT, PET/CT fusion. **b** From *left* to *right*: ^{68}Ga-DOTATATE PET maximum-intensity projection, ^{68}Ga-DOTATATE PET, CT, PET/CT fusion. *Arrow* Lymph node metastasis (SUV_{max} DOTATOC: 16.1; SUV_{max} DOTATATE: 36.8)

4 Discussion

This direct comparison demonstrates the good capability of both ^{68}Ga-DOTATATE and ^{68}Ga-DOTATOC to detect lesions from gastroenteropancreatic NET. However, ^{68}Ga-DOTATOC is potentially superior to ^{68}Ga-DOTATATE, presumably due to higher tumor uptake as indicated by SUV_{max}. Nonetheless, there was considerable variance in preferential tumor uptake of the two radiopeptides.

4.1 Lesion Detection

^{68}Ga-DOTATOC was marginally superior to ^{68}Ga-DOTATATE in detecting gastroenteropancreatic NET lesions. The advantage was "on the whole" and not limited to higher detection rates within one of the evaluated distinct body regions (head/neck, mediastinum, lung, liver, pancreas, abdomen/pelvis, bone, lymph nodes) or a distinct type of metastatic spread (lymphatic, hepatic, osseous, pulmonary). Four published studies compared both analogs (coupled to different radiometals) in patients (Forrer et al. 2004; Poeppel et al. 2011; Esser et al. 2006; Kwekkeboom et al. 2001), although mainly for dosimetric purposes. Forrer et al. (2004) provide some details about lesion detection. They investigated ^{111}In-DOTATOC and ^{111}In-DOTATATE in a small set of patients: The results obtained with both compounds were comparable; however, ^{111}In-DOTATOC enabled better visualization of some liver metastases (Forrer et al. 2004). The results of Poeppel et al. from different types of NET are in line with the actual results from sole gastroenteropancreatic NET.

Tumor differentiation influences the detection of NET lesions with radiolabeled somatostatin analogs owing to a varying capability of expressing sst (Kayani et al. 2008). Moreover, the origin of a NET influences its profile of expression of sst subtypes (Koopmans et al. 2009). We examined whether these parameters possessed differential influence on the rate of lesion detection with both tracers. However, we found no significant difference between the two imaging procedures in lesion detection with respect to grading (low, intermediate, high grade) or tumor origin (foregut, midgut, pancreas).

4.2 Tumor Uptake

SUV_{max} of concordant lesions obtained with ^{68}Ga-DOTATOC was significantly higher than that obtained with ^{68}Ga-DOTATATE. Normalization either to a tissue with moderate to high sst expression (liver) or to a tissue with low sst expression (muscle) was not able to reduce "interpeptide" variability and did not cause relevant changes of the results. According to Reubi and colleagues, bronchopulmonary and gastroenteropancreatic NET are mainly characterized by overexpression of sst1 and sst2 (Reubi and Waser 2003; Reubi et al. 2001). Neither ^{68}Ga-DOTATOC nor ^{68}Ga-DOTATATE show relevant binding to sst1 (Reubi et al. 2000). Hence, the higher SUV_{max} of ^{68}Ga-DOTATOC is surprising given that ^{68}Ga-DOTATATE possess an approximately tenfold higher in vitro affinity in binding sst2 [0.2 ± 0.04 versus 2.5 ± 0.5 nM (Reubi et al. 2000)]. However, some NET exhibit overexpression of sst5 (Reubi et al. 2001; Wild et al. 2005). ^{68}Ga-DOTATOC possesses a somewhat higher affinity for this receptor subtype in comparison with ^{68}Ga-DOTATATE (73 ± 21 versus 377 ± 18 nM) (Reubi et al. 2000). This difference in affinity profiles might explain the differential tumor uptake. However, this explanation remains hypothetical as no receptor staining of the NET lesions in question was performed.

Our results are in contrast to animal data: De Jong et al. compared ^{111}In-DTPA-octreotide and ^{111}In-DTPA-octreotate (and others) both in vitro and in vivo in the same rats bearing somatostatin receptor-expressing pancreatic tumors: ^{111}In-Octreotate possessed the highest uptake in tumors from all compounds tested (de Jong et al. 1998). Storch et al. reported similar results comparing ^{111}In-DTPA-octreotide and ^{111}In-DOTA-octreotate (and others) both in vitro and in vivo in rats (Storch et al. 2005). As aforementioned, there are four studies comparing biodistribution and dosimetry of both analogs in patients (Forrer et al. 2004; Poeppel et al. 2011; Esser et al. 2006; Kwekkeboom et al. 2001). Forrer et al. (2004) found no significant difference in mean residence times and estimated mean absorbed tumor doses for ^{90}Y-DOTATOC and

^{90}Y-DOTATATE, although mean doses derived from ^{111}In-DOTATOC were slightly higher. Poeppel et al. (2011) found the uptake of ^{68}Ga-DOTATOC to be higher than that of ^{68}Ga-DOTATATE in patients with different types of NET. In contrast to these results, Esser et al. reported ^{177}Lu-DOTATATE to possess higher affinity than ^{177}Lu-DOTATOC in the therapeutic setting. However, data are only provided for residence times (which were longer for ^{177}Lu-DOTATATE than ^{177}Lu-DOTATOC). Kwekkeboom et al. (2001) also reported higher tumor uptake of ^{177}Lu-DOTA-octreotate versus ^{111}In-DTPA-octreotide. However, they used both a different chelator and a different radiometal in their comparison, which exerts significant influence on receptor binding (Reubi et al. 2000).

The mean difference across all lesional SUV_{max} measurements between ^{68}Ga-DOTATATE and ^{68}Ga-DOTATOC tended to be small; however, there was considerable variance both within and between patients: nearly half of all patients displayed a mixture of lesions with either higher uptake of ^{68}Ga-DOTATATE or (predominantly) of ^{68}Ga-DOTATOC, most of the remaining patients displayed solely lesions with higher uptake of ^{68}Ga-DOTATOC, and a minority of patients displayed only lesions with higher uptake of ^{68}Ga-DOTATATE. Our findings are in line with those of Forrer et al. and Poeppel et al., who found sst expression to vary considerably between patients and tumor manifestations (Forrer et al. 2004; Poeppel et al. 2011). These variations imply a wide spectrum of cellular differentiation and receptor expression of NET. However, there was no significant relation between the differences of SUV_{max} measurements between ^{68}Ga-DOTATATE and ^{68}Ga-DOTATOC regarding tumor grading (low, intermediate, high grade) or tumor origin (foregut, midgut, pancreas).

In the case of receptor-active substances, the SUV_{max} represents a composite measure of specific receptor binding and internalization, unspecific binding, effects of tissue perfusion, and others (Koukouraki et al. 2006; Rodrigues et al. 2006). The intrapatient comparison approach in this study controls for most confounding factors, rendering differences in SUV_{max} to be most likely caused by differences in binding and internalization properties of the respective somatostatin analog. However, possible differences in attenuation correction between (predominantly) low-dose PET/CT in ^{68}Ga-DOTATATE scans and contrast-enhanced PET/CT in ^{68}Ga-DOTATOC scans may have influenced the results. However, those effects seem to be of negligible size (Antoch et al. 2002; Yau et al. 2005). In particular, relevant artificial differences are unlikely, since the ^{68}Ga-DOTATOC SUV_{max} of the combination of PET-only scans and low-dose PET/CT is still significantly higher than its ^{68}Ga-DOTATATE counterpart ($p < 0.05$). Also, a bias due to slightly longer uptake time of ^{68}Ga-DOTATOC than ^{68}Ga-DOTATATE scans cannot be excluded. However, there was no significant difference between the SUV_{max} of ^{68}Ga-DOTATATE scans with shorter versus longer uptake time than the corresponding ^{68}Ga-DOTATOC scans. Furthermore, somatostatin analog therapy may affect tumor uptake due to interacting factors such as partial saturation of sst-expressing nontarget tissues and competition of labeled and unlabeled somatostatin analog for the receptor on tumor tissue. On this account, the medication was discontinued before the imaging procedures. Consequently, no significant differences between measurements of SUV_{max} in patients with or without prior somatostatin analog therapy were found.

4.3 Renal Uptake

There was no significant difference between renal uptake of the two radiopeptides. However, the tumor-to-kidney ratio found in this study was significantly in favor of ^{68}Ga-DOTATOC. This finding is in contrast to aforementioned animal data on ^{111}In-DTPA-OC and ^{111}In-DTPA-TATE (Storch et al. 2005) but is in line with human data derived from a comparison of ^{111}In-DOTATOC and ^{111}In-DOTA-TATE (Forrer et al. 2004) as well as ^{68}Ga-DOTATOC and ^{68}Ga-DOTATATE (Poeppel et al. 2011). As nephrotoxicity is a major concern in PRRT (Bodei et al. 2008; Valkema et al. 2005), one might thus speculate about the peptide to prefer for therapy to receive optimal tumor doses while avoiding renal impairment (Rolleman et al. 2010). However, caution must be applied when translating this diagnostic investigation to a therapeutic setting, as significantly higher peptide concentrations are used in the latter case. The interplay of unspecific peptide binding, partial saturation of sst-expressing nontarget tissues, and competition of labeled and unlabeled peptide for the receptor on tumor tissue affects overall uptake in the tumor (de Jong et al. 1999; Velikyan et al. 2010). Hence, the uptake of radiolabeled somatostatin analogs in sst-expressing tumors is dependent on the amount of injected peptide mass (de Jong et al. 1999). Moreover, not only peptide uptake but also residence times are factors determining the target dose. Esser et al. (2006) found the residence times of ^{177}Lu-DOTATATE in comparison with ^{177}Lu-DOTATOC to be longer both in tumors and in the kidneys. However, division of the mean tumor residence time ratio by the mean kidney residence time ratio yielded a factor of 1.5 in favor of ^{177}Lu-DOTATATE. It is thus even more complicated to decide which peptide is to be preferred for radiotherapy. Moreover, tumor uptake shows high inter- and intraindividual variance, with unpredictable preferential of one radiopeptide. Only measurements with both radiopeptides reliably permit the choice of the optimal radiopeptide for therapy. Moreover, individual dosimetry seems advisable to decide whether a patient can be admitted for therapy with radiolabeled DOTATOC or DOTATATE.

5 Conclusion

^{68}Ga-DOTATOC and ^{68}Ga-DOTATATE possess comparable diagnostic value in detection of lesions of gastroenteropancreatic NET with a potential advantage of ^{68}Ga-DOTATOC. The approximately tenfold higher affinity in binding sst2 of ^{68}Ga-DOTATATE does not prove to be diagnostically relevant. Quite unexpectedly, maximal uptake of ^{68}Ga-DOTATOC tended to be higher than its ^{68}Ga-DOTATATE counterpart.

Nevertheless, there is significant inter- and intraindividual variance regarding which radiopeptide has maximal lesional uptake. Thus, our data encourage the application of different sst ligands to enable personalized imaging and therapy of gastroenteropancreatic NET with optimal targeting of tumor receptors.

References

Antoch G, Freudenberg LS, Stattaus J, Jentzen W, Mueller SP, Debatin JF et al (2002) Whole-body positron emission tomography-CT: optimized CT using oral and IV contrast materials. AJR Am J Roentgenol 179:1555–1560

Antoch G, Kuehl H, Kanja J, Lauenstein TC, Schneemann H, Hauth E et al (2004) Dual-modality PET/CT scanning with negative oral contrast agent to avoid artifacts: introduction and evaluation. Radiology 230:879–885. doi:10.1148/radiol.2303021287

Binderup T, Knigge U, Loft A, Mortensen J, Pfeifer A, Federspiel B et al (2010) Functional imaging of neuroendocrine tumors: a head-to-head comparison of somatostatin receptor scintigraphy, 123I-MIBG scintigraphy, and 18F-FDG PET. J Nucl Med 51:704–712. doi: 10.2967/jnumed.109.069765

Bodei L, Cremonesi M, Ferrari M, Pacifici M, Grana CM, Bartolomei M et al (2008) Long-term evaluation of renal toxicity after peptide receptor radionuclide therapy with 90Y-DOTATOC and 177Lu-DOTATATE: the role of associated risk factors. Eur J Nucl Med Mol Imaging 35:1847–1856. doi:10.1007/s00259-008-0778-1

Boy C, Heusner TA, Poeppel TD, Redmann-Bischofs A, Unger N, Jentzen W et al (2011) (68)Ga-DOTATOC PET/CT and somatostatin receptor (sst1–sst5) expression in normal human tissue: correlation of sst2 mRNA and SUV(max). Eur J Nucl Med Mol Imaging. doi: 10.1007/s00259-011-1760-x

Buchmann I, Henze M, Engelbrecht S, Eisenhut M, Runz A, Schafer M et al (2007) Comparison of 68Ga-DOTATOC PET and 111In-DTPAOC (octreoscan) SPECT in patients with neuroendocrine tumours. Eur J Nucl Med Mol Imaging 34:1617–1626. doi: 10.1007/s00259-007-0450-1

de Jong M, Breeman WA, Bakker WH, Kooij PP, Bernard BF, Hofland LJ et al (1998) Comparison of (111)In-labeled somatostatin analogues for tumor scintigraphy and radionuclide therapy. Cancer Res 58:437–441

de Jong M, Breeman WA, Bernard BF, van Gameren A, de Bruin E, Bakker WH et al (1999) Tumour uptake of the radiolabelled somatostatin analogue [DOTA0, TYR3]octreotide is dependent on the peptide amount. Eur J Nucl Med 26:693–698

Esser JP, Krenning EP, Teunissen JJ, Kooij PP, van Gameren AL, Bakker WH et al (2006) Comparison of [(177)Lu-DOTA(0), Tyr(3)]octreotate and [(177)Lu-DOTA(0), Tyr(3)]octreotide: which peptide is preferable for PRRT? Eur J Nucl Med Mol Imaging 33:1346–1351. doi:10.1007/s00259-006-0172-9

Forrer F, Uusijarvi H, Waldherr C, Cremonesi M, Bernhardt P, Mueller-Brand J et al (2004) A comparison of (111)In-DOTATOC and (111)In-DOTATATE: biodistribution and dosimetry in the same patients with metastatic neuroendocrine tumours. Eur J Nucl Med Mol Imaging 31:1257–1262. doi:10.1007/s00259-004-1553-6

Gabriel M, Decristoforo C, Kendler D, Dobrozemsky G, Heute D, Uprimny C et al (2007) 68Ga-DOTA-Tyr3-octreotide PET in neuroendocrine tumors: comparison with somatostatin receptor scintigraphy and CT. J Nucl Med 48:508–518.

Hoyer D, Bell GI, Berelowitz M, Epelbaum J, Feniuk W, Humphrey PP et al (1995) Classification and nomenclature of somatostatin receptors. Trends Pharmacol Sci 16:86–88. doi: S0165614700889889

Kayani I, Bomanji JB, Groves A, Conway G, Gacinovic S, Win T et al (2008) Functional imaging of neuroendocrine tumors with combined PET/CT using 68Ga-DOTATATE (DOTA-DPhe1, Tyr3-octreotate) and 18F-FDG. Cancer 112:2447–2455. doi:10.1002/cncr.23469

Koopmans KP, Neels ON, Kema IP, Elsinga PH, Links TP, de Vries EG et al (2009) Molecular imaging in neuroendocrine tumors: molecular uptake mechanisms and clinical results. Crit Rev Oncol Hematol 71:199–213. doi:10.1016/j.critrevonc.2009.02.009

Koukouraki S, Strauss LG, Georgoulias V, Schuhmacher J, Haberkorn U, Karkavitsas N et al (2006) Evaluation of the pharmacokinetics of 68Ga-DOTATOC in patients with metastatic neuroendocrine tumours scheduled for 90Y-DOTATOC therapy. Eur J Nucl Med Mol Imaging 33:460–466. doi:10.1007/s00259-005-0006-1

Kwekkeboom DJ, Bakker WH, Kooij PP, Konijnenberg MW, Srinivasan A, Erion JL et al (2001) [177Lu-DOTAOTyr3]octreotate: comparison with [111In-DTPAo]octreotide in patients. Eur J Nucl Med 28:1319–1325

Plockinger U, Rindi G, Arnold R, Eriksson B, Krenning EP, de Herder WW et al (2004) Guidelines for the diagnosis and treatment of neuroendocrine gastrointestinal tumours. A consensus statement on behalf of the European neuroendocrine tumour society (ENETS). Neuroendocrinology 80: 394–424. doi: 10.1159/000085237

Poeppel TD, Binse I, Petersenn S, Lahner H, Schott M, Antoch G et al (2011) 68Ga-DOTATOC vs. 68Ga-DOTATATE PET/CT in functional imaging of Neuroendocrine Tumours. J Nucl Med 52:1864–1870

Reubi JC, Waser B (2003) Concomitant expression of several peptide receptors in neuroendocrine tumours: molecular basis for in vivo multireceptor tumour targeting. Eur J Nucl Med Mol Imaging 30:781–793. doi:10.1007/s00259-003-1184-3

Reubi JC, Schar JC, Waser B, Wenger S, Heppeler A, Schmitt JS et al (2000) Affinity profiles for human somatostatin receptor subtypes SST1-SST5 of somatostatin radiotracers selected for scintigraphic and radiotherapeutic use. Eur J Nucl Med 27:273–282

Reubi JC, Waser B, Schaer JC, Laissue JA (2001) Somatostatin receptor sst1–sst5 expression in normal and neoplastic human tissues using receptor autoradiography with subtype-selective ligands. Eur J Nucl Med 28:836–846

Rodrigues M, Traub-Weidinger T, Li S, Ibi B, Virgolini I (2006) Comparison of 111In-DOTA-DPhe1-Tyr3-octreotide and 111In-DOTA-lanreotide scintigraphy and dosimetry in patients with neuroendocrine tumours. Eur J Nucl Med Mol Imaging 33:532–540. doi: 10.1007/s00259-005-0020-3

Rolleman EJ, Melis M, Valkema R, Boerman OC, Krenning EP, de Jong M (2010) Kidney protection during peptide receptor radionuclide therapy with somatostatin analogues. Eur J Nucl Med Mol Imaging 37:1018–1031. doi:10.1007/s00259-009-1282-y

Storch D, Behe M, Walter MA, Chen J, Powell P, Mikolajczak R et al (2005) Evaluation of [99mTc/EDDA/HYNIC0]octreotide derivatives compared with [111In-DOTA0, Tyr3, Thr8]octreotide and [111In-DTPA0]octreotide: does tumor or pancreas uptake correlate with the rate of internalization? J Nucl Med 46:1561–1569

Therasse P, Arbuck SG, Eisenhauer EA, Wanders J, Kaplan RS, Rubinstein L et al (2000) New guidelines to evaluate the response to treatment in solid tumors. European Organization for Research and Treatment of Cancer, National Cancer Institute of the United States, National Cancer Institute of Canada. J Natl Cancer Inst 92:205–216

Valkema R, Pauwels SA, Kvols LK, Kwekkeboom DJ, Jamar F, de Jong M et al (2005) Long-term follow-up of renal function after peptide receptor radiation therapy with (90)Y-DOTA(0), Tyr(3)-octreotide and (177)Lu-DOTA(0), Tyr(3)-octreotate. J Nucl Med 46(Suppl 1):83S–91S

Velikyan I, Sundin A, Eriksson B, Lundqvist H, Sorensen J, Bergstrom M et al (2010) In vivo binding of [68Ga]-DOTATOC to somatostatin receptors in neuroendocrine tumours–impact of peptide mass. Nucl Med Biol 37:265–275. doi:10.1016/j.nucmedbio.2009.11.008

Wild D, Macke HR, Waser B, Reubi JC, Ginj M, Rasch H et al (2005) 68Ga-DOTANOC: a first compound for PET imaging with high affinity for somatostatin receptor subtypes 2 and 5. Eur J Nucl Med Mol Imaging 32:724. doi:10.1007/s00259-004-1697-4

Yau YY, Chan WS, Tam YM, Vernon P, Wong S, Coel M et al (2005) Application of intravenous contrast in PET/CT: does it really introduce significant attenuation correction error? J Nucl Med 46:283–291

Zhernosekov KP, Filosofov DV, Baum RP, Aschoff P, Bihl H, Razbash AA et al (2007) Processing of generator-produced 68Ga for medical application. J Nucl Med 48:1741–1748. doi:10.2967/jnumed.107.040378

High Uptake of ^{68}Ga-DOTATOC in Spleen as Compared to Splenosis: Measurement by PET/CT

Harshad R. Kulkarni, Vikas Prasad, Daniel Kaemmerer, Merten Hommann and Richard P. Baum

Abstract

Aim: The aim of this study is to ascertain the high somatostatin receptor (SSTR) uptake in spleen and to compare the uptake in spleen and splenosis using SSTR PET/CT using ^{68}Ga-DOTATOC. *Materials and Methods*: SUV_{max} of spleen on ^{68}Ga-DOTATOC SSTR PET/CT (acquired for initial staging) in 10 patients with known neuroendocrine neoplasm of pancreatic tail was analyzed. All patients underwent left pancreatectomy and splenectomy. Diagnosis of splenosis was confirmed on CT, and SUV_{max} was noted on follow-up SSTR PET/CT. *Results*: $SUV_{max}$was 28.8 ± 12.5 in normal spleen and 10.5 ± 4.3 in splenosis. *Conclusion*: The high uptake of ^{68}Ga-DOTATOC (which has a high affinity to SSTR 2) in the spleen as compared to splenosis, which has a different histology, suggests white pulp as the probable site of high SSTR 2 expression.

Keywords

Somatostatin receptor · ^{68}Ga-DOTATOC · PET/CT · Splenosis

H. R. Kulkarni · V. Prasad · R. P. Baum (✉)
Department of Nuclear Medicine/Center for PET/CT, ENETS Center of Excellence, Zentralklinik Bad Berka, 99437 Bad Berka, Germany
e-mail: richard.baum@zentralklinik.de

D. Kaemmerer · M. Hommann
Department of General and Visceral Surgery, Zentralklinik Bad Berka, Bad Berka, Germany

R. P. Baum and F. Rösch (eds.), *Theranostics, Gallium-68, and Other Radionuclides*, Recent Results in Cancer Research 194, DOI: 10.1007/978-3-642-27994-2_19,

Contents

1 Introduction

The spleen shows very high uptake of somatostatin analogs (SA) as known from imaging using ^{111}In-pentetreotide (Lamberts et al. 1994). It also receives a significant radiation dose during peptide receptor radionuclide therapy (PRRNT) for neuroendocrine tumors using radiolabeled peptides such as DOTATOC or DOTATATE which mainly target somatostatin receptor (SSTR) 2 (Wehrmann et al. 2007). The high uptake of SA has been previously postulated to be related to the presence of somatostatin receptors on lymphocytes in the spleen (Lamberts et al. 1994). However, to the best of our knowledge, the exact site and mechanism of uptake of radiolabeled SA in the spleen have not been clearly elucidated.

Splenosis is an acquired condition involving autotransplantation of normal viable splenic tissue which occurs after rupture of the spleen, either traumatic or iatrogenic (during splenectomy) (Jacobson and De Nardo 1971). Accessory spleens on the other hand, are congenital, arising from the left side of the dorsal mesogastrium during the embryological period of development (Standring 2008).

The aim of this study is to ascertain the high uptake in spleen on somatostatin receptor PET/CT (SSTR PET/CT) and to compare the uptake in normal spleen with that in splenosis.

2 Materials and Methods

This study was a retrospective analysis of 10 patients (age 58 $\pm$ 11 years; five males, five females) diagnosed with neuroendocrine neoplasm of the tail of the pancreas at time of first presentation at our hospital. All of these patients had undergone SSTR PET/CT (Biograph Duo, Siemens) using ^{68}Ga-DOTATOC for the purpose of staging before treatment. Imaging was performed according to European Association of Nuclear Medicine (EANM) guidelines [injected activity of ^{68}Ga-DOTATOC 126 $\pm$ 16 MBq (mean $\pm$ SD), acquisition time 65 $\pm$ 10 min after injection, attenuation correction by spiral CT]. Maximum standardized uptake values (SUV_{max}) were determined by drawing manual region of interest

Table 1 SUV_{max} of normal organs on ^{68}Ga-DOTATOC PET/CT

Organ/region of interest	SUV_{max} (mean ± SD)
Spleen	28.8 ± 12.5
Renal cortex	12.8 ± 3.4
Liver	11.6 ± 3.8
Blood pool	2.3 ± 1.1

(ROI) around the entire spleen. Additionally, SUV_{max} of the kidney cortex, normal liver, and blood pool activity (over left ventricle) were also measured. All patients had undergone left pancreatectomy and splenectomy, accessory spleens having been ruled out on preoperative CT and also intraoperatively. The decision for resection of the primary tumor was based on individual discussion of each case in our interdisciplinary neuroendocrine tumor board.

Diagnosis of splenosis in left hypochondrium was first suspected on postpancreatectomy SSTR PET/CT showing a new, irregularly shaped mass lesion in the left hypochondrium with mildly increased ^{68}Ga-DOTATOC uptake. Restaging SSTR PET/CT 4–7 months after a subsequent cycle of PRRNT was available in 7 out of the 10 patients at time of the analysis. SUV_{max} of splenosis in each patient was noted on follow-up SSTR PET/CT using ^{68}Ga-DOTATOC.

3 Results

3.1 Initial Staging SSTR PET/CT

The spleen showed the highest uptake of all normal organs. Blood pool activity, measured in the left ventricle, was very low (Table 1).

3.2 Postpancreatectomy SSTR PET/CT Pre PRRNT

The mean SUV_{max} of the splenosis (10.5 ± 4.3) measured in 10 patients was found to be about one-third of that of normal spleen (as measured on initial staging SSTR PET/CT).

3.3 Restaging SSTR PET/CT Post PRRNT

The results of restaging SSTR PET/CT performed 4–7 months after a subsequent cycle of PRRNT were available in seven patients at time of this study. Three of these patients had stable disease, two had partial remission, and two had progressive disease. The size and SUV_{max} of splenosis and previously known metastases in the abdomen (abdominal lymph nodes and liver lesions) on

Table 2 Comparison between size (longest diameter) and SUV_{max} of metastases and splenosis on pre- and post-PRRNT SSTR PET/CT

Region of interest	No.	Pretherapy size (mean ± SD) cm	Posttherapy size (mean ± SD) cm	*p*-Value (size)	Pretherapy SUV_{max} (mean ± SD)	Posttherapy SUV_{max} (mean ± SD)	*p*-Value (SUV_{max})
Metastases	33	5.3 ± 2.1	4.7 ± 2.2	0.034	29.2 ± 13.8	21.8 ± 12.4	0.018
Splenosis	7	2.8 ± 1.3	2.9 ± 1.2	>0.05	10.5 ± 4.3	11.2 ± 5.6	>0.05

pretherapy SSTR PET/CT were compared with the values on posttherapy SSTR PET/CT in seven patients (Table 2). While there was a significant change in the size and SUV_{max} of the metastases in the abdominal lymph nodes and liver, there was no significant change in the size or SUV_{max} of splenosis, on the posttherapy follow-up SSTR PET/CT in seven patients (Fig. 1).

4 Discussion

The highest uptake of ^{68}Ga-DOTATOC amongst all normal tissues was noted in the spleen, confirming the results of a previous study (Prasad and Baum 2010). A strong correlation between uptake (SUV) of ^{68}Ga-DOTATOC and SSTR 2 expression had been proven earlier (Miederer et al. 2009; Boy et al. 2011). The exclusive correlation between SUV_{max} and SSTR 2 expression at the level of mRNA in normal human tissues has also been proven (Boy et al. 2011). Our study corroborates the evidence for high SSTR PET/CT uptake in the spleen.

Analysis of splenosis in 10 patients revealed low SUV_{max} on ^{68}Ga-DOTATOC PET/CT (about one-third), when compared with that in normal spleen. This finding may be attributed to the fact that the histological structure of splenosis is different from that of normal spleen. Previous reports have shown that the tissues in splenosis lack trabecular structures and have less elastic tissue than normal spleen. Splenosis also lacks the hilum and has a poorly formed capsule. Furthermore, our finding of low uptake in splenosis on SSTR PET/CT could be related to the histological finding that splenosis has poorly formed or deficient white pulp with normal-appearing red pulp (Buchino 1998; Carr and Turk 1992). This study therefore suggests that white pulp could be the site of predominant SSTR 2 expression. On the other hand, a previous study more than 20 years ago described high somatostatin receptor density in red pulp of the spleen (Reubi et al. 1990). It must also be pointed out, however, that two cases have been reported by Carr and Turk where the histology and immunohistochemistry of splenosis were indistinguishable from that of normal splenic tissue (Carr and Turk 1992).

Lack of histopathological confirmation of the diagnosis of splenosis was one of the limitations of our study. The diagnosis was retrospective, being first suspected on SSTR PET/CT and confirmed on morphological imaging (CT) (Short et al.

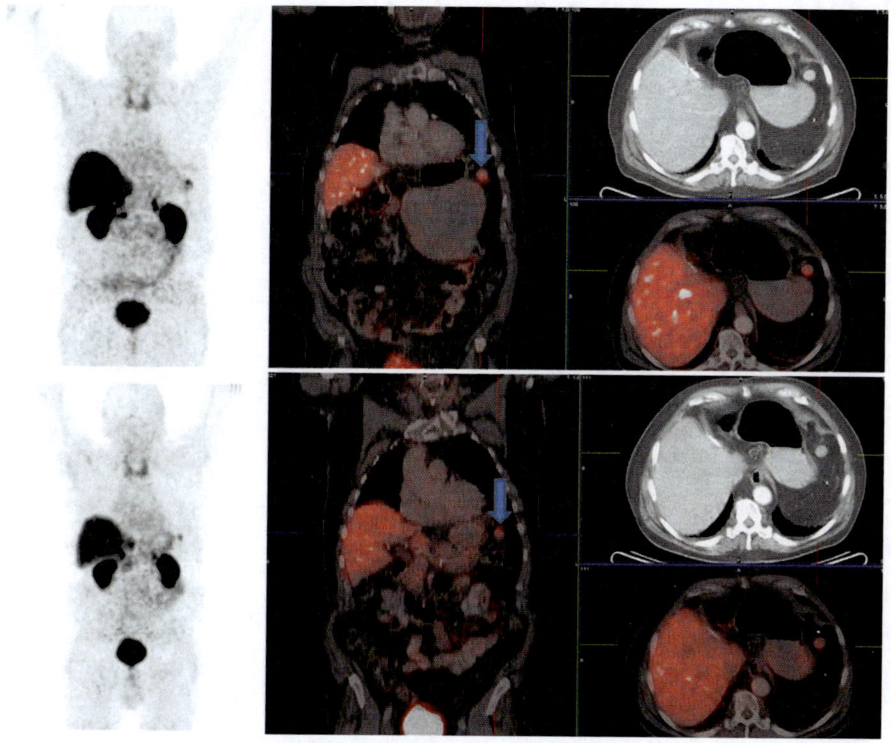

Fig. 1 ^{68}Ga-DOTATOC PET/CT (MIP image on the *left*, coronal fused image in the *middle*, and transverse CT and fused images on the *right*; *upper* row shows images acquired before PRRNT, and *lower* row shows images acquired 4 months after a cycle of PRRNT) in a patient after splenectomy demonstrating splenosis (*arrows*); no change in size and no significant change in SUV_{max} of splenosis was noted before and after PRRNT

2011). However, corroborating evidence in favor of the diagnosis of splenosis was that there was no significant change in size or SUV_{max} of splenosis as seen on subsequent follow-up SSTR PET/CT, whereas metastases showed a significant response to PRRNT. This could not have been the case had the uptake been due to peritoneal metastasis in left hypochondrium.

5 Conclusions

Somatostatin receptor 2 is probably expressed by T and B lymphocytes, predominantly distributed in white pulp of spleen, resulting in high splenic uptake on somatostatin receptor PET/CT using ^{68}Ga-DOTATOC. The low somatostatin receptor PET/CT uptake seen in splenosis could be attributed to the fact that splenosis has poorly formed or deficient white pulp, as described in previous histological studies, and therefore possibly lower somatostatin receptor 2 expression as compared with normal spleen.

References

Boy C, Heusner TA, Poeppel TD, Redmann-Bischofs A, Unger N, Jentzen W, Brandau W, Mann K, Antochs G, Bockisch A, Petersenn S (2011) ^{68}Ga-DOTATOC PET/CT and somatostatin receptor (sst1–sst5) expression in normal human tissue: correlation of sst2 mRNA and SUV_{max}. Eur J Nucl Med Mol Imaging 38(7):1224–1236

Buchino JJ (1998) Thoracic splenosis. South Med J 91:1054–1056

Carr NJ, Turk EP (1992) The histological features of splenosis. Histopathology 21:549–553

Jacobson SJ, De Nardo GL (1971) Splenosis demonstrated by splenic scan. J Nucl Med 12:570–572

Lamberts SWJ, Reubi JC, Krenning EP (1994) Somatostatin and the concept of peptide receptor scintigraphy in oncology. Semin Oncol 21:13–15

Miederer M, Seidl S, Buck A, Scheidhauer K, Wester HJ, Schwaiger M, Perren A (2009) Correlation of immunohistopathological expression of somatostatin receptor 2 with standardised uptake values in ^{68}Ga-DOTATOC PET/CT. Eur J Nucl Med Mol Imaging 36:48–52

Prasad V, Baum RP (2010) Biodistribution of the Ga-68 labeled somatostatin analogue DOTA-NOC in patients with neuroendocrine tumors: characterization of uptake in normal organs and tumor lesions. Q J Nucl Med Mol Imaging 54:61–67

Reubi JC, Kvols L, Krenning EP, Lamberts SWJ (1990) Distribution of somatostatin receptor in normal and tumour tissue. Metabolism 302(Suppl 2):78–81

Standring S (2008) Gray's anatomy: the anatomical basis of clinical practice, 40th edn. Elsevier, Churchill-Livingstone

Short NJ, Hayes TG, Bhargava P (2011) Intra-abdominal splenosis mimicking metastatic cancer. Am J Med Sci 341:246–249

Wehrmann C, Senftleben S, Zachert C, Müller D, Baum RP (2007) Results of individual patient dosimetry in peptide receptor radionuclide therapy with ^{177}Lu DOTA-TATE and ^{177}Lu DOTA-NOC. Cancer Biother Radiopharm 22:406–416

Rare Metastases Detected by ^{68}Ga-Somatostatin Receptor PET/CT in Patients with Neuroendocrine Tumors

Cecilia Carreras, Harshad R. Kulkarni and Richard P. Baum

Abstract

Aim: The most common sites of metastasis in neuroendocrine tumors are liver, lymph nodes, and bone. The aim of this study is to determine the prevalence and location of other sites of metastasis. *Methods*: 4,210 Ga-68 somatostatin-receptor PET/CT studies were performed at our center between July 2004 and December 2009. We retrospectively reviewed the reports of patients to check rare sites of metastasis other than liver, bone, and lymph nodes. Lesions were confirmed on follow-up and/or other imaging methods (MRI, echocardiography, and ultrasound). *Results*: The different sites of metastasis according to frequency of occurrence were: cardiac ($n = 29$), breast ($n = 21$), retro-orbital ($n = 9$), uterus ($n = 7$), skin ($n = 8$), brain ($n = 6$), spleen ($n = 3$), testes ($n = 1$), seminal vesicle ($n = 1$), and intramuscular in psoas muscle ($n = 4$). *Conclusions*: Cardiac and breast metastases appear to be not infrequent in neuroendocrine tumor patients. Ga-68 somatostatin-receptor PET/CT enables detection of these and other rare sites of metastasis.

Contents

C. Carreras · H. R. Kulkarni · R. P. Baum (✉)
Department of Nuclear Medicine/Center for PET/CT, ENETS Center of Excellence, Zentralklinik Bad Berka, 99437 Bad Berka, Germany
e-mail: richard.baum@zentralklinik.de
URL: www.zentralklinik-bad-berka.de

R. P. Baum and F. Rösch (eds.), *Theranostics, Gallium-68, and Other Radionuclides*, Recent Results in Cancer Research 194, DOI: 10.1007/978-3-642-27994-2_20,

1 Introduction

Neuroendocrine tumors (NETs) are a heterogeneous group of neoplasms which are characterized by their endocrine metabolism and histology pattern. It has been shown that liver is the most common site of metastasis from NETs, followed by lymph nodes and bone (Scarsbrook et al. 2007).

To the best of our knowledge, no data from a large series of patients is available to accurately define the prevalence of rare metastases of NETs. Approximately 20% of patients with carcinoid tumors have metastatic disease at time of diagnosis, and in half of those patients the primary tumor is not located at initial imaging (Zuetenhorst and Taal 2005). Detection of these sites could have a significant impact on the available treatment options and therefore on survival and quality of life in long-term outcome of patients with NETs (Srirajaskanthan et al. 2009).

The aim of this chapter is to review the prevalence and location of rare neuroendocrine tumor metastases.

2 Prevalence and Location of Rare Metastases of Neuroendocrine Tumors

We retrospectively reviewed the reports of 4,210 ^{68}Ga-somatostatin receptor PET/CT studies to check rare sites of metastasis other than liver, bone, and lymph nodes. All lesions were confirmed on follow-up and/or other imaging methods (MRI, echocardiography, and ultrasound). We found 95 rare metastasis, indicating prevalence in this series of 2.25%.

The different sites of metastasis according to frequency of occurrence were: cardiac ($n = 35$), breast ($n = 21$), retro-orbital ($n = 9$), uterus ($n = 7$), skin ($n = 8$), intramuscular ($n = 4$), brain ($n = 6$), spleen ($n = 3$), testes ($n = 1$), and seminal vesicle ($n = 1$) (Fig. 1).

2.1 Cardiac Metastases

Cardiac metastases are rare in all primary neoplasms (Bussani et al. 2007). Although secondary cardiac tumors are rare, their reported incidence is between 1.6 and 20.6% (Rafajlovski et al. 2005). The commonest tumors related with cardiac metastasis are melanoma, lung, breast, lymphoreticular malignancies, and mediastinal primary tumors (Smith 1986). Neoplastic cells may disseminate to the

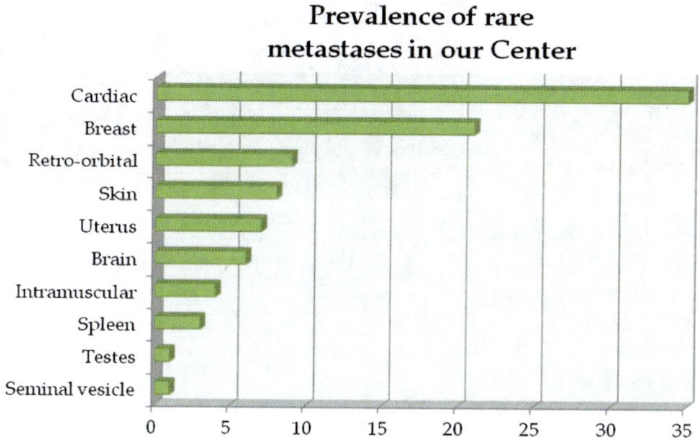

Fig. 1 Prevalence of rare metastases at the Bad Berka theranostics center

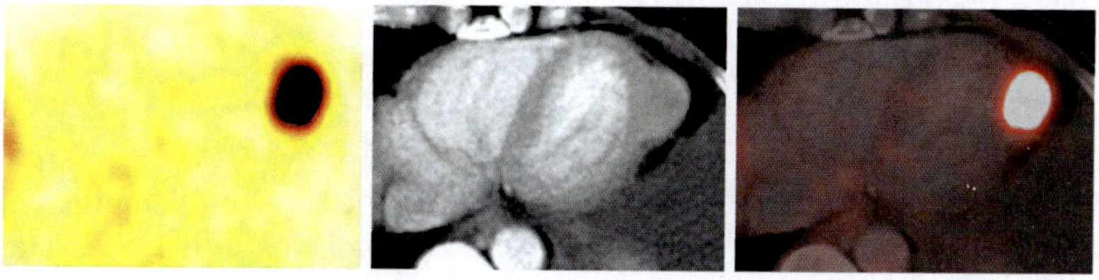

Fig. 2 A 70-year-old man with diagnosis of highly differentiated neuroendocrine carcinoma of unknown origin. The ^{68}Ga-DOTATATE PET/CT (PET, CT, and fused) transverse image shows a somatostatin receptor (SSTR)-positive lesion near the apex of the heart

heart by lymphatic or hematogenous pathways, local spread, or transvenous extension. Retrograde spread through lymphatic channels is the most common route of extension. Since most of the neoplastic cells are filtered by the hepatic and pulmonary microcirculation, hematogenous metastases to the heart are associated with metastases to these organs as well (Makhija et al. 2009). We detected 35 cases of cardiac metastasis (prevalence of 0.83%) (Fig. 2).

2.2 Breast Metastases

Metastases to the breast are also uncommon, fewer than 2% of all breast tumors. Of all metastatic tumors in the breast, most arise from contralateral breast primaries. Other reported primary solid tumors are melanoma, lung, gastric, renal cancers, and a few cases of neuroendocrine tumors (Geyer et al. 2010). In our series we detected 21 cases of breast metastasis (prevalence of 0.49%) (Fig. 3).

2.3 Retro-Orbital

Ocular metastases from carcinoid tumors are considered rare. Isidori et al. (2002) identified 6 of 40 patients (15%) with ocular metastases by [^{111}In]octreotide. We detected nine cases of retro-orbital metastasis (prevalence of 0.21%) (Fig. 4).

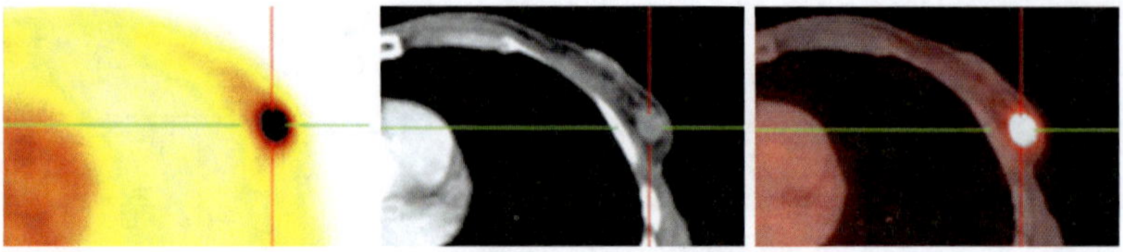

Fig. 3 A 49-year-old woman with diagnosis of neuroendocrine tumor of the pancreatic tail. The ^{68}Ga-DOTATATE PET/CT (PET, CT, and fused) transverse image shows a SSTR-positive solid lesion compatible with right breast metastasis

2.4 Soft Tissue

Soft tissue has been also reported as a possible location for uncommon metastasis of NETs. We detected eight cases of skin metastasis (prevalence of 0.19%) and four cases of intramuscular metastasis (prevalence of 0.09%) (Fig. 5).

2.5 Uterus, Testes, and Seminal Vesicles

Other uncommon localizations include uterus, testes, and seminal vesicles. We detected seven cases of uterine metastasis (prevalence of 0.16%), one case of testicular metastasis (prevalence of 0.02%), and one case of seminal vesicle metastasis (prevalence of 0.02%) (Fig. 6).

2.6 Brain

It is also described that NETs can metastasize to the brain (Scarsbrook et al. 2007). We detected six cases of brain metastasis (prevalence of 0.14%) (Fig. 7).

2.7 Spleen

The spleen is a rare location of metastasis from solid tumors. In a recent review of 6,137 patients with metastatic malignant tumors, only 59 (0.96%) involved the spleen. Carcinoid metastasis involving the spleen is extremely rare with only a few isolated cases being reported to date (Balmforth et al. 2011). We detected three cases of spleen metastasis (prevalence of 0.07%).

3 Discussion

As is well known, survival of patients with cancer has increased due to the development of new drugs for treatment of neoplasms and improved diagnostic methods. As patient survival increases and the natural history of cancer is modified by the multiple treatments received, it is not uncommon to find new sites of

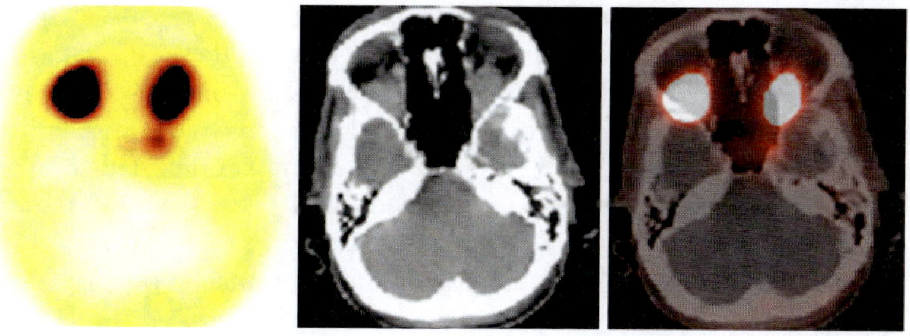

Fig. 4 A 66-year-old man with diagnosis of well-differentiated rectal neuroendocrine tumor. The ^{68}Ga-DOTATATE PET/CT (PET, CT, and fused) transverse image shows bilateral retro-orbital SSTR-positive metastases (SUV_{max} 15.2)

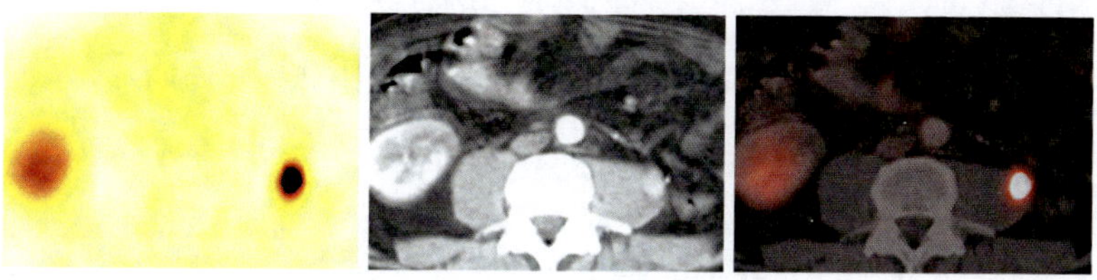

Fig. 5 A 50-year-old man with diagnosis of functional VIPoma of the pancreatic tail. The ^{68}Ga-DOTATATE PET/CT (transverse image) shows an intense SSTR-positive lesion in the left psoas muscle

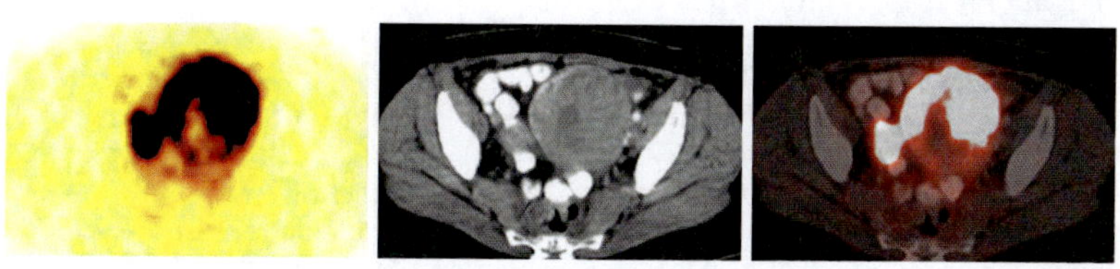

Fig. 6 A 61-year-old woman with diagnosis of neuroendocrine tumor of the pancreas. The SSTR PET/CT (PET, CT, and fused) transverse image shows uterine metastasis with high SSTR expression

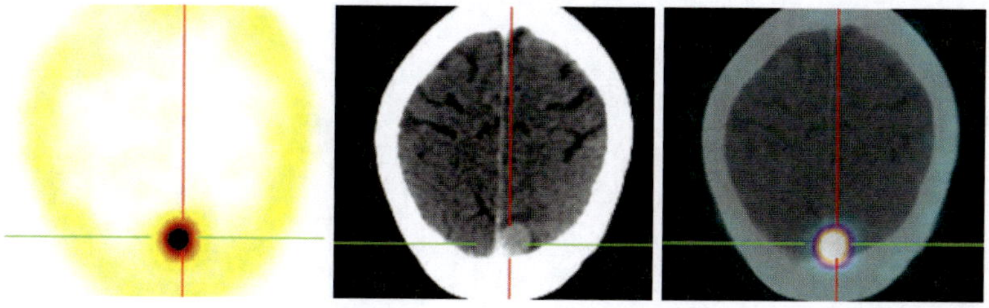

Fig. 7 A 72-year-old man with diagnosis of neuroendocrine tumor in the pancreatic uncinate process. The SSTR PET/CT (PET, CT, and fused) transverse image shows a SSTR-positive brain metastasis

metastasis. For these reasons it is important to have sensitive and specific diagnostic methods for diagnosis and follow-up of these metastatic lesions. ^{68}Ga-somatostatin receptor PET/CT is a unique tool for diagnosis and monitoring of patients with neuroendocrine tumors. It is highly sensitive and specific and has the advantage of whole-body imaging. In this study, we reported the prevalence and location of rare metastases in a large group of patients with neuroendocrine tumors. Many studies have discussed isolated cases of rare metastases; however, a multicenter study with larger number of patients is mandatory to establish the prevalence of rare metastases from neuroendocrine tumors.

References

Balmforth D, Skouras C, Palazzo F, Zacharakis E (2011) Laparoscopic management for carcinoid metastasis to the spleen. HPB Surg 2011(346507):4

Bussani R, De-Giorgio F, Abbate A, Silvestri F (2007) Cardiac metastases. J Clin Pathol 60(1):27–34

Geyer HL, Viney J, Karlin N (2010) Metastatic carcinoid presenting as a breast lesion. Curr Oncol 17(6):73–77

Isidori AM, Kaltsas G, Frajese V, Kola B, Whitelocke RA, Plowman PN, Britton KE, Monson JP, Grossman AB, Besser GM (2002) Ocular metastases secondary to carcinoid tumors: the utility of imaging with ^{123}I-MIBG and ^{111}In-DTPA pentetreotide. J Clin Endocrinol Metab 87: 1627–1633

Makhija Z, Deshpande R, Desai J (2009) Unusual tumors of the heart: diagnostic and prognostic implications. J Cardiothorac Surg 4:4

Rafajlovski S, Tatić V, Ilić S, Kanjuh V (2005) Frequency of metastatic tumors in the heart. Vojnosanit Pregl 62(12):915–920

Smith C (1986) Tumors of the heart. Arch 110(5):371–374

Scarsbrook AF, Ganeshan A, Statham J, Thakker RV, Weaver A, Talbot D, Boardman P, Bradley KM, Gleeson FV, Phillips RR (2007) Anatomic and functional imaging of metastatic carcinoid tumors. Radio Graphics 27:455–477

Srirajaskanthan R, Desai K, Jayaratnam A, Carras E, Toumpanakis C, Meyer T, Caplin M (2009) Uncommon sites for metastasis of neuroendocrine tumor in adults. J Clin Oncol 27:4656

Zuetenhorst JM, Taal BG (2005) Metastatic carcinoid tumors: a clinical review. Oncologist 10:123–131

Comparison of Different Positron Emission Tomography Tracers in Patients with Recurrent Medullary Thyroid Carcinoma: Our Experience and a Review of the Literature

Giorgio Treglia, Paola Castaldi, Maria Felicia Villani, Germano Perotti, Angelina Filice, Valentina Ambrosini, Nadia Cremonini, Annibale Versari, Stefano Fanti, Alessandro Giordano and Vittoria Rufini

Abstract

Several morphological and functional imaging techniques are usually used to detect residual/recurrent medullary thyroid carcinoma (MTC) with variable results; currently, there is growing interest in positron emission tomography (PET) methodology. Herein, we report our experience of and a literature review about the comparison of different positron emission tomography (PET) tracers in patients with residual/recurrent MTC. ^{18}F-DOPA PET/CT seems to be the most useful imaging method to detect recurrent MTC lesions, performing better than ^{18}F-FDG and ^{68}Ga-somatostatin analogs PET/CT. ^{18}F-FDG may complement ^{18}F-DOPA in patients with aggressive tumors. ^{68}Ga-somatostatin analogs PET/CT may be useful to select patients who could benefit from radioreceptor therapy. The information provided by the various PET tracers reflects different metabolic pathways, and may help to select the most appropriate treatment.

G. Treglia (✉) · P. Castaldi · M. F. Villani · G. Perotti · A. Giordano · V. Rufini
Institute of Nuclear Medicine, Catholic University of the Sacred Heart,
Largo Gemelli 8, 00168 Rome, Italy
e-mail: giorgiomednuc@libero.it

A. Filice · A. Versari
Nuclear Medicine Unit, Santa Maria Nuova Hospital,
Reggio Emilia, Italy

V. Ambrosini · S. Fanti
Nuclear Medicine Unit, Sant'Orsola-Malpighi Hospital,
University of Bologna, Bologna, Italy

N. Cremonini
Unit of Endocrinology, Ospedale Maggiore, Bologna, Italy

R. P. Baum and F. Rösch (eds.), *Theranostics, Gallium-68, and Other Radionuclides*, 385
Recent Results in Cancer Research 194, DOI: 10.1007/978-3-642-27994-2_21,

Keywords
Positron emission tomography · Medullary thyroid carcinoma · PET/CT · Diagnosis · Neuroendocrine tumors

Contents

1 Introduction

Medullary thyroid carcinoma (MTC) derives from neuroendocrine parafollicular C thyroid cells, accounting for only 5–8% of all thyroid malignancies. It mostly occurs sporadically (70–80% of cases), but familial forms (occurring alone or as part of MEN 2A and MEN 2B syndromes) have also been described (20–30% of cases) (Pacini et al. 2010).

First-line treatment is radical thyroidectomy with associated cervical lymphadenectomy. Surgery is curative in the vast majority of patients with MTC; however, disease can persist or recur, and early detection of malignant lesions is a crucial step in the therapeutic management of these patients. Tumor recurrence after surgery, either locally or with metastatic spread (typically to lungs, liver, bone), is associated with rising levels of blood calcitonin and/or CEA (Kebebew et al. 2000; Pellegriti et al. 2003).

Several morphological and functional imaging techniques have been used to detect recurrent MTC with variable results (Rufini et al. 2006; Rufini et al. 2008a, b). Among nuclear medicine techniques, currently there is growing interest in positron emission tomography (PET) methodology, which offers higher image quality and higher spatial resolution, and in PET tracers such as ^{18}F-fluorodeoxyglucose (^{18}F-FDG), which is the most used PET tracer in oncology and reflects tumor glucose metabolism and proliferative activity; ^{18}F-fluorodihydroxyphenylalanine (^{18}F-DOPA), which reflects a typical metabolic pathway (amine decarboxylation) of neuroendocrine tumors; and ^{68}Ga-somatostatin analogs, which reflect the expression of somatostatin receptors (Rufini et al. 2008a, b; Ambrosini et al. 2010).

We report our experience of the comparison of different PET tracers in patients with residual/recurrent MTC suspected on the basis of increased serum calcitonin levels. We also report the results of other authors who performed PET/CT with different tracers in patients with residual/recurrent MTC.

2 Our Experience

2.1 Patients

Inclusion criteria for our study were: early surgery for MTC, availability of serum calcitonin and carcinoembryonic antigen (CEA) levels, increased serum calcitonin levels, availability of conventional imaging studies and functional imaging modalities (^{18}F-DOPA PET/CT, ^{18}F-FDG PET/CT, and ^{68}Ga-somatostatin analogs PET/CT performed within a 6-month interval), and availability of a cytohistological diagnosis or clinical information on follow-up (at least 12 months). Eighteen patients (6 men, 12 women, mean age 53 years, range 24–86 years) with residual/recurrent MTC were included. All patients had undergone total thyroidectomy with prophylactic central compartment neck dissection 12–192 months (median 90 months) before imaging; in 11 cases also lateral compartment neck dissection had been performed. In 5 cases (28%) the reason for the imaging study was to functionally assess known lesions detected at conventional imaging; in 13 cases (72%) the reason was to detect and localize recurrent disease suggested by biochemical data. In all cases neck ultrasonography (US) was performed. Additional imaging studies were available: whole-body contrast-enhanced CT in 16 cases, magnetic resonance imaging (MRI) of the abdomen in 2 cases, and bone scintigraphy in 2 cases. The use of ^{68}Ga-somatostatin analogs was approved by the local medical ethics committees. All patients gave written informed consent for the three PET/CT studies and for treatment of personal data.

2.2 PET/CT Protocol and Data Analysis

PET/CT studies were performed in three Italian centers: the PET/CT center of the Policlinico A. Gemelli, Università Cattolica del Sacro Cuore in Rome (center A), the PET/CT center of the Sant'Orsola-Malpighi Hospital in Bologna (center B), and the PET/CT center of Santa Maria Nuova Hospital in Reggio Emilia (center C). All ^{18}F-DOPA and ^{18}F-FDG PET/CT studies were performed in center A according to a previously described protocol (Rufini et al. 2011; Treglia et al. 2011). ^{68}Ga-somatostatin analogs PET/CT studies were performed in the three centers according to a previously described protocol (Castellucci et al. 2011; Versari et al. 2010).

Any focal accumulation of each tracer outside the normal distribution or higher than the surrounding physiological uptake was considered an abnormal finding.

Studies were classified as positive if at least one abnormal focus was found. Since increased calcitonin levels are related to residual and/or recurrent disease, any negative PET/CT result was interpreted as a false negative. The number and site of abnormal foci detected by all methods were also recorded. Comparison of the results of the three functional imaging modalities was made on a per-patient basis and on a per-lesion basis. At the end of the observational study, cytohistology was available in 8 of the 18 cases (44%). When a cytological or histological examination was not available, a combination of all morphologic and functional imaging modalities and clinical information at follow-up (at least 12 months) was used as a reference standard for the presence of tumoral lesions.

2.3 Statistical Analysis

For statistical analysis we used the Kruskal–Wallis test to compare the results of PET/CT methods. p-Value <0.05 was considered statistically significant. The statistical tests were performed using Statistix® software for Windows.

2.4 Results

2.4.1 Laboratory and Radiological Findings

Calcitonin levels were increased in all patients with a mean value of 2,580 pg/mL (range 66.7–14,186 pg/mL). CEA levels were increased in 14/18 patients (78%) with a mean value of 67.6 ng/mL (range 0.5–322 ng/mL). According to cytohistology and the combination of all imaging studies and clinical information at follow-up, locoregional disease was detected in 8 of 18 patients (44%), locoregional disease and distant metastases in 3 patients (17%), and distant disease alone in 2 (11%). In five patients (28%) the disease site was undetected at all imaging studies.

2.4.2 PET/CT Findings: Patient-Based Analysis

At least one focus of abnormal uptake was observed in 13/18 patients at ^{18}F-DOPA PET/CT [72.2% sensitivity, 95% confidence interval (CI) 48.8–87.8%], in 3/18 at ^{18}F-FDG PET/CT (16.7% sensitivity, CI 5.0–40.0%), and in 6/18 at ^{68}Ga-somatostatin analogs PET/CT (33.3% sensitivity, CI 16.1–56.4%) ($p = 0.001$). Seven patients were positive at ^{18}F-DOPA PET/CT alone. No patient was positive at ^{68}Ga-somatostatin analogs or ^{18}F-FDG PET/CT alone. In 5 of 18 patients (28%) there were known lesions at conventional imaging; ^{18}F-DOPA PET/CT was positive in all five and showed new sites of involvement in three cases; both ^{18}F-FDG PET/CT and ^{68}Ga-somatostatin analogs PET/CT were positive in three cases and showed new sites of involvement in two of them. In 13 of 18 patients (72%) conventional imaging was negative or inconclusive: ^{18}F-DOPA PET/CT was positive in 8, ^{68}Ga-somatostatin analogs PET/CT in 3, whereas ^{18}F-FDG PET/CT was negative in all 13 patients. In five patients the three PET/CT studies gave negative results. The statistical analysis showed a significant difference between ^{18}F-DOPA PET/CT and ^{18}F-FDG PET/CT results ($p = 0.005$) and between ^{18}F-DOPA PET/CT and ^{68}Ga-somatostatin analogs PET/CT results ($p = 0.02$). No significant differences between ^{68}Ga-somatostatin analogs PET/CT and ^{18}F-FDG PET/CT were found.

2.4.3 PET/CT Findings: Lesion-Based Analysis

Overall, 72 lesions were identified with the three PET/CT studies. ^{18}F-DOPA PET/CT detected 85% of lesions (61/72), ^{68}Ga-somatostatin analogs PET/CT 20% of lesions (14/72), and ^{18}F-FDG PET/CT 28% of lesions (20/72) ($p = 0.002$). In 10 cases ^{18}F-DOPA PET/CT identified more lesions than ^{68}Ga-somatostatin analogs and ^{18}F-FDG PET/CT, whereas in 1 case ^{18}F-FDG PET/CT revealed multiple liver lesions missed by the other two methods, as well as two additional locoregional lymph nodes. No additional lesions were identified by ^{68}Ga-somatostatin analogs PET/CT. According to the site of involvement, there were 12 bone lesions, 32 liver lesions, 26 locoregional lymph nodes, and 1 local recurrence. The statistical analysis showed a significant difference between the number of lymph nodes detected by ^{18}F-DOPA PET/CT and ^{18}F-FDG PET/CT ($p = 0.02$) and between ^{18}F-DOPA PET/CT and ^{68}Ga-somatostatin analogs PET/CT ($p = 0.009$), while there was no difference between ^{68}Ga-somatostatin analogs PET/CT and ^{18}F-FDG PET/CT results (p: ns). Even though ^{18}F-DOPA PET/CT detected more liver and bone lesions than the other two PET/CT studies, the difference was not statistically significant.

3 Literature Review

A search for articles comparing PET or PET/CT findings with different tracers in patients with residual/recurrent MTC was also performed; Pubmed and Embase databases were investigated, and the literature search was updated until August 2011. Some articles compared ^{18}F-DOPA with ^{18}F-FDG PET or PET/CT (Hoegerle et al. 2001; Beuthien-Baumann et al. 2007; Koopmans et al. 2008; Beheshti et al. 2009; Marzola et al. 2010) and ^{68}Ga-somatostatin analogs with ^{18}F-FDG PET/CT (Conry et al. 2010; Pałyga et al. 2010) in patients with residual/recurrent MTC. Nevertheless, comparison between ^{18}F-DOPA and ^{68}Ga-somatostatin analogs PET/CT in patients with residual/recurrent MTC was lacking. Only one article compared ^{11}C-methionine and ^{18}F-FDG (Jang et al. 2010).

4 Discussion

In our experience, we compared ^{18}F-DOPA, ^{18}F-FDG, and ^{68}Ga-somatostatin analogs PET/CT findings in a group of patients with residual/recurrent MTC on the basis of increased serum calcitonin levels. Both patients with known lesions and patients with negative or inconclusive conventional imaging results were included, the latter representing the greatest number. Early detection of residual/recurrent MTC is a crucial step in the selection of patients who may benefit from curative surgery. Our study confirmed that ^{18}F-DOPA PET/CT is a valuable tool in the evaluation of patients with residual/recurrent MTC, providing better results than the other functional imaging methods, on both a per-patient and a per-lesion basis.

The different behavior of ^{18}F-DOPA, ^{18}F-FDG, and ^{68}Ga-somatostatin analogs can be explained by their different uptake mechanisms that reflect the different metabolic pathways of neuroendocrine cells, including MTC cells. L-DOPA is an amino acid that enters the cell by the larger amino acid transporter (LAT) and is converted to dopamine by aromatic amino-acid decarboxylase; labeled with ^{18}F, L-DOPA is retained in the cells owing to intracellular decarboxylation, which is a feature of the neuroendocrine origin of MTC. So, it is assumed that higher ^{18}F-DOPA uptake is related to a higher degree of cell differentiation, and this might explain the high sensitivity of ^{18}F-DOPA PET/CT in the detection of small lymph node lesions, so-called minimal or occult disease (Hoegerle et al. 2001; Beuthien-Baumann et al. 2007; Koopmans et al. 2008; Beheshti et al. 2009; Marzola et al. 2010).

^{18}F-FDG, the glucose analog most used in oncology, accumulates in neoplastic cells, allowing scintigraphic visualization of those tumors that use glucose as an energy source according to their proliferative activity. Neuroendocrine tumors usually show an indolent course, and consequently low ^{18}F-FDG uptake. These tumors, however, when undergoing dedifferentiation, become more aggressive and may show increased ^{18}F-FDG uptake (Adams et al. 1998).

Due to their neuroendocrine origin, MTC cells express somatostatin receptors on their surface; however, immunohistochemical studies have produced generally low estimates for somatostatin receptor density in MTC cells (Reubi et al. 1991; Papotti et al. 2001). In vivo detection of expression of somatostatin receptors has been the molecular basis for tumor imaging with radiolabeled somatostatin analogs in PET imaging (Conry et al. 2010; Pałyga et al. 2010).

Previous studies comparing ^{18}F-DOPA and ^{18}F-FDG in the assessment of residual/recurrent MTC patients showed either better results of ^{18}F-DOPA (Beheshti et al. 2009; Koopmans et al. 2008) or a complementary role of the two tracers (Marzola et al. 2010; Beuthien-Baumann et al. 2007). First of all, in 2001, Hoegerle et al. reported 11 MTC patients who underwent both PET modalities, reporting a per-lesion sensitivity of 63% for ^{18}F-DOPA PET versus 44% for ^{18}F-FDG PET (Hoegerle et al. 2001). Our findings are in line with those reported by Hoegerle et al. who obtained the best results with ^{18}F-DOPA PET for detection of lymph node involvement and locoregional relapse. Beheshti et al. found superiority of ^{18}F-DOPA PET/CT with respect to the other imaging modalities in 26 patients with residual/recurrent MTC, and proposed this technique as a one-stop procedure to provide both functional and morphological information in order to select those patients who may benefit from reoperation with curative intent. These authors reported per-patient sensitivity of 81% for ^{18}F-DOPA PET/CT versus 58% for ^{18}F-FDG PET/CT, and per-lesion sensitivity of 94% for ^{18}F-DOPA PET/CT versus 62% for ^{18}F-FDG PET/CT (Beheshti et al. 2009). Koopmans et al. in their study reported per-patient sensitivity of 62% for ^{18}F-DOPA PET versus 23% for ^{18}F-FDG PET, and per-lesion sensitivity of 71% for ^{18}F-DOPA PET versus 30% for ^{18}F-FDG PET (Koopmans et al. 2008). In 18 patients with aggressive MTC and rapidly increasing calcitonin levels, Marzola et al. found slightly higher sensitivity of ^{18}F-DOPA than ^{18}F-FDG PET/CT on per-patient analysis (83 versus 61% respectively); nevertheless, in some cases the ^{18}F-FDG scan was superior to the ^{18}F-DOPA PET/CT results, thus suggesting a complementary role of the two modalities, in order to gain the maximum benefit from their combined sensitivity (Marzola et al. 2010). The complementary role of these two PET modalities in patients with recurrent MTC has been also suggested by Beuthien-Baumann et al. who reported the same per-patient sensitivity with both methods (47%), which, however, detected different metastatic lesions (Beuthien-Baumann et al. 2007).

The experience with ^{68}Ga-somatostatin analogs in MTC is very limited (Conry et al. 2010; Pałyga et al. 2010). In particular, Conry et al. compared ^{68}Ga-DOTATATE PET/CT versus ^{18}F-FDG PET/CT in 18 MTC patients; these authors found similar per-patient sensitivity of these methods (78 and 72% respectively); nevertheless, ^{18}F-FDG PET/CT showed more lesions than ^{68}Ga-somatostatin analogs PET/CT, mainly in the liver (Conry et al. 2010). In a similar way, in our series ^{68}Ga-somatostatin analogs PET/CT missed all liver lesions detected by ^{18}F-FDG PET/CT and ^{18}F-DOPA PET/CT, a finding that may be explained by the low lesion-to-background ratio due to the low expression of the somatostatin receptors and the physiological uptake of the tracer in the liver.

Up to now, there are no published data comparing ^{18}F-DOPA and ^{68}Ga-somatostatin analogs in patients with residual/recurrent MTC. In our study, PET/CT with ^{68}Ga-somatostatin analogs showed lower sensitivity than ^{18}F-DOPA PET/CT (33.3 versus 72.2% respectively), providing no additional information on any patient, except for the feasibility of ^{90}Y/^{177}Lu-radioreceptor therapy to treat metastatic lesions showing high uptake (Bodei et al. 2004).

Preliminary data about ^{11}C-methionine PET/CT in residual/recurrent MTC showed that, despite its similar sensitivity to ^{18}F-FDG PET/CT for detecting residual or metastatic MTC lesions, ^{11}C-methionine PET/CT provided minimal additional information compared with combined ^{18}F-FDG PET/CT and neck US (Jang et al. 2010).

5 Conclusion

^{18}F-DOPA PET/CT, whose distinctive characteristic is the specific uptake mechanism reflecting the metabolic pathways of neuroendocrine cells, seems to be the most useful imaging method to detect persistent or recurrent lesions in patients with MTC. ^{18}F-FDG positivity is a sign of aggressive tumor behavior and may complement ^{18}F-DOPA PET/CT. ^{68}Ga-somatostatin analogs PET/CT does not provide any additional information except for the feasibility of radioreceptor therapy to treat metastatic lesions showing high uptake. In any case, the different uptake patterns observed with the various PET tracers reflect different metabolic pathways such as the uptake of hormone precursors, glucose metabolism, and receptor expression; this information may help to broaden the knowledge of MTC and potentially to select the most appropriate treatment.

Acknowledgments This manuscript was awarded as "Best Oral Presentation" at the 1st World Congress on Gallium-68 and Peptide Receptor Radionuclide Therapy, Bad Berka (Germany), June 23–26, 2011

References

Adams S, Baum RP, Hertel A et al (1998) Metabolic (PET) and receptor (SPET) imaging of welland less well-differentiated tumours: comparison with the expression of the Ki-67 antigen. Nucl Med Commun 19:641–647

Ambrosini V, Marzola MC, Rubello D et al (2010) (68)Ga-somatostatin analogues PET and (18)F-DOPA PET in medullary thyroid carcinoma. Eur J Nucl Med Mol Imaging 37:46–48

Beheshti M, Pöcher S, Vali R et al (2009) The value of 18F-DOPA PET-CT in patients with medullary thyroid carcinoma: comparison with 18F-FDG PET-CT. Eur Radiol 19:1425–1434

Beuthien-Baumann B, Strumpf A, Zessin J et al (2007) Diagnostic impact of PET with ^{18}F-FDG, ^{18}F-DOPA and 3-O-methyl-6-[^{18}F]fluoro-DOPA in recurrent or metastatic medullary thyroid carcinoma. Eur J Nucl Med Mol Imaging 34:1604–1609

Bodei L, Handkiewicz-Junak D, Grana C et al (2004) Receptor radionuclide therapy with ^{90}Y-DOTATOC in patients with medullary thyroid carcinomas. Cancer Biother Radiopharm 19:65–71

Castellucci P, Pou Ucha J, Fuccio C et al (2011) Incidence of increased ^{68}Ga-DOTANOC uptake in the pancreatic head in a large series of extrapancreatic NET patients studied with sequential PET/CT. J Nucl Med 52:886–890

Conry BG, Papathanasiou ND, Prakash V et al (2010) Comparison of (68)Ga-DOTATATE and (18)F-fluorodeoxyglucose PET/CT in the detection of recurrent medullary thyroid carcinoma. Eur J Nucl Med Mol Imaging 37:49–57

Hoegerle S, Altehoefer C, Ghanem N et al (2001) ^{18}F-DOPA positron emission tomography for tumour detection in patients with medullary thyroid carcinoma and elevated calcitonin levels. Eur J Nucl Med 28:64–71

Jang HW, Choi JY, Lee JI et al (2010) Localization of medullary thyroid carcinoma after surgery using (11)C-methionine PET/CT: comparison with (18)F-FDG PET/CT. Endocr J 57:1045–1054

Kebebew E, Ituarte PH, Siperstein AE et al (2000) Medullary thyroid carcinoma: clinical characteristics, treatment, prognostic factors, and a comparison of staging systems. Cancer 88:1139–1148

Koopmans KP, de Groot JW, Plukker JT et al (2008) 18F-dihydroxyphenylalanine PET in patients with biochemical evidence of medullary thyroid cancer: relation to tumor differentiation. J Nucl Med 49:524–531

Marzola MC, Pelizzo MR, Ferdeghini M et al (2010) Dual PET/CT with (18)F-DOPA and (18)F-FDG in metastatic medullary thyroid carcinoma and rapidly increasing calcitonin levels: Comparison with conventional imaging. Eur J Surg Oncol 36:414–421

Pacini F, Castagna MG, Cipri C et al (2010) Medullary thyroid carcinoma. Clin Oncol 22: 475–485

Pałyga I, Kowalska A, Gąsior-Perczak D et al (2010) The role of PET-CT scan with somatostatin analogue labelled with gallium-68 (^{68}Ga-DOTA-TATE PET-CT) in diagnosing patients with disseminated medullary thyroid carcinoma (MTC). Endokrynol Pol 61:507–511

Papotti M, Kumar U, Volante M et al (2001) Immunohistochemical detection of somatostatin receptor types 1–5 in medullary carcinoma of the thyroid. Clin Endocrinol 54: 641–649

Pellegriti G, Leboulleux S, Baudin E et al (2003) Long-term outcome of medullary thyroid carcinoma in patients with normal postoperative medical imaging. Br J Cancer 88:1537–1542

Reubi JC, Chayvialle JA, Franc B et al (1991) Somatostatin receptors and somatostatin content in medullary thyroid carcinomas. Lab Invest 64:567–573

Rufini V, Calcagni ML, Baum RP (2006) Imaging of neuroendocrine tumours. Semin Nucl Med 36:228–247

Rufini V, Castaldi P, Treglia G et al (2008a) Nuclear medicine procedures in the diagnosis and therapy of medullary thyroid carcinoma. Biomed Pharmacother 62:139–146

Rufini V, Treglia G, Perotti G et al (2008b) Role of PET in medullary thyroid carcinoma. Minerva Endocrinol 33:67–73

Rufini V, Treglia G, Castaldi P et al (2011) Comparison of 123I-MIBG SPECT-CT and ^{18}F-DOPA PET-CT in the evaluation of patients with known or suspected recurrent paraganglioma. Nucl Med Commun 32:575–82

Treglia G, Calcagni ML, Rufini V et al (2011) Clinical significance of incidental focal colorectal [(18) F]FDG uptake: our experience and a review of the literature. Colorectal Dis. doi:10.1111/j.1463-1318.2011.02588.x

Versari A, Camellini L, Carlinfante G et al (2010) Ga-68 DOTATOC PET, endoscopic ultrasonography, and multidetector CT in the diagnosis of duodenopancreatic neuroendocrine tumors: a single-centre retrospective study. Clin Nucl Med 35:321–328

PET Lung Ventilation/Perfusion Imaging Using ^{68}Ga Aerosol (Galligas) and ^{68}Ga-Labeled Macroaggregated Albumin

S. J. Ament, S. Maus, H. Reber, H. G. Buchholz, N. Bausbacher, C. Brochhausen, F. Graf, M. Miederer and M. Schreckenberger

Abstract

Pulmonary imaging using ventilation/perfusion (V/P) single-photon emission tomography (V/P scan) with Tc-99m-labeled radiotracers is a well-established diagnostic tool for clinically suspected pulmonary embolism (PE). Ga-68 aerosol (Galligas) and Ga-68-labeled macroaggregated albumin (MAA) are potential tracers for positron emission tomography (PET) lung V/P imaging and could display an advantage over conventional V/P scans in terms of sensitivity and specificity. After radiochemical and animal studies, the clinical applicability of Ga-68 aerosol (Galligas) and Ga-68-labeled MAA was investigated in an exploratory study in patients with clinical suspicion of PE. PET scans were acquired using a 16-slice Gemini TF positron emission tomography/computed tomography (PET/CT) scanner. The acquisition protocol included low-dose computed tomography (CT) for attenuation correction (AC). Dosimetry calculations and continuative phantom measurements were performed. Structural analyses showed no modification of the particles due to the labeling process. In addition, in vitro experiments showed stability of Ga-68 MAA in various media. As expected, Ga-68-labeled human serum albumin microspheres (HSAM) were completely retained in the lung of the animals. In clinical use,

S. J. Ament (✉) · S. Maus · H. Reber · H. G. Buchholz · N. Bausbacher · F. Graf · M. Miederer · M. Schreckenberger
Department of Nuclear Medicine, University Medical Centre, Johannes Gutenberg-University, Langenbeckstraße 1, 55131 Mainz, Germany
e-mail: stephan-johann.ament@unimedizin-mainz.de; stephan.ament@gmx.de

C. Brochhausen
Institute of Pathology, University Medical Centre, Johannes Gutenberg-University, Mainz, Germany

R. P. Baum and F. Rösch (eds.), *Theranostics, Gallium-68, and Other Radionuclides*, Recent Results in Cancer Research 194, DOI: 10.1007/978-3-642-27994-2_22,

PET lung ventilation and perfusion imaging using Ga-68 aerosol (Galligas) and Ga-68-labeled MAA was successful in all cases. In one case a clinically suspected PE could be detected and verified. The administered activity of Ga-68 aerosol (Galligas) and Ga-68-labeled MAA may be reduced by more than 50%, resulting in comparable radiation exposure to conventional V/P scans. In conclusion, Ga-68 aerosol (Galligas) and Ga-68-labeled MAA are efficient substitutes for clinical use and could be an interesting alternative with high accuracy for lung V/P imaging with Tc-99m-labeled radiotracers, especially in times of Mo-99 shortages and increasing use and spread of PET/CT scanners and Ga-68 generators, respectively.

Abbreviations

AC	Attenuation correction
CT	Computed tomography
CTA	Computed tomography angiography
cGMP	Current good manufacturing practice
DLP	Dose–length product
DOTA	1,4,7,10-Tetraazacyclododecane-1,4,7,10-tetraacetic acid (chelate)
DVT	Deep vein thrombosis
EANM	European Association of Nuclear Medicine
HSA	Human serum albumin
HSAM	Human serum albumin microspheres
HU	Hounsfield unit
ICRP	International Commission on Radiological Protection
ITLC	Instant thin-layer chromatography
MAA	Macroaggregated albumin
NEC	Noise-equivalent count
OSEM	Ordered-subsets expectation maximization (reconstruction)
PE	Pulmonary embolism
PET	Positron emission tomography
PET/CT	Positron emission tomography/computed tomography
RNP	Radionuclide purity
ROI	Region of interest
rpm	Revolutions per minute
SEM	Scanning electron microscopy
SPECT	Single-photon emission computed tomography
SUV	Standardized uptake value
VOI	Volumes of interest
V/P	Ventilation/perfusion

Contents

1 Introduction

1.1 Background

Since being introduced to clinical medicine in the mid 1960s, pulmonary ventilation and perfusion imaging with single-photon emission tomography (V/P scan) has become a widely used method and a well-established diagnostic tool in the diagnosis of clinically suspected pulmonary embolism (PE) (Stein et al. 2009). Knipping et al. (1955) used xenon-133 to measure lung ventilation. Lung perfusion imaging was first performed by Wagner et al. (1964) using iodine-131-labeled macroaggregated albumin (MAA). Meanwhile, the standard technique for assessing lung ventilation and perfusion distribution is the use of an ultrafine aerosol of Tc-99m-labeled carbon particles (Technegas®) and Tc-99m-labeled MAA.

Used clinically since 1960, Tc-99m is the most widely available isotope in diagnostic nuclear medicine, firstly because of its attractive physical characteristics (half-life: 6 h, energy: 140 keV), and secondly because of the convenience of onsite supply via a molybdenum (Mo-99) generator. The daughter nuclide technetium (Tc-99m) is used in approximately 600,000 medical imaging procedures worldwide every week, corresponding to a demand of 450 TBq of Mo-99 (Ballinger 2010).

The majority of the Mo-99 produced for Tc-99m medical use is covered by U-235 fission, mostly in highly enriched uranium nuclear reactors. Only five of these reactors are available around the world, and all of them are more than 40 years old, approaching the end of their lifetime. The now-frequent shutdowns are evidence of this. Consequently, any interruption in the routine operation of any of these reactors leads to supply shortages of Mo-99/Tc-99m in days, because of the short half-life of Mo-99 of 66 h (Ballinger 2010).

To be prepared for the future, it is necessary to seek suitable alternatives to be more independent from any lack of Mo-99/Tc-99m.

Use of an alternative γ-emitting radionuclide (e.g., thallium-201, iodine-123, or indium-111) is associated with higher radiation exposure. In terms of sensitivity and specificity, PET scans, which provide quantitative images with high spatial resolution in three dimensions, could display an advantage over conventional V/P scans using single-photon emission computed tomography (SPECT).

Cyclotron-produced positron-emitting fluorine-18 (F-18, half-life: 110 min) is the most used radionuclide in PET. FDA approval of sodium fluoride F-18 (F-18-NaF) as a substitute for Tc-99m-labeled radiotracer for bone scans is one answer to the Mo-99 supply problems. Otherwise, the dependence upon a cyclotron is a logistical and economical disadvantage of F-18-labeled radiotracers.

Against this background, use of a generator-produced positron emitter instead of a cyclotron product could reduce cost effectively. Commercially available Ge-68/Ga-68 (271 days, 68 min) generators provide a decent lifetime of approximately 6 months and could be a potential alternative source (Ballinger 2010; Fani et al. 2008). In the past decade, one example using this source has been imaging of neuroendocrine tumors with Ga-68-labeled somatostatin receptor binding peptides as efficient substitutes for octreotide scintigraphy using SPECT (Baum et al. 2008).

Consequently, in times of Mo-99/Tc-99m shortage, the renaissance of gallium-68 aerosol and gallium-68-labeled MAA for lung ventilation/perfusion (V/P) imaging was a question of time.

1.2 Objective

The feasibility of producing an ultrafine dispersion of Ga-68-labeled carbon particles using a Technegas® generator was already published by Nozaki et al. (1995). Meanwhile, clinical use of PET aerosol lung scintigraphy was described and proposed for lung ventilation imaging by Kotzerke et al. (2010). These human studies could prove a constant activity over the lung (half-time corrected) and thus the stability of the deposition of Ga-68-labeled carbon particles (Galligas) over 3.5 h.

Several methods for labeling of human serum albumin (HSA) microspheres with Ga-68 were described. An early approach was hydrolysis and precipitation of Ga(III)-68 ion in the presence of albumin particles (Hnatowich in 1976). PET scans were performed in dogs following intravenous administration of the microspheres (Chesler et al. 1975). Images obtained 6 h after injection showed that the Ga-68 activity was retained in the lung during this period, with negligible activity appearing in the liver. Wagner and Welch (1979) modified these method and used HSA microspheres as a model compound to attach Ga-68 by covalent conjugation via bifunctional high-affinity gallium chelation. The same group could detect deposition of Ga-68-DTPA-HSA in the lung of dogs over the entire PET study period. Even and Green (1989) performed the first direct labeling of MAA with Ga-68. They obtained radiochemical purities of $98.4 \pm 0.3\%$ and labeling yield of $97.0 \pm 0.5\%$.

Consequently, Ga-68 aerosol (Galligas) and Ga-68-labeled MAA are potential tracers for positron emission tomography (PET) lung V/P imaging and could display an advantage over conventional V/P scans in terms of sensitivity and specificity. After own radiochemical and animal studies, the clinical applicability of Ga-68 aerosol (Galligas) and Ga-68-labeled MAA was investigated in an exploratory study in patients with clinical suspicion of PE.

2 Materials and Methods

2.1 Materials

2.1.1 Chemicals

MAA was purchased from GE Healthcare Buchler (Braunschweig, Germany) and HSA from ROTOP Pharmaka AG (Radeberg, Germany). HCl (0.6 N) for generator elution was prepared from TraceSELECT® Ultra HCl (30%) and sterile pyrogen-free water, both purchased from Sigma-Aldrich Chemie GmbH (Taufkirchen, Germany). Aseptic ethanol (99.5%) was obtained from the central pharmacy of the University Medical Center of the Johannes Gutenberg University (Mainz, Germany). TLC was carried out on ITLC-SG glass-fiber sheets from PALL Life Sciences (Port Washington, NY, USA), recorded with Gina Star TLC, and analyzed using miniGita software from Raytest (Straubenhardt, Germany).

2.1.2 Ge-68/Ga-68 Generator

The short-half-life positron-emitting radionuclide Ga-68 (half-life: 68 min) was obtained as [Ga-68]Ga-chloride from a commercially available 30-mCi (1,110-MBq) Ge-68/Ga-68 generator produced by iThemba LABS (Somerset West, South Africa) under current good manufacturing practice (cGMP) and distributed by IDB Holland (Baarle-Nassau, The Netherlands). The generator is a ready-to-use, closed system. The system contains a tin dioxide (SnO_2) column in a polyethylene column with polyethylene tubing and no metal parts for the parent Ge-68 (half-life: 271 days) (Operating Instructions, ^{68}Ga Generator iThemba LABS[1]).

2.2 Methods

2.2.1 Elution Characteristics

The generator was eluted six times a week, one time per day. The equilibration time between elution was 4 h to allow regeneration of the Ge-68/Ga-68 generator. Ga-68 was obtained as [Ga-68]Ga-chloride. In analogy to Breeman et al. (2005) and the manufacturer instructions, fractionated elution of 10 fractions, each fraction composed of 0.5 mL 0.6 N HCl, was performed to concentrate and purify the eluate of metal impurities. The first eluate was discarded and served only to rinse the generator (Maus et al. 2011). Only fractions 3–5 containing the main activity (>80%) and a Ge-68 breakthrough less than 0.001% were used for radiopharmaceutical production. The same technique was performed to evaluate Ge-68 breakthrough after 24 and 48 h.

[1] Operating Instructions GMP Produced ^{68}Ga Generator iThemba LABS (Somerset West, South Africa), distributed by IDB Holland (Baarle-Nassau, The Netherlands).

2.2.2 Preparation of MAA and HSA Human Serum Albumin Kits

Each kit was resuspended in 5 mL 0.9% sodium chloride and vigorously mixed for 0.5 h to wash the particles free of compounds such as stannous chloride, polysorbate, and hydrochloric acid (Maus et al. 2011). These steps were repeated three times before the microspheres were used for labeling with Ga-68. After centrifugation, the supernatants were discarded and the retained particles were reconstituted in 0.5 mL sterile water (B.Braun Melsungen AG, Melsungen, Germany).

2.2.3 Labeling With Ga-68

The reconstituted spheres were mixed in 0.5 mL sterile water with 1.5 mL generator eluate corresponding to the middle fraction and containing 600–1,200 MBq Ga-68. The mixture was adjusted to pH 4 with 265 mg HEPES buffer (GERBU Biochemicals GmbH, Gaiberg, Germany). The mixture was allowed to react for 20 min at 75°C under gentle agitation. This is the optimum reaction time indicated by the time–activity curve obtained (Maus et al. 2011). The volume of the reaction mixture was increased to 10 mL with sterile water and then purified for the application by a threefold centrifugation at 1,500 rpm for 10 min.

2.2.4 Determination of Labeling Yields

Two different methods could be used to determine the labeling yield. First, instant thin-layer chromatography (ITLC) was performed using silica gel impregnated glass-fiber sheets and 0.9% NaCl solution as mobile phase. The Ga-68-labeled MAA and HSA microspheres remain at the start position, while free Ga-68 moves with the solvent front. The percentages of each fraction were determined relative to the total activity of the chromatogram (Maus et al. 2011). The second method was based on separation by centrifugation. Sterile water (10 mL) was added to the reaction mixture and centrifuged for 10 min at 1,500 rpm. Here, the activity of supernatant was defined as the free Ga-68 activity and the Ga-68-labeled microspheres as the labeled product (Maus et al. 2011).

2.2.5 Stability Experiments of Ga-68-MAA in Various Media

To prove the stability of the Ga-68-MAA, tests in sterile water, 0.9% NaCl, and human plasma were performed. The plasma was obtained by taking blood samples from a human individual with immediate centrifugation at 2,700 rpm for 5 min over EDTA K monovettes from Sarstedt, Nümbrecht. Aliquots of the labeled particles containing activities between 100 and 120 MBq were added to 1 mL sterile water, 0.9% NaCl, and plasma obtained as described.

After incubation for 1 h, each mixture was centrifuged for 5 min at 2,700 rpm, and the supernatants were removed and measured in a dose calibrator. The whole procedure was repeated three times.

2.2.6 Structural Analyses of Microspheres by Scanning Electron Microscopy (SEM)

Particles were placed on a SEM specimen holder with a self-adhesive graphite pad for scanning electron microscopy. The microspheres were sputter-coated (Edward Sputter Coater S150B) with gold according to laboratory standard. The microspheres were imaged using a Zeiss DSM 962 scanning electron microscope with a voltage of 15 KV in case of macroaggregated albumin and 5 KV in case of HSA spheres.

2.3 Exploratory Studies

2.3.1 Animal Studies

The animal study was approved by the animal study authority.

For each formulation, two Sprague–Dawley rats (400–500 g) were anesthetized with 2% isoflurane/100% pure oxygen gas mixture. The biodistribution of the Ga-68-labeled MAA and HSA microspheres was visualized and quantified using a dedicated microPET scanner Focus 120 (Siemens, Knoxville, TN). The scanner has axial field of view of 7.6 cm. The rats ($n = 2 + 2$) were positioned on the scanner bed in supine position covering the lungs and the proximal part of the abdomen. The scans started simultaneously with i.v. application of about 10.3 $\pm$ 1.5 MBq via the tail vein. List-mode acquisition lasted 60 min, and in addition, a transmission scan using a Co-57 point source was performed for attenuation correction (AC). Data were histogrammed into 19 frames (3 $\times$ 20, 3 $\times$ 60, 3 $\times$ 120, and 10 $\times$ 600 s) and reconstructed iteratively with the ordered-subsets expectation-maximization (OSEM 2D) algorithm. Volumes-of-interest (VOI) analyses were performed using the PMOD 2.95 image analysis software package. VOIs for lung, liver, and unspecific binding were defined, and time–activity curves were derived from the VOI statistics. Taking into account the different amounts of injected activity and the different weights of the rats, standardized uptake values (SUV) were calculated (Maus et al. 2011). Additionally, lung ventilation and perfusion imaging with Ga-68 aerosol (Galligas) and Ga-68-labeled MAA were performed ($n = 1$) using a Gemini TF positron emission tomography/computed tomography (PET/CT) scanner (Philips, Best, The Netherlands) before clinical use. An ultrafine dispersion of Ga-68-labeled carbon particles was generated using a commercially available Technegas® generator (Tetley Manufacturing Ltd., Sydney, Australia) for lung ventilation imaging. A concentrated Ga-68 generator eluate solution (20 MBq/0.1 mL) was loaded into a graphite crucible (Pulmotec™) prefilled with ethanol using a 1-mL syringe. In analogy to the production of Technegas®, the combination of graphite and an argon atmosphere was used for vaporization and subsequent generation of Ga-68 aerosol (Galligas).

2.3.2 Clinical Studies

Due to the absence of alternatives in the Mo-99 crisis, the clinical applicability of Ga-68 aerosol (Galligas) and Ga-68-labeled MAA was investigated in an exploratory study in patients with clinical suspicion of PE. After detailed explanation and written consent, five patients (two male, three female; median age 75 years, range 66–83 years) with suspicion of PE each underwent PET/CT scan after inhalation of Ga-68-labeled carbon particles (3.4–12.6 MBq) and subsequent application of 42–105 MBq Ga-68-labeled MAA (injected activity calculated based on assessment of inhaled activity).

According to European Association of Nuclear Medicine (EANM) guidelines for V/P scintigraphy and its key recommendations for investigation of regional pulmonary perfusion in PE diagnosis, Tc-99m-labeled MAA is the agent recommended for perfusion scintigraphy with evidence level IIa, grade B (Bajc et al. 2009b). Consequently, perfusion imaging was performed with Ga-68-labeled MAA microspheres (200,000–400,000 particles). In analogy to the administration of Tc-99m-labeled MAA, the vial was shaken gently before use and withdrawal of blood into the syringe during application was avoided (Bajc et al. 2009a). The suspension was given as intravenous bolus injection over 30 s while the patient breathed at normal tidal volume to ensure that the particles were infused over several respiratory cycles, facilitating uniform distribution within the pulmonary circulation (Bajc et al. 2009a).

Analogously to the standard method for production of Technegas®, an aerosol of Ga-68-labeled carbon particles was generated by vaporization of Ga-68 generator eluate solution (80–100 MBq/0.1 mL). Ga-68 aerosol (Galligas) was used within 10 min of generation to avoid aggregation of the particles. Administration was performed according to the manufacturer's instructions for Tc-99m-labeled carbon particles (Technegas® generator user manual 2005).

PET scans were acquired using a 16-slice Gemini TF PET/CT scanner (Philips, Best, The Netherlands) with axial field of view of 18 cm and transverse and axial resolution of 4.8 mm. Further specifications were published by Surti et al. (2007). The scatter fraction and noise-equivalent count (NEC) were measured by NEMA cylinder (20 cm diameter). The absolute sensitivity is 6.6 cps/kBq, whereas the scatter fraction is 27% and the peak NEC rate is 125 kcps at activity concentration of 17.4 kBq/mL. The system coincidence timing resolution is denoted by 585 ps (Surti et al. 2007).

Lung ventilation and perfusion imaging was performed in 3D acquisition mode in two bed positions (from neck to abdomen, in one case three bed positions) with acquisition time of 5 min per bed position.

Image reconstructions were performed using the standard Philips time-of-flight ordered-subsets expectation-maximization reconstruction (OSEM: 33 subsets, 3 iterations), and corrections for random events, scatter and attenuation were applied (Surti et al. 2007).

The acquisition protocol included low-dose computed tomography (CT) [120 kV, 0.5 s/rotation, 5 mm slices, max. 60 mAs, dose–length product (DLP) 98–142 mGy·cm, field of view 600 mm] for AC with dose modulation and anatomic orientation.

Additionally, dosimetry calculations using OLINDA (version 1.1; Vanderbilt University, 2007) and continuative phantom measurements were performed.

3 Results

3.1 ^{68}Ga-Labeled Human Serum Albumin Microspheres

The experimental results for the labeling yields of both compounds with Ga-68 showed a dependence on the heating time as demonstrated exemplarily in Fig. 1. The determined labeling efficiency of MAA was 85 $\pm$ 2%, and of HSA was

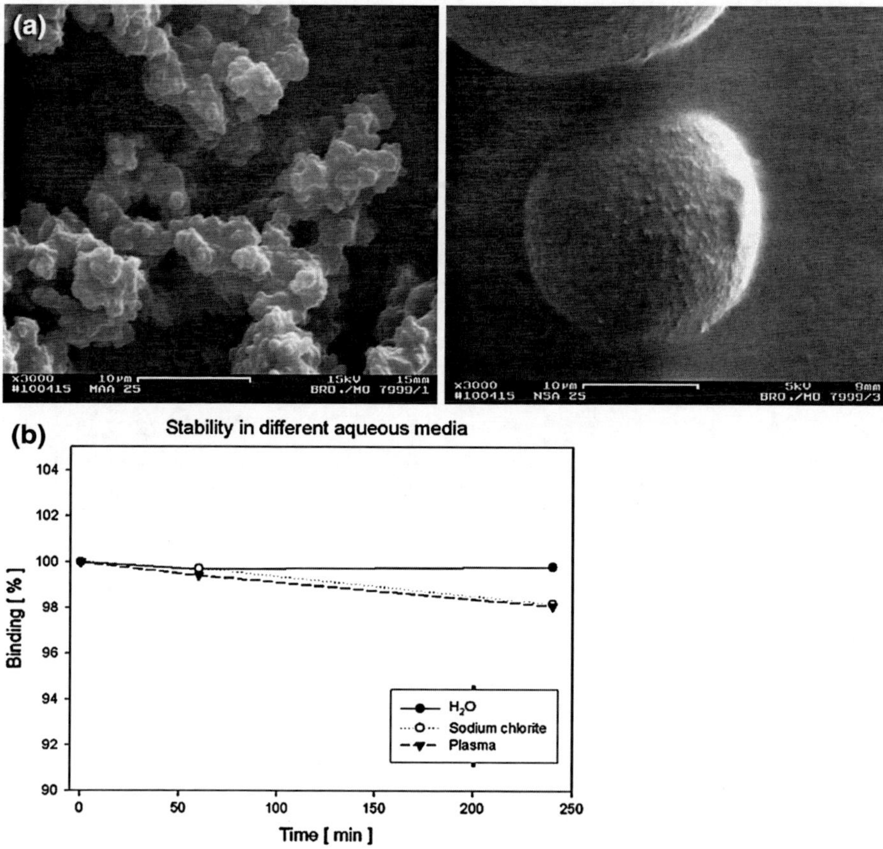

Fig. 1 **a** SEM images after the labeling procedure: *left* MAA, *right* HSA spheres, ultrastructural analysis (Maus et al. 2011). **b** Stability tests in sterile water, 0.9% sodium chloride (NaCl), and human plasma were performed (Sect. 2.2.5). No significant release of Ga-68 could be detected during the measurement period of 240 min

80 ± 5%. After washing with sterile water, the radiochemical purity for both was higher than 97% (Maus et al. 2011).

MAA used for pulmonary perfusion scintigraphy contained approximately 2×10^6 microspheres with particle sizes between 3 and 150 μm. However, approximately 95% particles were specified within the range of 3–40 μm. HSA spheres, also used for perfusion diagnostics, contained $3–5 \times 10^5$ microspheres in the narrower size range of 10–30 μm (Maus et al. 2011). Structural analyses of MAA and HSA by SEM showed no modification of the particles due to the labeling process (Fig. 1a). In addition, in vitro experiments showed stability of Ga-68-labeled MAA in sterile water, 0.9% NaCl, and human plasma. No significant release of Ga-68 could be detected during the measurement period (Fig. 1b).

Table 1 Clinical data and results of lung V/P imaging using PET/CT

Clinical symptoms	Ventilation	Perfusion	Pulmonary embolism (PE)	Additional information from low-dose CT
77-year-old male with dizziness, decreased oxygen pressure, diabetic kidney disease, D-dimer at 5.66 μg/l	Homogeneous	Homogeneous	Excluded	Coronary atherosclerosis, calcification of the aortic valve, axial hiatal hernia, solitary gallstone, degenerative changes in the spine
66-year-old female with heart failure NYHA class III, chronic obstructive pulmonary disease, extreme obesity, type II diabetes, previous artificial pacemaker implantation, previous acute kidney failure, previous PE and DVT, increasing dyspnea since 1 week, D-dimer at 1.24 μg/l	Inhomogeneous with central depositions and defects left lateral and in projection to horizontal fissure of right lung (Fig. 3a)	Inhomogeneous with defects left lateral and in projection to horizontal fissure of right lung (Fig. 3b)	Excluded, combined V/P defects left lateral with suspicion of pneumonia and in projection to horizontal fissure of right lung	Pleural effusion, ground-glass opacities particularly in left lower lobe, coronary atherosclerosis and severe aortic sclerosis, left ventricular dilatation, artificial pacemaker in the left upper chest
70-year-old female with chronic asthma with acute dyspnea, D-dimer at 8.0 μg/l, creatinine at 2.02 mg/dL	Inhomogeneous with central radionuclide depositions (Fig. 3c)	Inhomogeneous, hypoperfusion in the right lower lobe dorsolateral (Fig. 3d)	Mismatch in terms of a PE	Pleural effusion, axillary lymph nodes increased but not enlarged, degenerative changes in the spine, calcification on the left lobe of the thyroid, enlarged left adrenal gland
83-year-old male with acute dyspnea, two-level DVT, D-dimer at 4.4 μg/l, creatinine at 1.75 mg/dL, known prostate carcinoma	Homogeneous	Homogeneous	Excluded	Small pleural nodules, coronary atherosclerosis aortic sclerosis, multiple gallstones, suspect metastatic lesion in L1 vertebral body (Fig. 3f)
80-year-old female with acute dyspnea, tachycardia, known thrombosis, renal insufficiency, D-dimer at 2.06 μg/l	Inhomogeneous with central and peripheral radionuclide depositions and defect in the left lower lobe	Homogeneous	Excluded, reverse mismatch in terms of pleural effusion with adjacent ventilation failure and suspicion of pneumonia	Severe pleural effusion with adjacent ventilation failure, dystelectasis and signs of lung infiltrate in the left lower lobe, severe aortic sclerosis and carotid artery stenosis, degenerative changes in the spine, calcified, right dorsal flexed uterus (Fig. 3i)

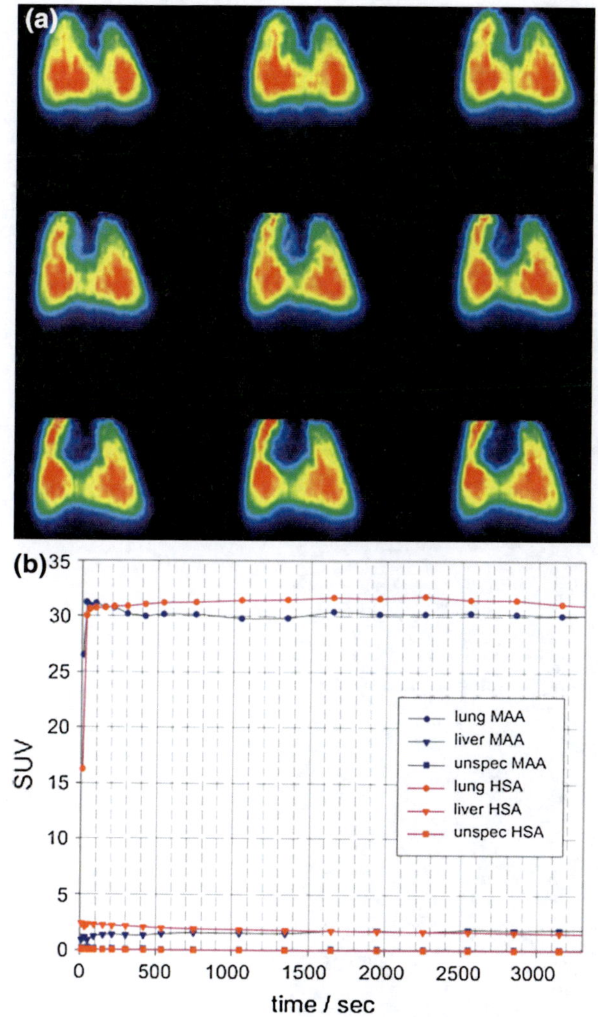

Fig. 2a, b **a** PET images (coronal slices) of the lung 30–60 min after i.v. injection of Ga-68-labeled MAA using a dedicated microPET scanner Focus 120 (Sect. 2.3.1, Maus et al. 2011). **b** SUV curves after i.v. injection of Ga-68-labeled MAA and Ga-68-labeled HSA (Maus et al. 2011)

3.2 Exploratory Studies

3.2.1 Animal Study

MAA and HSA particles were completely retained in the lung of the animals as demonstrated by the animal PET analyses (Fig. 2a). No significant differences in retention in the lung could be found. The time–activity curve indicated high in vivo stability, since no decrease of activity or migration of particles was observed within the

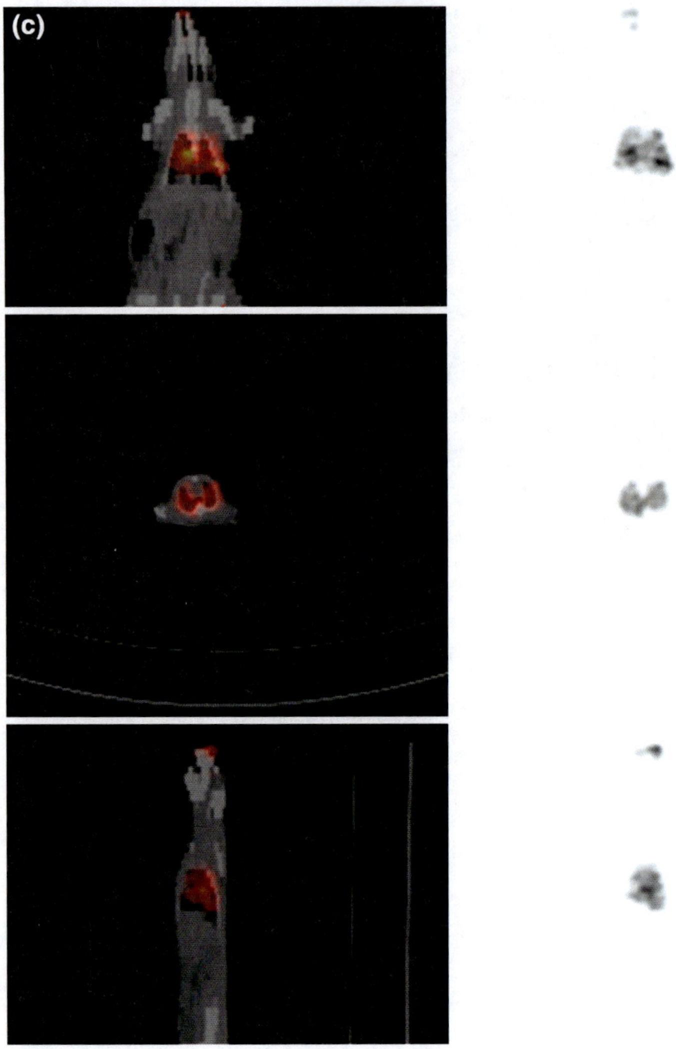

Fig. 2c, d Lung (**c**) ventilation (*top* coronal slices, *middle* transaxial slices, *bottom* sagittal slices) and (**d**) perfusion (*top* coronal slices, *middle* transaxial slices, *bottom* sagittal slices) scan with an aerosol of Ga-68-labeled carbon particles (Galligas) and Ga-68-labeled MAA performed ($n = 1$) using a Gemini TF PET/CT scanner (Philips, Best, The Netherlands) showing complete incorporation in the lung of a Sprague–Dawley rat without any extrapulmonary activity being visualized

(d)

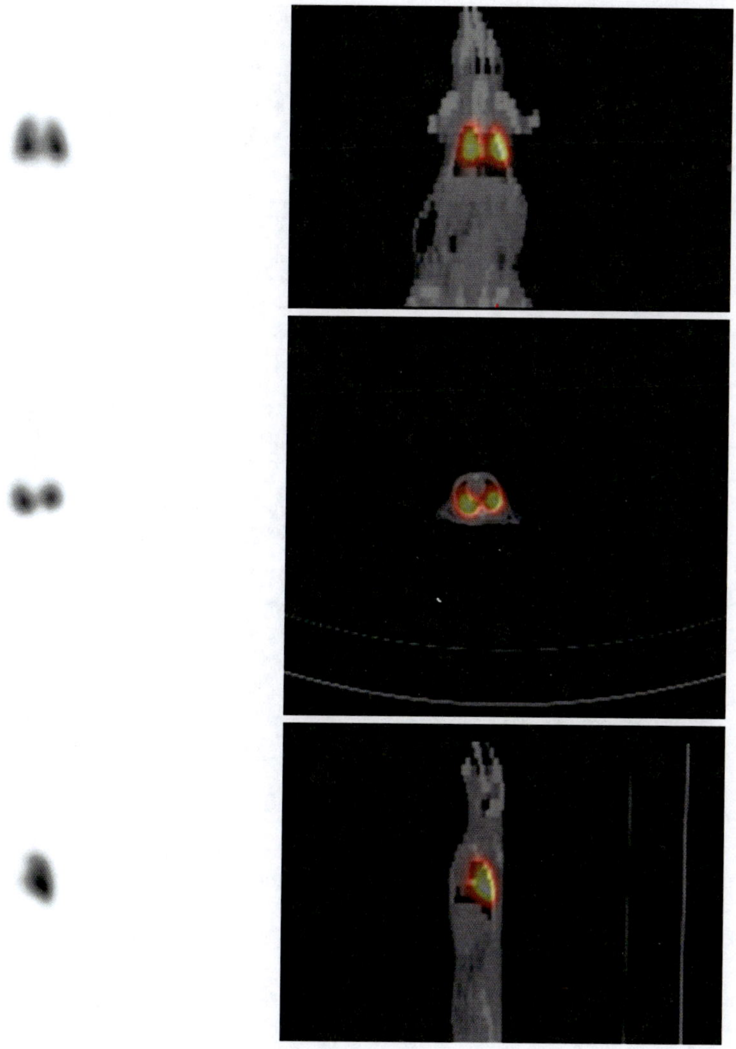

Fig. 2c, d (continued)

first hour (Fig. 2b). No significant retention of Ga-68 MAA or Ga-68 HSA particles in the liver was detected (Maus et al. 2011). Additionally, we could demonstrate complete incorporation of Ga-68-labeled carbon particles (Galligas) in the lung of a Sprague–Dawley rat without any extrapulmonary activity being visualized (Fig. 2c, d).

3.2.2 Clinical Study

In clinical use, PET lung ventilation and perfusion imaging using Ga-68 aerosol (Galligas) and Ga-68-labeled MAA was successful in all cases.

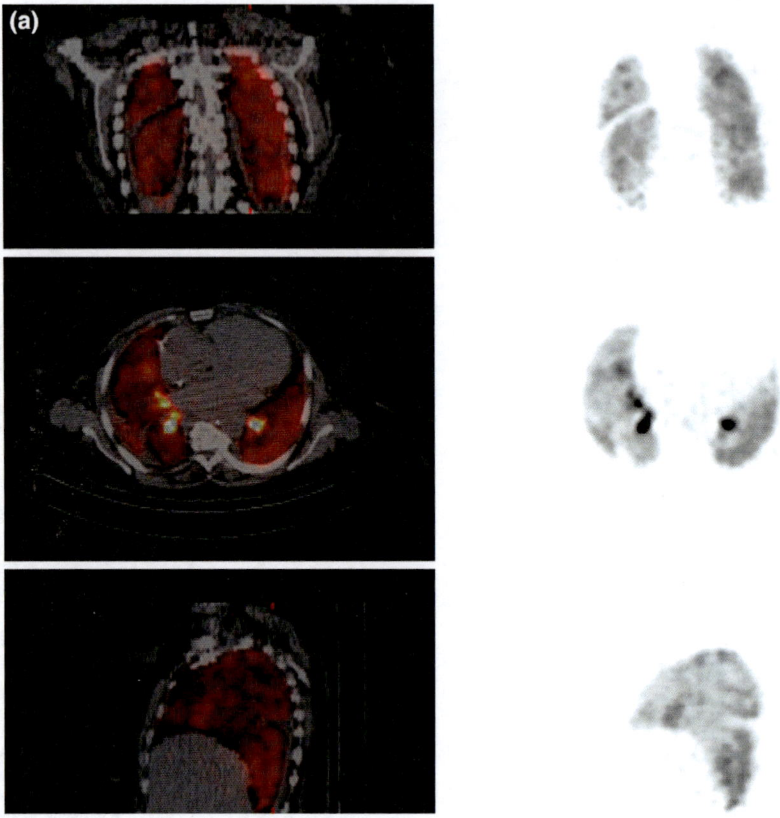

Fig. 3a, b PET lung (**a**) ventilation and (**b**) perfusion imaging using Ga-68 aerosol (Galligas) and Ga-68-labeled MAA showing combined ventilation (*top* coronal slices, *middle* transaxial slices, *bottom* sagittal slices)/perfusion (*top* coronal slices, *middle* transaxial slices, *bottom* sagittal slices) defects left lateral and in projection to the horizontal fissure of right lung PET lung

Ventilation imaging was homogeneous in two cases. In three cases, inhomogeneous accumulation with central deposition of radionuclide could be observed (Table 1).

The perfusion imaging was homogeneous in three cases. In one case, perfusion defects with corresponding ventilation defects were found (Fig. 3a, b).

Case 1. 70-year-old female with acute dyspnea, elevated D-dimer to 8.0 μg/l, and creatinine to 2.02 mg/dL showed an inhomogeneous nuclide accumulation with a hypoperfusion in the right lower lobe dorsolateral (especially segment 6) and preserved ventilation in the same region in terms of PE (mismatch defect) (Fig. 3c, d). A follow-up study was performed with Tc-99m aerosol (Technegas®) and Tc-99m-labeled MAA 3 days later (Fig. 3e).

(b)

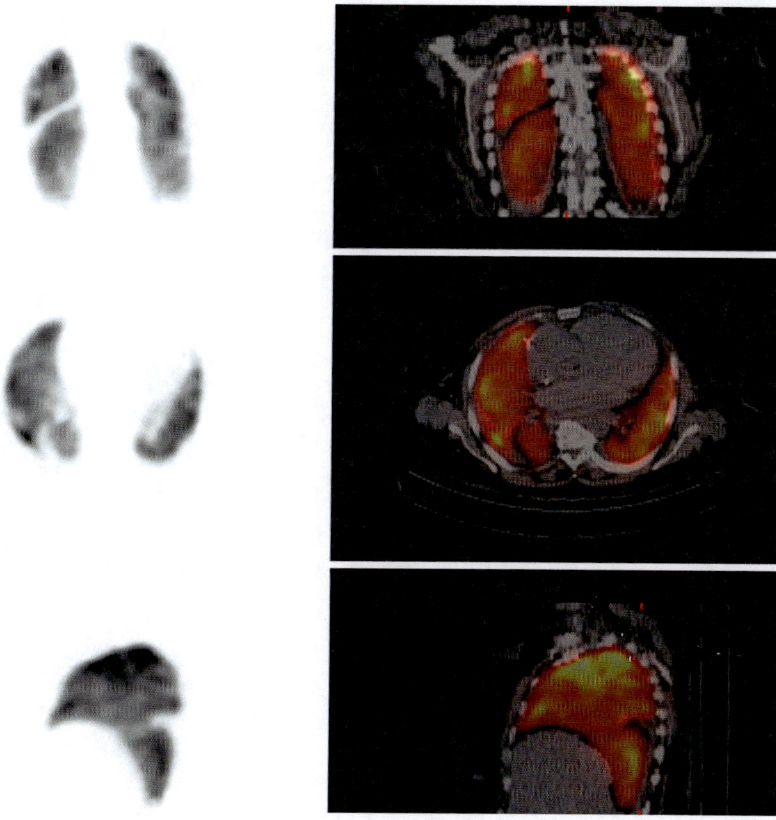

Fig. 3a, b (continued)

In all other cases PE as reason for the clinical symptoms could be excluded. Due to the low-dose CT performed for AC there was additional diagnostic information, for example, pleural effusion, infiltrates, dystelectasis, and more (Table 1).

Case 2. 83-year-old male with acute dyspnea, known two-level deep vein thrombosis (DVT), elevated D-dimer to 4.4 μg/l, and subsequent suspicion of PE. CT angiography (CTA) was not applicable in regard of creatinine elevated to 1.75 mg/dL. The V/P imaging showed homogeneous accumulation in both scans without any signs for PE. Nevertheless, low-dose CT showed a significant metastatic suspect lesion in L1 vertebral body (Fig. 3f) especially in the knowledge of an operated prostate

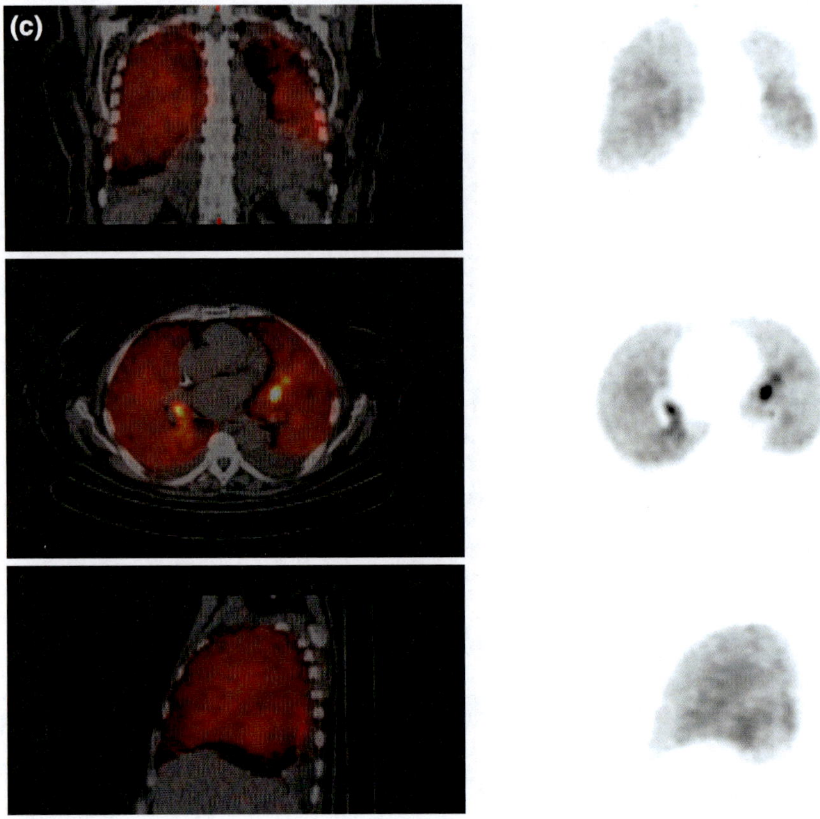

Fig. 3c, d c Ventilation (*top* coronal slices, *middle* transaxial slices, *bottom* sagittal slices) and (**d**) perfusion (*top* coronal slices, *middle* transaxial slices, *bottom* sagittal slices) imaging using Ga-68 aerosol (Galligas) and Ga-68-labeled MAA showing a hypoperfusion in the right lower lobe dorsolateral (especially segment 6) and preserved ventilation in the same region in terms of PE (mismatch defect)

carcinoma 2 years ago. Additional bone scintigraphy revealed multifocal metastatic bone disease (Fig. 3g).

Case 3. 80-year-old female with acute dyspnea, known thrombosis, renal insufficiency, and elevated D-dimer to 2.06 µg/l. PE as reason for the clinical symptoms could be excluded. The V/P imagings showed a reversed mismatch according to morphological signs of pneumonia. In this patient a third bed position was performed with the lower abdomen. No activity in the urinary bladder could be observed (Fig. 3h). Concomitant low-dose CT revealed a calcified, right dorsal flexed uterus with suspicion of uterine myomatosis (Fig. 3i).

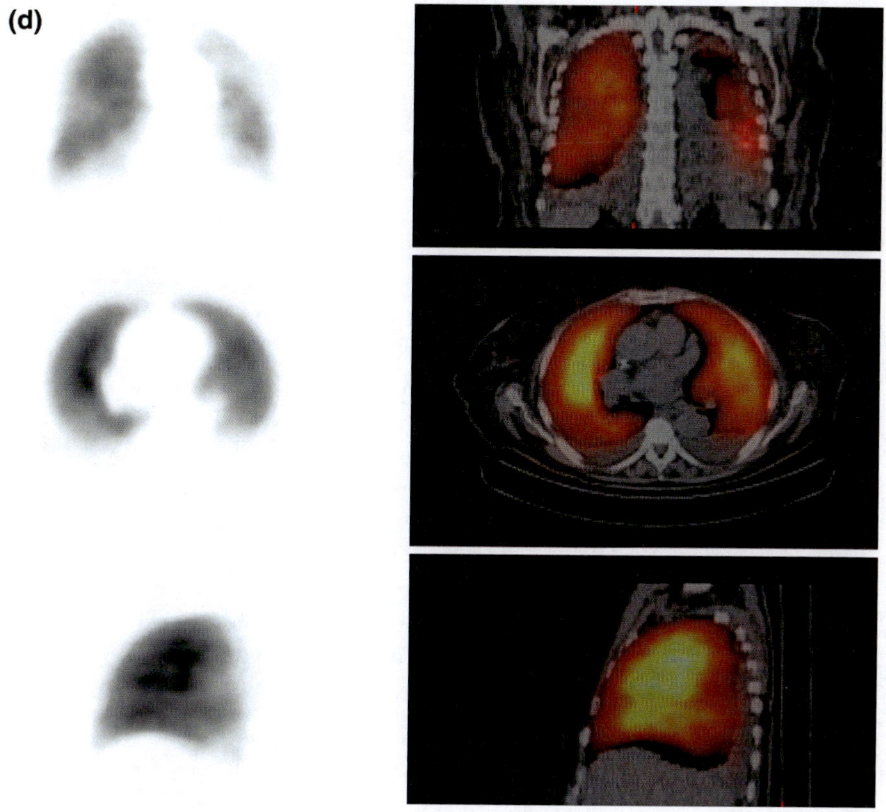

Fig. 3c, d (continued)

3.3 Dosimetry

Dosimetry calculations were performed using OLINDA (version 1.1, Vanderbilt University, 2007). Residence times were calculated assuming purely physical disintegration of activity in the lung. Administered activity was recovered almost fully in the "whole-body" region of interest (ROI) of the PET images (in two or three bed positions) except for in one patient, in whom activity in the liver was detectable but not completely in the visual field.

On average, 7.5 MBq Ga-68 aerosol (Galligas) was inhaled (3.4–12.6 MBq), determined from the "whole-body" ROI (two or three bed positions). Previously, validation with a Ge-68/Ga-68 homogeneous cylinder phantom (27 MBq) was obtained.

The mean application activity for perfusion imaging was 70.4 MBq (42–105 MBq) as determined by decay-corrected measurement of the syringe

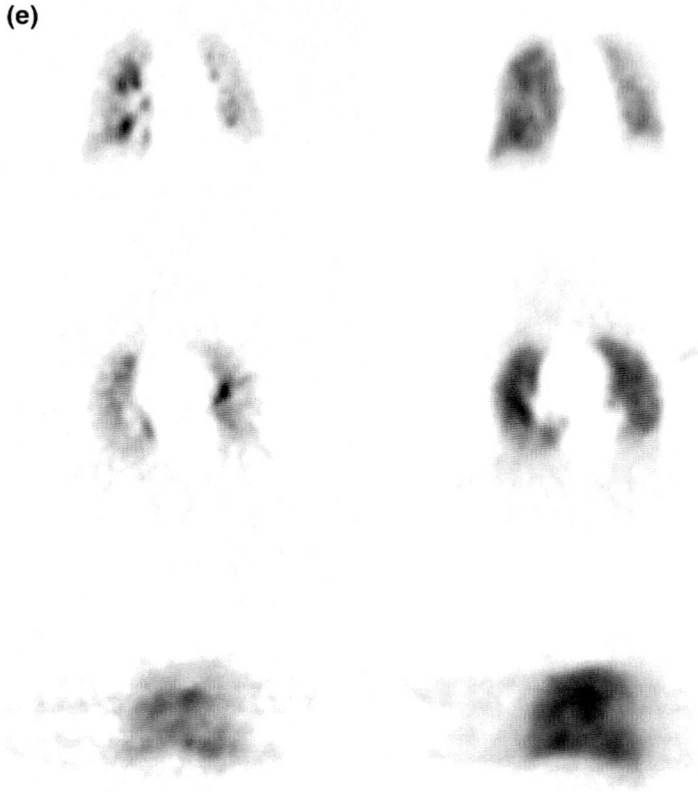

Fig. 3e Follow-up 3 days later (case 1). *Left* Ventilation imaging with Tc-99m aerosol (Technegas®); *Right* Perfusion imaging with Tc-99m-labeled MAA

before and after injection. The remaining activities were adjusted to the time difference between ventilation and perfusion imaging (19.6–23.7 min) and were included in the dosimetry calculations for perfusion imaging. This activity correction was 6 MBq on average.

Ventilation studies with Ga-68 aerosol (Galligas) showed a radiation exposure for the lung of 0.85 mSv/MBq and an effective dose of 0.11 mSv/MBq. According to the mean administered activity of 7.5 MBq, a lung dose of 6.4 mSv and an effective dose of 0.8 mSv could be calculated, respectively. In regard to image quality, 3.4 MBq inhaled Ga-68 aerosol (Galligas) was sufficient for ventilation imaging (Fig. 4a).

The lung perfusion scans provided a lung dose of 0.71 mSv/MBq (0.09 mSv/MBq effective dose). With the mean administered activity of 70.4 MBq, a lung dose of 49.4 mSv and an effective dose of 6.6 mSv were calculated.

"Extrapulmonary activity" could be visualized and verified in dosimetry calculations in the rib skeleton (Fig. 4) and in one case in the liver but not completely

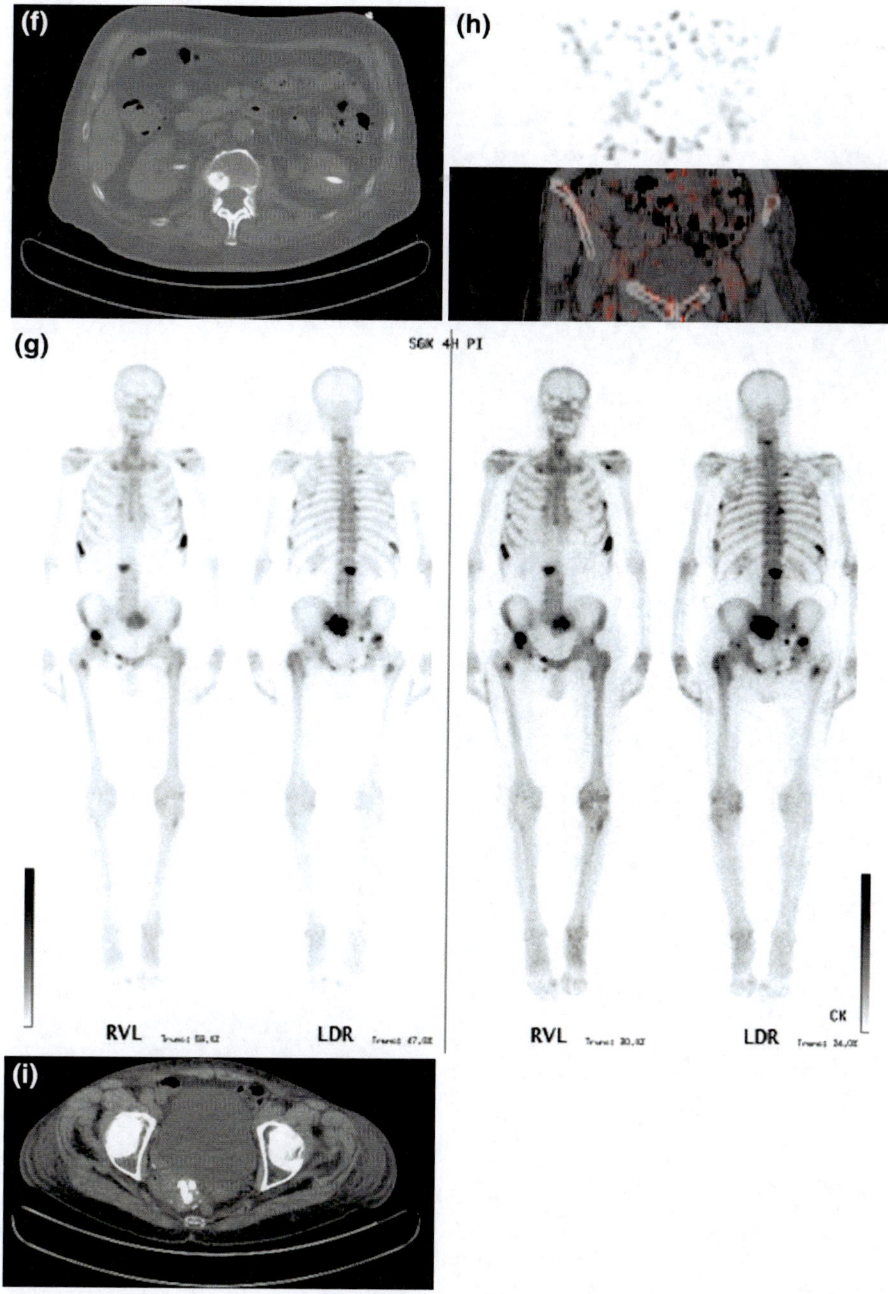

Fig. 3f–i **f** Low-dose CT with significant metastatic suspect lesions in L1 vertebral body (case 2). **g** Bone scintigraphy with multifocal metastatic bone disease (case 2). **h** PET scan of lower abdomen without visible activity in the urinary bladder (case 3). **i** Low-dose CT showing a calcified, right dorsal flexed uterus (case 3)

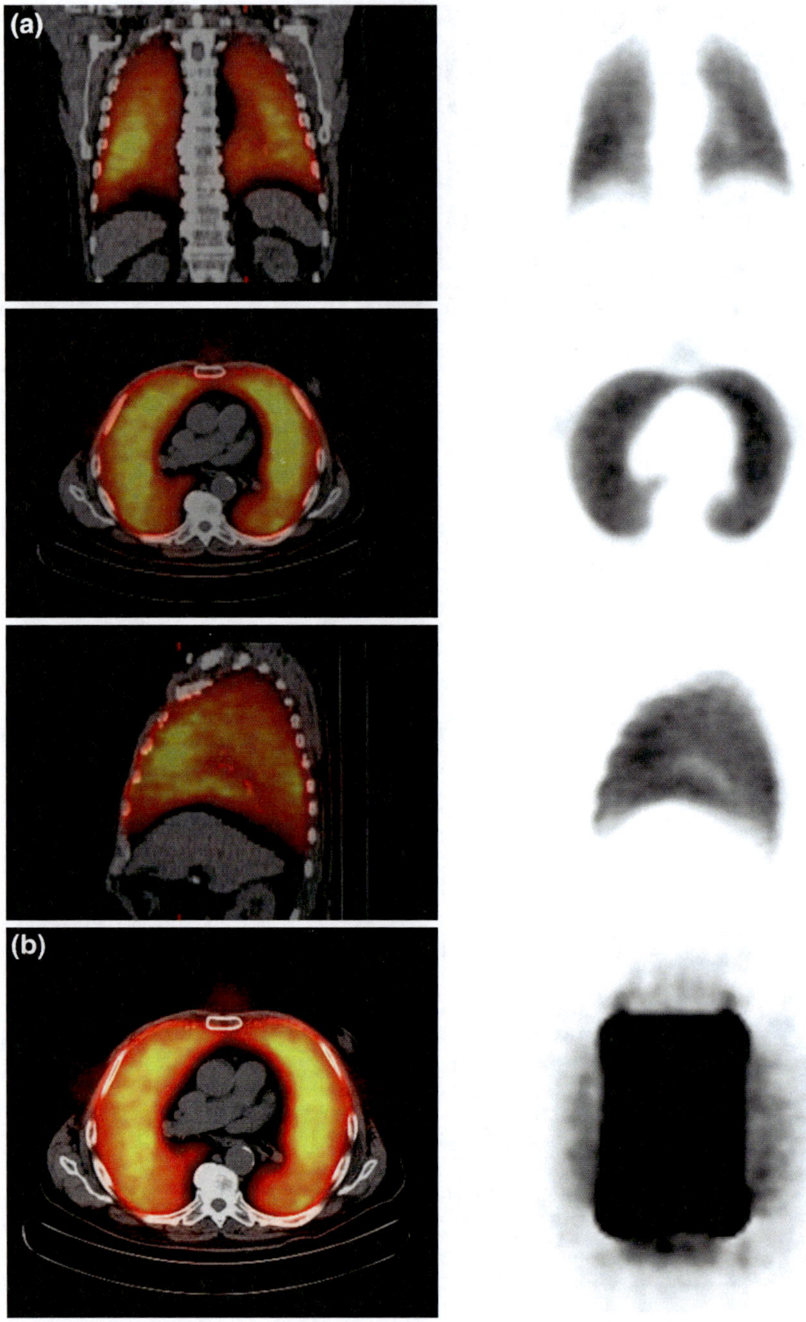
(a)
(b)

◀ **Fig. 4** **a** Ventilation imaging (*top* coronal slices, *middle* transaxial slices, *bottom* sagittal slices) performed with 3.4 MBq inhaled Ga-68 aerosol (Galligas). **b** *Left* "Extrapulmonary activity" could be visualized (ventilation imaging, transaxial slices; see **a** for coronal and sagittal slices) and verified in dosimetry calculations in the rib skeleton. *Right* Phantom measurements with lung mass density equivalent material (−850 HU, healthy lung: −910 to −700 HU) in a closed hollow cylinder showing inhomogeneous Ga-68 tracer accumulation. The hollow cylinder was in a torso phantom filled with (Ga-68-free) water. The quantification showed that 15% of the total applied activity dose was measurable (but "not existing") in the water

in the visual field for further quantification. Further phantom measurements showed that quantification of Ga-68 could be difficult. Of the administered activity in a closed hollow cylinder with lung mass density equivalent material (Fig. 4) 15% was recovered outside in activity-free water (inside of the torso phantom).

Low-dose CT (120 kV, 0.5 s/rotation, 5 m slices, max. 60 mAs, DLP 73.9–132.9 mGy·cm, field of view 600 mm) were obtained for AC with additional radiation exposure of 1.5 mSv on average.

4 Discussion

4.1 ^{68}Ga-Labeled Radiotracer for Lung Ventilation and Perfusion Imaging

4.1.1 Ga-68 Aerosol (Galligas)

The feasibility of producing radioactive-labeled carbon aerosol with other radionuclides (F-18, K-42, Cu-64, Ga-68) using a Technegas® generator was already investigated by Nozaki et al. in 1995. The latest preparation and assessment of F-18 fluorogas for lung scintigraphy was presented by Henriksen et al. (2011). Three healthy male volunteers underwent PET/CT scan after inhalation of >37 MBq fluorogas (185 MBq loaded into the crucible). Homogeneous distribution of activity over the entire lung parenchyma was described. These findings correlate with the data of Nozaki et al. (1995), who demonstrated a good distribution of F-18-labeled carbon particles in the lung periphery, but also rapid elimination from the lungs with half-life of 10 min. F-18 had labeling yield of 20–25%. In contrast, Ga-68 and Tc-99m showed similar labeling yields of 30–45% and a similar washout fraction in cold water of 5–15% and <15%, respectively. The combination of graphite and an argon atmosphere was used to vaporize generator-eluted [Ga-68]Ga-chloride for generating Ga-68-labeled particles. The assumption was that charged Ga-68 binds by adsorption to the carrier particles (carbon particles) in the aerosol (Nozaki et al. 1995). The physical and chemical nature of Technegas® were described in detail by Senden et al. (1997). The generated particles consist of hexagonal platelets of metallic Tc-99m, which are tightly enclosed by a thin layer of carbon. The average size of the particles is about 30–60 nm with approximately 80% of particles smaller than 100 nm. The ratio of thickness to diameter is approximately 1:10. Similar findings are expected for Ga-68-labeled carbon particles (Galligas).

Animal studies using "Gallgas" (Ga-68-labeled pseudogas) showed greater differences between poorly and well-ventilated regions, suggesting higher resolution using PET/CT (Borges et al. 2011). In comparative studies on healthy piglets and piglets with diffuse airway obstructions induced by methacholine infusion, ventilation scans were performed using Technegas® (SPECT) and Ga-68 aerosol (PET/CT). Good visualization was obtained with both techniques. However, the distribution of Ga-68-labeled pseudogas in the ventilated lung tissue was more detailed in the PET image. No additional stability analyses were performed. In analogy, we could demonstrate complete incorporation of Ga-68 aerosol (Galligas) in the lung of a Sprague–Dawley rat using a PET/CT scanner (Fig. 2c). No activity in the abdomen, urinary bladder, or blood pool could be detected.

Human studies with 20 healthy subjects using Ga-68 aerosol Galligas (named by Kotzerke et al. 2010a) could prove constant activity over the lung (half-time corrected) and thus the stability of the deposition of Ga-68-labeled carbon particles over 3.5 h without elimination via blood, urine, or feces being observed. Nevertheless, our results only allow information over the measurement period in clinical routine; later images are not available.

In consequence, first clinical studies were performed by Kotzerke et al. (2010b). Fifteen patients with clinical suspicion of PE were investigated after inhalation of Galligas for ventilation imaging and subsequent administration of Ga-68-labeled HSAM for perfusion imaging (Sect. 4.1.2). In correlation to these clinical studies and the previously described animal studies (Borges et al. 2011), ventilation imaging with Ga-68 aerosol (Galligas) revealed inhomogeneous distribution with central and peripheral depositions of the radionuclide observed in cases with severe obstructive ventilation disorders or pneumonic infiltrate (Table 1, Fig. 3a, c).

However, the automated Technegas® generator does not allow researchers to change the operating conditions according to the experimental setup. Consequently a series of questions remain unanswered. Further studies on the physical and chemical properties of Ga-68 aerosol (Galligas) are awaited.

4.1.2 Ga-68-Labeled HSAM

Due to the high binding affinity of Ga(III)-68 to the blood serum protein transferrin (given by log K1 = 20.3), the main requirement is thermodynamic stability towards hydrolysis and formation of $Ga(OH)_3$ (Harris and Pecoraro 1983). A prerequisite for a radiopharmaceutical, especially when used as a perfusion tracer, is avoidance of ligand exchange with human transferrin (Fani et al. 2008). For this reason, an early approach was to attach bifunctional metal chelating agents to macromolecules such as human serum albumin. Wagner and Welch (1979) used HSA as a model compound to attach In-111 and Ga-68 to albumin by covalent conjugation via a bifunctional high-affinity Ga-68 chelating ligand because of the high stability constant of Ga-68 to transferrin. Deposition of Ga-68-DTPA-HSA in the lungs of dogs could be demonstrated over the entire PET study period.

Recently, Wunderlich et al. (2010) compared the stability of Y-90-, Lu-177-, and Ga-68-labeled HSAM using DOTA as a high-affinity Ga-68 chelating ligand. Animal studies with Ga-68-DOTA-HSA microspheres showed that PET could detect and quantify regional pulmonary blood flow in animals as small as the rat (Richter et al. 2010).

First human studies were performed by Kotzerke et al. (2010b). Fifteen patients with clinical suspicion of PE were investigated after inhalation of 5–20 MBq Galligas and subsequent administration of Ga-68-labeled HSAM [injected activity four to eight times higher than the activity deposition (5–20 MBq) from the previous ventilation study with Galligas]. The deposition of Galligas was homogeneous in 11 cases and slightly inhomogeneous in 2 cases. In two other cases, inhomogeneous accumulation could be observed. For the production of Galligas, 100 MBq [Ga-68]Ga-chloride was loaded into the graphite crucible of a commercially available Technegas® generator. Subsequently, the program for Technegas® generation was initiated to produce an ultrafine dispersion of Ga-68-labeled carbon particles. In three patients the lung perfusion scan showed perfusion defects with preserved ventilation in the same region in terms of PE. Another five patients had inhomogeneous deposition of the Ga-68-labeled HSA microspheres and a homogeneous ventilation scan.

Perfusion imaging was obtained in this study with Ga-68-labeled HSA microspheres (Rotop Pharmaka GmbH, Radeberg, Germany). In contrast to our animal studies using same HSA microspheres (Sect. 3.2.1), labeling of HSA with Ga-68 was performed using a high-affinity Ga-68 chelating ligand for stabilization of the product. Nevertheless, using a chelator results in additional purification steps to remove unbounded chelator from the matrix.

Another labeling procedure was described by Hnatowich in 1976. Labeling of tin-soaked albumin microspheres with Ga-68 was performed by hydrolysis and precipitation of Ga(III)-68 ions in the presence of albumin particles. The labeling procedure itself is simple, since gallium forms complexes without use of reducing agents. Even and Green (1989) and Maziere et al. (1986) first described direct labeling of commercial MAA kits with Ga-68. They used a generator with a tin dioxide column as carrier for the mother nuclide Ge-68. The generator was eluted with 2–2.5 mL 1 N HCl and provided [Ga-68]Ga-chloride. Due to the solvent volume, this method includes an evaporating step under nitrogen gas. Mathias and Green (2008) described a method using a TiO_2-based generator which could be eluted with 0.1 N HCl, which made an evaporating step unnecessary. The final Ga-68-labeled MAA product was obtained with $81.6 \pm 5.3\%$ decay-corrected radiochemical yield and radiochemical purity of $99.8 \pm 0.1\%$.

We could verify the results of Even and Green (1989) and Mathias and Green (2008), especially the prewashing step to free the particles of compounds such as stannous chloride, polysorbate, and hydrochloric acid. Conscientious preparation could increase the labeling yield up to 10%. MAA was labeled with efficiency of $85 \pm 2\%$, and HSA with $80 \pm 5\%$. The minor differences are caused by leakages during the process of purification as a consequence of the differences in particle size. After washing with sterile water, the radiochemical purity for both kits was higher than 97%. The whole procedure from elution up to the final product takes a total of less than 30 min (Maus et al. 2011). In contrast, we used a SnO_2-based generator eluted with 0.6 N HCl. In the past, SnO_2 showed the best parameters in terms of Ge-68 breakthrough and Ga-68 elution (Rösch and Knapp 2003). The major requirement for clinical use of Ga-68 is a specified Ge-68 breakthrough of <0.001%. We could show that our final Ga-68 solution had radionuclide purity (RNP), expressed as the ratio of activities of Ge-68 over Ga-68, of 0.0005%. It was already demonstrated that the eluate of the iThemba Labs SnO_2-based generator has low metal impurities (de Blois et al. 2011). Consequently, the eluate could be used directly for labeling with DOTA peptides and showed full incorporation in radiopeptides.

As expected, both MAA and HSA particles were retained in the lungs of animals as demonstrated by the animal PET analyses. No significant differences in retention in the lung could be found. Time–activity curves suggested high in vivo stability, since no decrease of activity or migration of particles was observed within the first hour (Fig. 2b). No significant retention and no visual uptake of Ga-68 MAA or Ga-68 HSA particles in the liver were detectable (Fig. 2b, c).

In conclusion, we could demonstrate that HSAM could be successful and stably labeled with Ga-68 by a simple and fast preparation method. Adapted to an automatic synthesis unit and produced in compliance with GMP guidelines, Ga-68-labeled MAA or HSA spheres are an effective substitute as PET perfusion tracer for human use.

According to EANM guidelines for V/P scintigraphy and its key recommendations for investigation of regional pulmonary perfusion in PE diagnosis, 99 mTc-MAA is the agent recommended for perfusion scintigraphy with evidence level IIa, grade B (Bajc et al. 2009b). Consequently, perfusion imaging was performed with Ga-68-labeled MAA. Our findings showed correlated and complementary results to previously described studies. Although for a very small group of patients, our results show that Ga-68 aerosol (Galligas) and Ga-68-labeled MAA are efficient for clinical use and could be an interesting alternative with high accuracy to lung V/P imaging with Tc-99m-labeled radiotracers. The image quality of PET lung ventilation and perfusion scans using Ga-68 aerosol (Galligas) and Ga-68-labeled MAA was excellent, succeeding in safe diagnosis of PE (Fig. 3c, d). A follow-up 3 days later with Tc-99m aerosol (Technegas®) and Tc-99m MAA (Fig. 3e) enables an implicit comparison of the two methods, showing the advantage of the PET/CT scan in providing images with high spatial resolution. In one case a third bed position was performed with the lower abdomen, but no activity in the urinary bladder could be detected (Fig. 3h). In addition, in vitro experiments showed high stability of Ga-68-labeled MAA in sterile water, 0.9% NaCl, and human plasma. No significant release of Ga-68 could be detected during the measurement period of 4 h (Fig. 1). The complexes seemed to be more stable than the Ga(III)-68-transferrin complex, or kinetically inert. In result there is no exchange with this protein, which in turn would also lead to an accumulation in the blood pool that could not be visualized in our studies.

Nevertheless, in contrast to our animal studies, activity in the liver was visually detectable in one patient, but not completely in the visual field for further quantification. After exclusion of other sources, an arteriovenous shunt was most likely the reason for this. However, the detailed chemical nature of the Ga-68 binding to the MAA particles is still unknown. Mathias and Green (2008) hypothesized that Ga-68 adsorbs to the surface of the MAA particles after hydrolysis to insoluble gallium hydroxide.

Another example of efficient clinical use of Ga-68-labeled MAA is provided by its intraarterial application into the hepatic artery as an integral part of patient evaluation before selective intraarterial radioembolization (SIRT) of hepatic neoplasm to quantify the hepatopulmonary shunt, possible dystopic extrahepatic flow, and regional intrahepatic distribution of particles (Gartenschlaeger et al. 2011).

4.2 Dosimetry

4.2.1 V/P Ratio

Dosimetry calculations showed higher radiation exposure in comparison with SPECT using Tc-99m-labeled radiotracers for lung V/P imaging. Due to the heterogeneity in the V/P ratio (coincidence rate 37,040–118,810 for ventilation scans; coincidence rate 409,230–811,680 for perfusion scans, V/P ratio from 1:4 up to 1:16) and taking into account the influence of the true coincidence, an additional exemplary dosimetry calculation was performed in the case with a reliable V/P ratio.

In this case (patient with PE) the radiation exposure for 6 MBq inhaled Ga-68 aerosol (Galligas) (lung dose 5.7 mSv, effective dose 0.7 mSv, coincidence rate 71,000) was comparable to that for 40 MBq inhaled Technegas® for lung ventilation imaging (lung dose 4.4 mSv, effective dose 0.6 mSv, International Commission on Radiological Protection 1998) and 50% higher for the application of 42 MBq Ga-68-labeled MAA (lung dose 28.7 mSv, effective dose 3.7 mSv, coincidence rate 415,000) compared with 200 MBq Tc-99m-labeled MAA for lung perfusion imaging (lung dose 13.2 mSv, effective dose 2.2 mSv, International Commission on Radiological Protection 1998). Formally, the administrated activity could still have been reduced up to 50% without any influence on image resolution.

In the study of Kotzereke et al. (2010b), the administered activity of Ga-68-labeled HSAM for perfusion imaging was four to eight times higher than the activity deposition (5–20 MBq) from the previous ventilation study with Galligas. The image quality was so good that use of 3 MBq administered activity for ventilation imaging was proposed. In comparison, we could exemplarily show very good results in terms of image quality in ventilation imaging performed with

3.4 MBq inhaled Ga-68 aerosol (Galligas) (Fig. 4a). In this case, the radiation exposure (0.31 mSv/3.4 MBq, coincidence rate 37,040) was even 50% lower than with Technegas® (0.6 mSv/40 MBq, ICRP 80) for lung ventilation imaging (Fig. 4a).

Further phantom measurements with Ga-68 revealed a possible reduction of the acquisition time to 90 s for each scan without any influence on image quality and subsequent reduction of the additional radiation exposure of the obtained low-dose CT.

4.2.2 Ga-68 Properties

The visualized "extrapulmonary activity" in the rib skeleton (Fig. 4b, left) as a result of free Ga-68 is predicted to be implausibly as it is well established that Ga(III)-68 distributes through the circulatory system bound to the serum iron-transport protein transferrin (Harris and Pecoraro 1983).

The high kinetic energy and consecutive high positron range of Ga-68 (max 1.9 MeV, median 0.84 MeV) could have an unwanted effect on PET imaging, especially in regard to quantification of Ga-68. Kemerink et al. (2011) could show in phantom measurements that Ga-68 sources are visualized sharply in air but tail with a large fraction of annihilations extending over several centimeters. Nevertheless, the central peak of Ga-68 was even slightly narrower in lung-like material than in soft tissue. They proposed that only annihilations in the source could be detected, because once a positron leaves the source in air it is likely to be lost from detection, its range being about 800 times larger than in water (i.e., several metres). Otherwise, in medium with increasing density (e.g., bone), positrons that escape in air are increasingly scattered, stopped, and annihilated in a region outside the source, making the volume with annihilations larger than in air and visualizable by the scanner (Kemerink et al. 2011). This phenomenon was also described with another high-energy positron emitter I-124 with similar profile to Ga-68 (Kemerink et al. 2011).

In human studies with patients with differentiated thyroid cancer and lesions around the air-filled trachea, shine-through artifacts were described due to annihilations of I-124 in the opposite wall of the trachea, incorrectly suggesting activity at that location (Adul-Fatah et al. 2009). In terms of sensitivity and specificity of the performed lung ventilation and perfusion imaging, this aspect is mostly neglected. Nevertheless, for quantification of Ga-68, large VOI are needed for complete activity recovery (Kemerink et al. 2011).

With VOI around the lung excluding the rib skeleton, extrapulmonary activity could be detected. Analogously, in our phantom measurements, 15% of activity administered in a closed hollow cylinder with lung mass density equivalent material (Fig. 4b, right) was recovered outside in activity-free water (inside of a torso phantom).

In our clinical study, iterative reconstruction using ordered-subset expectation maximization (OSEM) with 33 subsets and 3 iterations was performed. However, other reconstruction algorithms did not show any effects on the visualized "extrapulmonary activity."

4.3 Perspectives

Currently, CT angiography (CTA) and multidetector CT angiography have replaced ventilation/perfusion (V/P) scintigraphy as the primary imaging modality for PE in many centers (Pipavath and Godwin 2008; Strashun 2007). However, in comparison, CTA is more expensive and the radiation exposure is much higher. Radiation exposure should always follow the "as low as reasonably achievable" (ALARA) principle, and CT pulmonary angiography delivers a nonnegligible radiation dose of at least, e.g., 20 mGy to the breasts of an average-sized woman (Parker et al. 2005). Moreover, it is not applicable in patients who have contra-indications to iodinated contrast material (Freeman et al. 2007; Sostmann et al. 2008). Consequently, V/P scans will continue to retain a high priority in diagnosis of PE (Gutte et al. 2009; Zöpfel et al. 2009).

To be equipped for the future, especially in times of Mo-99 shortages and increasing use and spread of PET/CT scanners and Ga-68 generators, it is worth performing further studies on Ga-68-labeled radiotracers for ventilation and perfusion imaging. Further information on the binding affinities and complete biodistribution of Ga-68-labeled HSAM needs to be obtained. In terms of reconstruction artifacts, further investigation on the broad range of positrons due to the high kinetic energy of Ga-68 and the possible direct effects of both on the quantification of PET lung V/P imaging should be performed.

Nevertheless, the higher resolution of PET imaging and additional information from the low-dose CT performed for AC could display an advantage over conventional V/P scans in terms of sensitivity and specificity. Although the radiation exposure of a low-dose CT for a lung scan is 1.5 mSv on average, the morphological imaging can provide a different specific diagnosis such as, e.g., pneumonia, pleural effusion, and dystelectasis (Table 1). Gutte et al. (2009) also found better estimation in a subset of 81 patients using V/P SPECT and low-dose CT (sensitivity 97%, specificity 100%) than in a subset of 77 patients using V/P SPECT alone (sensitivity 97%, specificity 88%). In comparison, multidetector CT angiography alone (81 patients) had sensitivity of 68% and specificity of 100% (Gutte et al. 2009).

However, a comparative study of Ga-68-labeled radiotracers using PET/CT and Tc-99m-labeled radiotracers using SPECT/CT for lung ventilation and perfusion imaging with a larger group of patients is necessary to ensure clinical utility.

References

Abdul-Fatah SB, Zamburlini M, Halders SG et al (2009) Identification of a shine through artifact in the trachea with I-124 PET/CT. J Nucl Med 50:909–911

Bajc M, Neilly JB, Miniati M et al (2009a) EANM guidelines for ventilation/perfusion scintigraphy, part 1-pulmonary imaging with ventilation/perfusion single photon emission tomography. Eur J Nucl Med Mol Imaging 36:1356–1370

Bajc M, Neilly JB, Miniati M et al (2009b) EANM guidelines for ventilation/perfusion scintigraphy, part 2-algorithms and clinical considerations for diagnosis of pulmonary emboli with V/PSPECT and MDCT. Eur J Nucl Med Mol Imaging 36:1528–1538

Ballinger JR (2010) Mo-99 shortage in nuclear medicine: crisis or challenge? J Labelled Compd Radiopharm 53:167–168

Baum RP, Prasad V, Hommann M et al (2008) Receptor PET/CT imaging of neuroendocrine tumors. Recent Results Cancer Res 170:225–242

Borges JB, Velikyan I, Langström B et al (2011) Ventilation distribution studies comparing technegas and "gallgas" using $^{68}GaCl_3$ as the label. J Nucl Med 52:206–209

Breeman WA, de Jong M, de Blois E et al (2005) Radiolabelling DOTA-peptides with ^{68}Ga. Eur J Nucl Med Mol Imaging 32:478–485

Chesler DA, Hales C, Hnatowich DJ et al (1975) Three-dimensional reconstruction of lung perfusion image. J Nucl Med 16:80–82

de Blois E, Sze Chan H, Naidoo C et al (2011) Characteristics of SnO_2 based Ge-68/Ga-68 generator and aspects of radiolabelling DOTA-peptides. Appl Radiat Isot 69:308–315

Even GA, Green MA (1989) Gallium-68-labeled macro aggregated human serum albumin, ^{68}Ga-MAA. Nucl Med Biol 16:319–321

Fani M, Andreé JP, Maecke HR et al (2008) ^{68}Ga-PET: a powerful generator-based alternative to cyclotron-based PET radiopharmaceuticals. Contrast Media Mol Imaging 3:67–77

Freeman LM (2007) Don't bury the V/P Scan: it's as good as multidetector CT angiograms with a lot less radiation exposure. J Nucl Med 49:5–8

Gartenschlaeger M, Maus S, Buchholz H et al (2011) Investigation for extrahepatic shunt before SIRT by PET/CT with ^{68}Ga-. Nuklearmedizin 50(4):N37–N38 (in German)

Gutte H, Mortensen J, Jensen CV et al (2009) Detection of pulmonary embolism with combined ventilation-perfusion SPECT and low-dose-CT: Head-to-head comparison with multidetector CT angiography. J Nucl Med 50:1987–1992

Harris WR, Pecoraro VL (1983) Thermodynamic binding constants for gallium transferrin. Biochemistry 22(2):292–299

Henriksen G, Scheidhauer K, Schwaiger M et al. (2011) Preparation and assessment of F-18 fluorogas for lung scintigraphy. J Nucl Med 52(1):315P(1493)

Hnatowich DJ (1976) Labeling of tin-soaked albumin microspheres with ^{68}Ga. J Nucl Med 17:57–60

International Commission on Radiological Protection (1998) Radiation dose to patients from radiopharmaceuticals (addendum to ICRP publication 53). Ann ICRP 28(3):1–126 (ICRP Publication 80)

Kemerink GJ, Visser MG, Franssen R et al (2011) Effect of the positron range of ^{18}F, ^{68}Ga, ^{124}I on PET/CT in lung–equivalent materials. Eur J Nucl Med Mol Imaging 38:940–948

Knipping HW, Bolt W, Venrath H et al (1955) A new method of heart and lung function testing, the regional functional analysis in the lung and heart clinic by the radioactive noble gas xenon 133 (isotope thoracography). Dtsch Med Wochenschr 80(31–32):1146–1147 (in German)

Kotzerke J, Andreeff M, Wunderlich G (2010a) PET aerosol lung scintigraphy using galligas. Eur J Nucl Mol Imaging 37:175–177

Kotzerke J, Andreeff M, Wunderlich G et al (2010b) Ventilation/perfusion lung scintigraphy using PET and ^{68}Ga-labeled radiopharmaceuticals. Nuklearmedizin 49:203–208 (in German)

Mathias CJ, Green MA (2008) A convenient rote to [^{68}Ga]Ga-MAA for use as a particulate PET perfusion tracer. Appl Radiat Isot 66:1910–1912

Maus S, Buchholz HG, Ament S et al (2011) Labelling of commercially available human serum albumin kits with ^{68}Ga as surrogates for ^{99m}Tc-MAA microspheres. Appl Radiat Isot 69(1):171–175

Maziere B, Loc'h C, Steinling M et al (1986) Stable labeling of serum albumin microspheres with gallium-68. Appl Radiat Isot 37:360–361

Nozaki T, Muraoka H, Hara T et al (1995) Production of fine aerosols labelled with various radionuclides by sublimation from a graphite boat, and their properties an tracer use. Appl Radiat Isot 46(3):157–165

Parker MS, Hui FK, Camacho MA, Chung JK, Broga DW, Sethi N (2005) Female breast radiation exposure during CT pulmonary angiography. Am J Roentgenol 185(5):1228–1233

Pipavath SNJ, Godwin JD (2008) Acute pulmonary thromboembolism: a historical perspective. Am J Roentgenol 191(3):639–641

Richter T, Bergmann R, Pietzsch J et al (2010) Effects of posture on regional pulmonary blood flow in rats as measured by PET. J Appl Physiol 108(2):422–429

Rösch F, Knapp FF (2003) Radionuclide generators. In: Vértes A, Nagy S, Klencsár Z, Rösch F (eds) Handbook of nuclear chemistry, vol 4. Kluwer Academic, The Netherlands

Senden TJ, Moock KH, Gerald JF et al (1997) The physical and chemical nature of technegas. J Nucl Med 38:1327–1333

Sostmann DH, Miniati M, Gottschalk A et al (2008) Sensitivity and specificity of perfusion scintigraphy combined with chest radiography for acute pulmonary embolism in PIOPED II. J Nucl Med 49:1741–1748

Stein PD, Freeman LM, Sostman HD et al (2009) SPECT in acute pulmonary embolism. J Nucl Med 50(12):1999–2007

Strashun AM (2007) A reduced role of V/Q scintigraphy in the diagnosis of acute pulmonary embolism. J Nucl Med 48:1405–1407

Surti S, Kuhn A, Werner ME et al (2007) Performance of philips gemini TF PET/CT scanner with special consideration for its time of flight imaging capabilities. J Nucl Med 48:471–480

Technegas® generator user manual (2005) European english version/revision A http://www.cyclopharm.com/system/asset/location/95/TGP_Manual_Euro_-8_06.qxp.pdf. Last accessed 12 Aug 2011

Wagner HN Jr, Sabiston DC Jr, Ilo M et al (1964) Regional pulmonary blood flow in man by radioisotope scanning. J Am Med Assoc 187:601–603

Wagner SJ, Welch MJ (1979) Gallium-68 labeling of albumin and albumin microspheres. J Nucl Med 20:428–433

Wunderlich G, Schiller E, Bergmann R et al (2010) Comparison of the stability of Y-90-, Lu-177- and Ga-68-labeled human serum albumin microspheres (DOTA-HSAM). Nucl Med Biol 37(8):861–867

Zöpfel K, Bacher-Stier C, Pinkert J et al (2009) Ventilation/perfusion lung scintigraphy: what is still needed? A review considering technetium-99 m-labeled macro-aggregates of albumin. Ann Nucl Med 23(1):1–16

Combined PET/MR Imaging Using ^{68}Ga-DOTATOC for Radiotherapy Treatment Planning in Meningioma Patients

Daniela Thorwarth, Arndt-Christian Müller,
Christina Pfannenberg and Thomas Beyer

Abstract

Hybrid imaging is beneficial for improved medical diagnosis and therapy planning today. Hybrid imaging describes the prospective correlation of two or more complementary sets of imaging information, such as functional and anatomical image volumes. Correlation can be performed through physically combined imaging modalities, such as PET/CT, SPECT/CT, or PET/MR. Here we present first results from employing fully integrated PET/MR tomography for intensity-modulated radiotherapy (IMRT) treatment planning in patients with meningioma using [^{68}Ga]-DOTATOC as the biomarker of choice. Combined PET/MR offers higher soft tissue contrast and the ability to add functional information to the plain combination of MR-based anatomy and PET-based metabolic and molecular information. Furthermore, fully integrated PET/MR employs novel PET technology that is neither available in PET-only nor PET/CT systems. Despite the current lack of broad clinical evidence, integrated PET/MR may become particularly important and clinically

D. Thorwarth (✉)
Section for Biomedical Physics, University Hospital for Radiation Oncology,
Eberhard-Karls-University Tübingen, Hoppe-Seyler-Str. 3,
72076 Tübingen, Germany
e-mail: daniela.thorwarth@med.uni-tuebingen.de

A.-C. Müller
University Hospital for Radiation Oncology, Eberhard-Karls-University,
Tübingen, Germany

C. Pfannenberg
Department for Diagnostic and Interventional Radiology, Division of Radiology,
Eberhard-Karls-University, Tübingen, Germany

T. Beyer
CMI Experts GmbH, Pestalozzistr. 3, CH - 8032 Zürich, Switzerland

R. P. Baum and F. Rösch (eds.), *Theranostics, Gallium-68, and Other Radionuclides*,
Recent Results in Cancer Research 194, DOI: 10.1007/978-3-642-27994-2_23,

useful for improved, individualized RT therapy planning for brain lesions. In particular, logistical and diagnostic benefits of integrated PET/MR-based treatment planning over treatment planning based on PET/CT data may be expected in meningioma patients.

Keywords

PET · ^{68}Ga tracer · Combined PET/MR · Meningioma

Abbreviations

APD	Avalanche photodiode
CT	Computed tomography
DCE	Dynamic contrast enhanced
DOTATOC	1,4,7,10-Tetraazacyclododecane-1,4,7,10-tetraacetic acid (DOTA)-D-Phe1-Tyr3-octreotide (TOC)
DWI	Diffusion-weighted imaging
FDG	[^{18}F]-Fluorodeoxyglucose
FET	*O*-(2-[^{18}F]-Fluoroethyl)-L-tyrosine
GTV	Gross target volume
IMRT	Intensity-modulated radiation therapy
MET	Methionine
MI	Mutual information
mL	Milliliter
MRI	Magnetic resonance imaging
MRS	Magnetic resonance spectroscopy
OSEM	Ordered-subsets expectation maximization
p.i.	Post injection
PET	Positron emission tomography
PTV	Planning target volume
RT	Radiation therapy
SNR	Signal-to-noise ratio
SPECT	Single-photon emission computed tomography
TBR	Tumor-to-blood ratio
TV	Target volume

Contents

1 Introduction

Noninvasive medical imaging is an integral part of state-of-the-art patient management. Medical imaging can be categorized broadly into anatomical and functional imaging, making reference, respectively, to the ability to acquire information of the anatomy such as bone and soft tissue structures through the use of computed tomography (CT) or magnetic resonance imaging (MRI), and to acquire information on molecular or biochemical processes such as hypermetabolism as a criterion for potential cancerous tissue infiltration (Warburg 1956) through the use of positron emission tomography (PET).

Historically, medical devices to image either anatomical structure or functional processes have developed along somewhat independent paths, but the usefulness of combining anatomical and functional planar images was evident to physicians as early as the 1960s. The recognition that combining images from different modalities offers significant diagnostic advantages gave rise to sophisticated software techniques to co-register structure and function (Townsend 2008). For relatively rigid objects such as the brain, software can successfully align images from MR, CT, and PET, whereas in regions of the body outside the brain, accurate alignment is difficult owing to the large number of possible degrees of freedom.

Alternatives to software-based fusion have now become available through hardware fusion (Beyer et al. 2011). Combined, or hybrid, tomographs such as SPECT/CT or PET/CT can acquire co-registered structural and functional information sequentially within a single study. The data are complementary, allowing CT to accurately localize functional abnormalities and SPECT or PET to highlight areas of abnormal tracer uptake. This is of particular importance in case PET (or SPECT) images of the distribution of highly specific tracers reveal very little anatomical background information. Figure 1 illustrates this with the example of a highly specific tracer ([^{68}Ga]-labeled somatostatin-receptor ligand: [^{68}Ga]-DOTATOC), which specifically binds to somatostatin-expressing receptors. Several studies are available today demonstrating the utility and efficacy of combined PET/CT imaging using a variety of tracers (Czernin et al. 2007; Nestle et al. 2009). As a consequence, following their recent introduction into the clinic, combined PET/CT and SPECT/CT devices are now playing an increasing role in diagnosis and staging of patients with oncological and inflammatory diseases.

However, despite the success and wide distribution of PET/CT, there are some shortcomings in use of CT as the anatomical complement to PET. CT uses a source of ionizing radiation for imaging and, therefore, adds significant radiation dose to

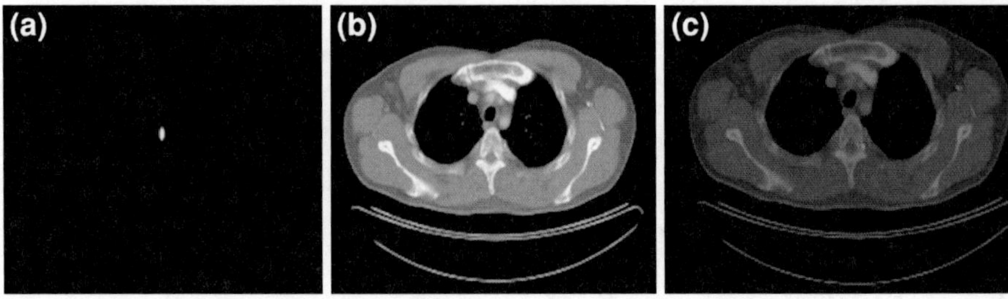

Fig. 1 [^{68}Ga]-DOTATOC study of a patient with neuroendocrine tumor. From *left* to *right* axial images of: **a** attenuation-corrected PET, **b** CT, and **c** PET/CT. Without any anatomical correlated uptake, highly specific PET tracer uptake cannot be localized sufficiently; here, combined imaging becomes mandatory. Data courtesy of Hofmann (Hannover) and Bockisch (Essen)

the overall examination (Brix et al. 2005), which may raise concern in selected populations such as adolescents, females, and patients with benign diseases. Further, CT provides comparatively low soft tissue contrast unless additional CT contrast agent are used. MR, on the other hand, does not suffer from these two major disadvantages and, in addition, offers more advanced functional imaging information, such as dynamic contrast-enhanced (DCE), diffusion-weighted imaging (DWI), or magnetic resonance spectroscopy (MRS), without adding to the overall radiation exposure burden.

The combination of PET and MR in a single imaging system has the potential to become a multimodality imaging technology of choice combining anatomical, functional, and molecular information into a single multiparametric imaging modality. Nonetheless, it is hard to make hypotheses on the main clinical applications of combined PET/MR at this stage (Beyer and Pichler 2009), where first prototype systems are being validated in clinical and research settings (Pichler et al. 2010). The potential areas of application of combined PET/MR imaging in brain imaging, for example, benefit greatly from the additional morphologic information provided by MRI. Combined amino acid PET and MR imaging is likely to enhance diagnostic sensitivity for gliomas and may allow closer correlation between tracer uptake and metabolic changes (e.g., choline peaks in MR spectroscopy) in neoplastic tissue (Bisdas et al. 2009). Likewise, arterial spin-labeling estimations of perfusion and diffusion changes occurring in low-grade gliomas may be studied in conjunction with different PET tracers to establish reliable disease markers. Boss and colleagues recently evaluated simultaneous PET/MRI for assessing intracranial tumors using [^{11}C]-methionine for glioma or [^{68}Ga]-DOTATOC for meningioma. They demonstrated image quality and quantitative data achieved from PET/MRI to be similar to that of PET/CT (Boss et al. 2010).

Given the availability of combined PET/MR systems, functional MRI and molecular PET image data can be acquired simultaneously, thus offering much improved spatial and temporal co-registration, which may become beneficial for image-guided radiotherapy (RT) treatment planning of various oncological diseases (Werner et al. 2011).

2 Methods

2.1 PET/MR Tomography

MR requires very high field homogeneity. Furthermore, the presence of PET detectors within the field could interfere with MR imaging. In contrast, PET detectors have to withstand not only a high static field level (up to 3 T for clinical MR) but also the rapidly changing field gradients required by the imaging process. PET/MR was destined to remain in the preclinical arena for another decade until, in 2006, the first simultaneous MR and PET images of the human brain were acquired (Schmand et al. 2007).

Existing hardware concepts for clinical PET/MR imaging essentially fall into three categories (Fig. 2): (a) separate gantries operated in different rooms, (b) gantries arranged in the direction of the main scanner axis with a patient-handling system mounted in between, and (c) fully integrated systems. The first design, presented in 2006 and also being the most challenging (Fig. 2c), is based on a PET detector ring designed as an insert that can be placed inside a Siemens 3-T Trio MR scanner (Siemens Healthcare). This prototype system (BrainPET) was anticipated for brain imaging only (Schlemmer et al. 2008). A similar design was replicated and made available for whole-body applications in late 2010 by the same company.

The coplanar PET/MR concept (Fig. 2b), first presented in 2010, is based on a tandem design of a whole-body time-of-flight (TOF) (Budinger 1983) PET system and a 3-T Philips Achieva MR system (Philips Healthcare, Cleveland, USA) with a rotating table platform in between. Through minor modifications of the PET detector system (e.g., orientation of the photomultiplier tube (PMT), minor shielding) the PET gantry can be operated in close proximity to the 3-T MRI system.

The third design was proposed by GE Healthcare in late 2010 and is available as prototype technology only. This design is based on a combination of a dual-modality PET/CT and a 3-T MR system that are operated side-by-side in separate rooms next to each other; patients are shuttled from one system to the other without getting off the bed. This approach substitutes the challenges of hardware integration for immense logistical challenges in timing access to the two systems while minimizing patient motion in between examinations. However, this approach has been argued as the most cost-effective compared with fully integrated PET/MR based on workflow aspects and machine utilization (Schulthess and Burger 2010).

In addition to the technical challenges of combining PET and MRI, which increase with the amount of PET and MR system integration, the necessary attenuation correction factors for the PET emission data must be derived from PET/MR measurements (Hofmann et al. 2009). While in PET/CT PET attenuation data can be derived from transforming available CT transmission images into maps of attenuation coefficients at 511 keV (Kinahan et al. 2003), no such transmission data are available in PET/MR. This is primarily due to the lack of physical space to host a

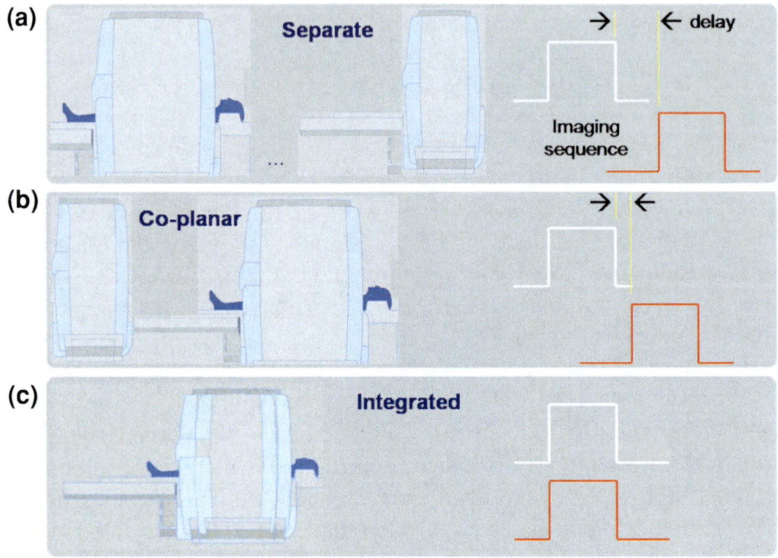

Fig. 2 System designs for combined PET/MR tomography: **a** PET (or PET/CT) and MR are situated in separate rooms and combined via a mobile, docking table platform, **b** PET and MR are within the same room with a joint table platform, and **c** integrated design where the PET component fits within the MRI gantry, and data are acquired simultaneously

transmission source. Therefore, PET/MR requires novel approaches to MR-based attenuation correction (MR-AC). While segmentation-based approaches have been proposed to classify tissues on MR images and to assign respective attenuation coefficients, which work well in brain imaging (Zaidi 2007); MR-AC in extracerebral applications is, however, much more challenging (Beyer et al. 2008).

2.2 Diagnosis and RT Treatment Planning of Meningioma

Meningiomas are mesodermal tumors originating from the arachnoid membrane and represent one of the most frequently diagnosed types of brain tumor. Incidence is about 25 per million people, peaking in patients between 40 and 70 years and increasing with age. Henze et al. (2001) demonstrated for the first time that PET imaging using [^{68}Ga]-DOTATOC [1,4,7,10-tetraazacyclododecane-1,4,7,10-tetraacetic acid (DOTA)-D-Phe1-Tyr3-octreotide (TOC)] is a promising diagnostic test for meningioma patients. This is due to the fact that meningiomas are known to express somatostatin receptor subtype 2 (SSTR2) for which, consequently, [^{68}Ga]-DOTATOC can be used as a biomarker to visualize the extension of meningiomas in PET or PET/CT studies. Henze et al. (2001) showed good correlation of tracer boundaries with anatomical delineation obtained from (co-registered) CT and MR image volumes, even for small meningiomas of 7 mm.

Treatment of meningiomas can be difficult due to their proximity to organs at risk (e.g., brainstem, cranial nerves). Although surgical resection is the main treatment approach, RT has been reported to be a highly effective treatment modality (Milker-Zabel et al. 2007). Until now, RT treatment planning has been based mainly on CT and contrast-enhanced MRI (Debus et al. 2001). However, in the case of quasiplanar growth, these imaging techniques have limitations concerning visualization of the exact tumor extension. Thus, PET or PET/CT is highly valuable as an additional imaging modality for more accurate target volume (TV) delineation (Milker-Zabel et al. 2006).

Intensity-modulated radiation therapy (IMRT) is an effective technique for treating meningiomas with high levels of conformality. A combination of CT, MR, and [^{68}Ga]-DOTATOC-PET imaging has been reported to improve TV delineation for IMRT treatment planning (Gehler et al. 2009; Thorwarth et al. 2011).

2.3 ^{68}Ga-DOTATOC PET/MR Protocol

Here we present three cases of patients with meningiomas undergoing [^{68}Ga]-DOTATOC PET/MR imaging. All patients had a clinical indication for a PET/CT study, which was performed prior to the PET/MR study.

The PET/CT examination was performed with a Biograph HiRez 16 unit (Siemens Healthcare, Knoxville, USA), which is equipped with $4 \times 4 \times 16$ mm^3 lutetium oxyorthosilicate (LSO) scintillation crystals in combination with a 16-slice CT. Patients were injected intravenously with an average activity of 150 MBq of [^{68}Ga]-DOTATOC. Static emission scans of two overlapping bed positions in the tumor region were acquired 40 min post injection (p.i.), with acquisition time of 4 min per bed position. PET images were reconstructed iteratively using a two-dimensional (2D) ordered-subset expectation-maximization (OSEM) algorithm with 4 iterations and 8 subsets. CT-based attenuation and scatter correction was performed. Reconstructed PET data had in-plane resolution of 6 mm and slice thickness of 5 mm.

PET/MR imaging commenced immediately after the completion of the PET/CT acquisition in a different part of the hospital. A prototype PET/MR system dedicated to brain imaging (BrainPET; Siemens Healthcare, Knoxville, USA) was used (Schmand et al. 2007). Briefly, a clinical 3-T MR system (Magnetom Trio; Siemens Healthcare, Erlangen, Germany) is equipped with an MR-compatible brain PET insert. The PET detector ring consists of $2.5 \times 2.5 \times 20$ mm^3 LSO scintillation crystals in combination with avalanche photodiodes (APD). The PET resolution is less than 3 mm in the center of the field of view. PET data acquisition started approximately 100 min p.i. List-mode data were acquired over a period of 30 min to compensate for the longer uptake time. PET reconstruction was performed using a 3D ordinary Poisson OSEM resolution-modeling algorithm with 6 iterations and 16 subsets, 3D scatter correction, and MRI-based attenuation correction (Hofmann et al. 2008).

MRI was performed using the birdcage transmit/receive coil, which is suitable for all routine clinical examinations. The MR sequences used for examinations of the brain with combined PET/MR are described in detail elsewhere (Boss et al. 2010). The combined PET/MR machine allows PET and MR acquisition of data not only in the same geometrical localization but also simultaneously.

2.4 Radiotherapy Treatment Planning

For all patients, IMRT treatment planning was performed using 6 MV photons from seven different beam angles. IMRT was planned with a dynamic delivery technique using a linear accelerator equipped with a multileaf collimator with leaf widths of 4 mm in the isocenter plane (Elekta Synergy S, Crawley, UK). For accurate patient positioning, a thermoplastic mask system was used in addition to onboard position verification with the cone-beam CT system.

First, IMRT TVs were delineated manually based on a combination of CT, [^{68}Ga]-DOTATOC PET, and separately acquired MR data (Gehler et al. 2009). A second set of contours was created using only combined PET/MR imaging data in addition to the planning CT required for RT dose calculation. IMRT treatment planning was performed using the PET/CT-based TVs as reference, which was then cross-evaluated for the PET/MR-based TVs to evaluate the dosimetric differences imposed by PET/MR-guided IMRT planning.

2.5 Clinical Examples

Case 1

A 73-year-old female presented with recurrence of an atypical meningioma (WHO II) in the right anterior central region 15 months after complete resection. Clinical findings before first resection were left-sided gait abnormality and disease progression on MR imaging. Postoperative imaging consisting of MRI and [^{68}Ga]-DOTATOC-PET/CT did not determine any residual tumor. Due to aggravation of the pre-existing gait abnormality 15 months after surgery, another set of MRI and [^{68}Ga]-DOTATOC-PET/CT examinations was performed, and recurrent disease was detected. This case was discussed in an interdisciplinary neurooncology tumor board, and radiation treatment was recommended.

First, TV delineation was performed separately on PET/CT and MR image volumes. Fusion of these two TVs resulted in a total gross target volume ($GTV_{PET/CT+MR}$) of 12.7 mL. In a second step, a corresponding $GTV_{PET/MR}$ was defined exclusively based on simultaneous PET/MR, which had size of 13.5 mL. Subsequently, both GTVs were expanded isotropically by 4 mm to create the respective planning target volumes (PTVs). Figure 3 shows the TVs defined on the basis of PET/CT and MR ($PTV_{PET/CT+MR}$ and $GTV_{PET/CT+MR}$) (Fig. 3b) and PET/MR ($PTV_{PET/MR}$ and $GTV_{PET/MR}$) (Fig. 3d) superimposed on the planning CT.

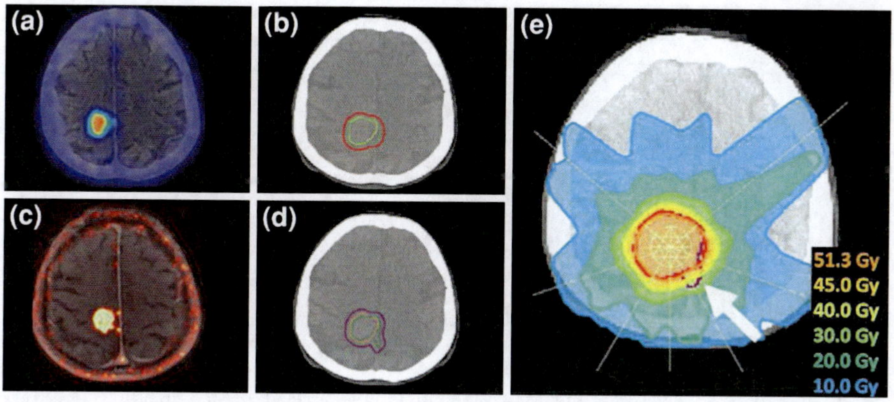

Fig. 3 Patient 1: 73-year-old female with meningioma WHO grade II following [^{68}Ga]-DOTATOC PET/CT and PET/MR: axial PET/CT (**a**) and PET/MR image (**c**), GTVs based on PET/CT (*yellow*) and additional MR (*green*) data in addition to the resulting PTV (*red*) (**b**), and after TV delineation based solely on hybrid PET/MR (PET: *green*, simultaneously acquired MR: *orange*, PTV: *purple*) (**d**). IMRT plan created for TVs based on PET/CT only (*red*) and cross-evaluated for TVs delineated on simultaneous PET/MR image data (*purple*) shown in (**d**). The *arrow* shows an infiltrated tumor region only visualized on hybrid PET/MR, which would have been significantly underdosed after TV delineated based solely on combined PET/CT

PET/CT- and PET/MR-based TV delineation resulted in PTVs of 28.0 and 31.5 mL, respectively.

When using PET/MR for TV delineation, the TV was slightly enlarged compared with that derived from PET/CT images. Tumor parts infiltrating into critical regions were visible more clearly on PET/MR, thanks to the higher signal-to-noise ratio (SNR) on the simultaneously acquired PET/MR data. As a consequence, the IMRT plan designed on the basis of PET/CT imaging would have significantly underdosed these specific regions of the tumor only visible on the hybrid PET/MR data (Fig. 3d, arrow) (Thorwarth et al. 2011).

Case 2

A 72-year-old female patient presented 17 years ago with dizziness and focal signs of a parasagittal cortex syndrome including sensory disturbance of the right side and headache. After complete resection of a left-sided parasagittal meningioma (WHO I) the symptoms resolved. In 2010, increasing paraesthesia of the right hand and right side of face were observed. Two left-sided subdural recurrences were detected by CT and MRI, extending from frontal to parietal parts of trepanation. Within 3 months, one of the two manifestations progressed from 23×18 to 29×25 mm. The other lesion did not change with 19×15 mm. Hybrid [^{68}Ga]-DOTATOC-PET/CT and PET/MR confirmed both manifestations. Radiation treatment options were recommended, in particular in view of the proximity of the lesion to the sinus sagittalis superior.

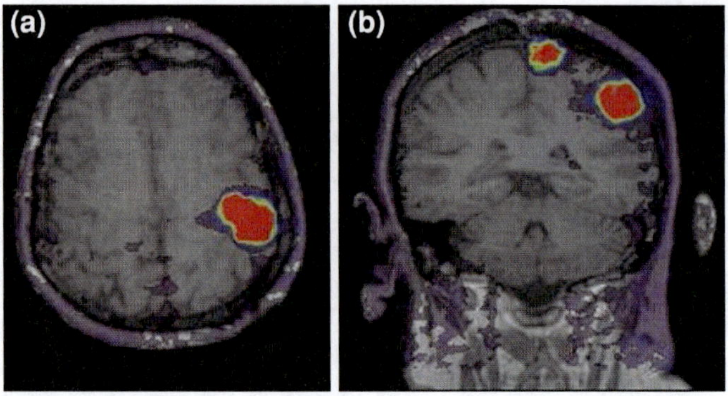

Fig. 4 Patient 2: 72-year-old female with meningioma WHO I treated in 1993. Transverse (**a**) and coronal (**b**) hybrid [^{68}Ga]-DOTATOC PET/MR images showing tumor recurrence in frontal-parietal region with hybrid PET/MR imaging performed in 2010

PET/CT-based TV delineation yielded a GTV of 18.0 mL, whereas the PET/MR-based TV was slightly larger (19.0 mL). Nevertheless, both GTVs were located within the same geographical area and did not show any significant difference. IMRT treatment planning did not differ significantly (Fig. 4).

Case 3

A 69-year-old female treated with surgery for a 46 × 47 mm^2 atypical meningioma (WHO II) in the right frontal region. The initial signs were weakness of the left hand and sensory disturbance of the seventh cranial nerve. One year later, a 9 × 14 × 13 mm^3-sized recurrence was diagnosed on MRI in the right frontal region. On additional MRI 3 months later, a smaller lesion of 8 mm diameter was detected close to the main tumor mass in the right frontal area, which had progressed in size to 16 × 25 × 14 mm^3 (Fig. 6a, b). An additional satellite lesion close to the sinus frontalis showed only very moderate tracer uptake on the [^{68}Ga]-DOTATOC PET/CT 60 min p.i. (Fig. 5), but was clearly visible on the combined [^{68}Ga]-DOTATOC PET/MR (Fig. 6c, d). Taking prior complications after the first surgery into account (bony infection followed by repeated surgery with duraplasty), the interdisciplinary recommendation for treatment of recurrence was RT.

At the time, the hybrid PET/MR data originating from this system could not be used for diagnostic and therapeutic decisions. Therefore, this patient was treated based on PET/CT information only. However, due to the very moderate tracer uptake in the small frontal satellite lesion, which was not taken into account during PET/CT-based target contouring, PET/MR-based TVs were significantly larger. In contrast, delayed PET/MR images reveal higher resolution (Fig. 6). The IMRT treatment plan for this patient, taking into account the frontal satellite lesion detected on PET/MR only, is shown in Fig. 7.

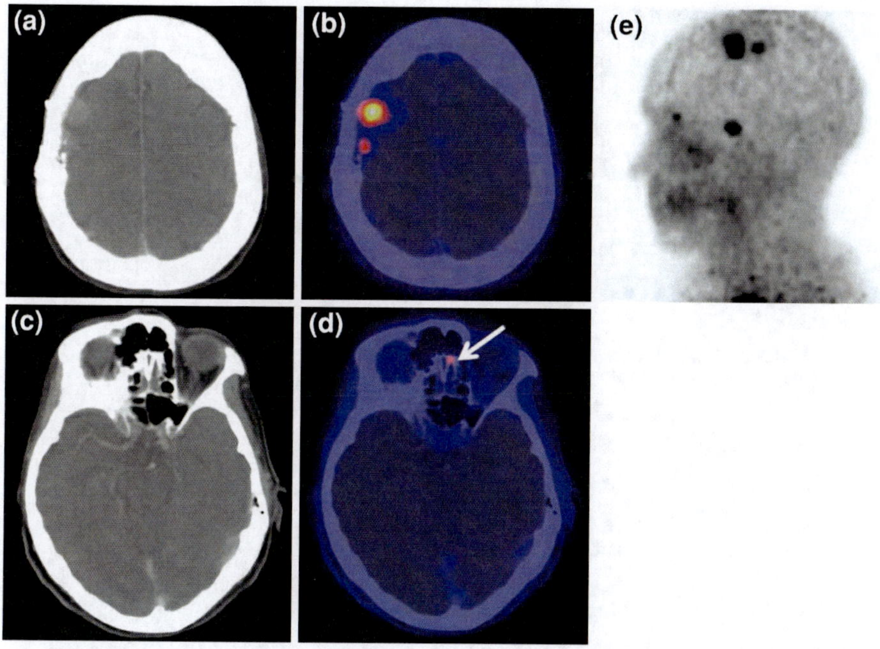

Fig. 5 [^{68}Ga]-DOTATOC PET/CT image data of patient 3. Axial CT (**a**) and PET/CT (**b**) image show the main tumor mass. Offset axial CT (**c**) and PET/CT (**d**) show the small satellite lesion in the frontal region. Comparatively low tracer retention can be seen in this lesion (*arrow*). PET maximum-intensity projection is shown in (**e**)

3 Discussion

The three cases presented here illustrate the practical application of [^{68}Ga]-DOTATOC PET/MR in a clinical setting. In two cases (patients 1 and 3) the tumor identified on PET/MR was not completely covered with the prescribed radiation dose derived from prior PET/CT imaging. As a consequence, PET/MR imaging with improved PET resolution might be highly beneficial for improved TV delineation for RT treatment of meningioma, although further studies with histology verification or long-time outcome are required.

Somatostatin receptor (SSTR) imaging was shown to provide improved characterization of tumors near the skull base in case of unclear diagnosis and anatomical information on MR imaging data. Also for patients being considered for stereotactic RT, [^{68}Ga]-DOTATOC PET imaging is beneficial to differentiate between meningiomas/neurinomas and optical nerve gliomas (Henze et al. 2001). Furthermore, SSTR imaging using [^{68}Ga]-DOTATOC results in extremely high tumor-to-blood ratios (TBR) even in very small regions (Henze et al. 2005). On the one hand such high TBRs yield high diagnostic quality, but on the other

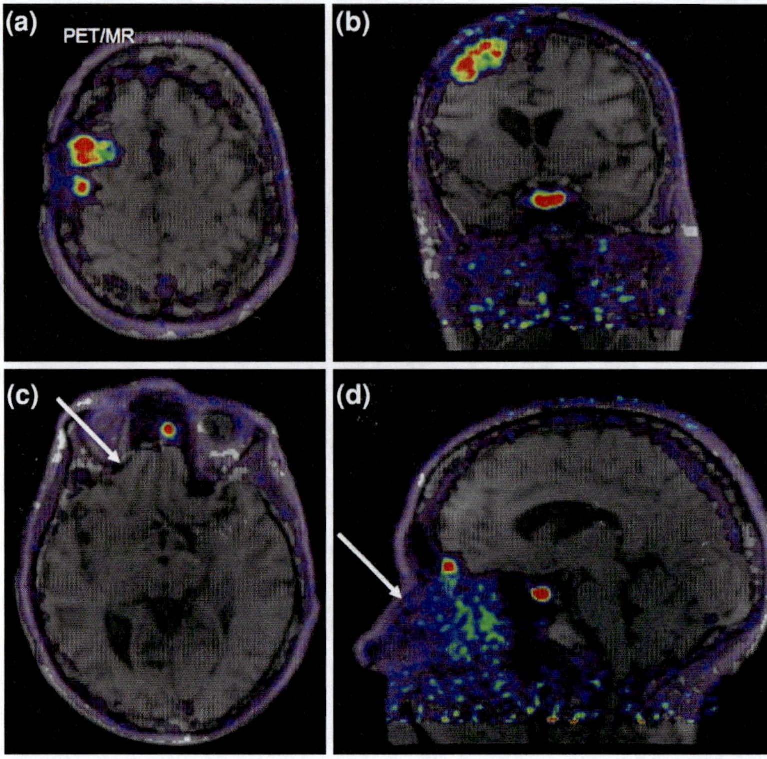

Fig. 6 Patient 3: 69-year-old female with meningioma WHO II in right frontal region. In addition to the two lesions detected on PET/CT (Fig. 5), PET/MR reveals third satellite lesion in the frontal sinus: transverse (**a**) and coronal (**b**) view of the main tumor mass, transverse (**c**) and sagittal (**d**) view of a small satellite lesion in the dorsal region of the frontal sinus (*arrow*)

hand they require anatomical correlates and—potentially—simultaneous PET/MR imaging for improved target localization.

Alternatively, a number of different PET tracers can be used to accurately visualize meningiomas for improved TV definition, such as [^{18}F]-fluorodeoxyglucose ([^{18}F]-FDG (Lee et al. 2009), *O*-(2-[^{18}F]-fluoroethyl)-L-tyrosine ([^{18}F]-FET) (Rutten et al. 2007), [^{11}C]-acetate (Liu et al. 2010), [^{11}C]-choline (Fallanca et al. 2009), or [^{11}C]-methionine ([^{11}C]-MET) (Astner et al. 2008; Grosu et al. 2006). More specifically, Lee et al. demonstrate that FDG uptake in meningiomas was predictive of tumor recurrence (Lee et al. 2009). Rutten et al. (2007) showed that meningiomas are visualized clearly after RT using [^{18}F]-FET but report discrepancies between PET- and MR-based TV. Grosu et al. (2006) showed that [11C]-MET helps to reduce interobserver variability in TV delineation of meningiomas.

Improved TV definition using [^{68}Ga]-DOTATOC PET/CT was demonstrated by several studies, but nevertheless PET information as obtained from PET/CT imaging was reported to be of limited value in certain tumor regions such as the

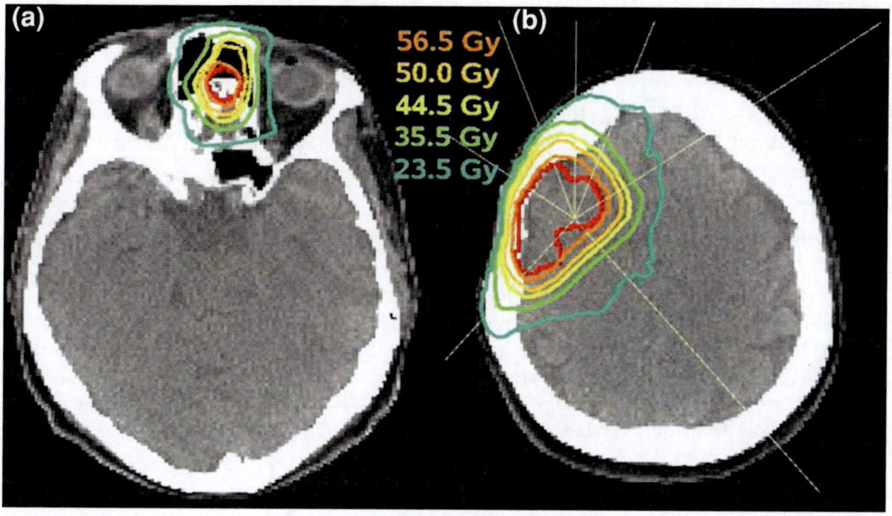

Fig. 7 Patient 3: 69-year-old female with meningioma WHO II in right frontal region. IMRT plan taking into account the small tumor satellite in the frontal region which had been visualized on [^{68}Ga]-DOTATOC PET/MR only (**a**). Dose distribution in the main tumor region (**b**), PTV is outlined in *red*. Seven beam angles for IMRT delivery are schematically represented by *yellow lines*

pituitary gland and lesions next to the cavernous sinus (Milker-Zabel et al. 2006; Hyun et al. 2011). Here, PET/MR might be advantageous, as simultaneously acquired functional MR data may help to further differentiate tumor diagnosis based on PET.

Another advantage for PET/MR is intrinsic co-registration that dismisses retro-registration, for which more background information would be required. Therefore, [^{68}Ga]-DOTATOC can be used with PET/MR as well as MET and FET, which are reported to contain more background information useful for mutual information (MI)-based registration, which is no longer required in PET/MR (Astner et al. 2008).

Co-registered MR information can be used to define microscopic tumor growth (Nyuyki et al. 2010) that is known to be a problem for PET/CT-guided RT in meningioma (Gehler et al. 2009). Here, accurate image matching is absolutely necessary to accurately locate infiltrative regions of the tumor by means of high-precision RT.

4 Conclusion

Simultaneous [^{68}Ga]-DOTATOC-PET/MR imaging is clinically feasible in brain applications. It may be beneficial for more accurate TV delineation of meningioma, thus benefiting IMRT treatment planning and other highly conformal RT techniques. Simultaneous brain PET/MR imaging may allow more detailed visualization and functional–anatomical co-registration of meningiomas, especially in small infiltrated regions that may not be detected with larger PET detector systems. In addition, combined PET/MR imaging helps expedite clinical workflow.

In general, within the next years, we may expect to see PET/MR gaining momentum and find a place in clinical routine. This advance can be fostered by the adoption of highly specific PET tracers that contain less anatomical background information on PET only, for example. Hybrid imaging by means of PET/CT and PET/MR will be mandatory when using [^{68}Ga]-labeled tracers.

Acknowledgments NS, SW, GH, MR, AK, BP for help with patient management, data acquisition, image analysis and data interpretation. DT is supported by the European Social Fund and the Ministry of Science, Research, and the Arts Baden-Württemberg. This work was supported by the Imaging Science Institute (ISI) Tübingen. Mirada Imaging, UK (w3.mirada-medical.com): Software fusion and image display. *Duality-of-Interest* T.B. is president and founder of Switzerland-based cmi-experts GmbH. The Imaging Science Institute of Tübingen is supported by Siemens Healthcare.

References

Astner ST, Dobrei-Ciuchendea M, Essler M et al (2008) Effect of 11C-methionine-positron emission tomography on gross tumor volume delineation in stereotactic radiotherapy of skull base meningiomas. Int J Radiat Oncol Biol Phys 72(4):1161–1167

Beyer T, Pichler B (2009) A decade of combined imaging: from a PET attached to a CT to a PET inside an MR. Eur J Nucl Med Mol Imaging 36(Suppl 1):S1–S2

Beyer T, Weigert M, Quick HH et al (2008) MR-based attenuation correction for torso-PET/MR imaging: pitfalls in mapping MR to CT data. Eur J Nucl Med Mol Imaging 35(6):1142–1146

Beyer T, Freudenberg LS, Townsend DW et al (2011) The future of hybrid imaging—part 3: combined PET/MR and small animal imaging, other imaging combinations and additional concerns. Insights Imaging 2(3):235–246

Bisdas S, Nägele T, Schlemmer HP et al (2009) Switching on the lights for real-time multimodality tumor neuroimaging: the integrated positron-emission tomography/MR imaging system. AJNR Am J Neuroradiol 31(4):610–614

Boss A, Bisdas S, Kolb A et al (2010) Hybrid PET/MRI of intracranial masses: initial experiences and comparison to PET/CT. J Nucl Med 51(8):1198–1205

Brix G, Lechel U, Glatting G et al (2005) Radiation exposure of patients undergoing whole-body dual-modality FDG-PET/CT examinations. J Nucl Med 46(4):608–613

Budinger T (1983) Time-of-flight positron emission tomography: status relative to conventional PET. J Nucl Med 24(1):73–78

Czernin J, Allen-Auerbach M, Schelbert HR (2007) Improvements in cancer staging with PET/CT: literature-based evidence as of September 2006. J Nucl Med 48(Suppl 1):78S–88S

Debus J, Wuendrich M, Pirzkall A et al (2001) High efficacy of fractionated stereotactic radiotherapy of large base-of-skull meningiomas: long-term result. J Clin Oncol 19(15):3547–3553

Fallanca F, Giovacchini G, Picchio M et al (2009) Incidental detection by [11C]choline PET/CT of meningiomas in prostate cancer patients. Q J Nucl Med Mol Imaging 53(4):417–421

Gehler B, Paulsen F, Öksüz MÖ et al (2009) [68Ga]-DOTATOC-PET/CT for meningioma IMRT treatment planning. Radiat Oncol 4:56

Grosu AL, Weber WA, Astner ST et al (2006) 11C-methionine PET improves the target volume delineation of meningiomas treated with stereotactic fractionated radiotherapy. Int J Radiat Oncol Biol Phys 66(2):339–344

Henze M, Schuhmacher J, Hipp P et al (2001) PET imaging of somatostatin receptors using [68GA]DOTA-D-Phe1-Tyr3-octreotide: first results in patients with meningiomas. J Nucl Med 42(7):1053–1056
Henze M, Dimitrakopoulou-Strauss A, Milker-Zabel S et al (2005) Characterization of 68Ga-DOTA-D-Phe1-Tyr3-octreotide kinetics in patients with meningiomas. J Nucl Med 46(5): 763–769
Hofmann M, Steinke F, Scheel V et al (2008) MRI-based attenuation correction for PET/MRI: a novel approach combining pattern recognition and atlas registration. J Nucl Med 49(11): 1875–1883
Hofmann M, Pichler B, Schölkopf B et al (2009) Towards quantitative PET/MRI: a review of MR-based attenuation correction techniques. Eur J Nucl Med Mol Imaging 36(Suppl 1): S93–S103
Hyun SH, Choi JY, Lee KH et al (2011) Incidental focal 18F-FDG uptake in the pituitary gland: clinical significance and differential diagnostic criteria. J Nucl Med 52(4):547–550
Kinahan PE, Hasegawa BH, Beyer T (2003) X-ray-based attenuation correction for positron emission tomography/computed tomography scanners. Semin Nucl Med 33(3):166–179
Lee JW, Kang KW, Park SH et al (2009) 18F-FDG PET in the assessment of tumor grade and prediction of tumor recurrence in intracranial meningioma. Eur J Nucl Med Mol Imaging 36(10):1574–1582
Liu RS, Chang CP, Guo WY et al (2010) 1–11C-acetate versus 18F-FDG PET in detection of meningioma and monitoring the effect of gamma-knife radiosurgery. J Nucl Med 51(6): 883–891
Milker-Zabel S, Zabel-du Bois A, Henze M et al (2006) Improved target volume definition for fractionated stereotactic radiotherapy in patients with intracranial meningiomas by correlation of CT, MRI, and [68Ga]-DOTATOC-PET. Int J Radiat Oncol Biol Phys 65(1):222–227
Milker-Zabel S, Zabel-du Bois A, Huber P et al (2007) Intensity-modulated radiotherapy for complex-shaped meningioma of the skull base: long-term experience of a single institution. Int J Radiat Oncol Biol Phys 68(3):858–863
Nestle U, Weber W, Hentschel M, Grosu AL (2009) Biological imaging in radiation therapy: role of positron emission tomography. Phys Med Biol 54(1):R1–R25
Nyuyki F, Plotkin M, Graf R et al (2010) Potential impact of (68)Ga-DOTATOC PET/CT on stereotactic radiotherapy planning of meningiomas. Eur J Nucl Med Mol Imaging 37(2): 310–318
Pichler B, Kolb A, Nägele T et al (2010) PET/MRI: paving the way for the next generation of clinical multimodality imaging applications. J Nucl Med 51(3):333–336
Rutten I, Cabay JE, Withofs N et al (2007) PET/CT of skull base meningiomas using 2-18F-fluoro-L-tyrosine: initial report. J Nucl Med 48(5):720–725
Schlemmer HP, Pichler BJ, Schmand M et al (2008) Simultaneous MR/PET imaging of the human brain: feasibility study. Radiology 248(3):1028–1035
Schmand M, Burbar Z, Corbeil JL et al (2007) BrainPET: first human tomograph for simultaneous (functional) PET and MR imaging. J Nucl Med 48(6):45P
Schulthess G, Burger C (2010) Integrating imaging modalities: what makes sense from a workflow perspective? Eur J Nucl Med Mol Imaging 37(5):980–990
Thorwarth D, Henke G, Müller AC et al (2011) Simultaneous [^{68}Ga]DOTATOC PET/MR for IMRT treatment planning of meningeoma: first experience. Int J Radiat Oncol Biol Phys 81(1):277–283
Townsend DW (2008) Multimodality imaging of structure and function. Phys Med Biol 53(4): R1–R39
Warburg O (1956) On the origin of cancer cells. Science 123:306–314
Werner MK, Schwenzer NF, Thorwarth D (2011) Hybrid MR/PET imaging: principles, problems and potential for radiotherapy. Der Nuklearmediziner 34:108–113
Zaidi H (2007) Is MR-guided attenuation correction a viable option for dual-modality PET/MR imaging? Radiology 244(3):639–642

Part IV
Targeted Radiotherapy (Peptide Receptor Radionuclide Therapy) and Dosimetry

A Rare Case of a Large Spinal Meningioma with Mediastinal Extension and Malignant Behavior Classified Histologically as Benign

S. Dahdal, R. H. Andres, E. Hewer, J. C. Reubi, B. Klaeser, A. Raabe, N. Cihoric, R. Schmid, K. Tänzler, T. Krause, D. M. Aebersold and M. Schmuecking

S. Dahdal · K. Tänzler
Department of Internal Medicine, Inselspital, Bern University Hospital, and University of Bern, Bern, Switzerland

R. H. Andres · A. Raabe
Department of Neurosurgery, Inselspital, Bern University Hospital and University of Bern, Bern, Switzerland

E. Hewer · J. C. Reubi
Department of Pathology, Inselspital, Bern University Hospital and University of Bern, Bern, Switzerland

B. Klaeser · T. Krause
Department of Nuclear Medicine, Inselspital, Bern University Hospital, and University of Bern, Bern, Switzerland

N. Cihoric · D. M. Aebersold · M. Schmuecking (✉)
Department of Radiation Oncology, Inselspital, Bern University Hospital, and University of Bern, Freiburger Street 18, 3010 Bern, Switzerland
e-mail: michael.schmuecking@insel.ch

R. Schmid
Department of Thoracic Surgery, Inselspital, Bern University Hospital, and University of Bern, Freiburger Street 18, 3010 Bern, Switzerland

R. P. Baum and F. Rösch (eds.), *Theranostics, Gallium-68, and Other Radionuclides*, Recent Results in Cancer Research 194, DOI: 10.1007/978-3-642-27994-2_24,

Abstract

Aim: To report a rare case of a spinal WHO grade I meningioma extending through intervertebral foramina C7 to D4 with an extensive mediastinal mass and infiltration of the vertebrae, and to discuss the malignant behavior of a tumor classified as benign. *Methods* (*Clinical Presentation, Histology, and Imaging*): A 54-year-old man suffered from increasing lower back pain with gait difficulties, weakness and numbness of the lower extremities, as well as urge incontinence. CT scan of the thorax and MRI scan of the spine revealed a large prevertebral tumor, which extended to the spinal canal and caused compression of the spinal cord at the levels of C7 to D4 leading to myelopathy with hyperintense signal alteration on T2-weighted MRI images. The signal constellation (T1 with and without contrast, T2, TIR) was highly suspicious for infiltration of vertebrae C7 to D5. Somatostatin receptor SPECT/CT with ^{111}In-DTPA-D-Phe-1-octreotide detected a somatostatin receptor-positive mediastinal tumor with infiltration of multiple vertebrae, dura, and intervertebral foramina C7–D4, partially with Krenning score >2. Percutaneous biopsies of the mediastinal mass led to histopathological findings of WHO grade I meningioma of meningothelial subtype. *Results* (*Therapy*): C7 to D4 laminoplasty was performed, and the intraspinal, extradural part of the tumor was microsurgically removed. Postoperative stereotactic radiation therapy was done using the volumetric modulated arc therapy (VMAT) technique (RapidArc). No PRRNT with ^{90}Y-DOTA-TOC was done. *Conclusions*: Due to the rare incidence and complex presentation of this disease not amenable to complete surgical resection, an individualized treatment approach should be worked out interdisciplinarily. The treatment approach should be based not only on histology but also on clinical and imaging findings. Close clinical and radiological follow-up may be mandatory even for benign tumors.

Contents

1 Case Presentation

1.1 Clinical Findings

A 54-year-old man suffered from increasing lower back pain for 5 months. Due to increasing gait difficulties, the patient had resorted to a walking frame, with which he could move well for a while. The gait difficulties increased steadily; additionally, weakness and numbness of lower extremities occurred, as well as urge incontinence. Finally, the patient was admitted to our hospital by the family doctor. At admission, the patient presented with right-oriented paraparesis and loss of sensation up to dermatome D5. Because of overflow incontinence, a suprapubic urine catheter (Cystofix) was inserted. The neurological deficits were rapidly progressive, so that the patient was bedridden within 2 weeks. After primary treatment the patient was transferred to a neurological rehabilitation unit and showed good clinical recovery with gradual recovery from paraparesis. Eight months after surgery followed by radiation therapy, he was independently living at home, ambulating with a walker, and had normal bowel function. He still relied on a suprapubic urine catheter. Clinical examination revealed marked recovery of sensory as well as motor function (M4–5) in the lower extremity, however prominent gait ataxia persisted.

1.2 Histology and Genetic Analyses

Percutaneous biopsies of the mediastinal mass led to histopathological findings of WHO grade I meningioma of meningothelial subtype. Immunohistochemically, the tumor was positive for epithelial membrane antigen (EMA) and vimentin, infrequently positive for S-100, and negative for glial fibrillary acidic protein (GFAP), pancytokeratin, synaptophysin, chromogranin A, and serotonin, excluding paraganglioma and neuroendocrine tumor. The proliferation rate (MIB-1) was 3–5%. The tumor presented intense expression of somatostatin receptor (SSTR) type 2A (Figs. 1, 2). Meningiomas are the next most common tumor type after vestibular schwannoma in neurofibromatosis type 2. Due to the presence of multiple cranial meningiomas, genetic examination was performed, which could exclude neurofibromatosis type 2 in our patient.

1.3 Pretherapeutic Imaging

CT scan of the thorax and MRI scan of the spine revealed a large prevertebral tumor, which extended to the spinal canal. This tumor caused compression of the spinal cord at levels C7 to D4, leading to myelopathy with hyperintense signal alteration on T2-weighted MRI images (Figs. 3, 4, 5). CT scan of the skull revealed, in addition to the spinal meningioma, several cranial meningiomas with typical contrast enhancement, partially with calcification. To verify the histological SSTR expression and evaluate the possibility of peptide receptor radionuclide therapy (PRRNT) with ^{90}Y-DOTA-TOC, somatostatin receptor SPECT/CT was done (Fig. 6). The somatostatin receptor SPECT/CT with ^{111}In-DTPA-D-Phe-1-octreotide detected a somatostatin receptor-positive mediastinal tumor with infiltration of multiple vertebrae, dura, and intervertebral foramina C7–D4, partially with Krenning score >2 (1 = lower than liver uptake; 2 = equivalent to liver uptake; 3 = higher than liver uptake). No other SSTR-positive lesions were visible; especially, the intracranial lesions showed no SSTR expression.

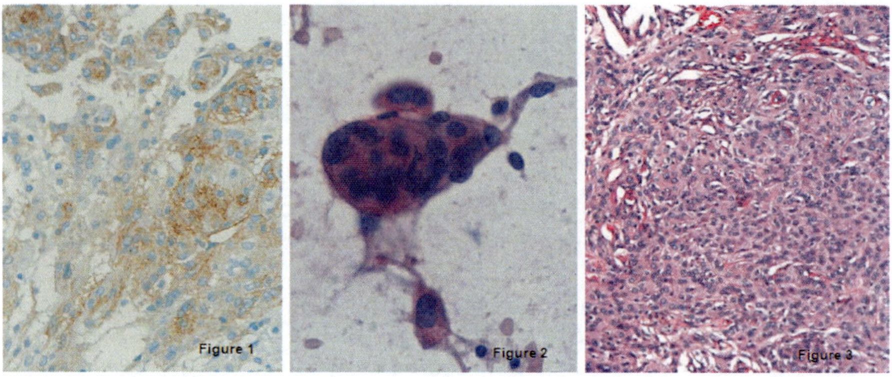

Fig. 1 CT-guided core-needle biopsy of the mediastinal tumor showed a moderately differentiated cellular neoplasm with syncytial growth pattern lacking mitotic activity. Immunohistochemically the tumor was positive for EMA (Fig. 1) while lacking immunoreactivity for cytokeratin, S100, chromogranin A, or synaptophysin. Intraoperative smear preparation of the spinal part of the tumor showed neoplastic cells that were partially arranged in whorls and displayed indistinct cell borders and monotonous round to oval nuclei with finely granular chromation and occasional intranuclear pseudoinclusions (Fig. 2). On hematoxylin-eosin-stained paraffin sections, occasional mitotic figures and rare foci of necrosis were identified (Fig. 3). Both histologic tumor type and immunohistochemical profile corresponded to that of the mediastinal tumor. Proliferation index as assessed by immunohistochemistry for MIB-1 (Ki67) reached up to 3–5%. Based upon these findings, a diagnosis of meningotheliomatous meningioma was issued. It was commented that, although the tumor fell short of formal criteria of atypical meningioma (WHO grade I), the borderline increased mitotic and proliferative activity as well as the focal presence of necrosis possibly indicated increased risk of progression or recurrence, and close follow-up was suggested

1.4 Therapy

C7 to D4 laminoplasty was performed, and the intraspinal, extradural part of the well-vascularized tumor was microsurgically removed using a diode-pumped solid-state (DPSS) laser system (RevoLix). Small amounts of tumor located ventral to the dural sac and in the neural foramina were not amenable to surgical resection. Intraoperative ultrasound demonstrated no residual compression of the spinal cord. Combined motor evoked potential (MEP) and somatosensory evoked potential (SEP) neuromonitoring during spine surgery detected no significant intraoperative MEP/SEP changes, and no new postoperative neurological deficits were noted. Due to secondary bleeding with compression of the myelon and worsening of the neurological deficits, reoperation to evacuate hematoma had to be done in an emergency situation. No other postoperative complications occurred (Figs. 7, 8, 9).

Postoperative fractionated stereotactic radiation therapy using the volumetric modulated arc therapy (VMAT) technique (RapidArc) was started to prevent further paraparesis by tumor progression. 6D image guidance was done with the ExacTrac X-ray system. The residual intraspinal and intraforaminal parts of the

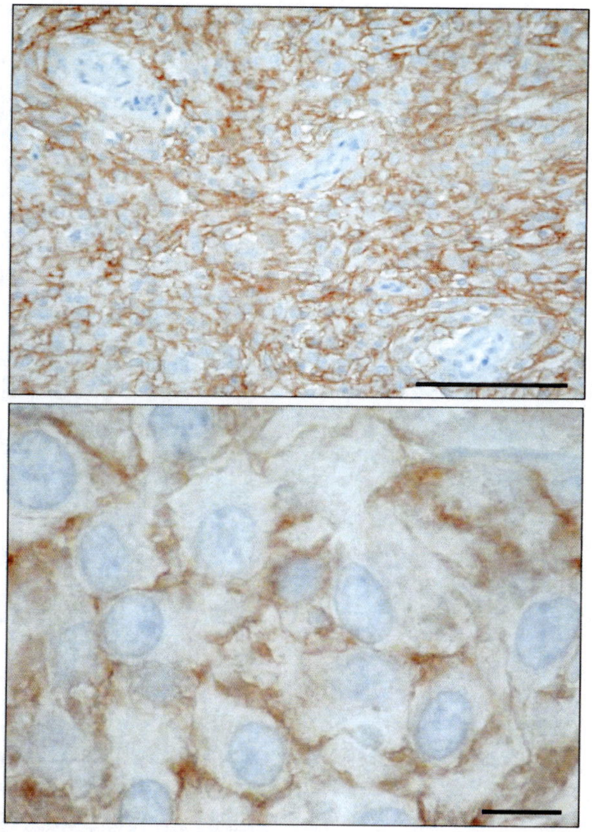

Fig. 2 SSTR type 2 immunohistochemical staining showing strong positivity, preferably membranous, in the majority of tumor cells. Bars = 0.1 mm (*above*) and 0.01 mm (*below*)

tumor received up to 51 Gy, and the mediastinal mass up to 55 Gy. The spinal cord (organ at risk) received less than 48 Gy. For the lung (organ at risk), V20 Gy was 25% and the mean lung dose was 18.6 Gy. (Figs. 10, 11, 12, 13).

2 Discussion

Primary tumors of the spinal cord are uncommon; only about 5% are primary intramedullary tumors or arise from the spinal meninges. The most common tumor types are meningioma, ependymoma, and schwannoma (CBTRUS 2000; Mawrin and Perry 2010; Perry et al. 1999; Nakasu et al. 2009; Lee et al. 2010; Engelhard et al. 2010). Our case is even more exceptional because the meningioma grew out of the spinal canal through the intervertebral foramina and so presented with a manifestation in the spinal canal and in the posterior mediastinum as well. Only a few cases similar to ours have been reported (Buchfelder et al. 2001; Barbanera et al. 2007; Incarbone et al. 2008). Most of the authors of these case reports

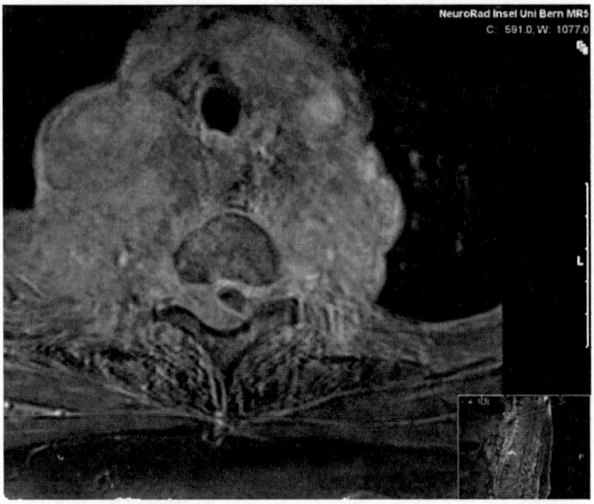

Fig. 3 MRI of the spine: large intraspinal tumor, which extended to the mediastinum. MRI: T1 GRE (FLASH) with contrast

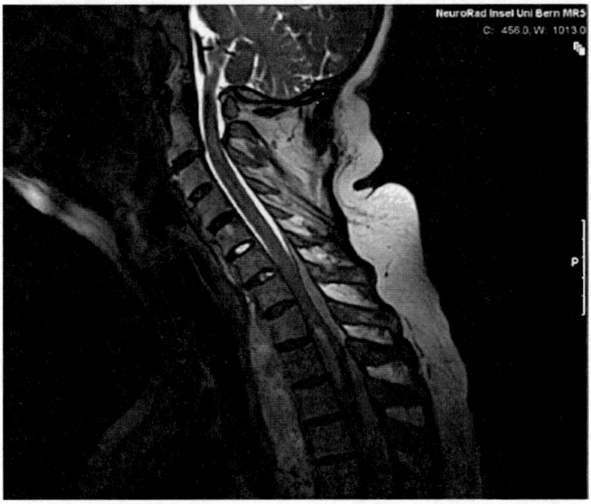

Fig. 4 MRI of the spine: large intraspinal tumor, which extended to the mediastinum. MRI: T2* GRE (FLASH)

recommend surgical therapy, sometimes with a two-stage approach (Mimoto et al. 1991; Yoon et al. 2007; Goldsmith et al. 1994; Jenkinson et al. 2006; Gambardella et al. 2003).

Meningiomas are generally slowly growing and produce neurological signs and symptoms by compression on adjacent structures. The classic and common variant is the meningothelial meningioma. It is known that the clinical course is often difficult to predict; even histopathologically benign meningiomas (WHO grade I) can recur despite seemingly complete surgical resection. The major clinical factors in recurrence are extent of resection and the grading. However, at least for WHO grade I cranial meningioma, no significant influence of extent of resection (Simpson grade I-IV) on tumor recurrence has been found (Sughrue et al. 2010).

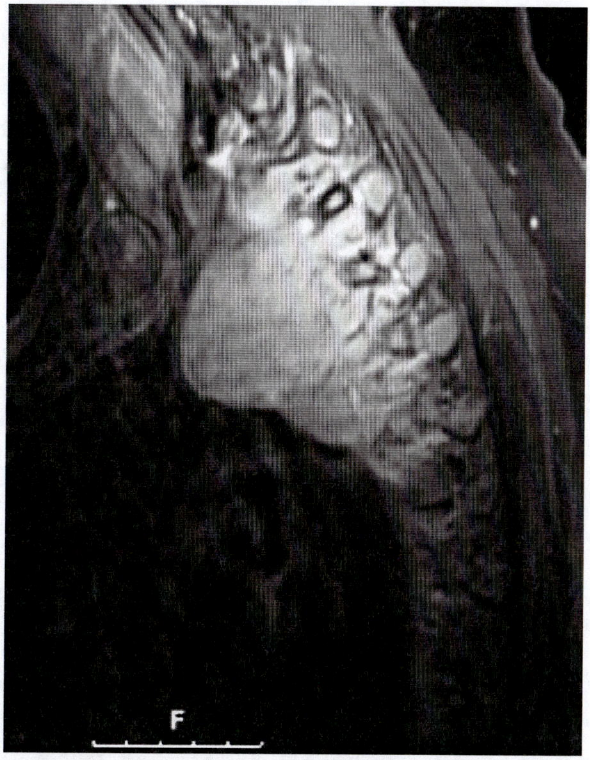

Fig. 5 MRI of the spine: large intraspinal tumor, which extended to the mediastinum. MRI: T1 TSE-fs with contrast

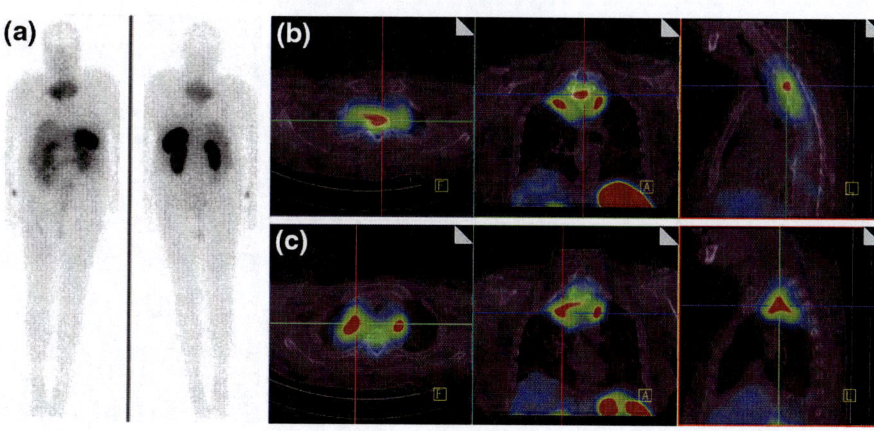

Fig. 6 Somatostatin receptor SPECT/CT and whole-body scan with ^{111}In-DTPA-D-Phe-1-octreotide: somatostatin receptor-positive mediastinal tumor with infiltration of multiple vertebrae, dura, and intervertebral foramina C7–D4, partially with Krenning score >2

Figs. 7–9 C7 to D4 laminoplasty was performed, and the intraspinal, extradural part of the well-vascularized tumor was microsurgically removed using a diode-pumped solid-state (DPSS) laser system

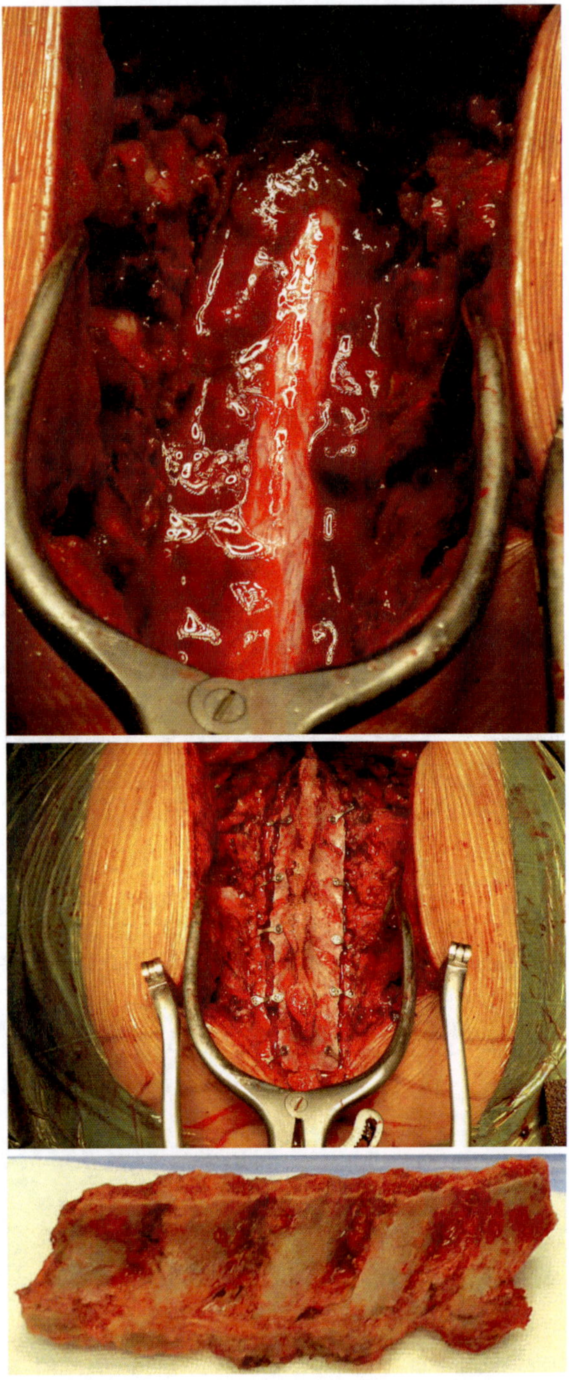

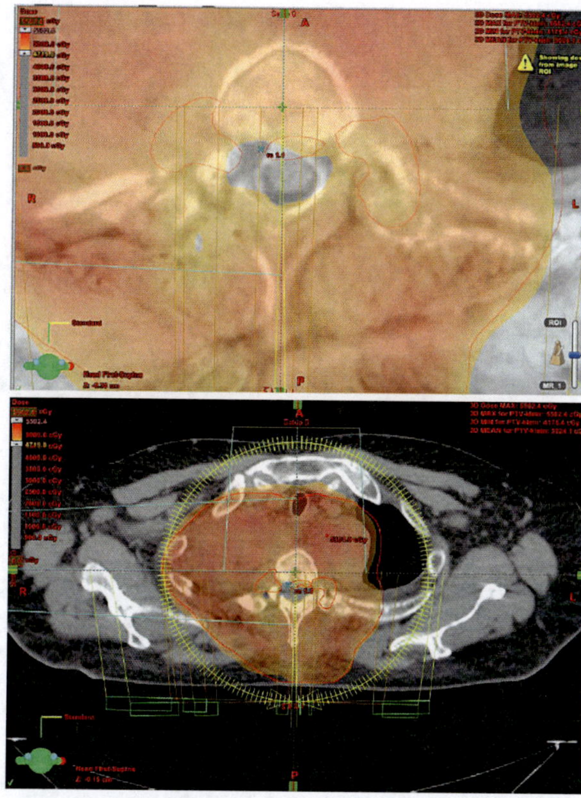

Figs. 10–11 Outer *red* line: planning target volume receiving up to 55 Gy; inner *red* lines: SSTR-positive intraspinal lesions with Krenning score >2, receiving up to 51 Gy; the myelon received less than 48 Gy, possible with VMAT technique

Atypical (WHO grade II) and anaplastic meningioma (WHO grade III) have a higher recurrence rate than benign meningioma. Levy et al. (1982) holds that the presence of an extradural component in spinal meningiomas is associated with more aggressive behavior and higher recurrence rate. Solero et al. (1989), analyzing a series of 174 patients operated on for spinal meningiomas, drew the conclusion that extradural component is not associated with higher incidence of recurrence. None of the aspects used in the WHO grading to define malignancy in meningiomas (hypercellularity, loss of architecture, nuclear pleomorphism, high mitotic index, focal necrosis, and brain invasion) were present in our reported case. However, MR imaging and somatostatin receptor imaging showed infiltration of multiple vertebrae, a criterion for malignancy and aggressiveness.

Somatostatin receptors are expressed in neuroendocrine tumors; so far, six subtypes have been identified (SSTR types 1, 2A, 2B, 3, 4, and 5). Meningiomas express preferential SSTR2 (Prasad et al. 2007). Expression of somatostatin receptors is an indicator for well-differentiated tumors, while undifferentiated tumors may not express somatostatin receptors (Reubi 2004; Reubi et al. 2000; Kaemmerer et al. 2011; Rufini et al. 2006; Baum et al. 2004a, b; Kwekkeboom et al. 2000; Imhof et al. 2011; Menda et al. 2010; Forrer et al. 2006). In our case,

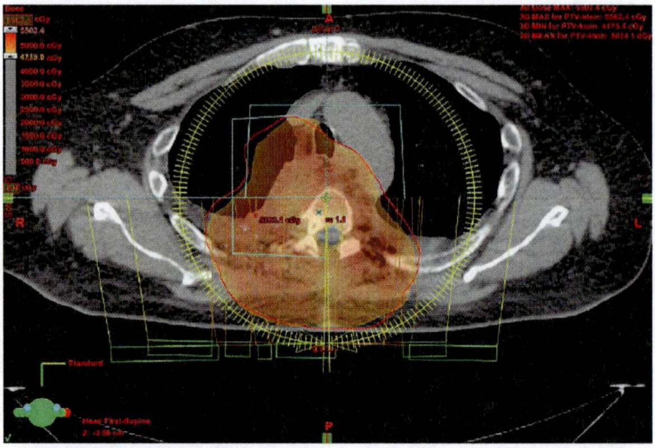

Fig. 12 *Red* line: planning target volume receiving up to 55 Gy; the myelon received less than 48 Gy, possible with VMAT technique

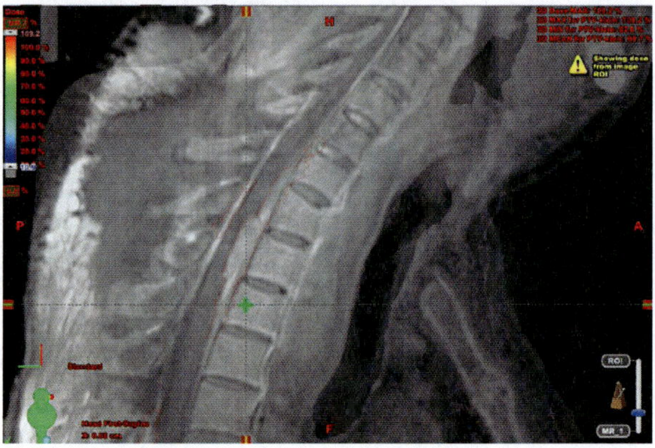

Fig. 13 Image fusion of sagittal MRI with sagittal CT for radiation treatment planning (*red* line: intraspinal gross tumor volume with intense somatostatin receptor expression, Krenning score >2)

somatostatin receptor scintigraphy showed a somatostatin-positive lesion with inhomogeneous receptor expression, only partially with Krenning score >2 (1 = lower than liver uptake; 2 = equivalent to liver uptake; 3 = higher than liver uptake), possibly a hint of dedifferentiation (Krenning et al. 1993). Due to the inhomogeneous SSTR expression and Krenning score of 1, partially detected in the intraspinal part of the tumor, PRRNT with ^{90}Y-DOTA-TOC was not performed. In contrast, with external-beam radiation therapy a more homogeneous dose distribution could be achieved in this case as compared with the dose distribution of PRRNT with ^{90}Y-DOTA-TOC. Furthermore, there are not yet enough experience and data to know the dose dependence and incidence of radiation-induced spinal cord toxicity due to PRRNT with ^{90}Y-DOTA-TOC and whether radioisotope-induced myelopathy would be comparable to the delayed radiation-induced myelopathy caused by excessive external-beam radiation therapy.

The mediastinal manifestation of the meningioma in our case did not lead to any respiratory symptoms such as shortness of breath. Because of that and the high tendency of the tumor to bleed, the mediastinal manifestation of the meningioma was not surgically approached (Palimento and Picchio 2006). The impossibility of complete resection in our case was the reason why finally postoperative radiotherapy was performed to prevent further paraparesis by tumor progression. To deliver as much dose as possible, the patient was positioned in an immobilization device to deliver fractionated stereotactic radiation therapy (SRT) using the VMAT technique. 6D image guidance was done with the ExacTrac X-ray system. Due to the large target volume, a single-dose radiosurgical approach could not be performed (Gerszten et al. 2008).

Close follow-up in this particular case is crucial. First, the inhomogeneous SSTR expression pattern on scintigraphy may be an indicator that this meningioma is partially less differentiated. Potentially, these parts belong to a higher WHO grading with a higher tendency for recurrence. Second, MR imaging and SSTR imaging showed infiltration of multiple vertebrae, a criterion for malignant behavior and aggressiveness. Third, intraoperatively the tumor showed high tendency to bleed, which could indicate a more aggressive clinical course. Guevara et al. (2010) showed that, besides the extent of resection, there is an association between vascular density index and local recurrence of meningiomas. Furthermore, our patient had nontotal resection of the tumor. Due to the rare incidence and complex presentation of this disease not amenable to complete surgical resection, an individualized treatment approach should be worked out interdisciplinarily. The treatment approach should be based not only on histology but also on clinical and imaging findings.

References

Barbanera A, Nina P, Serchi E, Ascanio F (2007) Aggressive recurrence of intra-extradural cervico-thoracic meningothelial meningioma. Acta Neurochir (Wien) 149:83–86

Baum RP, Söldner J, Schmücking M, Niesen A (2004a) Peptidrezeptorvermittelte Radiotherapie (PRRT) neuroendokriner Tumoren. Klinische Indikationen und Erfahrung mit 90Yttrium-markierten Somatostatinanaloga. Onkologe 10:1098–1110

Baum RP, Soeldner J, Schmuecking M (2004b) Clinical results of peptide receptor radionuclide therapy (PRRT) with yttrium-90-DOTA-TYR3-OCTREOTATE (Y-90 DOTA-TATE) in patients with neuroendocrine tumors. J Nucl Med 45:90P

Buchfelder M Nomikos P, Paulus W, Rupprecht H (2001) Spinal-thoracic dumbbell meningioma: a case report. Spine (Phila Pa 1976) 26:1500–1504

Central Brain Tumor Registry of the United States (CBTRUS): Statistical report: Primary brain tumors in the United States, 2000–2004

Engelhard HH et al (2010) Clinical presentation, histology, and treatment in 430 patients with primary tumors of the spinal cord, spinal meninges, or cauda equina. J Neurosurg Spine 13(1):67–77

Forrer F et al (2006) Targeted radionuclide therapy with ^{90}Y-DOTATOC in patients with neuroendocrine tumors. Anticancer Res 26(1B):703–707

Gambardella G, Gervasio O, Zaccone C (2003) Approaches and surgical results in the treatment of ventral thoracic meningiomas. Review of our experience with a postero-lateral combined transpedicular-transarticular approach. Acta Neurochir (Wien) 145:385–392

Gerszten PC, Burton SA, Ozhasoglu C, McCue KJ, Quinn AE (2008) Radiosurgery for benign intradural spinal tumors. Neurosurgery 62:887–895

Goldsmith BJ, Wara WM, Wilson CB, Larson DA (1994) Postoperative irradiation for subtotally resected meningiomas. A retrospective analysis of 140 patients treated from 1967 to 1990. J Neurosurg 80:195–201

Guevara P, Escobar-Arriaga E, Saavedra-Perez D, Martinez-Rumavor A, Flores-Estrada D, Rembao D, Calderon A, Sotelo J, Arrieta O (2010) Angiogenesis and expression of estrogen and progesterone receptors as predictive factors for recurrence of meningioma. J Neurooncol 98:379–384

Imhof Anna, Brunner Philippe, Marincek Nicolas, Briel Matthias, Schindler Christian, Rasch Helmut, Maecke HelmutR, Rochlitz Christoph, Mueller-Brand Jan, Walter MartinA (2011) Response, survival, and long-term toxicity after therapy with the radiolabeled somatostatin analogue ^{90}Y-DOTA-TOC in metastasized neuroendocrine cancers. J Clin Oncol 29:2416–2423

Incarbone M, Ceresoli GL, Di Tommaso L, Cappuzzo F, Inzirillo F, Infante M, Alloisio M (2008) Primary pulmonary meningioma: report of a case and review of the literature. Lung Cancer 62:401–407

Jenkinson MD, Simpson C, Nicholas RS, Miles J, Findlay GF, Pigott TJ (2006) Outcome predictors and complications in the management of intradural spinal tumours. Eur Spine J 15:203–210

Kaemmerer D, Peter L, Lupp A, Schulz S, Sänger J, Prasad V, Kulkarni H, Haugvik SP, Hommann M, Baum RP (2011) Molecular imaging with ^{68}Ga-SSTR PET/CT and correlation to immunohistochemistry of somatostatin receptors in neuroendocrine tumours. Eur J Nucl Med Mol Imaging. 38:1659–1668

Krenning EP, Kwekkeboom DJ, Bakker WH, Breeman WA, Kooij PP, Oei HY, van Hagen M, Postema PT, de Jong M, Reubi JC (1993) Somatostatin receptor scintigraphy with (^{111}In-DTPA-D-Phe1)- and (^{123}I-Tyr3)-octreotide: The Rotterdam experience with more than 1,000 patients. Eur J Nucl Med 20:716–731

Kwekkeboom D, Krenning EP, de Jong M (2000) Peptide receptor imaging and therapy. J Nucl Med 41:1704–1713

Lee Y, Liu J, Patel S, Cloughesy T, Lai A, Farooqi H, Seligson D, Dong J, Liau L, Becker D, Mischel P, Shams S, Nelson S (2010) Genomic landscape of meningiomas. Brain Pathol 20:751–762

Levy W, Bay J, Dohn D (1982) Spinal cord meningioma. J Neurosurg 57:804–812

Mawrin C, Perry A (2010) Pathological classification and molecular genetics of meningiomas. J Neurooncol 99:379–391

Menda Y, O'Dorisio M, Kao S, Khanna G, Michael S, Connolly M, Babich J, O'Dorisio T, Bushnell D, Madsen M (2010) Phase I trial of ^{90}Y-DOTATOC therapy in children and young adults with refractory solid tumors that express somatostatin receptors. J Nucl Med 51:1524–1531

Mimoto H, Tomita R, Nakahara K, Tanaka H, Hada J, Noguchi K (1991) A case of dumbbell-shaped type extradural spinal meningioma. Kyobu Geka 44:961–964

Nakasu S, Fukami T, Jito J, Nozaki K (2009) Recurrence and regrowth of benign meningiomas. Brain Tumor Pathol 26:69–72

Palimento D, Picchio M (2006) Meningioma of the mediastinum causing spontaneous hemothorax. Ann Thorac Surg 81:1903–1904

Perry A, Scheithauer BW, Stafford SL, Lohse CM, Wollan PC (1999) "Malignancy" in meningiomas: a clinicopathologic study of 116 patients, with grading implications. Cancer 85:2046–2056

Prasad V, Fetscher S, Baum RP (2007) Changing role of somatostatin receptor targeted drugs in NET: Nuclear Medicine's view. J Pharm Pharm Sci 10:321s–337s

Reubi JC (2004) Somatostatin and other peptide receptors as tools for tumor diagnosis and treatment. Neuroendocrinology 80(Suppl 1):51–56

Reubi JC, Schär JC, Waser B, Wenger S, Heppeler A, Schmitt JS, Mäcke HR (2000) Affinity profiles for human somatostatin receptor subtypes SST1-SST5 of somatostatin radiotracers selected for scintigraphic and radiotherapeutic use. Eur J Nucl Med 27:273–282

Rufini V, Calcagni ML, Baum RP (2006) Imaging of neuroendocrine tumors. In: Semin in Nucl Med 36:228–247

Solero CL, Fornari M, Giombini S, Lasio G, Oliveri G, Cimio C, Pluchino F (1989) Spinal meningiomas: review of 174 operated cases. Neurosurgery 125:153–160

Sughrue ME et al (2010) The relevance of simpson grade I and II resection in modern neurosurgical treatment of World Health Organization Grade I meningiomas. J Neurosurg 113:1029–1035

Yoon SH, Chung CK, Jahng TA (2007) Surgical outcome of spinal canal meningiomas. J Korean Neurosurg Soc 42:300–304

Peptide Receptor Radionuclide Therapy for Neuroendocrine Tumors in Germany: First Results of a Multi-institutional Cancer Registry

Dieter Hörsch, Samer Ezziddin, Alexander Haug, Klaus Friedrich Gratz, Simone Dunkelmann, Bernd Joachim Krause, Carl Schümichen, Frank M. Bengel, Wolfram H. Knapp, Peter Bartenstein, Hans-Jürgen Biersack, Ursula Plöckinger, Sabine Schwartz-Fuchs and R. P. Baum

D. Hörsch (✉)
Department of Gastroenterology and Endocrinology,
Center of Neuroendocrine Tumors Bad Berka–ENETS Center of Excellence,
Zentralklinik Bad Berka GmbH, Robert-Koch-Allee 9, 99437 Bad Berka, Germany
e-mail: dieter.hoersch@zentralklinik.de
URL: http://www.zentralklinik-bad-berka.de; http://www.neuroendokrin.de

S. Ezziddin · H.-J. Biersack
Klinik und Poliklinik für Nuklearmedizin am Universitätsklinikum Bonn,
Sigmund-Freud-Street 25, 53127 Bonn, Germany

A. Haug · P. Bartenstein
Klinik und Poliklinik für Nuklearmedizin, Ludwig Maximilian Universität München,
Ziemsenstraße 1, 80336 München, Germany

K. F. Gratz · F. M. Bengel · W. H. Knapp
Klinik für Nuklearmedizin, Medizinische Hochschule Hannover,
Carl-Neuberg-Straße 1, 30625 Hannover, Germany

S. Dunkelmann · B. J. Krause · C. Schümichen
Klinik und Poliklinik für Nuklearmedizin, Universitätsklinikum Rostock,
Gertrudenplatz 1, 18057 Rostock, Germany

U. Plöckinger
Charité, Campus Virchow-Klinikum, Universitätsmedizin Berlin,
Augustenburger Platz 1, 13353 Berlin, Germany

S. Schwartz-Fuchs
Städtisches Klinikum München, Klinikum München Bogenhausen,
Klinik für Gastroenterologie, Hepatologie und gast,
Onkologie, Englschalkinger Street 77, 81925 München, Germany

R. P. Baum
PET Center/Department of Nuclear Medicine,
Zentralklinik Bad Berka GmbH, Bad Berka, Germany

R. P. Baum and F. Rösch (eds.), *Theranostics, Gallium-68, and Other Radionuclides*,
Recent Results in Cancer Research 194, DOI: 10.1007/978-3-642-27994-2_25,

Abstract

Peptide receptor radionuclide therapy is an effective treatment option for patients with well-differentiated somatostatin receptor-expressing neuroendocrine tumors. However, published data result mainly from retrospective monocentric studies. We initiated a multi-institutional, prospective, board-reviewed registry for patients treated with peptide receptor radionuclide therapy in Germany in 2009. In five centers, 297 patients were registered. Primary tumors were mainly derived from pancreas (117/297) and small intestine (80/297), whereas 56 were of unknown primary. Most tumors were well differentiated with median Ki67 proliferation rate of 5% (range 0.9–70%). Peptide receptor radionuclide therapy was performed using mainly yttrium-90 and/or lutetium-177 as radionuclides in 1–8 cycles. Mean overall survival was estimated at 213 months with follow-up between 1 and 230 months after initial diagnosis, and 87 months with follow-up between 1 and 92 months after start of peptide receptor radionuclide therapy. Median overall survival was not yet reached. Subgroup analysis demonstrated that best results were obtained in neuroendocrine tumors with proliferation rate below 20%. Our results indicate that peptide receptor radionuclide therapy is an effective treatment for well- and moderately differentiated neuroendocrine tumors irrespective of previous therapies and should be regarded as one of the primary treatment options for patients with somatostatin receptor-expressing neuroendocrine tumors.

Contents

1 Introduction

Expression of somatostatin receptors on cellular membranes of neuroendocrine tumor cells is the basis for imaging of these tumors by somatostatin receptor-based scintigraphy and PET/CT methods (Rufini et al. 2006; Kwekkeboom et al. 2010). In addition, linkage of beta- and gamma-emitting radionuclides to somatostatin analogs has been successfully used to treat somatostatin receptor-expressing tumors (de Jong et al. 1999; Valkema et al. 2006; Kwekkeboom et al. 2008; Imhof et al. 2011).

However, reported results are hampered by retrospective and monocentric data accumulation, with the exception of one multicentric, multinational prospective study using yttrium-90 edotreotide (Bushnell et al. 2010). Progression-free survival data and overall survival indicate superiority of peptide receptor radionuclide therapy compared with other treatment modalities. The largest study using lutetium-177 DOTATATE in 310 patients with neuroendocrine tumors of different origins reported median overall survival of all patients of 46 months. Median overall survival increased to more than 48 months in patients responding with any kind of remission or stable disease, whereas patients with progressive disease survived only 11 months in median. These results were recently updated in 263 Dutch patients followed from 2000 to 2010. In these patients, overall median survival was 51 months for patients responding with any kind of remission or stable disease, whereas patients with progressive disease survived only 10 months in median (Kwekkeboom et al. 2008; Kwekkeboom, personal communication June 2010). These groups reported a median of about 60 months overall survival for patients with a different kind of neuroendocrine tumors, namely 136 patients with pancreatic neuroendocrine tumors. When these results are compared to the results of the Surveillance, Epidemiology, and End Results (SEER) database, the 5-year survival rate of locally advanced or metastasised well-differentiated neuroendocrine tumors of the pancreas was 22% (Yao et al. 2008). In a recent placebo-controlled trial, overall survival of patients treated with placebo was 22 months (Raymond et al. 2011). Newer databases from Berlin, Germany and Tampa, FL, USA reported longer median overall survival times, however results cannot be compared since overall survival was measured from time of initial diagnosis (Pape et al. 2008; Strosberg et al. 2011). As such, peptide receptor radionuclide therapy translates into survival advantages of several years in patients responding to the therapy (Kwekkeboom et al. 2008).

However, these results have to be weighed against known side-effects of peptide receptor radionuclide therapy such as kidney and bone marrow toxicity (Merola et al. 2010; Imhof et al. 2011). To circumvent side-effects of peptide receptor radionuclide therapy, meticulous selection of patients, dosimetry of tumor dose compared with radiation of other organs, and application of suitable protocols developed to protect kidneys and other organs can be used (Wehrmann et al. 2007; Rollman et al. 2010; Zaknun et al. in press).

We initiated a prospective, multicentric registry for patients treated with peptide receptor radionuclide therapy in Germany in 2009 and report here the first interim analysis of 297 registered patients.

2 Patients and Methods

In 2009, a multi-institutional cancer registry for neuroendocrine tumor patients treated with peptide receptor radionuclide therapy was initiated by U. Plöckinger in Berlin, Germany. Approval of the local ethical committee was obtained on the basis of informed consent. To date, 297 patients have been registered at five institutions in Germany (four university hospitals and one academic hospital). All patients had signed informed consent for prospective evaluation during and after peptide receptor radionuclide therapy. Registry of patients was performed by trained medical documentaries on site at the university hospitals and is ongoing in Bad Berka. Registered items were, among others, origin of primary tumors, number of previous therapies, dose and repetitions of peptide receptor radionuclide therapy, and side-effects on bone marrow and kidney function. Response status was registered at every visit and after discontinuation of peptide receptor radionuclide therapy. Repeated visits are planned at 2-year intervals to document long-term effects of peptide receptor radionuclide therapy.

3 Results

In five centers between 17 and 149 patients each were registered in 2009 and 2010 (total 297). Most patients were of male sex (156 male and 141 female patients) with a median age of 58 years (mean 57 years, standard deviation 12 years, range 12–86 years). Proliferation rate was determined in 164 patients. Median proliferation rate was 5% (mean 9.8%, standard deviation 10%, range 0.9–70%). G1, G2, and G3 tumors were present in 13%, 33%, and 5%, respectively. Proliferation rate was not known in 142/293 patients (48%). Origin of neuroendocrine tumor could be determined in 80% of patients (233/297). The majority of the neuroendocrine tumors derived from pancreas (39%, 117/297), small intestine (26%, 80/297), cecum, colon, and rectum (5%, 15/297), lung (3%, 9/297), and stomach (2%, 6/297). Duodenal neuroendocrine tumors were present in four cases, and one metastasized neuroendocrine tumor of appendix was included (Fig. 1).

Patients were heavily pretreated. In 218 patients, number and kind of previous therapies were documented and included in the registry. Of these 218 patients, 44 (20%) experienced no previous therapy, while the rest had undergone between one and eight previous therapies. Most patients were treated by 1–2 therapies (122 patients, 55%), 20% (45 patients) by 3–4 therapies, whereas 5–8 therapies had seldom been used and performed in only 7 patients (3%). Mostly surgery (125/218 patients, 57%) or medical therapy (114/218 patients, 52%) was performed, while local ablative therapies were used as pretreatment in 20/218 patients (9%) and radiotherapy (external beam) in 14/218 patients (6%).

Between 1 and 8 cycles of peptide receptor radionuclide therapy were administered (median 3, mean 3.07, standard deviation 1.5) using mainly lutetium-177 (53%, 160/297) and yttrium-90 (46%, 137/297). Two patients were treated with gallium-67 radionuclide. As somatostatin analogs and chelators, mostly [DOTA0, Tyr3] octreotate (DOTATATE) and [DOTA0, Tyr3] octreotide (DOTATOC) were applied, in 91% and 8% of therapy cycles, respectively, whereas in 1% of cycles other ligands and chelators were used.

For the first cycle of peptide receptor radionuclide therapy, median activity was 3.75 GBq in 134 patients treated with yttrium-90 (mean 3.79 GBq, range 1.5–8.14 GBq) and 7.4 GBq in the 160 patients treated with lutetium-177 (mean 6.93 GBq, range 0.629–7.4 GBq). Cumulative dose was in median 7.35 GBq in 66 patients treated solely with yttrium-90 (mean 7.9 GBq, range 2–19 GBq) and 22 GBq for the 133 patients treated exclusively with lutetium-177 (mean 21.2 GBq, range 2.6–51.9 GBq).

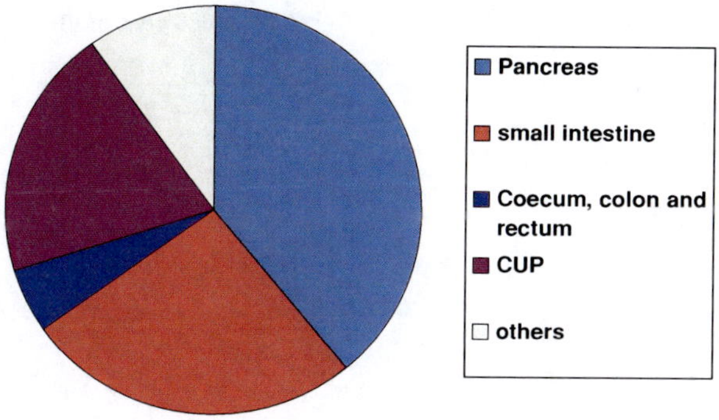

Fig. 1 Origin of registered neuroendocrine tumors

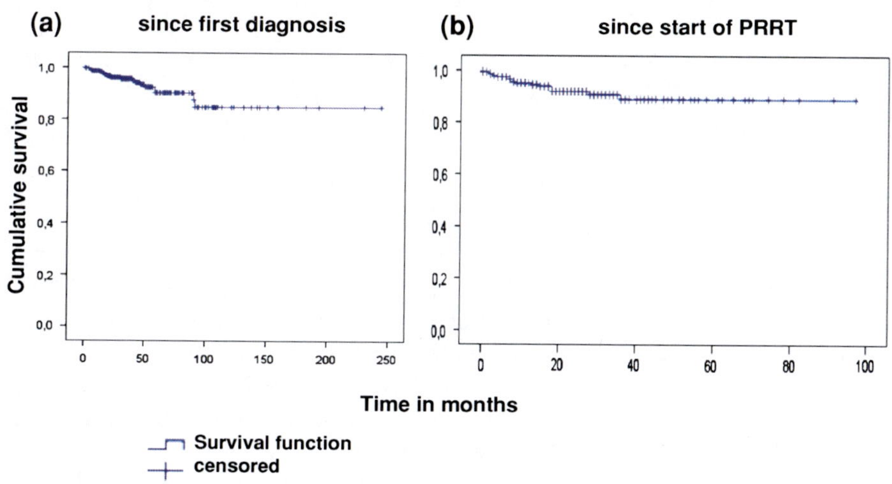

Fig. 2 Overall survival of all patients after initial diagnosis (**a**) and after start of peptide receptor radionuclide therapy (**b**)

Peptide receptor radionuclide therapy was not continued in 190 of 297 patients. Of these patients, response status was known in 151 patients. Any kind of remission was noted in 20% of patients (5% complete remission, 14% partial remission, 0.5% minor remission), stable disease in 48%, and progressive disease in 10% of patients. Among all 297 patients, 19 deaths were noted. Mean overall survival was estimated at 213 months with follow-up between 1 and 230 months after initial diagnosis, and 87 months with follow-up between 1 and 92 months after start of peptide receptor radionuclide therapy. Median overall survival was not yet reached (Fig. 2a, b).

Subgroup analysis was performed according to tumor grade, number of previous therapies, and grading of the neuroendocrine tumors by Ki67-based proliferation rate. Of 293 patients, 38 had proliferation index <2% (G1; 13%), 97 had

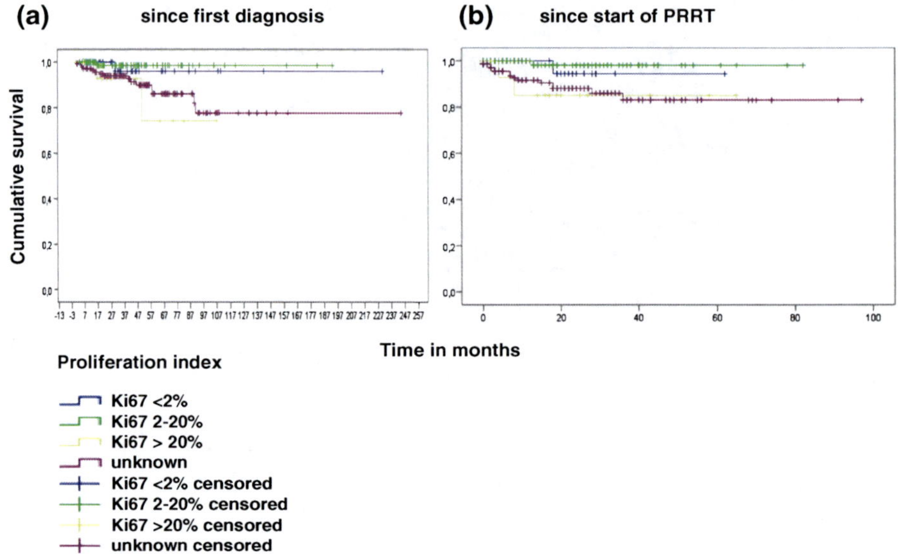

Fig. 3 Overall survival according to tumor grading determined by Ki67 index after initial diagnosis (**a**) and after start of peptide receptor radionuclide therapy (**b**)

proliferation index 2–20% (G2; 33%), and 16 had proliferation index >20% (G3; 5%). In almost half of cases, proliferation rates were not documented (142/293; 48%). Subgroup analysis demonstrated that best results were obtained in grade 1 and 2 neuroendocrine tumors with proliferation rate below 20%. Interestingly, results were similar in the group without known proliferation rate and the group with proliferation rate higher than 20% (G3; Fig. 3a, b).

Overall survival was not dependent upon number of previous therapies. Most patients with documented previous therapies had had two or three therapies (90/293; 30%). No previous therapy was noted in 43/293 patients (14%), 66 (22%) had had one previous therapy, and 17/293 (5%) more than three previous therapies. No information could be assessed for 77/293 (26%). Although most patients were pretreated, no difference in survival could be documented depending on the number of pretreatments (Fig. 4a, b). Best results were obtained in patients with documented previous therapies, whereas unknown pretreatments appeared to be a risk factor in survival analysis.

4 Discussion

Our results indicate that peptide receptor radionuclide therapy is effective and safe for treatment of well- and moderately differentiated neuroendocrine tumors. Although, the registry so far does not contain long-term follow-up, mean follow-up of registered patients was 19.6 months, resulting in long mean survival times of

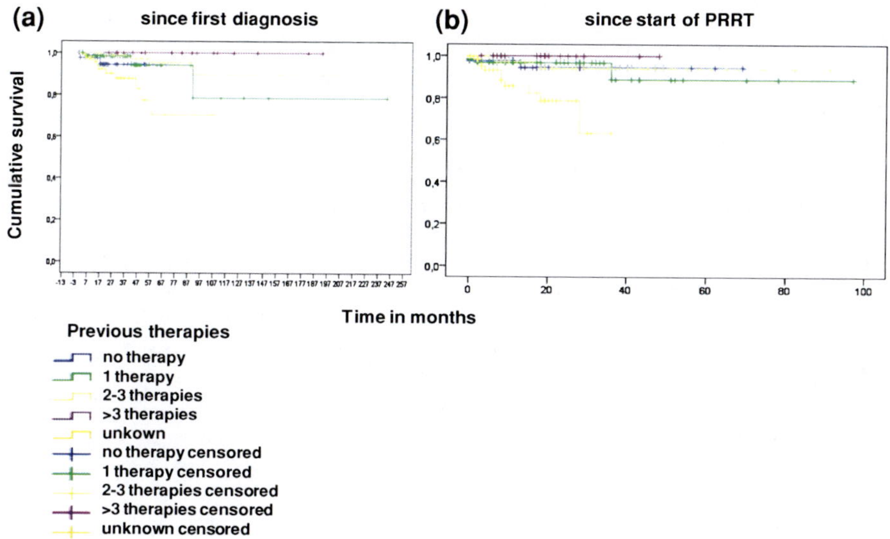

Fig. 4 Overall survival according to previous therapies after initial diagnosis (**a**) and after start of peptide receptor radionuclide therapy (**b**)

more than 200 months after first diagnosis and more than 80 months after start of peptide receptor radionuclide therapy. Scheduled follow-ups at 24-month intervals will complete these promising data in the next years. Survival curves presented in this preliminary analysis indicate that prognosis of neuroendocrine tumor patients treated by peptide receptor radionuclide therapy is excellent. Since patients treated by peptide receptor radionuclide therapy undergo a selection process prior to therapy, these data may represent positive selection according to slow tumor progression as well as effects of peptide receptor radionuclide therapy on tumor progression. To date, registered data on side-effects of peptide receptor radionuclide therapy do not indicate serious side-effects on kidney and bone marrow function, data which are especially sensitive to close follow-up of treated patients in the coming years.

Subgroup analysis indicates that peptide receptor radionuclide therapy is especially sensitive to meticulous selection of patients by complete pathological reports and history of previous therapies. Although survival curves did not differ between patients with different number of previous therapies, results were better when these data were documented. Likewise, results were superior in patients with proliferation rate by Ki67 index of lower than 20% compared with proliferation indices above 20%. Patients with missing proliferation rate showed a survival curve similar to patients with proliferation rate higher than 20%, indicating that preselection of patients for peptide receptor radionuclide therapy by complete pathological report is essential for success of this innovative treatment.

Our results show that peptide receptor radionuclide therapy is an effective and safe treatment option for G1 and G2 neuroendocrine tumors irrespective of previous therapies and should be regarded as one of the primary treatment options for patients with somatostatin receptor-expressing neuroendocrine tumors. We intend to use this register not only for documentation of current therapy protocols but also as an innovation platform for prospective studies/evaluations of new treatment modalities and combination therapies (Hörsch et al. 2010; Seregni et al. 2010).

Acknowledgments We are indebted to all patients who agreed to be registered. The registry of peptide receptor radionuclide therapy was founded in 2009 by U. Plöckinger and S. Schwartz-Fuchs with great enthusiasm. Data collection and analysis were performed by S. Skrobek-Engel and H. Franz of Lohmann and Birkner in Berlin, Germany. Supported by Covidien Inc., ITG, MDS Nordion, and Eckert and Ziegler Radiopharma GmbH.

References

Bushnell DL Jr, O'Dorisio TM, O'Dorisio MS et al (2010) ^{90}Y-edotreotide for metastatic carcinoid refractory to octreotide. J Clin Oncol 28:1652–1659

de Jong M, Breeman WA, Bernard HF et al (1999) Therapy of neuroendocrine tumours with radiolabeled somatostatin-analogues. Q J Nucl Med 43:356–366

Hörsch D, Prasad V, Petrovitch A, Baum RB (2010) Combined treatment of rapidly progressing neuroendocrine tumors by transcatheter arterial chemoembolisation of the liver and peptide-receptor radiotherapy is safe and effective: Report of 30 consecutive patients. J Clin Oncol 28(suppl):e14634 (abstr)

Imhof A, Brunner P, Marincek N et al (2011) Response, survival, and long-term toxicity after therapy with the radiolabeled somatostatin analogue [^{90}Y-DOTA]-TOC in metastasized neuroendocrine cancers. J Clin Oncol 22:2416–2423

Kwekkeboom D, de Herder W, Kam B et al (2008) Treatment with the radiolabeled somatostatin analog [^{177}Lu-DOTA0, Tyr3] octreotate: toxicity, efficacy, and survival. J Clin Oncol 26:2124–2130

Kwekkeboom DJ, Kam Bl, van Essen M et al (2010) Somatostatin receptor based imaging and therapy of gastroenteropancreatic neuroendocrine tumors. Endocr Relat Cancer 17:R53–R73

Merola E, Capurso G, Campana D (2010) Acute leukaemia following low dose peptide receptor radionuclide therapy for an intestinal carcinoid. Dig Liver Dis 42:457–458

Pape UF, Jann H, Müller-Nordhorn J et al (2008) Prognostic relevance of a novel TNM classification system for upper gastroenteropancreatic neuroendocrine tumors. Cancer 113:256–265

Raymond E, Niccoli P, Raoul J et al (2011) Updated overall survival (OS) and progression-free survival (PFS) by blinded independent central review (BICR) of sunitinib (SU) versus placebo (PBO) for patients (Pts) with advanced unresectable pancreatic neuroendocrine tumors (NET). J Clin Oncol 29(suppl):4008 (abstr)

Rollman EJ, Melis M, Valkema R (2010) Kidney protection during peptide receptor radionuclide therapy with somatostatin analoques. Eur J Nucl Mol Imaging 37:1018–1031

Rufini V, Calcagni ML, Baum RP (2006) Imaging of neuroendocrine tumors. Semin Nucl Med 36:228–247

Seregni E, Maccauro M, Coliva A et al (2010) Treatment with tandem [(90)Y] DOTA-TATE and [(177)Lu] DOTA-TATE of neuroendocrine tumors refractory to conventional therapy: preliminary results. Q J Nucl Med Mol Imaging 54(1):84–91

Strosberg J, Cheema A, Weber J et al (2011) Prognostic validity of a novel American joint committee on cancer staging classification for pancreatic neuroendocrine tumors. J Clin Oncol 29:3044–3049

Valkema R, Pauwels S, Kvols LK et al (2006) Survival and response after peptide receptor radionuclide therapy with [^{90}Y-DOTA0, Tyr3] octreotide in patients with advanced gastroenteropancreatic neuroendocrine tumors. Semin Nucl Med 36:147–156

Wehrmann C, Senftleben S, Zachert C (2007) Results of individual patient dosimetry in peptide receptor radionuclide therapy with ^{177}Lu DOTA-TATE and ^{177}Lu DOTA-NOC. Cancer Biother Radiopharm 22:406–416

Yao JC, Hassan M, Phan A et al (2008) One hundred years after "carcinoid": epidemiology of and prognostic factors for neuroendocrine tumors in 35,825 cases in the United States. J Clin Oncol 26:3063–3072

Zaknun JJ et al. (eds) Practical guidance on peptide receptor radionuclide therapy (PRRNT) for neuroendocrine tumors. (in press IAEA)

Polish Experience in Peptide Receptor Radionuclide Therapy

Jolanta Kunikowska, Leszek Królicki, Anna Sowa-Staszczak, Alicja Hubalewska-Dydejczyk, Dariusz Pawlak, Renata Mikolajczak, Daria Handkiewicz-Junak, Norbert Szaluś, Grzegorz Kamiński, Jaroslaw Cwikla, Maciej Jakuciński, Anna Lukiewicz, Aldona Kowalska and Pawel Gut

J. Kunikowska (✉) · L. Królicki
Nuclear Medicine Department, Medical University of Warsaw,
Ul.Banacha 1 A, 02-097, Warsaw, Poland
e-mail: jolanta.kunikowska@wum.edu.pl

A. Sowa-Staszczak · A. Hubalewska-Dydejczyk
Chair and Department of Endocrinology and Nuclear Medicine,
Jagiellonian University Collegium Medicum, Cracow, Poland

D. Pawlak · R. Mikolajczak
Institute of Atomic Energy POLATOM, Świerk-Otwock, Poland

D. Handkiewicz-Junak
Department of Nuclear Medicine and Endocrine Oncology,
Maria Skłodowska-Curie Memorial Cancer Center,
Institute of Oncology Gliwice Branch, Gliwice, Poland

N. Szaluś · G. Kamiński
Nuclear Medicine Department, Military Institute of Medicine, Warsaw, Poland

J. Cwikla
Department of Radiology and Diagnostic Imaging,
Medical Centre for Postgraduate Education and Central Clinical
Hospital of Ministry of Internal Affairs and Administration, Warsaw, Poland

M. Jakuciński
Nuclear Medicine Department Brodnowski Hospital, Warsaw, Poland

A. Lukiewicz
Department of Nuclear Medicine and Endocrine Oncology,
Maria Skłodowska-Curie Memorial Cancer Center, Institute of Oncology,
Warsaw Branch, Warsaw, Poland

A. Kowalska
Department of Endocrinology and Nuclear Medicine Holycross Cancer Centre (HCC),
Kielce, Poland

P. Gut
Department of Endocrinology, Metabolism and Internal Diseases,
Poznań University of Medical Sciences, Poznań, Poland

R. P. Baum and F. Rösch (eds.), *Theranostics, Gallium-68, and Other Radionuclides*,
Recent Results in Cancer Research 194, DOI: 10.1007/978-3-642-27994-2_26,

Abstract

Patients and Methods: During the period from April 2004 to December 2010, 358 patients underwent peptide receptor radionuclide therapy (PRRT) (^{90}Y–DOTATATE, ^{177}Lu–DOTATATE, and ^{90}Y/^{177}Lu–DOTATATE) in Poland. *Results*: The majority of patients underwent ^{90}Y–DOTATATE therapy ($n = 177$) with progression-free survival (PFS)/time to progression (TTP) of 17–44 months and overall survival (OS) of 22–34.2 months. Twelve-month follow-up revealed stable disease (SD) in 46–60%, disease regression (RD) in 16–35%, disease progression (PD) in 7–17%, and complete remission (CR) in 3% of patients. In patients treated with ^{90}Y/^{177}Lu–DOTATATE ($n = 44$), PFS/TTP was 24.2–28.3 months and OS was 49.8–52.8 months. Twelve-month follow-up showed SD in 62–70%, RD in 15–20%, and PD in 10–12% of patients. The treatment was well tolerated. No severe adverse events occurred. Grade 3 toxicity [in leucocytes (WBC) and thrombocytes (PLT)] was seen in 6–20% of patients treated with ^{90}Y–DOTATATE. In that group, renal toxicity grade 3 was seen in 5–12% and grade 4 in 3–8%. In patients treated with tandem therapy with ^{90}Y/^{177}Lu–DOTATATE or ^{177}Lu–DOTATATE alone, hematological and renal toxicity grade 3 or 4 was not observed. *Conclusions*: The results indicate that PRRT with the procedures and isotopes used is an effective and safe therapy option for patients with metastatic or inoperable neuroendocrine tumors (NETs). Our results suggest that tandem therapy with ^{90}Y/^{177}Lu–DOTATATE provides longer overall survival than single-isotope treatment. Hematological toxicity was rare in all treated patients. Renal toxicity grade 3 and 4 was observed only in the group treated with ^{90}Y–DOTATATE.

Keywords

Somatostatin receptor · Peptide receptor radionuclide therapy · Neuroendocrine tumors · ^{90}Y–DOTATATE · ^{177}Lu–DOTATATE

Contents

1 Introduction

Neuroendocrine tumors, defined as epithelial neoplasms with predominant neuroendocrine differentiation, can arise in most organs of the body. Because of this and the possibility of excretion of some hormones, only combined effort by multiple specialists may lead to implementation of new management of patients suffering from NET. The choice of an appropriate treatment option for patients with inoperable or metastatic neuroendocrine tumors is limited. Knowledge of overexpression of somatostatin analogs leads to the possibility of its use in diagnosis and radiolabeled therapy. Peptide receptor radionuclide therapy (PRRT) with ^{90}Y–DOTA-octreotide and ^{177}Lu–DOTA-octreotate in neuroendocrine tumors (NETs) results in symptomatic improvement, prolonged survival, and enhanced quality of life.

First peptide radionuclide therapy with radiolabeled somatostatin analogs (PRRT) was performed in April 2004 in Nuclear Medicine Department Warsaw Medical University (Kunikowska et al. 2005).

In the past, neuroendocrine tumors (NET) were diagnosed too rarely in Poland, but great effort by the Polish Society of Neuroendocrine Tumors has provided improved knowledge about this disease in multidisciplinary specialization. PRRT started with well-known therapy with ^{90}Y–DOTATATE, and after that, based on experience by de Jong et al. (2002a, 2002b, 2005), with tandem therapy with ^{90}Y and ^{177}Lu.

2 Materials and Methods

PRRT is performed in 10 nuclear departments in Poland:

- Nuclear Medicine Department Warsaw Medical University (52 patients)
- Chair and Department of Endocrinology and Nuclear Medicine, Jagiellonian University Collegium Medicum, Cracow (62 patients)
- Nuclear Medicine Department, Military Institute of Medicine (47 patients)
- Department of Radiology and Diagnostic Imaging, Medical Centre for Postgraduate Education and Central Clinical Hospital of Ministry of Internal Affairs and Administration, Warsaw (79 patients)
- Department of Nuclear Medicine and Endocrine Oncology, Maria Skłodowska-Curie Memorial Cancer Center, Institute of Oncology, Gliwice Branch, Gliwice (75 patients)
- Nuclear Medicine Department, Brodnowski Hospital (20 patients)
- Department of Nuclear Medicine and Endocrine Oncology, Maria Skłodowska-Curie Memorial Cancer Center, Institute of Oncology, Warsaw Branch, Warsaw (12 patients)
- Department of Endocrinology and Nuclear Medicine Holycross Cancer Centre (HCC), Kielce (6 patients)
- Department of Endocrinology, Metabolism and Internal Diseases, Poznań University of Medical Sciences (5 patients)

In 10 nuclear medicine departments, 358 patients underwent PRRT between April 2004 and December 2010. Data were available for 299 patients.

Two hundred sixty-nine patients had histological confirmation of metastatic or inoperable neuroendocrine tumors, including foregut tumors (126 patients), midgut tumors (96 patients), hindgut neuroendocrine tumors (11), and cancer of unknown primary (CUP, 36).

Thirty patients were treated with other diseases, including astrocytoma in 20 patients, medullary thyroid carcinoma in 4 patients, malignant pheochromocytoma in 1 patient, multiple endocrine neoplasia (MEN1) in 1 patient, Hippel–Landau syndrome in 1 patient, small pelvis in 1 patient, and retroperitoneum in 1 patient.

At time of treatment, all patients with NET showed progressive disease confirmed by CT examination and receptor imaging using ^{99m}Tc HYNIC-TOC (Tektrotyd, Polatom, Świerk) or ^{68}Ga–DOTATATE. For patients with neuroendocrine tumors additionally increasing blood concentration of chromogranin A (CgA).

The major criterion for inclusion in this study was benefit from PRRT therapy. Karnofsky index was used to estimate the patients' general condition.

The following inclusion criteria to therapy were used:

- Somatostatin receptor imaging-positive disease with uptake in the tumor and metastases evaluated within 3 months before inclusion (qualitative analysis)
- For NET tumor histological confirmation, inoperable or metastatic disease
- For other tumors, histological confirmation of neoplasm, progression after conventional other treatment methods, and somatostatin receptor imaging-positive disease
- Hemoglobin level (Hb) $\geq$10 g/dL, leucocytes (WBC) $\geq 2 \times 10^9$/L, thrombocytes (PLT) $\geq 90 \times 10^9$/L
- Calculated creatinine clearance (CrCl) >40 mL/min
- Karnofsky Performance Status $\geq$60
- Life expectancy >3 months
- No pregnancy or lactation

Only in the Department of Radiology and Diagnostic Imaging in Warsaw, the following other qualifications were used:

- Hemoglobin level (Hb) $\geq$8 g/dL, thrombocytes (PLT) $\geq 80 \times 10^9$/L
- Calculated creatinine clearance (CrCl) >30 mL/min

All patients underwent blood tests (full blood count, kidney, liver functions tests, and CgA) and staging prior to therapy with the use of CT and somatostatin receptor imaging.

For patients receiving cold long-acting somatostatin analogs, the radionuclide therapy was performed 4–5 weeks after completion of octreotide (Sandostatin LAR; Novartis) and 3–5 weeks after lanreotide (Somatuline; Ipsen).

In patients with WHO grade III glioma, the following inclusion criteria for locoregional administration of ^{90}Y–DOTATATE were used:

- Previous traditional treatment, including surgical excision and external-beam radiotherapy

- Recurrence of brain tumor, confirmed by tissue sampling during biopsy and/or recraniotomy
- Karnofsky Performance Status ≥70
- High tumor uptake of ^{99m}Tc HYNIC-TOC (Tektrotyd, Polatom, Świerk) tumor/brain (T/B) ratio >3
- Life expectancy >5 months
- No pregnancy or lactation

2.1 Radiopharmaceuticals

The labeling procedures and quality control were performed in the Institute of Atomic Energy POLATOM, Świerk-Otwock. Between April 2004 and December 2010, about 1,200 therapeutic doses of DOTATATE labeled with ^{90}Y, ^{177}Lu, and ^{90}Y/^{177}Lu were prepared (71% ^{90}Y–DOTATATE, 17% ^{177}Lu–DOTATATE, and 12% ^{90}Y/^{177}Lu–DOTATATE).

The radioactivity of doses was 3.7, 2.96 or 2.22 GBq for ^{90}Y–DOTATATE, 7.4 or 3.7 GBq for ^{177}Lu–DOTATATE, and 1.85 GBq ^{90}Y + 5.55 GBq ^{177}Lu or 1.85 GBq ^{90}Y + 1.85 GBq ^{177}Lu for ^{90}Y/^{177}Lu. Specific activity for ^{90}Y–DOTATATE was in the range 33.7 to 74.0 GBq/mg DOTATATE and from 18.5 to 48.8 GBq/mg DOTATATE for ^{90}Y and ^{177}Lu–DOTATATE, respectively. Radiochemical purity for all doses was >99%.

2.2 Treatment Procedure

Therapy was performed on an out- and inpatient basis.

Mixed amino acid (1,000–1,500 mL Vamin 18; Nephroprotect Fresenius Kabi or Aminotel) was infused over 8–10 h for kidney protection, with infusion of 200 mL prior to administration of the treatment (Behr et al. 1998; Rolleman et al. 2003; Jamar et al. 2003; Bernhardt et al. 2001). Before administration of radiopharmaceutical, ondansetron (8 mg, Zofran; Glaxo Wellcome, Atossa, Anpharm S.A.) was injected intravenously or given orally to prevent nausea and vomiting.

The following protocols were used for patients with NET:

- Calculated doses in three departments
  $7.4\,\mathrm{GBq/m^2}$ in 3–5 cycles, 4–8 interval
- Fixed doses
  3–4 × 2.96 GBq each 6–8 weeks
  4 × 3.7 GBq each 6–8 weeks
  4 × 2.96 GBq ^{90}Y–DOTATATE every 12 weeks + 3.7 GBq ^{177}Lu–DOTATATE after 6 weeks
  For ^{177}Lu–DOTATATE, 3–5× 7.4 GBq each 8–12 weeks

The injected activity per one course was 2.2–7.4 GBq.

For tandem therapy with ^{90}Y/^{177}Lu–DOTATATE, two protocols were used:

– 50% activity of ^{90}Y–DOTATATE and 50% activity of ^{177}Lu–DOTATATE (1.85 GBq ^{90}Y + 1.85 GBq ^{177}Lu)
– 75% activity of ^{177}Lu–DOTATATE and 25% activity of ^{90}Y–DOTATATE (1.85 GBq ^{90}Y + 5.55 GBq ^{177}Lu)

For patients with gliomas, ^{90}Y–DOTATATE was directly injected into a port-a-cath, the capsule of which had been permanently implanted into postsurgical cavity by stereotactic navigation. The radioactivity of ^{90}Y–DOTATATE was 1.1 GBq per injection, with a 4–6-week interval.

2.3 Evaluation of Results and Assessment of Clinical Benefit

Disease staging and treatment response in patients with NET were evaluated on 12-month follow-up (except at Department of Nuclear Medicine and Endocrine Oncology, Gliwice Branch, where they performed response 6–8 weeks after treatment completion). Response of treatment on CT was defined according to Response Evaluation Criteria in Solid Tumors (RECIST) criteria. Side-effects were scored according to WHO criteria.

Progression-free survival/time to progression (PFS/TTP) and overall survival (OS) were calculated by Kaplan–Meier estimation and used for treatment response.

Treatment response in patients with gliomas was defined according to RECIST criteria. MRI was performed 7, 21, and 30 days after ^{90}Y–DOTATATE injection. Side effects were scored according to WHO criteria.

3 Results

Considering the number of treated patients, we included the results of therapy in patients with NET from five departments ($n = 233$) in the analysis (Kunikowska et al. 2011; Cwikla et al. 2010).

The majority of patients underwent ^{90}Y–DOTATATE therapy ($n = 177$) with PFS/TTP of 17–37 months and OS of 22–34.2 months.

The observed results were as follows:

- Nuclear Medicine Department Warsaw Medical University
  $n = 18$ patients; PFS/TTP 27.8 months; OS 34.2 months
- Chair and Department of Endocrinology and Nuclear Medicine, Jagiellonian University Collegium Medicum, Cracow
  $n = 39$ patients; PFS/TTP 37.6 months; OS not reached
- Nuclear Medicine Department, Military Institute of Medicine
  $n = 25$ patients; PFS/TTP 22 months; OS 24.5 months
- Department of Radiology and Diagnostic Imaging, Medical Centre for Post-graduate Education and Central Clinical Hospital of Ministry of Internal Affairs and Administration, Warsaw
  $n = 57$ patients; PFS/TTP 17 months; OS 22 months

Table 1 WHO response to treatment in 12-month follow-up after ^{90}Y–DOTATATE

12-Month follow-up	Nuclear Medicine Department Warsaw Medical University, $n = 18$ (%)	Chair and Department of Endocrinology and Nuclear Medicine, Jagiellonian University, $n = 39$ patients (%)	Nuclear Medicine Department, Military Institute of Medicine $n = 25$ patients (%)	Central Hospital of Ministry of Internal Affairs and Administration, $n = 60$ patients (%)
Regression (RD)	16	31	20	35
Stable (SD)	57	47	60	56
Progression (PD)	10	4	10	9
Death	17	18	10	

- Department of Nuclear Medicine and Endocrine Oncology, Maria Skłodowska-Curie Memorial Cancer Center, Institute of Oncology, Gliwice Branch, Gliwice,

  $n = 35$ patients; PFS/TTP 44 months; OS not reached

Among these patients, 12-month follow-up revealed stable disease (SD) in 47–60%, disease regression (RD) in 16–35%, and disease progression (PD) in 4–10%; 10–18% of patients died.

Detailed response after 1 year is listed in Table 1.

Only at the Department of Nuclear Medicine and Endocrine Oncology, Gliwice Branch was the response evaluated 6–8 weeks after completed therapy, with the following results: complete remission (CR) in 3%, SD in 60%, RD in 20%, and disease progression in 17%.

In patients treated with ^{90}Y/^{177}Lu–DOTATATE ($n = 44$), PFS/TTP was 24.2–28.3 months and OS was 49.8–52.8 months. Twelve-month follow-up revealed SD in 62–70% of patients, RD in 15–20% of patients, and PD in 10–12% of patients.

Only 12 patients were treated with ^{177}Lu–DOTATATE with the following results: PFS/TTP of 25.2 months and OS of 42.1 months. Twelve-month follow-up revealed SD in 50% of patients, RD in 25% of patients, and PD in 25% of patients.

In the group treated with sequential treatment (4× ^{90}Y–DOTATATE and one dose of ^{90}Y/^{177}Lu–DOTATATE) the data are not available.

Results of treatment of patients with gliomas are being developed.

Table 2 Hematological and renal grade 3 and 4 toxicities after ^{90}Y–DOTATATE

12-Month follow-up	Nuclear Medicine Department Warsaw Medical University, $n = 18$	Chair and Department of Endocrinology and Nuclear Medicine, Jagiellonian University $n = 39$ patients	Nuclear Medicine Department, Military Institute of Medicine, $n = 25$ patients	Central Hospital of Ministry of Internal Affairs and Administration, $n = 60$ patients
Hematological toxicity grade 3	6%	Not observed	Not observed	3–5%
Hematological toxicity grade 4	Not observed	Not observed	Not observed	Not observed
Renal toxicity grade 3	Not observed	Not observed	12%	5%
Renal toxicity grade 4	Not observed	5%	8%	Not observed

3.1 Side-Effects of Treatment

The treatment was well tolerated. No severe adverse events occurred.

Nausea and vomiting during administration of treatment and amino acids were observed in 15–40%. All cases of nausea and vomiting were successfully treated with ondansetron.

Mild pain (no treatment required) at the site of the tumor was observed in 12–16% within the first 48–72 h post treatment.

According to WHO hematological toxicity criteria, grade 3 toxicity (in WBC and PLT) during therapy was seen in 6–20% of patients treated with ^{90}Y–DOTATATE, but on 12-month follow-up in only 3–8% of patients. In patients treated with tandem therapy with ^{90}Y/^{177}Lu–DOTATATE or ^{177}Lu–DOTATATE alone, toxicity grade 3 or 4 was not seen.

WBC and PLT decrease after therapy was only measured by blood test without clinical symptoms. Hematological toxicity was seen mainly in patients who received chemotherapy before PRRT.

Hemoglobin level showed grade 3 toxicity in only 5–8% of patients treated with ^{90}Y–DOTATATE; in the others, toxicity of this parameter was mild (grade 1 or 2).

According to renal toxicity as defined by the National Cancer Institute, in patients treated with ^{90}Y–DOTATATE renal toxicity grade 3 was seen in 5–12% and grade 4 in 3–8%. In patients treated with tandem therapy with ^{90}Y/^{177}Lu–DOTATATE or ^{177}Lu–DOTATATE alone, toxicity grade 3 or 4 was not seen. Mean glomerular filtration rate (GFR) decrease was 6.1–7.2 mL/min per year in patients treated with ^{90}Y–DOTATATE, 2.7–3.4 mL/min per year in patients treated with ^{90}Y/^{177}Lu–DOTATATE, and 1.7 ml/min per year in patients treated with ^{177}Lu–DOTATATE.

Detailed renal and hematological grade 3 and 4 toxicities are listed in Table 2.

Locoregional treatment of gliomas was well tolerated. No severe adverse events occurred. Side-effects were mostly transient without neurological deficits. In two patients epilepsy seizure and in few cases transient headache was observed. There was no observed hematological, endocrinological, or renal toxicity during the follow-up period.

4 Discussion

PRRT using radiolabeled somatostatin analogs is a promising new treatment option for patients with metastatic or inoperable somatostatin receptor-positive tumors. In Poland, the majority of treated patients were suffering from neuroendocrine tumors, whereas some underwent locoregional treatment for astrocytoma, and other indications were rare.

Clinical publications in the literature and radiochemistry examinations using the β-emitters ^{90}Y and ^{177}Lu in PRRT have developed over the past 11 years (de Jong et al. 2002b; Otte et al. 1999; Breeman et al. 2001). ^{90}Y emits β-particles with longer path lengths and higher energies, while ^{177}Lu emits β-particles with shorter range and has a longer half-life. The fact that ^{177}Lu has a longer half-life means that it takes longer to deliver the same dose as ^{90}Y (Bernhardt et al. 2001; de Jong et al. 2001; Capello et al. 2003).

Another option discussed is sequential administration of isotopes, with initial administration of ^{90}Y-labeled analog followed by ^{177}Lu-labeled analog in the next treatment cycle(s). This option has been used in one department for 3 years, but data are not yet available.

Polish results of PRRT revealed good response to therapy in all treated patients, irrespective of the procedures used. Observed OS and PFS as primary end points were similar to in other published studies using ^{90}Y (Valkema et al. 2006) and ^{177}Lu (Kwekkeboom et al. 2008). Most of the published data on PRRT of neuroendocrine tumors using ^{90}Y–DOTATOC show an objective response with tumor size reduction of 22–34% and 60–65% in case of disease stabilization (Kunikowska et al. 2011; Cwikla et al. 2010; de Jong et al. 2002b; Valkema et al. 2006; Kwekkeboom et al. 2008; Waldherr et al. 2001; Paganelli et al. 2001; Kloeppel et al. 2007). Similar results, irrespective of the administration procedures used, were obtained in the Polish experience.

We first started tandem ^{90}Y/^{177}Lu–DOTATATE therapy to evaluate the role of combined PRRT in disseminated NETs. We obtained very similar results in two departments using two different isotope proportions in tandem therapy.

PRRT was well tolerated in most patients, and the most frequently reported side-effects of nausea and vomiting were probably related to coadministration of amino acid infusions. The rate was similar to that reported in previous trials (de Jong et al. 2002b; Otte et al. 1999; Breeman et al. 2001; Waldherr et al. 2001; Paganelli et al. 2001; Waldherr et al. 2002; Baum et al. 2004; Baum et al. 2007).

The reported hematological toxicity as assessed according to WHO criteria was limited and without clinical manifestation in all treated patients. Renal toxicity provided to dialysis was observed only in patients treated with ^{90}Y–DOTATATE, at the same frequency as previously published in the literature (Chinol et al. 2002). Therefore, we conclude that treatment with ^{90}Y–DOTATATE, ^{90}Y/^{177}Lu–DOTATATE, or ^{177}Lu–DOTATATE in patients with disseminated or inoperable NET is feasible and safe. Clinical improvement could be observed, and most patients benefited from the treatment. In addition, labeling and administration of DOTATATE in combined therapy was straightforward, and its application was safe. No serious adverse events occurred after treatment with either ^{90}Y/^{177}Lu–DOTATATE or ^{90}Y–DOTATATE.

The major limitation of all examinations, as in other published PRRT studies in the literature, is the lack of randomization and the many different protocols used. In single department, the reported data includes not more than 100 patients, as in most other published studies (Otte et al. 1999; Waldherr et al. 2001; Paganelli et al. 2001; Eriksson et al. 2008; Waldherr et al. 2002; Kwekkeboom et al. 2003), except that by Baum et al. (2007) (360 patients) and the Rotterdam trial (380 patients) (Capello et al. 2003).

5 Conclusions

The results indicate that PRRT with the procedures and isotopes used is an effective and safe therapy option for patients with metastatic or inoperable neuroendocrine tumors.

Our results suggest that tandem therapy with ^{90}Y/^{177}Lu–DOTATATE provides longer overall survival time than single-isotope treatment.

Hematological toxicity was rare in all treated patients. Renal toxicity grade 3 and 4 was observed only in the group treated with ^{90}Y–DOTATATE.

However, more extensive studies with a larger number of patients in the same protocol are required to evaluate PFS and OS, and to establish the proportion of each isotope to be used in tandem therapy.

Acknowledgments Special thanks are due to all co-authors for their very good cooperation in data analysis.

Conflict of Interest The authors declare that they have no conflicts of interest.

References

Baum RP, Soldner J, Schmucking M, Niesen A (2004) Intravenous and intra-arterial peptide receptor radionuclide therapy (PRRT) using ^{90}Y-DOTA-TYR3-OCTREOTATE (^{90}Y DOTATATE) in patients with metastatic neuroendocrine tumors. Eur J Nucl Med Mol Imaging 31 (Suppl 2):S238

Baum RP, Wehrmann C, Zachert C et al (2007) Long-term results of peptide receptor radionuclide therapy (PRRT): 5-year follow-up of 1,150 courses in 360 patients with progressive, somatostatin receptor positive neuroendocrine tumors in one clinical center. J Nucl Med 48 (Suppl 2):37P

Behr TM, Goldenberg DM, Becker W (1998) Reducing the renal uptake of radiolabeled antibody fragments and peptides for diagnosis and therapy: present status, future prospects and limitations. Eur J Nucl Med 25:201–212

Bernhardt P, Forssell-Aronsson E, Jacobsson L et al (2001) Low-energy electron emitters for targeted radiotherapy of small tumours. Acta Oncol 40:602–608

Breeman WA, de Jong M, Kwekkeboom DJ et al (2001) Somatostatin receptormediated imaging and therapy: basic science, current knowledge, limitations and future perspectives. Eur J Nucl Med 28:1421–1429

Capello A, Krenning EP, Breeman WA et al (2003) Tyr^3-octreotide and Tyr^3-octreotate radiolabeled with ^{177}Lu or ^{90}Y: peptide receptor radionuclide therapy results in vitro. Cancer Biother Radiopharm 18:761–768

Chinol M, Bodei L, Cremonesi M et al (2002) Receptor-mediated radiotherapy with YDOTA-DPhe-Tyr-octreotide: the experience of the European Institute of Oncology Group. Semin Nucl Med 32:141–147

Cwikla JB, Sankowski A, Seklecka N et al (2010) Efficacy of radionuclide treatment DOTATATE Y-90 in patients with progressive metastatic gastroenteropancreatic neuroendocrine carcinomas (GEP-NETs): a phase II study. Ann Oncol 21:787–794

de Jong M, Breeman WA, Bernard BF et al (2001) [^{177}Lu-DOTA0, Tyr3] octreotate for somatostatin receptor-targeted radionuclide therapy. Int J Cancer 92:628–633

de Jong M, Bernard HF, Breeman WA et al (2002a) Combination of ^{90}Y- and ^{177}Lu- labeled somatostatin analogs is superior for radionuclide therapy compared to ^{90}Y- or ^{177}Lu-labeled analogs only. J Nucl Med 43:123P–124P

de Jong M, Valkema R, Jamar F et al (2002b) Somatostatin receptor-targeted radionuclide therapy of tumors: preclinical and clinical findings. Semin Nucl Med 32:133–140

de Jong M, Breeman WA, Valkema R, Bernard BF (2005) Krenning EP Combination radionuclide therapy using ^{177}Lu- and ^{90}Y-labeled somatostatin analogs. J Nucl Med 46(Suppl 1): 13S–17S

Eriksson B, Kloeppel G, Krenning EP et al (2008) Consensus guidelines for the management of patients with digestive neuroendocrine tumors—well differentiated jejunal–ileal tumor/ carcinoma. Neuroendocrinology 87:8–19

Jamar F, Barone R, Mathieu I et al (2003) ^{86}Y-$DOTA^0$-D-Phe^1-Tyr^3-octreotide (SMT487): a phase 1 clinical study—pharmacokinetics, biodistribution and renal protective effect of different regimens of amino acid co-infusion. Eur J Nucl Med Mol Imaging 30:510–518

Kloeppel G, Rindi G, Anlauf M et al (2007) Site-specific biology and pathology of gastroenteropancreatic neuroendocrine tumours. Virchows Arch 451:S9–S27

Kunikowska J, Królicki L et al (2005) Radioisotope therapy with somatostatin analogues in neuroendocrine tumours (case report)]. Endokrynol Pol 56:46–54

Kunikowska J, Królicki L, Hubalewska-Dydejczyk A, Mikołajczak R, Sowa-Staszczak A, Pawlak D (2011) Clinical results of radionuclide therapy of neuroendocrine tumours with (90)Y-DOTATATE and tandem (90)Y/(177)Lu-DOTATATE: which is a better therapy option? Eur J Nucl Med Mol Imaging 38:1788–1797

Kwekkeboom DJ, Bakker WH, Kam BL et al (2003) Treatment of patients with gastroentero-pancreatic (GEP) tumours with the novel radiolabelled somatostatin analogue [^{177}Lu-DOTA0, Tyr 3]octreotate. Eur J Nucl Med Mol Imaging 30:417–422

Kwekkeboom DJ, de Herder WW, Kam BL et al (2008) Treatment with the radiolabeled somatostatin analog [177Lu-DOTA0, Tyr3]octreotate: toxicity, efficacy, and survival. J Clin Oncol 26:2124–2130

Otte A, Herrmann R, Heppeler A et al (1999) Yttrium-90 DOTATOC: first clinical results. Eur J Nucl Med 26:1439–1447

Paganelli G, Zoboli S, Cremonesi M et al (2001) Receptor-mediated radiotherapy with ^{90}Y-DOTA-D-Phe1-Tyr3-octreotide. Eur J Nucl Med 28:426–431

Rolleman EJ, Valkema R, de Jong M et al (2003) Safe and effective inhibition of renal uptake of radiolabelled octreotide by a combination of lysine and arginine. Eur J Nucl Med Mol Imaging 30:9–15

Valkema R, Pauwels S, Kvols LK, Barone R, Jamar F, Bakker WH, Kwekkeboom DJ, Bouterfa H, Krenning EP (2006) Survival and response after peptide receptor radionuclide therapy with [^{90}Y-DOTA0, Tyr3]octreotide in patients with advanced gastroenteropancreatic neuroendocrine tumors. Semin Nucl Med 36:147–156

Waldherr C, Pless M, Maecke HR et al (2001) The clinical value of [^{90}Y-DOTA]-DPhe1-Tyr3-octreotide(90Y-DOTATOC) in the treatment of neuroendocrine tumors: a clinical phase II study. Ann Oncol 12:941–945

Waldherr C, Pless M, Maecke HR et al (2002) Tumor response and clinical benefit in neuroendocrine tumors after 7.4 GBq ^{90}Y-DOTATOC. J Nucl Med 43:610–616

PRRT as Neoadjuvant Treatment in NET

Anna Sowa-Staszczak, Alicja Hubalewska-Dydejczyk and Monika Tomaszuk

Abstract

This chapter describes the possibility of using peptide receptor radionuclide therapy (PRRT) as neoadjuvant treatment. PRRT is acknowledged to be a palliative treatment. Recently it has been reported that tumor size decrease followed by surgical intervention might be achieved in patients with neuroendocrine tumors (NETs) treated with somatostatin analogs labeled with beta emitters. Such outcome of therapy has been described in a relatively small group of patients. In those patients, the treatment enabled total or partial excision of the tumor, also with liver metastases. Reduction of tumor dimensions or total excision of the tumor corresponded with prolongation of overall survival. The discussed papers on this subject differ in details of treatment (utilization of various isotopes, total activity of the isotope, or combination with radiosensitizing chemotherapy). The chapter presents a brief review of recently published manuscripts.

Abbreviations

CT	Computed tomography
Ki index	Proliferation index

A. Sowa-Staszczak (✉) · A. Hubalewska-Dydejczyk · M. Tomaszuk
Department of Endocrinology, Jagiellonian University Medical College, ul. Kopernika 17, 31-501 Krakow, Poland
e-mail: sowiana@gmail.com

A. Hubalewska-Dydejczyk
e-mail: alahub@cm-uj.krakow.pl

M. Tomaszuk
e-mail: m.tomaszuk@gmail.com

R. P. Baum and F. Rösch (eds.), *Theranostics, Gallium-68, and Other Radionuclides*, Recent Results in Cancer Research 194, DOI: 10.1007/978-3-642-27994-2_27,

NET	Neuroendocrine tumor
PET/CT	Positron emission tomography/computed tomography
PNT	Pancreatic neuroendocrine tumor
PRRT	Peptide receptor radionuclide therapy
RECIST	Response evaluation criteria for solid tumors
SPECT-CT	Single-photon emission computed tomography
$T_{1/2}$	Physical half-life
5FU	5-Fluorouracil

Contents

1 Introduction

Recently, the subject of neuroendocrine tumors (NETs) has been widely discussed by different groups of specialists. We know that neuroendocrine tumors overexpress somatostatin receptors on their surface. This effect has become the molecular basis for the application of somatostatin analogs in diagnosis and therapy of these tumors. Unfortunately, in some cases, early diagnosis of NETs is impossible despite the availability of many different sophisticated imaging techniques, including SPECT-CT/PET-CT. As a consequence, proper evaluation of a patient's state is delayed. The diagnosis is often made when the disease is too advanced and distant metastases are present.

Currently, the only way to cure a patient with NET is radical surgery, enabling a prolonged time without progression of the disease. Unfortunately, when the tumor is too advanced, its total excision is generally impossible due to infiltration of other tissues and/or important blood vessels (Oberg et al. 2004). Recently, the benefit from tumor resection in patients with advanced malignant NETs has been described in the literature. The other therapeutic option in different malignant tumors is chemotherapy, but this kind of treatment has rather low efficacy in NETs. Other main problems with such systemic therapy are lack of selectivity and relatively high toxicity for healthy cells. Combined chemotherapy (e.g., cisplatin with etoposide) together with incomplete surgical eradication might be considered also in patients with disseminated disease (Sowa-Staszczak et al. 2011).

It has been shown for pancreatic neuroendocrine tumors that postoperative actuarial 5-year survival rates increase by 80% after extended tumor resection, even in patients with synchronous metastasis (Kaemmerer et al. 2009; Kazanjian et al. 2006). Aggressive surgical resection can be performed safely and may improve both symptomatic disease and overall survival (Kazanjian et al. 2006; Nomura et al. 2009). Therefore, treatment of patients with NETs should lead to surgical intervention.

To decrease tumor size, changing it from untreatable to removable and therefore enabling surgical intervention, neoadjuvant therapy is performed in different neoplasms. Also in NETs, neoadjuvant treatment might be helpful in decreasing tumor size to lead us to the point where an initially inoperable tumor becomes operable (Sowa-Staszczak et al. 2011). Systemic chemotherapy provides only modest benefit in down-sizing the tumor. Other therapies such as long-acting somatostatin analogs or interferon-alpha can decrease symptoms of the disease and lengthen time to tumor progression, but rarely result in objective tumor response (Rinke et al. 2009; Faiss et al. 2003). The advantage of targeted radionuclide therapy is its selective treatment effect due to the use of an appropriate ligand carrying the isotope directly to the malignant cell population. Peptide receptor radionuclide therapy (PRRT) is usually used as palliative treatment, but recently it has been reported that PRRT might be used as neoadjuvant treatment to decrease tumor size and enable surgical intervention. So far, only a few cases of utilization of PRRT to down-size the tumor have been described in literature.

2 Methods and Results

Two groups from Germany and one from Poland have described PRRT with use of somatostatin analogs labeled with yttrium-90 (^{90}Y) as neoadjuvant therapy. ^{90}Y (physical half-life $t_{1/2}$ of 64 h) is a pure beta emitter with maximum range of tissue irradiation of 10 mm. The high energy of this radioisotope (935 keV) is sufficient to achieve direct tumor effects. Due to the characteristics of ^{90}Y, the isotope seems to be better when used in PRRT as neoadjuvant treatment (Cremonesi et al. 2006).

Kaemmerer et al. (2009) described the case of a patient with pancreatic tumor (PNT) treated with PRRT. The patient was admitted to the hospital due to abdominal pain, flush attacks, and diarrhea. CT revealed enlarged paraaortic lymph nodes assessed on biopsy as metastasis of highly differentiated neuroendocrine carcinoma. Primary tumor in the head of pancreas (more than 2 cm in diameter) was found on exploratory laparotomy. At the beginning, the patient was qualified to biotherapy with somatostatin analogs, without any results. Based on the expression of somatostatin receptors as evaluated in PET/CT with gallium-68 (^{68}Ga), the patient received two cycles of PRRT during 4 months with total activity of 10.05 GBq. After two cycles, the abdominal lymph node metastases regressed significantly. After 4 months, the patient was operable, and pylorus-preserving pancreatoduodenectomy with en bloc resection of parts of the jejunum, as well as its mesenterium and lymph nodes, was performed. Tumor tissue infiltrated the surrounding pancreatic and intestinal tissues and also showed perineural infiltration. Results showed that 5–10% of tumor cells, which secreted glucagon and somatostatin, were negative for insulin, serotonin, and pancreatic polypeptide. The final stage was pT2 pN1 pM1(LYM). Repeated ^{68}Ga-DOTANOC PET/CT revealed complete remission.

Stoeltzing et al. (2010) also reported the case of a patient with pancreatic neuroendocrine tumor and concomitant multifocal hepatic lesions affecting both liver lobes. The patient had noncharacteristic symptoms 2 months before the admittance which initiated diagnostic procedures. Results of imaging studies led to the diagnosis of NET of pancreatic tail (5×3 cm^2) and multiple liver metastases (<5 cm). CT-guided needle biopsy of one of the hepatic lesions revealed moderately differentiated G2 NET. Based on SRS scan, PRRT with ^{90}Y-DOTATOC was performed. ^{90}Y-DOTATOC treatment was planned as neoadjuvant therapy for achieving potential resectability of liver metastases. The authors proposed a therapy concept based on staged surgery with first resection of the tumor, followed by ^{90}Y-DOTATOC treatment of liver metastases, and a second approach for potential surgical resection of remaining hepatic lesions. At the beginning, surgical excision of the primary tumor ($6 \times 5 \times 5$ cm^3) by extended left en bloc resection of the pancreatic tail was performed. Histopathological examination defined this tumor as a malignant epithelial tumor of the endocrine pancreas with 10 mitoses per 10 high-power fields, indicating well-differentiated NET. Vascular invasion was also detected. Eight weeks after surgery, the patient received two courses of ^{90}Y-DOTATOC with total activity of 28.9 GBq/m^2 (390 mCi/m^2) with an 8-week interruption between administrations. The PRRT resulted in impressive regression of hepatic lesions, thus facilitating surgical removal of all remaining liver metastases in a second operation. In addition, one lesion was ablated using radiofrequency ablation. On histopathological examination, metastases of NET corresponded to the resected primary lesion in the pancreatic tail. On immunohistochemical analysis, the tumor was negative for glucagons, insulin, somatostatin, gastrin, and serotonin. The proliferation rate of the primary tumor localized in the pancreatic tail was similar to the proliferation rate of liver metastases. However, these lesions elicited a slightly higher proliferating fraction (60%) than the ^{90}Y-DOTATOC-naive primary tumor in the pancreas (50%). One year after hepatic resection, no evidence of tumor recurrence or extrahepatic metastases was observed.

Our group used PRRT as neoadjuvant treatment (Sowa-Staszczak et al. 2011) in six patients: five with foregut tumors, including three with pancreatic NET (one with liver metastases), and one with midgut tumor. The Ki index in one patient with pancreatic NET was 20%, but we did not observe distant metastases in this case. In the other five patients, the Ki index was less than 10%. The patients received 7.4 GBq/m^2 of ^{90}Y-DOTATATE in 4–5 cycles every 6–9 weeks. After the treatment, partial response was observed in two patients. In one of them, only partial removal of the tumor was possible due to infiltration of large vessels. The patient was qualified to additional PRRT cycles with further reduction of tumor

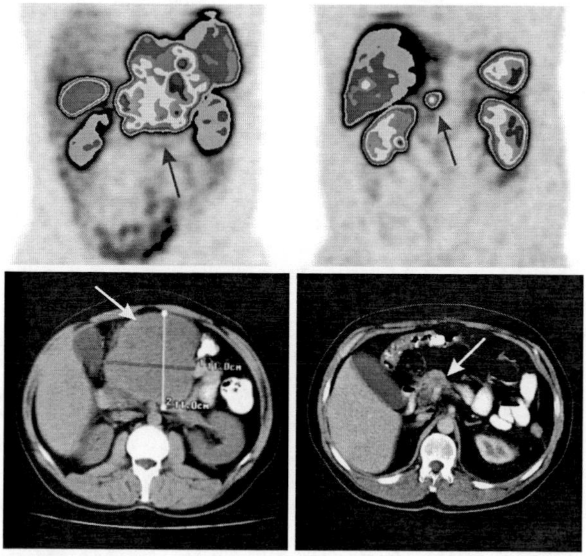

Fig. 1 ^{99m}Tc-EDDA/HYNIC-TOC SRS and CT before and after neoadjuvant therapy with PRRT in a patient with inoperable midgut tumor (male, 48 years old)

size, but it still remained inoperable (Fig. 1). The second patient with partial response after PRRT was qualified to surgery. In this patient, two lesions with pathological accumulation of tracer in liver disappeared after PRRT. The primary tumor decreased from 7.9 to 4.2 cm (Fig. 2). The remaining four cases were assessed as showing disease stabilization. It should be stressed that after PRRT not only the tumor size may change; we also observed attenuation changes, volume changes, and contrast enhancement changes in the course of treatment. According to RECIST, partial response requires a 30% decrease of the longest diameter of every measurable lesion, but sometimes other significant changes listed above can bear witness to the therapy response as a result of tumor tissue necrosis in NETs (Sowa-Staszczak et al. 2011).

A group from Australia (Barber et al. 2012) used ^{177}Lu-octreotate as neoadjuvant treatment. There were five patients, four with a primary nonfunctioning pancreatic neuroendocrine tumor and one with a locoregional recurrence of a duodenal tumor. Four patients had disease confined to local/locoregional sites, and one patient had also solitary liver metastases. Four patients with primary PNT were treated with four cycles of ^{177}Lu-DOTATATE with administered activity ranging from 7 to 10 GBq, at 6- to 8-week intervals. The subsequent three cycles of PRRT were administered with a concurrent radiosensitizing dose of infusional 5FU chemotherapy (200 mg/m^2/24 h) commencing 4 days prior and continuing for a total of 3 weeks. The remaining patient with a locoregional duodenal NET recurrence was treated with one cycle of ^{177}Lu-DOTATATE, which was

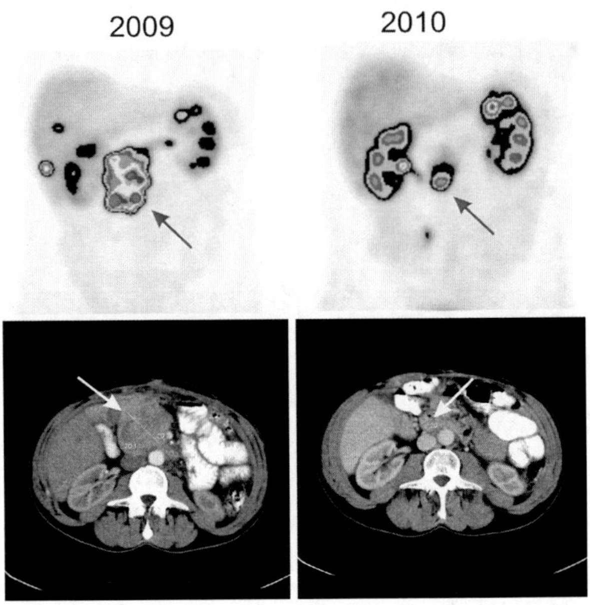

Fig. 2 ^{99m}Tc-EDDA/HYNIC-TOC SRS and CT before and after neoadjuvant therapy with PRRT in a patient with inoperable pancreatic NET (male, 56 years old)

administered 3 weeks prior to previously planned external-beam radiotherapy (45 Gy in 25 fractions) to maximize the radiation dose delivered to the tumor. The patient received also concurrent 5FU chemotherapy. At 3 months post treatment, all five patients had scintigraphic response, four had radiological response, and three of the four symptomatic patients responded clinically. All five patients had ongoing treatment response beyond 3 months, including the one whose further tumor shrinkage facilitated curative surgery (6 months after completion of treatment). Complete resection was performed subsequently. Histological examination demonstrated a Ki67 index of 5%, which was lower than in the biopsy before surgery. The patient with distant metastases had ongoing complete scintigraphic and radiological response of the solitary liver metastasis at 18-month follow-up. The remaining patients were deemed unsuitable for curative resection due to medical comorbidities (two patients), ongoing technical surgical difficulties (one patient), and patient choice (one patient).

3 Conclusion

These reports indicate the possibility of utilization of PRRT as neoadjuvant treatment. Most of the patients in those small groups suffered from pancreatic neuroendocrine tumors. The treatment may enable total or partial excision of the tumor, sometimes with liver metastases, despite diverse details of treatment such as different isotopes, total activity of the isotope, or combination with radiosensitizing chemotherapy. The treatment was safe, without significant hematological or renal toxicity. In cases where the tumor was still inoperable after PRRT or only partial response was assessed, the patients also had symptomatic response. Decreasing the tumor size or total excision of the tumor corresponded with prolongation of overall survival. The results of these studies suggest that PRRT may become the preferred approach for treatment of inoperable NETs. All authors stated that PRRT should be started early enough, before disease progression. All studies concluded that PRRT may be used as neoadjuvant treatment in patients with NETs.

References

Barber TW, Hofman MS, Thomson BN et al (2012) The potential for induction peptide receptor chemoradionuclide therapy to render inoperable pancreatic and duodenal neuroendocrine tumors resectable. Eur J Surg Oncol 38:64–71

Cremonesi M, Ferrari M, Bodei L et al (2006) Dosimetry in peptide radionuclide receptor therapy: a review. J Nucl Med 47:467–1475

Faiss S, Pape UF, Bohming M et al (2003) Prospective, randomized, multicenter trial on the antiproliferative effect of lanreotide, interferon alfa, and their combination for therapy of metastatic neuroendocrine gastroenteropancreatic tumors - the international lanreotide and interferon alfa study group. J Clin Oncol 21:2689–2696

Kaemmerer D, Prasad V, Daffner W et al (2009) Neoadjuvant peptide receptor radionuclide therapy for an inoperable neuroendocrine pancreatic tumor. World J Gastroenterol 15:5867–5870

Kazanjian KK, Reber HA, Hines OJ (2006) Resection of pancreatic neuroendocrine tumors: results of 70 cases. Arch Surg 141:765–769

Nomura N, Fujii T, Kanazumi N et al (2009) Nonfunctioning neuroendocrine pancreatic tumors: our experience and management. J Hepatobiliary Pancreat Surgery 16:639–647

Oberg K, Kvols L, Caplin M et al (2004) Consensus report on the use of somatostatin analogs for the management of neuroendocrine tumors of the gastroenteropancreatic system. Ann Oncol 15:966–973

Rinke A, Muller HH, Schade- Brittinger C et al (2009) Placebo-controlled, double-blind, prospective, randomized study on the effect of octreotide LAR in the control of tumor growth in patients with metastatic neuroendocrine midgut tumor: a report from the PROMID study group. J Clin Oncol 27:4656–4663

Sowa-Staszczak A, Pach D, Chrzan R et al (2011) Peptide receptor radionuclide therapy as a potential tool for neoadjuvant therapy in patients with inoperable neuroendocrine tumors (NETs). Eur J Nucl Med Mol Imaging 38:1669–1674

Stoeltzing O, Loss M, Huber M et al (2010) Staged surgery with neoadjuvant 90Y-DOTATOC therapy for down-sizing synchronous bilobular hepatic metastases from a neuroendocrine pancreatic tumor. Langenbecks Arch Surg 395:185–192

Intraoperative Somatostatin Receptor Detection After Peptide Receptor Radionuclide Therapy with ^{177}Lu- and ^{90}Y-DOTATOC (Tandem PRRNT) in a Patient with a Metastatic Neuroendocrine Tumor

Mila Todorović-Tirnanić, Daniel Kaemmerer, Vikas Prasad, Merten Hommann and Richard P. Baum

Abstract

Aim: The aim of this chapter is to present the results of the first intraoperative somatostatin receptor detection after peptide receptor radionuclide therapy (PRRNT) with ^{90}Y- and ^{177}Lu-DOTATOC using a handheld gamma probe and comparison with the findings of preoperative ^{68}Ga-DOTATOC PET/CT in a patient with a metastatic neuroendocrine tumor (NET) of the ileum. *Materials and Methods*: A 56-year-old female patient, treated twice by PRRNT, was admitted for the third cycle and subsequent surgery. Before operation, the following studies were performed for restaging after the second cycle of PRRNT: ^{99m}Tc-MAG3 + TER, ^{99m}Tc-DTPA + GFR, abdominal ultrasonography, MRI of the abdomen, ^{68}Ga-DOTATOC PET/CT as well as ^{18}F-fluoride PET/CT. Serum tumor markers were measured before and after PRRNT.

The first author was International Atomic Energy Agency (IAEA) fellow from February to April 2010 at the Department of Nuclear Medicine/PET Center, Zentralklinik Bad Berka when this work was prepared.

M. Todorović-Tirnanić
Center for Nuclear Medicine,
Clinical Center of Serbia and Faculty of Medicine,
University of Belgrade, Višegradska 26, 11000 Belgrade, Serbia
e-mail: t.t.mila@sezampro.rs

V. Prasad · R. P. Baum (✉)
Department of Nuclear Medicine, Center for P.E.T., Zentralklinik Bad Berka,
Robert-Koch-Allee 9, 99437 Bad Berka, Germany
e-mail: richard.baum@zentralklinik.de
URL: http://www.zentralklinik.de

D. Kaemmerer · M. Hommann
Department of General and Visceral Surgery,
Zentralklinik Bad Berka, Bad Berka, Germany

R. P. Baum and F. Rösch (eds.), *Theranostics, Gallium-68, and Other Radionuclides*,
Recent Results in Cancer Research 194, DOI: 10.1007/978-3-642-27994-2_28,

Tandem PRRNT was performed using 3000 MBq ^{90}Y-DOTATOC and 6000 MBq ^{177}Lu-DOTATOC. Whole-body scintigrams were obtained at 23 and 43 h. Five days after PRRNT, the patient was operated using a handheld gamma probe. Immunohistochemistry and histopathology of the resected tissue were performed. *Results*: Tandem PRRNT was very well tolerated by the patient. Before PRRNT, ^{68}Ga-DOTATOC PET/CT revealed the primary tumor in the ileocoecal region as well as bilobular liver metastases and a right iliac bone lesion (osteoblastic on ^{18}F-fluoride PET/CT). Compared with the previous findings, there was good therapy response (partial remission of the tumor lesions). No nephrotoxicity was observed. Serum chromogranin A (836 μg/l, $n < 100$) and serotonin (852 μg/l, $n < 200$) were strongly elevated. Posttherapy scans showed intense uptake in metastases and the primary tumor. Intraoperative gamma probe detected—in addition to the known lesions—bilateral ovarian metastases not visualized by ^{68}Ga-DOTATOC PET/CT. Bilateral adnexectomy, right hemicolectomy, excision of hepatic metastases in S3, and partial resection of peritoneum were performed. Histopathology confirmed metastases in both ovaries. *Conclusions*: Gamma probe-guided surgery after ^{177}Lu PRRNT is feasible and appears to be more sensitive than ^{68}Ga-DOTATOC PET/CT. This technique might aid the surgeon in achieving more complete tumor resection through intraoperative detection of very small lesions (<5 mm) directly after PRRNT.

Keywords

Intraoperative gamma probe detection • Peptide receptor radionuclide therapy (PRRNT) • Neuroendocrine tumor • Molecular imaging • ^{68}Ga-DOTATOC PET/CT

Abbreviations

PRRNT	Peptide receptor radionuclide therapy
GEP NET	Gastroenteropancreatic neuroendocrine tumor
MRI	Magnetic resonance imaging
CT	Computed tomography (X-ray)
SSTR	Somatostatin receptor
PET	Positron emission tomography
TER	Tubular extraction rate
GFR	Glomerular filtration rate
SUV	Standardized uptake value
S2, S3, S5, S7, S8	Liver segments

Contents

1 Introduction

Gastroenteropancreatic neuroendocrine tumors (GEP NETs) are rare neoplasms (2.5–5 cases per 100,000 inhabitants, 0.46% of all malignancies) that originate from the diffuse endocrine system of the gastrointestinal tract and the pancreas (Modlin et al. 2003). A wide spectrum of biologically active peptides is produced by NET cells (e.g., serotonin, gastrin, glucagon, and insulin) which are stored in vesicles, whose proteins (chromogranin A and synaptophysin) are common markers of GEP NETs (Wiedenmann et al. 1998).

The majority of GEP NETs express somatostatin receptors, five subgroups of which have been identified (all of them binding native somatostatin); however, they differ in their affinity for somatostatin analogs. In GEP NETs, somatostatin receptor 2 (SSTR2) is predominantly expressed, forming the basis for diagnostic application of radiolabeled somatostatin analogs such as ^{68}Ga-DOTATOC, ^{68}Ga-DOTANOC, ^{68}Ga-DOTATATE, etc. using SST receptor PET/CT, which has been proven to be the most sensitive of all imaging procedures.

Localization of ill-defined lesions in a scarred surgical field is facilitated by using intraoperative gamma probes (Gulec and Baum 2007). We speculated therefore that preoperative SSTR PET/CT, combined with an intraoperative handheld gamma probe approach, could increase the rate of successful surgical explorations, as it can identify very small lesions ($\leq$5 mm) with higher sensitivity than SSTR imaging alone (Adams et al. 1998; Adams and Baum 2000). We have shown already that intraoperative gamma probe exploration has 57% higher sensitivity as compared with manual exploration by the surgeon, and that additionally 36% of SSTR-positive lymph node metastases are detected by use of the intraoperative probe when compared with preoperative SSTR PET/CT (Kaemmerer et al. 2012). SSTR PET/CT combined with intraoperative gamma probe detection therefore improves the determination of disease extent, reduces the rate of negative laparotomies, and increases the rate of complete (R0) resections in surgical oncology.

Usually, detection of GEP NETs with a gamma probe is only possible when preoperative SSTR imaging demonstrates a lesion-to-background ratio of more than 1.5 (Gulec and Baum 2007).

In case of metastatic GEP NETs, cytoreductive therapeutic options are limited. A relatively new therapy approach is peptide receptor radionuclide therapy (PRRNT) with ^{90}Y- or ^{177}Lu-labeled somatostatin analogs.

Yttrium-90 PRRNT is thought to have better results when treating large tumors, while lutetium-177 PRRNT is commonly used for smaller lesions. The combination of ^{177}Lu- and ^{90}Y-labeled peptides (named by us tandem PRRNT) could be used in patients with both large and small metastatic deposits.

Lutetium-177 has a half-life of 6.7 days and emits beta and gamma radiation, allowing imaging and dosimetry after therapy (Kwekkeboom et al. 2008), while yttrium-90, as a pure beta emitter, does not allow proper imaging.

One factor predicting favorable treatment outcome with PRRNT is high uptake on the pretreatment SSTR imaging study. The benefit on overall survival from ^{177}Lu PRRNT ranges from 40 to 72 months (Kwekkeboom et al. 2008).

2 Materials and Methods

We present a 56-year-old female patient, presenting with a highly differentiated (grade G1) neuroendocrine neoplasm with bilobular liver metastases (overall 15 lesions up to 7 cm in diameter) with peritoneal involvement, who had already received two PRRNT cycles (10 GBq of ^{177}Lu-DOTATATE during the first cycle and 4 months later 8.3 GBq of ^{177}Lu-DOTATOC during the second PRRNT cycle).

The patient gained 5 kg after the second PRRNT and was admitted 4 months later for the third PRRNT cycle. Karnofsky index was 90%. The last subcutaneous injection of octreotide (Sandostatin 3 × 100 μg) had been given 3 months before the third cycle of PRRNT.

Examinations carried out on the first 2 days of hospitalization were blood chemistry, tumor markers (chromogranin A, serotonin), abdominal ultrasonography, ^{99m}Tc-MAG3 dynamic scintigraphy with TER calculation, SSTR PET/CT, abdominal MRI, GFR estimation using ^{99m}Tc-DTPA, and ^{18}F-fluoride PET/CT.

3 Results

^{68}Ga-DOTATOC PET/CT revealed bilobular, SSTR-positive liver metastases (target lesions were in segment S8 apical, S8 apicomedial/central, S2 medial, S5/S8/S7 with central necrosis, S4a, S3, S6 inferolateral, as described in Table 1). The primary tumor was detected in the ileocoecal region. A small SSTR-positive bone metastasis was present in the right iliac bone (Fig. 1). Uptake (SUV_{max}) in normal tissue was as follows: lung 1.0, liver 9.5, spleen 41.6, kidney 9.2, bone 2.1, gluteus muscle 1.4. Compared with the previous SSTR PET/CT results, the patient was found to have partial remission according to molecular imaging criteria (PERCIST).

Table 1 ^{68}Ga-DOTATOC PET/CT findings before the third, second, and first PRRNT cycle: site and standardized uptake values (SUV_{max}) of somatostatin receptor-positive target lesions

Site of SSTR-positive target lesions	Maximum SUV before PRRNT		
	Third	Second	First
Liver			
S8 apical	12.6	13.2	14.0
S8 apicomedial/central	11.0	14.0	12.2
S2 medial	13.7	15.2	12.9
S5/S8/S7 with central necrosis	16.6	18.1	16.8
S4a	11.6	14.0	12.2
S3	16.6	20.0	13,2
S6 inferolateral	16.2	18.4	15.2
Primary tumor			
Ileocoecal region	14.1	16.9	11.6
Iliac bone			
Right dorsal	8.0	10.8	–

Abdominal ultrasonography showed multiple focal hyperechogenic lesions in the steatotic liver, the largest being in segment S7 (7.4 cm × 6.7 cm in diameter) and in the left liver lobe with size of 2.3 × 1.9 cm. In the right lower abdomen, a hypoechogenic formation was found with diameter of 1.9 × 2.4 cm.

Kidney scintigraphy performed with ^{99m}Tc-MAG3 and tubular extraction rate (TER 219 ml/min, 82% of normal age-adjusted value, lower limit 186 ml/min) were normal and better than the initial value before first PRRNT. GFR (determined by using ^{99m}Tc-DTPA) was also normal (83 ml/min, 90% of normal age-adjusted value, lower limit 64 ml/min). Laboratory tests were unremarkable.

^{18}F-fluoride showed one osteoblastic metastasis in the right posterior iliac crest ($SUV_{max} = 21.1$) which was also SSTR positive.

Compared with the previous findings, MRI showed regression of liver metastases, particularly the largest ones located in S8 (maximum diameter 65 mm, previously 80 mm) and in S6 (downsized from 38 to 30 mm). Smaller liver metastases also showed regression (16 versus 20 mm).

Chromogranin A was elevated (770 μg/l, cutoff <100 μg/l), as was serotonin in serum (783 μg/l, normal range 40–200 μg/l).

The patient was treated intravenously with 3 GBq of ^{90}Y-DOTATOC and 6 GBq of ^{177}Lu-DOTATOC and tolerated the third PRRNT cycle very well. Whole-body scintigraphy was performed at 23 and 43 h after therapy using the gamma emission of ^{177}Lu (energy window set at 208 keV), and scintigraphic images showed very intense tumor uptake (Fig. 2).

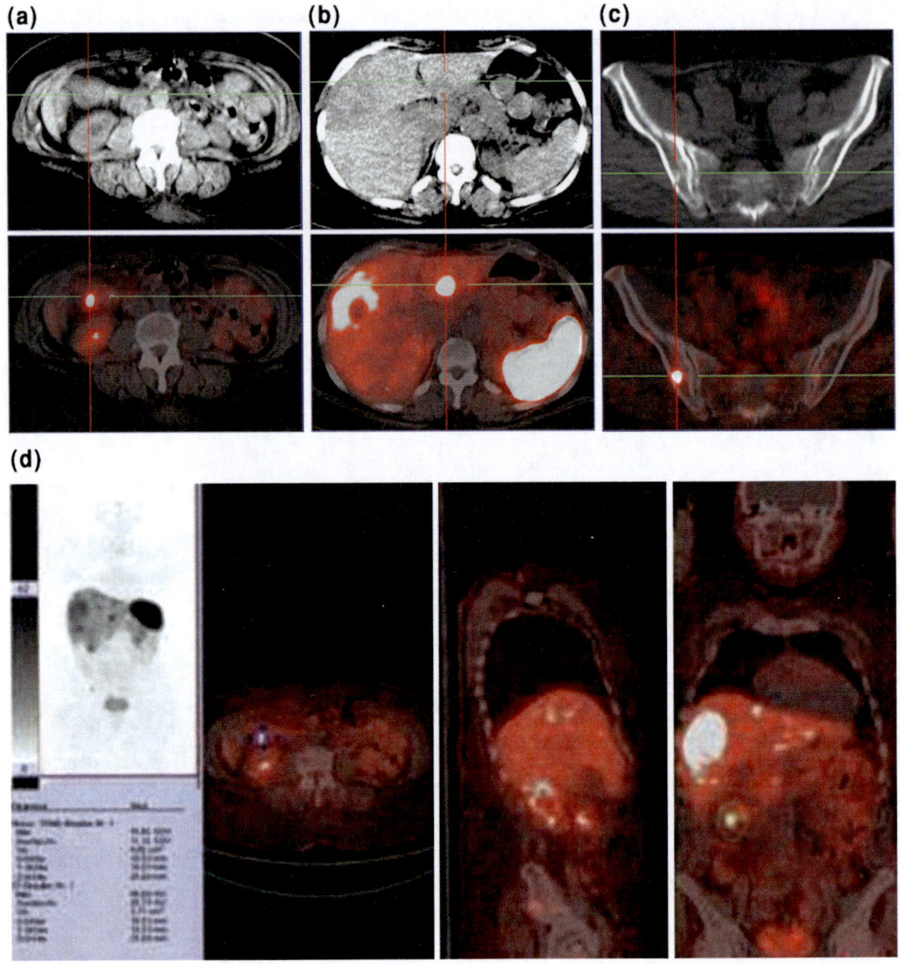

Fig. 1 ^{68}Ga-DOTATOC PET/CT showing the following somatostatin receptor-positive lesions: **a** primary tumor in the ileum (indicated by the *cross* on image "**a**" on transversal CT slice (*upper row*) and on fused PET/CT image (*lower row*); **b** in liver segment S3 (indicated by the *cross* on image "**b**" on transversal CT slice (*upper row*) and on fused PET/CT image (*lower row*); **c** in the posterior right iliac bone (indicated by the *cross* on image "**c**") on transversal CT slice (*upper row*), and on fused PET/CT image (*lower row*); **d** in the terminal ileum, primary tumor location (maximum-intensity projection, and fused transversal, sagittal, and coronal images)

Two days after PRRNT, the patient was transferred to the Department of General and Visceral Surgery, and operated 5 days after PRRNT using the intraoperative gamma probe (Tec Probe 2000). The probe consists of a cesium iodide crystal: 9.5 (diameter) × 15 mm (length), a photomultiplier (diameter 10 mm), and a collimator with aperture of 8 mm and length of 10 mm, and is connected to an electronic unit providing both visual and audible indication of the count rate (range 0–25,000 counts/s). The energy level was adjusted to the gamma

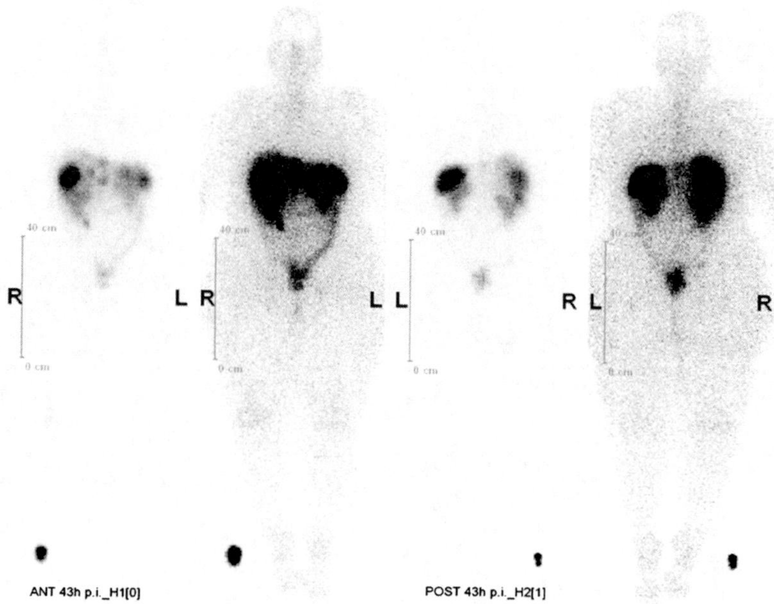

Fig. 2 Whole-body scans obtained 43 h after the third cycle of PRRNT using ^{177}Lu- and ^{90}Y-DOTATATE (double-intensity anterior and posterior projections) demonstrating intense somatostatin receptor binding of the therapeutic agent in the primary tumor and in the metastatic lesions in the liver as well as in the small metastasis in the right posterior iliac crest (faintly visible)

radiation energy of the ^{177}Lu (208 keV). Sterile latex covers, identical to those used for intraoperative ultrasound, were used to ensure sterility during surgery (Fig. 3). Results of intraoperative gamma probe measurements are presented in Table 2.

Tumor-to-background ratio was 2.0 for the primary tumor in the ileum and 3.7 for the liver metastases. Both values were higher than 1.5 (the lower limit for reliable detection of tumor lesions using the intraoperative gamma probe).

Besides the primary tumor and liver metastasis, bilateral ovarian metastases of the ileum NET were detected by the intraoperative gamma probe, which were previously not visualized by SSTR PET/CT, confirming the higher sensitivity of the probe as compared with PET/CT for lesions smaller than 5 mm.

The surgeons performed right hemicolectomy, excision of the hepatic S3 segment, bilateral adnexectomy, as well as partial peritoneal excision (Fig. 3). The absorbed dose that the surgeon received during the operation was 30.8 μSv in total.

Histopathological examination of the 8-cm-long resected segment of the ascending colon with coecum and an 8-cm-long segment of the terminal ileum was performed and revealed one centrally located NET in the mucosa at the ileocoecal

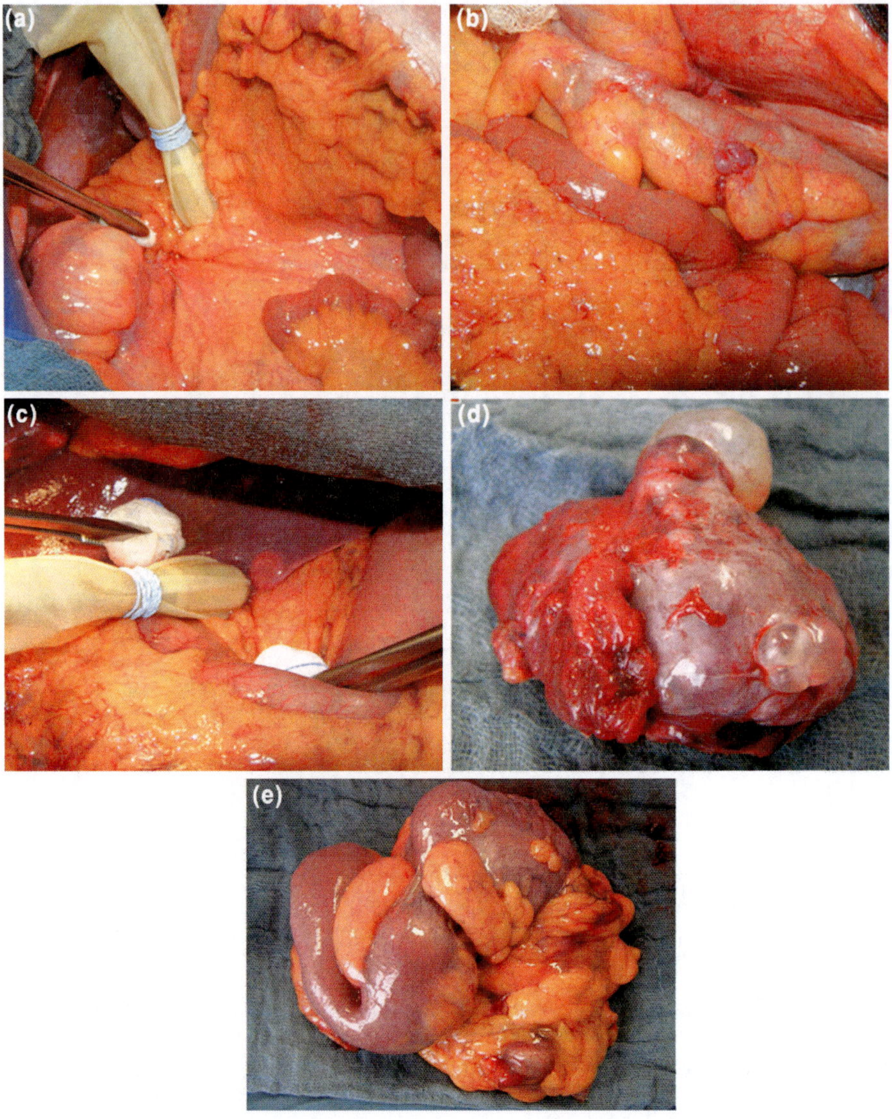

Fig. 3 **a** Intraoperative gamma probe in sterile latex cover directed towards the primary tumor in the ileum. **b** Peritoneal carcinosis in the sigmoidal region. **c** Intraoperative gamma probe in sterile latex cover pointing to a round-shaped liver metastasis. **d** Ovarian involvement with subperitoneal metastasis and coexisting benign serous cystadenoma. **e** Right hemicolon

region (Fig. 2). Immunohistochemical staining confirmed a NET with expression of chromogranin, synaptophysin, and SSTR2a in 90% of tumor cells. Proliferation rate (Ki-67/MIB-1) was low (1%) corresponding to highly differentiated NET (grade G1). Microscopic examination confirmed metastases of the neuroendocrine

Table 2 Intraoperative gamma probe measurement results

Gamma probe location	Radioactivity	
	Counts/s	Tumor/background
Liver (normal tissue)	135	–
Metastasis in the liver	500	3.7
Ileum (normal tissue)	72	–
Primary tumor in ileum	141	2.0
Right ovary	30	–
Left ovary	37	–

neoplasm in the region of the ileum and peritoneal metastases in both ovaries and the mesosalpinx (with coexisting benign serous cystadenoma). Peritoneal carcinosis was also found in the pelvic region.

Three days after operation, the chromogranin A level dropped from 836 (registered 1 day before operation) to 641 μg/l, and the serotonin value from 852 to 561 μg/l.

4 Discussion and Conclusions

Surgical resection is the most eminent curative treatment option for removing the primary tumor and extirpation of metastases; however, success of surgery heavily depends on the completeness of surgical excision. Therefore, it is very important to assess the exact location and extent of the primary tumor as well as of metastatic deposits. One of the locations of GEP NETs is the "gastrinoma triangle" (confluence of cystic duct, common hepatic duct, border of second and third portion of duodenum, and the neck of pancreas). Ectopic locations (the jejunum, stomach, mesentery, spleen, and ovaries) frequently result in failure of intraoperative localization (Gulec et al. 2002). It has been reported that negative laparotomies for small primary GEP NETs are as high as 30% (Sutton et al. 2003). Occult nodal metastasis may not be apparent during manual exploration. Recurrent metastatic disease poses additional problem to the surgeon. Due to the prior repeated explorations, the operative field may be obscured by scar tissue, which becomes a major problem in resecting small lymph nodes without breaching the vessels.

In surgically unresectable GEP NETs, neoadjuvant PRRNT is a novel approach for patients with SSTR-positive tumors, as first suggested and published by our group (Kaemmerer et al. 2009). This approach may be useful for down-staging of well-differentiated GEP NETs, thereby achieving a higher complete resection rate.

As reported here for the first time, the therapeutic activity of ^{177}Lu-DOTATOC administered for PRRNT can also be used for intraoperative gamma probe detection of neuroendocrine primary tumors and metastases. This technique, performed directly after PRRNT which is used to treat in addition nonresectable tumor deposits, appears to be more sensitive than ^{68}Ga-DOTATOC PET/CT alone for localization of lesions smaller than 5 mm and might aid the surgeon in finding the primary tumor more easily and achieving more complete tumor resection through intraoperative detection of small lesions of less than 5 mm.

References

Adams S, Baum RP (2000) Intraoperative use of gamma-detecting probes to localize neuroendocrine tumors. Q J Nucl Med 44:59–67

Adams S, Baum RP, Hertel A et al (1998) Intraoperative gamma probe detection of neuroendocrine tumors. J Nucl Med 39:1155–1160

Gulec SA, Baum RP (2007) Radio-guided surgery in neuroendocrine tumors. J Surg Oncol 96: 309–315

Gulec SA, Mountcastle TS, Frey D et al (2002) Cytoreductive surgery in patients with advanced stage carcinoid tumors. Am J Surg 68:667–671

Kaemmerer D, Prasad V, Daffner W et al (2009) Neoadjuvant peptide receptor radionuclide therapy for an inoperable neuroendocrine pancreatic tumor. World J Gastroenterol 46: 5867–5870

Kaemmerer D, Prasad V, Daffner W, Haugvik SP, Senftleben S, Baum RP, Hommann M (2012) Radioguided surgery in neuroendocrine tumours using Ga-68 labeled somatostatin analogues—a pilot study. Clin Nucl Med 37(2):142–147

Kwekkeboom DJ, De Herder WW, Kam BL et al (2008) Treatment with the radiolabelled somatostatin analog [^{177}Lu-DOTA^{0}, Tyr^{3}] octreotate: toxicity, efficacy, and survival. J Clin Oncol 26:2124–2130

Modlin IM, Lye KD, Kidd M (2003) A 5-decade analysis of 13,715 carcinoid tumors. Cancer 97:934–959

Sutton R, Doran HE, Williams EM et al (2003) Surgery for midgut carcinoid. Endocr Relat Cancer 10:469–481

Wiedenmann B, John M, Ahnert-Hilger G et al (1998) Molecular and cell biological aspects of neuroendocrine tumors of the gastroenteropancreatic system. J Mol Med 76:637–647

Personalized Image-Based Radiation Dosimetry for Routine Clinical Use in Peptide Receptor Radionuclide Therapy: Pretherapy Experience

Anna Celler, Joshua Grimes, Sergey Shcherbinin, Hanna Piwowarska-Bilska and Bozena Birkenfeld

Abstract

Patient-specific dose calculations are not routinely performed for targeted radionuclide therapy procedures, partly because they are time consuming and challenging to perform. However, it is becoming widely recognized that a personalized dosimetry approach can help plan treatment and improve understanding of the dose–response relationship. In this chapter, we review the procedures and essential elements of an accurate internal dose calculation and propose a simplified approach that is aimed to be practical for use in a busy nuclear medicine department.

Contents

A. Celler · J. Grimes · S. Shcherbinin
Medical Imaging Research Group, University of British Columbia, Vancouver Coastal Health Research Institute, 828 West 10th Avenue, Vancouver, BC V5Z 1M9, Canada

H. Piwowarska-Bilska · B. Birkenfeld (✉)
Department of Nuclear Medicine, Pomeranian Medical University, ul. Unii Lubelskiej 1, 71-252 Szczecin, Poland
e-mail: birka@pum.edu.pl

R. P. Baum and F. Rösch (eds.), *Theranostics, Gallium-68, and Other Radionuclides*,
Recent Results in Cancer Research 194, DOI: 10.1007/978-3-642-27994-2_29,

1 Introduction

Targeted radionuclide therapy (TRT) is the systemic administration of radiopharmaceuticals that are designed to specifically target tumor tissue (Williams et al. 2008). There are several benefits to this approach, which potentially allows for radiation dose to be delivered directly to tumors, while avoiding irradiation of healthy organs. Furthermore, in addition to already identified tumor sites, the radiopharmaceutical's affinity to a given receptor type allows it to target other, undiagnosed tumors that are expressing the same receptors and may be located anywhere in the body. An important advantage of TRT over other systemic treatments, such as chemotherapy, is the possibility to perform a pretreatment imaging study to plan patient-specific treatment, optimize the dose to be administered, and predict the effectiveness of the therapy for a given patient.

One of the most important applications of TRT is treatment of neuroendocrine tumors (NET) (van Essen et al. 2009; Nicolas et al. 2011). Since NETs have been shown to overexpress somatostatin receptors (SSTR), molecular imaging with radiolabeled somatostatin analogs has become widely used for staging and characterization of NET disease. In parallel, SSTR overexpression in NETs has been exploited for peptide receptor radionuclide therapy (PRRT) using particle-emitting radionuclides. Recent clinical studies, performed mostly in European centers, have reported very encouraging results of PRRT, with survival benefit of 40–72 months compared with historical controls (Kwekkeboom et al. 2008) as well as significant quality of life and symptom improvements (Khan et al. 2011). Unfortunately, there is large interpatient variability in treatment results and cure remains rare.

It is widely recognized that the large differences between individual patient responses to treatment may be related to the lack of patient-specific therapy planning, which should be based on accurate and personalized dose calculations (Brans et al. 2007; Cremonesi et al. 2010). Regrettably, in contrast to external-beam therapies, patient-specific treatment plans and dosimetry calculations are not routinely performed for TRT. Instead, administered activities follow the "one-size-fits-all" approach, constrained by the toxicity limits to critical organs. These are always low, as they are designed to not exceed dose estimates that are generally accepted to be associated with a 5% risk of complications with external-beam radiation therapy (EBRT) (Emami et al. 1991). However, due to the large interpatient variability in radiopharmaceutical uptake in both tumors and normal organs (Cremonesi et al. 2010; Bodei et al. 2008), many patients are not receiving the optimum activity for their specific case and are often underdosed.

This chapter discusses issues related to the methodology that is required for the development of a personalized image-based TRT dosimetry approach. The discussions are supplemented by the results from our phantom experiments and patient studies. Although the reported results are based on the analysis of studies performed with the diagnostic radioisotope ^{99m}Tc (diagnostic scans with ^{99m}Tc-HYNIC-Tyr^3-octreotide) (Grimes et al. 2011), our aim is to develop and optimize an image-based method that will allow us to perform personalized dose calculations for PRRT with therapeutic agents such as ^{177}Lu-octreotide. Although the techniques that would be necessary to achieve fully quantitative results are quite elaborate, our objective is to create a simple and practical method for pretherapeutic determination of the most appropriate treatment doses as well as for posttherapy dosimetry. Therefore, when analyzing the sophisticated and accurate approaches, we studied the relative contributions of different elements of the method to the accuracy of the final "product," with the objective to create a substantially simplified method, ready for routine clinical use in a busy nuclear medicine (NM) department.

2 Challenges in Patient-Specific Dosimetry for Radionuclide Therapy

One reason that is often given for not performing patient-specific dose calculations in current practice is the absence of a clear dose–response relationship in patients treated with radiopharmaceuticals. However, recent studies that employed more rigorous and patient-specific dosimetry calculations than conventionally used methods have demonstrated strong dose–response relationships (Pauwels et al. 2005; Wehrmann et al. 2007; Dewaraja et al. 2010). Similar studies must be performed in order to investigate the relationship between delivered doses and toxicity in normal (critical) organs.

Another reason for the lack of patient-specific considerations is that accurate dose calculations can be quite time consuming and difficult to perform. They must be based on imaging studies, as the absorbed radiation dose delivered to tissues depends on the fraction of administered activity that will accumulate and be subsequently retained in or cleared from the tissue (biodistribution). This fraction depends on the radiopharmaceutical kinetics and tissue properties, both of which are subject to many patient-specific factors that result in interpatient variability (often high) of the absorbed radiation dose per unit of administered activity. Personalized TRT dosimetry has to take all of these patient-related variables into account. Additionally, it must consider physics-related factors such as the type (particles or gammas) and the energy of radioactive emissions.

The main challenge in TRT dosimetry is to accurately determine the distribution of the injected radiopharmaceutical in different tissues. In principle, this information should be obtained from NM imaging studies prior to administration of the therapeutic radioactivity. This, however, would require the existence of molecular analogs that could be labeled with imaging isotopes that have biological behavior identical to the therapeutic agents (Rufini et al. 2006; Bombardieri et al. 2010; Ambrosini et al. 2010), and imaging methods allowing for quantitatively accurate determination of their biodistributions. Unfortunately, such radiopharmaceuticals are not readily available for patient studies. Additionally, quantitative NM imaging is technically difficult and currently not routinely performed in clinics (Chowdhury and Scarsbrook 2008). As a result, dose calculations commonly used in clinical studies suffer from several limitations, leading to large uncertainties (Garkavij et al. 2010).

In general, imaging studies use surrogate radiotracers which have biodistributions that only to a certain degree reflect those of the therapeutic agent (Brans et al. 2007; Pauwels et al. 2005; Rufini et al. 2006). In addition, the physical half-lives of many imaging radioisotopes (e.g., ^{99m}Tc and ^{68}Ga) are too short for meaningful biodistribution studies compared with longer-lived therapeutic radionuclides such as ^{90}Y or ^{177}Lu. Alternatively, dosimetry calculations based on posttherapy images have been proposed (Cremonesi et al. 2010). Unfortunately, most TRT procedures rely on ^{90}Y that only emits beta particles (electrons), which have a relatively short range in tissue and high "killing power" but cannot be directly imaged. The beta particle interactions with tissues result in bremsstrahlung (BRS) radiation, which potentially can be used to create images (Shen et al. 1994). These, however, have extremely poor resolution and cannot be easily translated into dose estimates, although some promising results have recently been reported when advanced data processing methods were applied (Minarik et al. 2010).

On the other hand, radiotracers such as ^{177}Lu and ^{188}Re, besides beta emissions, also emit gammas with energies that are appropriate for imaging with a standard gamma camera. Due to the presence of beta particles, these gamma lines are still accompanied by a strong BRS background, thus quantitative measurement of the activity distribution is not easy and requires advanced signal processing and corrections (Shcherbinin et al. 2011; Beauregard et al. 2011).

While dose estimates for tumors and organs (such as kidneys), with volumes of the order of several cubic centimeters, can rely on activity measurements from SPECT studies, the same approach cannot be applied to bone marrow due to its distribution in the body. However, methods have been described for estimating the red marrow absorbed dose from the activity measured in blood samples or from the total body dose (Siegel 2005; Stabin et al. 2011). This approach assumes that there is no specific uptake of radiotracer in the bone marrow, which has been shown to be the case for PRRT with ^{177}Lu-octreotate (Forrer et al. 2009).

3 General Concepts in Internal Dosimetry

The radiation absorbed dose is defined as the amount of energy deposited per unit mass. Thus, to estimate the dose, one must first specify the mass of the object of interest (m_{T}), the activity contained in that object, as well as the activity in the surrounding regions. The frequency (n) and energy (E) of each radiation type (i) emitted per nuclear decay of the administered radionuclide must also be known. Furthermore, a quantity referred to as the absorbed fraction (φ) is needed, which represents the fraction of energy emitted from the source (r_{S}) that is deposited in the target (r_{T}). These factors can be combined to form a generic equation for calculating the absorbed dose:

$$D(r_{\mathrm{T}} \leftarrow r_{\mathrm{S}}) = \tilde{A}(r_{\mathrm{S}}) \sum_i \frac{n_i E_i \varphi_i (r_{\mathrm{T}} \leftarrow r_{\mathrm{S}})}{m_{\mathrm{T}}}, \tag{1}$$

where $\tilde{A}(r_{\mathrm{S}})$ is the cumulated activity (total number of nuclear decays integrated over a time period measured from injection to infinity) of the source. This general equation for calculating the absorbed dose can be simplified using the Medical Internal Radiation Dose (MIRD) system, in which the dose to the target summed over all source regions is given by:

$$D(r_{\mathrm{T}}) = \sum_{r_{\mathrm{S}}} \tilde{A}(r_{\mathrm{S}}) S(r_{\mathrm{T}} \leftarrow r_{\mathrm{S}}), \tag{2}$$

where the S value, $S(r_{\mathrm{T}} \leftarrow r_{\mathrm{S}})$, represents the mean absorbed dose deposited in the target per unit of cumulated activity that is present in the source. Usually, S values at the organ level are employed, in which case these values are precalculated for reference phantoms representing average patients of given age and gender. One more quantity of interest that is utilized within the MIRD schema is the time-integrated activity coefficient $\tilde{a}(r_{\mathrm{S}})$, which is the cumulated activity in the source per unit of administered activity [traditionally, $\tilde{a}(r_{\mathrm{S}})$ was known as the residence time].

Additionally, to improve our understanding of the dose–response relationship, radiobiological information can be incorporated into TRT planning. This approach would allow us to better predict and account for radiation effects and toxicity. It is a well-established principle in EBRT that a given total dose, when delivered using different fractionation schemes, can result in different biological effects (Dale 1996). In radionuclide therapy, the absorbed dose rate depends on the amount and the type of the injected radionuclide. Furthermore, due to physical decay and biological elimination of the radiotracer, tissues are irradiated with a dose rate that decreases exponentially over time. The implications of these varying dose rates can be modeled using the biological effective dose (BED), which employs knowledge about radiosensitivity and repair rate for a given tissue type to predict total absorbed doses delivered at different dose rates.

Another relevant factor to consider is the spatial distribution of absorbed doses, which in TRT is typically more heterogeneous than in other forms of radiotherapy. Analogous to the BED model for comparing the effects of different dose rates, different spatial dose distributions can be compared using the equivalent uniform dose (EUD) (O'Donoghue 1999). As its name suggests, the EUD translates the heterogeneous 3D dose distribution into a uniform absorbed dose that would be expected to lead to the same biologic effects as the actual dose distribution.

4 Key Elements of Internal Dose Calculations

The procedure for performing patient-specific internal dose calculations can be broken down into several steps. First, a series of NM scans (planar and/or SPECT) must be acquired. Then, the planar and/or reconstructed SPECT images are analyzed to obtain volume and activity estimates of source regions of interest (ROI) inside the patient. Following this analysis, the cumulated activity in each ROI is determined and used to form the dose estimate. To complete each of these steps, dedicated software providing the necessary image analysis and dosimetry tools is required.

4.1 Imaging Protocol

A series of NM images are needed to identify source regions and to estimate cumulated activities in these regions. This is traditionally done using conjugate view analysis in which cumulated activities in source regions are estimated using a 2D imaging protocol (Matthay et al. 2001; Wiseman et al. 2003; Fisher et al. 2009). Simplified methods to correct for attenuation, scatter, and organ overlap in 2D images are then employed (Siegel et al. 1999). Using these approximate corrections, source activity data can be plotted versus time to generate the time–activity curve (TAC) for each of the regions and/or organs. Time-integrated activity coefficients are obtained through integration of the area under these TACs, divided by the injected activity.

The limitations of using a processing method based purely on planar studies have been explored, and large discrepancies between 2D and more advanced fully 3D approaches have been reported in simulations (He et al. 2008) and patient studies (Assie et al. 2008). These discrepancies can be attributed to the fact that in 2D studies it is impossible to properly compensate for organ overlap, attenuation, and scatter. Furthermore, dosimetry estimates based on 2D approaches usually do not consider patient-specific organ masses, instead using reference values based on the average patient. Given the inverse dependence of absorbed dose on mass, dose calculations that consider individual patient masses can vary considerably compared with calculations based on standard organ masses (Rajendran et al. 2004).

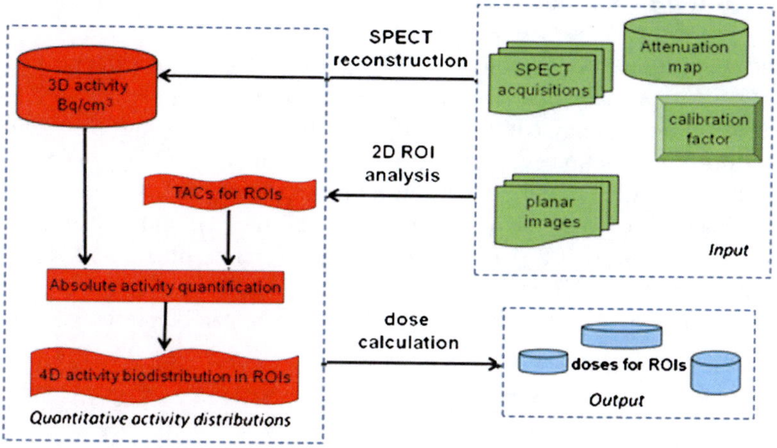

Fig. 1 Flowchart depicting general framework of hybrid planar/SPECT approach

To increase the accuracy of cumulated activity estimates for different areas in the body, hybrid planar/SPECT techniques have been proposed (Koral et al. 1994, 2000). In this approach (Fig. 1), the temporal changes in radiotracer concentration, represented by the TAC, are determined from a coregistered series of 2D whole-body (WB) images acquired over several hours or even days after radiotracer injection. Additionally, a single SPECT or SPECT/CT scan is acquired over the main area of interest to provide quantitation for this activity. The data acquired with any standard hybrid SPECT/CT camera allows the user to compensate for attenuation, creating images representing the 3D semiquantitative distribution of the radiotracer in the body. However, to obtain truly quantitative images, corrections for other effects (most importantly scatter, dead-time, and partial-volume effects) must be implemented (Shcherbinin et al. 2011; Beauregard et al. 2011). The resulting quantitative SPECT-based absolute activity measures can then be applied to rescale the TACs to obtain absolute values of time-integrated activity coefficients that are necessary for dosimetry calculations. The hybrid planar/SPECT method has been shown to perform much better than a purely planar approach, providing nearly the same accuracy as a purely SPECT-based method for estimating residence times (He et al. 2008, 2009).

The accuracy of the hybrid planar/SPECT technique makes it an attractive option for use as part of a practical dosimetry method for clinical use. In many clinics, a combination of planar and SPECT/CT scans are already acquired as part of the routine diagnostic procedure. There is a need for careful design of the imaging protocol to keep data acquisition acceptable for the patients and to limit the clinical burden in busy NM departments, while still acquiring all necessary temporal information.

4.2 Image Reconstruction

Although the filtered backprojection (FBP) algorithm is still extensively used in clinical studies, it does not reconstruct quantitative images. This is because FBP cannot accommodate any patient-specific quantitative corrections as it allows only for uniform attenuation correction with the Chang method. Therefore, for dosimetry calculations, more advanced iterative algorithms must be employed.

For advanced reconstruction of SPECT images, the maximum-likelihood expectation-maximization (MLEM), or its accelerated version, ordered-subsets expectation-maximization (OSEM) (Hudson and Larkin 1994), reconstruction algorithms are the most widely utilized. The iterative MLEM scheme can be presented as follows:

$$X_k^{(n-1)} \quad \Rightarrow \quad P_i^{(n-1)} = \sum_k C_{ik} X_k^{(n-1)} \quad \Rightarrow \quad X_j^{(n)} = \frac{X_j^{(n-1)}}{\sum_i C_{ij}} \sum_i C_{ij} \frac{Y_i}{P_i^{(n-1)}}, \qquad (3)$$

where $X_k^{(n)}$ is the image value generated in the kth voxel at the nth iteration, Y_i is the number of counts recorded in the ith pixel of the detector, $P_i^{(n)}$ is the number of counts in the ith pixel estimated in the projection of the image at the nth iteration, and C is the predetermined matrix formalizing the acquisition process for a particular imaging system (system matrix). In detail, the matrix element C_{ij} corresponds to the probability that a photon emitted from the jth voxel is recorded in the ith pixel. A system matrix that accurately models acquisition allows for calculation of realistic projections of the image, P. Furthermore, the consistency between the experimental Y_i and computed $P_i^{(n-1)}$ projections generally leads to improvement in the image estimate $X^{(n)}$, as the ratios $\frac{Y_i}{P_i^{(n-1)}}$ are included in Eq. 3.

To translate the reconstructed image $X^{(n)}$ to the distribution of activity expressed in absolute units (Bq or Ci), it must be multiplied by the camera sensitivity factor, which should be determined experimentally using a planar scan of a small point source.

The OSEM-based reconstructions that are currently used in clinics aim mostly at providing medical personnel with diagnostic rather than quantitatively accurate images. So, only a limited number of corrections for image-degrading factors (attenuation and, to some extent, detector response and scatter) are implemented into clinical OSEM algorithms. Therefore, in order to extract an absolute activity distribution from a standard SPECT scan, advanced data processing with more sophisticated corrections would be required. As recognized in the NM community (He et al. 2005; Du et al. 2006; Dewaraja et al. 2006; Ljungberg and Sjogreen-Gleisner 2011), attenuation correction, patient-specific modeling of scattered photons, and 3D resolution recovery must be incorporated. Additionally, the main photopeak photons for some radiotracers are accompanied by emissions of a different nature. Correspondingly, the acquired data are contaminated and additional corrections must be applied before reliable absolute quantification can be achieved; For example, when processing SPECT studies acquired with ^{123}I and ^{131}I, the collimator septal penetration of high-energy photons must be accounted for. For imaging therapeutic isotopes, such as ^{177}Lu or ^{188}Re, correction for the BRS component must be included into the reconstruction algorithm (Eq. 3).

Aiming to develop a quantitatively accurate, yet relatively simple and practical SPECT reconstruction, we pursue a "hybrid" tactic when adapting the standard OSEM reconstruction algorithm for dosimetry applications, with some corrections implemented directly into the system matrix and some included only in the projection step. First, we include a CT-based attenuation map and a 3D Gaussian model of the resolution loss into the system matrix C. Second, we acquire data in an additional energy window set above the main photopeak to estimate emissions corresponding to high-energy septal penetration and/or BRS. This simple approach allows us to avoid complex and time-consuming modeling of interactions of photons with the detector and collimator, and requires only minimal changes to the standard clinical protocols. Third, we accurately model the scatter component based on a standard clinical image and patient-specific CT-based density map (Vandervoort et al. 2005; Shcherbinin et al. 2008). Then, the combined corrections for scatter, BRS, and septal penetration are added in the denominator of Eq. 3 to the projections to get a more realistic estimate of P. Additionally, the final images obtained from this reconstruction can be corrected for the partial-volume effect (PVE) (Shcherbinin and Celler 2011).

To summarize, besides attenuation correction (which is now considered standard), we introduce additional corrections and build them into the reconstruction algorithm. Some of these corrections are based on measured rather than modeled data, in order to bypass time-consuming computations. However, the effects which may be critical for reconstructing the activity distribution in tumors (corrections for scatter and PVE) are modeled accurately.

Finally, injection of large therapeutic activities results in substantial dead-time and pulse pile-up effects in the camera. Furthermore, as count rates change during camera rotation (caused by different depths of tumors leading to different BRS components and attenuation effects), the dead-time may also vary. Therefore, if a therapeutic rather than diagnostic dose is injected, a dead-time correction (Beauregard et al. 2011; Koral et al. 1998; Delpon et al. 2002; Hobbs et al. 2010) must be performed. This correction should be determined from a time series of measurements of count-rate losses using phantom experiments containing insert(s) with high activities. The derived relationship between injected activity and detected counts is employed for correction of the reconstructed image.

4.3 Segmentation of Nuclear Medicine Images

The determination of total radiation absorbed dose in an ROI requires information about the activity accumulated in this region and its mass. Therefore, image segmentation is a crucial next step in the internal dose calculation process, as it is used to determine both region volume and activity. Since a CT scan is often acquired at the time of the SPECT acquisition, volumes of interest can be drawn manually on CT slices. Alternatively, organs and tumors may be segmented from SPECT images manually or by use of thresholds, which are defined as a percentage of the maximum number of counts inside a volume of interest. Use of thresholds ranging from 25% to 70% have been reported, while fixed thresholds set at around 40% of the maximum counts are most commonly employed (Erdi et al. 1995; Biehl et al. 2006). The problem with using a fixed threshold value is that the optimum threshold for volume determination depends on many factors such as the relative source-to-background activity, object size, and the reconstruction algorithm (Mut et al. 1988; Fleming and Alaamer 1998; Daisne et al. 2003). A more robust option is to use an adaptive threshold where the threshold value is calculated based on the source-to-background ratio (SBR), and different formulations with and without the need for a priori volume estimates from CT have been described (Daisne et al. 2003; Erdi et al. 1997).

To apply the adaptive threshold technique, a calibration phantom experiment must first be performed to obtain a threshold–SBR curve. This threshold–SBR curve relates the optimal threshold for segmentation of the object of interest to the measured SBR of that object. In the past, adaptive thresholds applied in this way have only been focused on exact volume estimates of organs and tumors. However, the total activity inside volumes segmented with this threshold will often underestimate the true activity because some activity will have spilled out of the object in the reconstructed image due to the partial-volume effect.

To correct for this problem, we recently proposed a modified adaptive threshold technique that utilizes two adaptive thresholds for each ROI (Grimes et al. 2011). The first threshold is employed in the standard way to estimate the volume of the object, while the second threshold is used to recover the true activity of the object.

A drawback of current adaptive threshold methods is that the background is typically defined using a manually selected region. This process can be tedious and may result in inconsistent results. To deal with this issue, we are currently working to further modify the adaptive threshold method so that the background is selected semi-automatically using an iterative approach.

4.4 Dose Calculation Method

Once the time-integrated activity coefficients for each ROI are determined, the corresponding dose distribution can be calculated. These calculations are most often performed using the OLINDA/EXM software, which calculates the total dose at the organ level (Stabin et al. 2005). Using OLINDA/EXM, the user inputs organ time-integrated activity coefficients and the program calculates the resulting absorbed dose for each organ, where the dose is assumed to be uniformly distributed throughout the organ volume. These doses are estimated based on the absorbed fractions calculated for standard phantoms representing the average male or female, so they are not patient specific. However, OLINDA/EXM allows the user to apply correction factors to account for individual patient organ masses.

Tumor doses are approximated using precalculated absorbed fractions to unit-density spheres of different sizes filled with uniform activity.

More advanced methods, such as the MIRD voxel S value approach and different Monte Carlo-based techniques, provide much better accuracy, but are currently used mostly in research studies (Bolch et al. 1999). As both of these methods use patient-specific information in their dose calculations, they constitute an important step towards personalized dosimetry.

The voxel S value approach uses lookup tables for absorbed dose fractions in a target voxel due to radiation emitted from a single source voxel. Unlike OLINDA/EXM, this method considers activity distributions at the voxel level (rather than at the organ level), and calculates the corresponding voxelized dose distribution. The drawback of this technique is that the lookup tables are calculated for a source material of uniform density and do not account for tissue inhomogeneities. The advantage of using voxel S values is that calculations are simple and fast.

Monte Carlo techniques involve the simulation of radioactive emissions, which are propagated through the body, and a dose distribution at the voxel level is determined. As a result, the computational times that they require are often substantial. Reconstructed SPECT images provide quantitative information about the activity distribution, and CT data are used to account for patient-specific anatomy and tissue density distributions. Monte Carlo simulation is the most robust method for dose estimation, but its use may be quite complicated, and as mentioned, it suffers from the drawback of long computation times. An example Monte Carlo code commonly used for radiotherapy applications is EGSnrc, which is accompanied by the user code DOSXYZnrc (Strigari et al. 2006).

It should be noted that, when estimating dose distributions using voxel S values or one of the Monte Carlo programs, one does not need to segment images, as the entire activity and tissue density distributions are used in calculations. However, in order to extract the total or mean dose for an organ or an ROI, segmentation of the dose distribution would be required, and thresholding methods analogous to those used for estimating total organ activity from an image could be used.

4.5 Software Tools for Dosimetry Calculations

As the discussion presented in the previous sections indicates, image-based dosimetry calculations require processing of a large body of data. To organize this data and to perform each of the steps necessary for dose estimation requires the use of various software tools. Currently, there is a lack of a generally accepted program that would be able to assist the user through the entire dose calculation process. Most existing software packages (e.g., Gardin et al. 2003; Glatting et al. 2005; Visser et al. 2007; Loudos et al. 2009) have limited functions and either do not provide enough tools to perform all of the necessary steps from image analysis to determination of time-integrated activity coefficients, to calculation of final dose estimates, or contain only specific tools that do not give enough versatility to account for different dosimetry protocols used in different centers. The need for a

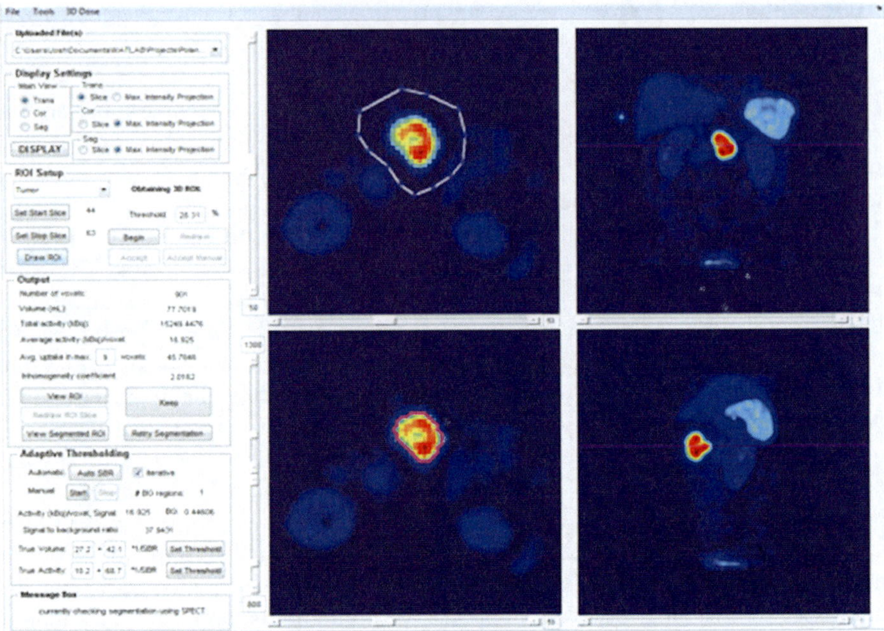

Fig. 2 GUI screenshot demonstrating how reconstructed SPECT images are analyzed. The user draws regions slice by slice in the *top left* window, with a choice of using a transaxial, coronal, or sagittal view. The remaining two views are displayed in the *top right* and *bottom* windows, which are used to check the slice position. The resulting segmented region (obtained, for example, by using the adaptive threshold method) is delineated in the *lower left* window

comprehensive yet versatile software package is particularly acute in busy clinics with limited time and programming skills, where the existence of a single program that could perform all of these tasks would encourage clinicians to perform dosimetry calculations for each individual patient.

We have developed a prototype of such a program. Our graphical user interface (GUI) is programed in MATLAB and features a single software environment for performing all steps in the dose calculation process. In particular, it provides options for considering different acquisition protocols (only planar scans or only SPECT scans or a hybrid planar/SPECT protocol). Additionally, it allows the user to coregister a series of images, perform image segmentation, and finally calculate the doses using one of three different dosimetry methods (OLINDA/EXM, voxel S values, or Monte Carlo). A screenshot of one window from this GUI is provided in Fig. 2, which shows an example of how the SPECT data are analyzed.

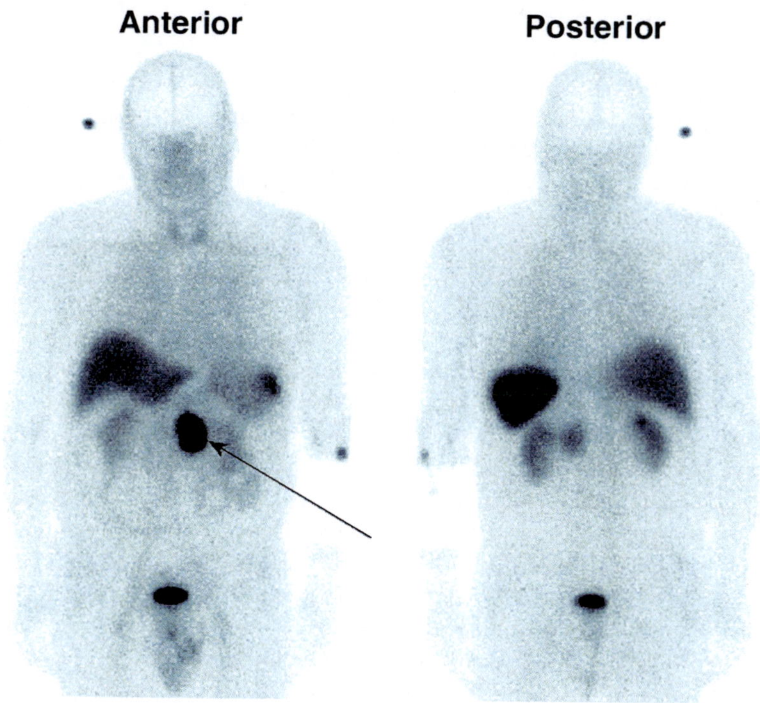

Fig. 3 Anterior and posterior views from a whole-body scan acquired at 2 h after injection, showing a neuroendocrine tumor in the small bowel

5 Clinical Implementation of the Proposed Dose Calculation Technique

As previously discussed, in order for patient-specific TRT treatment planning to be employed in routine clinical practice, a dose assessment technique that is simple and practical is needed. To address this need, we have implemented in our institution a patient-specific dose calculation approach that uses a hybrid planar/SPECT method combined with the adaptive thresholding technique for determination of volumes and activities in source regions of interest.

With the aim to optimize the parameters of different elements of the technique, the data from 45 patient studies were entered into this study, which was approved by the Ethics Review Board at our institution (Pomeranian Medical University). These 45 patients (23 males, 22 females) with median age of 57 years (range 7–78 years) were referred to our clinic for a diagnostic NET scan. Additionally, a number of phantom experiments were performed. These phantom experiments were used for normalization of the camera, calibration of the adaptive threshold technique, and investigation of BRS and camera dead-time effects.

5.1 Patient Image Acquisition

All patient scans were acquired using a dual-head Infinia Hawkeye 4 camera (GE Healthcare). For each patient, multiple (2–5) WB planar scans and one SPECT/CT scan were acquired over a period of 1–24 h following injection of 450–1,000 MBq of the somatostatin analog, ^{99m}Tc-HYNIC-Tyr^{3}-octreotide (Tektrotyd, IAE POLATOM, Poland).

The following imaging protocol was used: The WB anterior and posterior views used 256 × 1,024 matrixes with pixel size of 2.21 mm and scan speed of 20 cm/min. For quality control in all planar studies, a small ^{99m}Tc point source (marker) was placed beside the patient within the field of view (FOV) of the camera. An example WB scan of a patient with a NET in the small bowel is provided in Fig. 3.

For the SPECT scans, 60 projections were acquired over 360° with a noncircular orbit. All SPECT scans used high-resolution 128 × 128 projection matrixes with pixel size of 4.42 mm and 20 s per stop. The low-dose CT (Hawkeye) was used to create attenuation maps and, in a few cases, to determine organ boundaries.

Unfortunately, 11 patients from this group followed only a single-day protocol and therefore did not receive a 24-h WB scan. Additionally, the SPECT/CT scans for six patients did not include complete tumors or critical organs (kidney) in the FOV of the camera. Due to these deficiencies, both groups of patients had to be eliminated from consideration, leaving 28 patients in the study. This experience demonstrates the need for careful timing of the WB scans to ensure that all of the temporal information necessary for TAC determination is acquired, and the need for meticulous patient positioning during SPECT/CT imaging.

A general recommendation is to acquire scans over a time period covering at least three effective half-lives of the radiopharmaceutical (Stabin 2003), while the number of scans should be minimized for practical reasons. When analyzing our results, we found that for dosimetry studies with ^{99m}Tc-Tektrotyd, the following protocol is both practical and sufficient: Three WB scans should be performed at 2–3 and 4–6 h (to determine the shape of the rapid washout region of the TAC) and at 24 h (to determine the long-term retention behavior), and one SPECT/CT at 2–4 h to acquire sufficient count statistics for accurate quantification. Obviously, this protocol needs to be modified when another radionuclide with a different effective half-life is used.

5.2 Phantom Experiments to Calibrate Parameters for the Adaptive Threshold Technique

Volumes and activities were obtained from the SPECT images using our adaptive threshold technique. The calibration phantom SPECT/CT experiment, performed to obtain the threshold–SBR curves, consisted of 20 bottles varying in size from 12 to 200 mL. These bottles were filled with ^{99m}Tc activity concentrations ranging from 20 to 200 kBq and then placed inside large cylindrical phantoms filled with active water so that SBRs in the range of 2–10 could be modeled. These data were

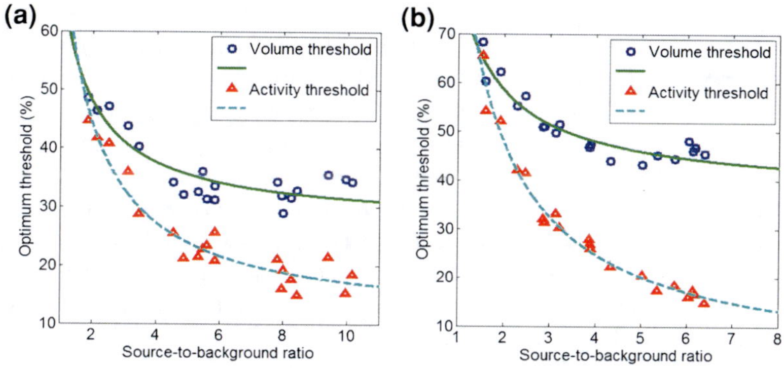

Fig. 4 Adaptive threshold curves relating optimal threshold for recovery of true volume and activity to the source-to-background ratio (SBR): **a** volume and activity threshold–SBR curves for the advanced reconstruction; **b** volume and activity threshold–SBR curves for the clinical reconstruction

reconstructed using two different reconstruction methods. The first method was a typical clinical reconstruction with attenuation correction. The second (advanced) reconstruction method featured resolution recovery, attenuation, and analytical scatter correction. For each bottle, the optimal threshold that recovered its true volume and activity was determined.

These optimal thresholds were plotted versus the measured SBR for each bottle (Fig. 4) for each of the reconstruction methods. This was done to assess how the complexity of the reconstruction method affected the accuracy of the final dose estimates obtained.

A second phantom experiment was performed to check the accuracy of the adaptive threshold method and the results of the calibration phantom curve fit. This validation phantom was also processed with the clinical and advanced reconstruction algorithms, and the corresponding adaptive thresholds were applied to estimate the volumes and activities of bottles placed in the phantom. On average, for both reconstruction methods, the estimated volumes and activities agreed within 4% of the known true values. This test demonstrated consistency of the results for the adaptive threshold technique, providing that the curve parameters are calibrated using the same reconstruction method as the one used for reconstruction of the analyzed data. This finding has important implications for the analysis of the patient studies.

5.3 Data Processing

For analysis of the patient data we used our GUI to perform each step of the hybrid planar/SPECT technique. First, the WB scans were used to determine the shape of the TACs. To accomplish this, 2D regions were manually drawn in the first WB scan around tumors and organs with significant uptake, which included the kidneys, liver, spleen, and in some cases the thyroid. These regions were drawn so that they included the tumor or organ of interest as well as some surrounding background.

Next, a 50% threshold of the maximum counts was applied inside each oversized region to define the boundaries of each object. These segmented regions were then manually registered to corresponding regions in the remaining WB scans.

To validate this approach, we tested the relationship between the threshold value that was used for this 2D analysis of a series of WB images and the shape of the TAC. Since cumulative activity is directly proportional to the integral of the area under the TAC curve, this area was considered to be a figure of merit in these tests. We found that, when the threshold was varied from 25% to 75%, the curve shape remained almost unchanged, and the area under the curve varied by only 1–2%. Based on these results, a relatively arbitrary threshold value of 50% was selected for use in TAC shape determination.

The geometric mean of count rates from the anterior and posterior views was multiplied by a background correction factor for each region of interest (Siegel et al. 1999). TACs were then obtained by fitting monoexponential functions through the background-corrected count rates, which were plotted versus time. Attenuation correction was not applied to the planar data since activity quantification was achieved using the SPECT/CT data.

Volumes and activities necessary for TAC normalization and subsequent dosimetry calculations were obtained from the 3D SPECT images using the adaptive threshold technique. In each case, these volumes and activities were determined from SPECT images reconstructed with the clinical and advanced methods, which were the same reconstruction algorithms used to obtain threshold–SBR curves in the calibration phantom experiment. SBRs were measured for each organ and tumor in the patient images. The measured SBRs were then related to the optimal thresholds for volume and activity determination based on the results from the calibration phantom experiment. For each SBR and reconstruction method the corresponding thresholds were read from the appropriate curve (Fig. 4). Finally, for each region, the TAC obtained from the WB analysis was normalized to pass through the absolute activity determined from the SPECT image at the time of the SPECT acquisition.

The final output from the GUI after performing each of these steps was the time-integrated activity coefficients (area under the TACs) for tumors and organs and the patient-specific masses for each of these regions. These values were used as inputs for the dose calculation with the OLINDA/EXM software.

5.4 Dosimetry Results

A sample of volume, activity, and dose estimates from three patients enrolled in this study is displayed in Table 1. For each region in Table 1, the estimates made from both reconstruction methods are displayed. Similar to the results obtained earlier in the phantom experiment performed to validate our adaptive threshold technique, the volumes, activities, and doses estimated from the clinical and advanced reconstruction methods agreed within 5%, on average. The agreement in doses between the two reconstruction algorithms was even slightly better than the

Table 1 Comparison of volume, activity, and dose estimates using clinical and advanced reconstruction methods from three patient studies

		Volume (mL)		Activity (MBq)		Dose (mSv/MBq)	
Patient	Region	Clinical	Advanced	Clinical	Advanced	Clinical	Advanced
1	Kidneys	461	421	29.0	27.9	1.96×10^{-2}	2.03×10^{-2}
	Liver	2,509	2,537	73.9	66.9	1.28×10^{-2}	1.15×10^{-2}
	Spleen	416	433	49.4	49.7	3.57×10^{-2}	3.46×10^{-2}
2	Kidneys	213	207	30.8	29.9	2.94×10^{-2}	2.92×10^{-2}
	Liver	1,442	1,503	61.3	59.6	1.23×10^{-2}	1.15×10^{-2}
	Spleen	127	132	13.3	13.6	2.28×10^{-2}	2.23×10^{-2}
	Tumor	23	23	2.0	1.8	1.45×10^{-2}	1.32×10^{-2}
3	Kidneys	311	296	16.3	15.5	1.61×10^{-2}	1.61×10^{-2}
	Liver	1,375	1,429	47.7	45.4	1.36×10^{-2}	1.25×10^{-2}
	Spleen	323	339	29.1	30.2	2.73×10^{-2}	2.71×10^{-2}
	Tumor	73	78	16.4	17.2	5.28×10^{-2}	5.25×10^{-2}
Average % difference (± SD)		4.3 ± 2.1%		4.7 ± 3.3%		4.2 ± 3.9%	

agreement in volumes and activities. This was probably due to the fact that, in many instances where the volume was overestimated in one reconstruction relative to the other, the activity was overestimated as well. Similarly, when the volume was underestimated, the activity was often underestimated too.

Based on all 28 patients in the study, the spleen received the highest average dose after injection with ^{99m}Tc-Tektrotyd. The average doses to the spleen, kidneys, and liver were 0.030, 0.021, and 0.012 mGy/MBq, respectively. Individual tumor doses were found to spread over a very wide range from 0.003 to 0.053 mGy/MBq.

The intrapatient ratio of tumor-to-kidney dose observed in this study ranged from 0.13 to 2.9. This disparity between patients is an indication of the importance of taking patient-specific biokinetics into consideration both for selecting suitable candidates for PRRT and for planning the therapeutic activities to administer.

5.5 Therapy

A subgroup of five patients with confirmed NETs is currently enrolled into PRRT using ^{177}Lu-octreotide. After each therapy cycle a series of WB scans and a SPECT/CT quantitative scan will be performed. Although for the initial, protocol optimization phase, more scans are being proposed (4–7 scanning sessions over a period of up to 10 days post PRRT), these numbers will be reduced once the minimal requirements for TAC measurement are determined. The proposed hybrid planar/SPECT dosimetry protocol will be employed. The results of these studies will be reported in a future publication.

Table 2 Summary of methods used for conventional and sophisticated dose calculations compared with the proposed patient-specific approach for practical clinical use

	Conventional	Advanced method for research use	Patient-specific approach for practical clinical use
Image protocol	Multiple planar scans	Multiple SPECT or hybrid planar/SPECT scans	Hybrid planar/ SPECT scans
Image reconstruction	(No SPECT)	Sophisticated SPECT image reconstruction	SPECT reconstruction using algorithms available on the camera
Image segmentation	Tumors/organs manually delineated in a series of planar images. Standard organ masses assumed	All kinds of sophisticated segmentation methods, often combining SPECT and CT images	Volumes and activities estimated using adaptive threshold approach
Dose calculation	OLINDA dose estimate	OLINDA, voxel S values, Monte Carlo dose estimate	OLINDA, voxel S values

6 Conclusions

In our effort to create a simple, practical, yet accurate method for personalized image-based dosimetry calculation for routine clinical use, we investigated all of the required elements of the procedure. Their relative contributions to the final dose estimate were evaluated, and in some situations, a simplified alternative version was proposed. A comprehensive GUI encompassing all elements of the dosimetry calculation, while giving the user substantial freedom to select the most appropriate approach, was developed. Table 2 summarizes and compares the conventional and sophisticated dose calculation methods discussed in this chapter.

The method was applied to and validated on 45 diagnostic patient studies performed with ^{99m}Tc-Tektrotyd. At the next stage, the developed protocols will be used for dosimetry calculation in therapy studies performed with ^{177}Lu, a beta+gamma-emitting isotope.

Based on our experience we expect that, when moving to this next stage, besides the obvious changes to the timing schedule of the scans, only a small adaptation of the protocol will be required. This will include acquiring data in two additional energy windows set above the two ^{177}Lu photopeaks, and including this information in the reconstruction. The modification to the algorithm to include correction for BRS and septal penetration based on the information acquired from these windows was discussed in Sect. 4.2. Additionally, a phantom experiment will be required to determine the dead-time of the camera. The necessary normalization factor will be included in the data scaling. New parameters for the adaptive threshold–SBR curve will have to be determined experimentally with the phantom data reconstructed with this new algorithm.

Although implementation of all elements of the dosimetry procedure, even in the proposed simplified version, will require some effort and a few calibration phantom studies, we believe that this effort is certainly worth doing as it will benefit the patients and contribute to better understanding of the disease and treatment.

References

Ambrosini V, Tomassetti P, Franchi R, Fanti S (2010) Imaging of NETs with PET radiopharmaceuti cals. Q J Nucl Med Mol Imaging 54:16–23

Assie K, Dieudonne A, Gardin I, Buvat I, Tilly H, Vera P (2008) Comparison between 2D and 3D dosimetry protocols in 90Y-ibritumomab tiuxetan radioimmunotherapy of patients with non-Hodgkin's lymphoma. Cancer Biother Radiopharm 23:53–64

Beauregard JM, Hofman MS, Pereira JM, Eu P, Hicks RJ (2011) Quantitative (177)Lu SPECT (QSPECT) imaging using a commercially available SPECT/CT system. Cancer Imaging 11:56–66

Biehl KJ, Kong F, Dehdashti F et al (2006) 18F-FDG PET definition of gross tumor volume for radiotherapy of non-small cell lung cancer: is a single standardized uptake value threshold approach appropriate? J Nucl Med 47:1808–1812

Bodei L, Cremonesi M, Ferrari M et al (2008) Long-term evaluation of renal toxicity after peptide receptor radionuclide therapy with 90Y-DOTATOC and 177Lu-DOTATATE: the role of associated risk factors. Eur J Nucl Med Mol Imaging 35:1847–1856

Bolch WE, Bouchet LG, Robertson JS et al (1999) MIRD pamphlet No. 17: the dosimetry of nonuniform activity distributions–radionuclide S values at the voxel level. J Nucl Med 40:11S–36S

Bombardieri E, Coliva A, Maccauro M et al (2010) Imaging of neuroendocrine tumours with gamma-emitting radiopharmaceuticals. Q J Nucl Med Mol Imaging 54:3–15

Brans B, Bodei L, Giammarile F et al (2007) Clinical radionuclide therapy dosimetry: the quest for the "Holy Gray". Eur J Nucl Med Mol Imaging 34:772–786

Chowdhury FU, Scarsbrook AF (2008) The role of hybrid SPECT-CT in oncology: current and emerging clinical applications. Clin Radiol 63:241–251

Cremonesi M, Botta F, Di Dia A et al (2010) Dosimetry for treatment with radiolabelled somatostatin analogues. A review. Q J Nucl Med Mol Imaging 54:37–51

Daisne J, Sibomana M, Bol A, Doumont T, Lonneux M, Grégoire V (2003) Tri-dimensional automatic segmentation of PET volumes based on measured source-to-background ratios: influence of reconstruction algorithms. Radiother Oncol 69:247–250

Dale RG (1996) Dose-rate effects in targeted radiotherapy. Phys Med Biol 41:1871–1884

Delpon G, Ferrer L, Lisbona A, Bardies M (2002) Correction of count losses due to deadtime on a DST-XLi (SmVi-GE) camera during dosimetric studies in patients injected with iodine-131. Phys Med Biol 47:N79–N90

Dewaraja YK, Ljungberg M, Fessler JA (2006) 3-D Monte carlo-based scatter compensation in quantitative I-131 SPECT reconstruction. IEEE Trans Nucl Sci 53:181

Dewaraja YK, Schipper MJ, Roberson PL et al (2010) 131I-tositumomab radioimmunotherapy: initial tumor dose-response results using 3-dimensional dosimetry including radiobiologic modeling. J Nucl Med 51:1155–1162

Du Y, Tsui BM, Frey EC (2006) Model-based compensation for quantitative 123I brain SPECT imaging. Phys Med Biol 51:1269–1282

Emami B, Lyman J, Brown A et al (1991) Tolerance of normal tissue to therapeutic irradiation. Int J Radiat Oncol Biol Phys 21:109–122

Erdi YE, Wessels BW, Loew MH, Erdi AK (1995) Threshold estimation in single photon emission computed tomography and planar imaging for clinical radioimmunotherapy. Cancer Res 55:5823s–5826s

Erdi YE, Mawlawi O, Larson SM et al (1997) Segmentation of lung lesion volume by adaptive positron emission tomography image thresholding. Cancer 80:2505–2509

Fisher DR, Shen S, Meredith RF (2009) MIRD Dose estimate report no. 20: radiation absorbed-dose estimates for 111In- and 90Y-Ibritumomab Tiuxetan. J Nucl Med 50:644–652
Fleming JS, Alaamer AS (1998) A rule based method for context sensitive threshold segmentation in SPECT using simulation. Phys Med Biol Med 43:2309
Forrer F, Krenning EP, Kooij PP et al (2009) Bone marrow dosimetry in peptide receptor radionuclide therapy with [177Lu-DOTA(0), Tyr(3)]octreotate. Eur J Nucl Med Mol Imaging 36:1138–1146
Gardin I, Bouchet LG, Assie K et al (2003) Voxeldose: a computer program for 3-D dose calculation in therapeutic nuclear medicine. Cancer Biother Radiopharm 18:109–115
Garkavij M, Nickel M, Sjogreen-Gleisner K et al (2010) 177Lu-[DOTA0, Tyr3] octreotate therapy in patients with disseminated neuroendocrine tumors: Analysis of dosimetry with impact on future therapeutic strategy. Cancer 116:1084–1092
Glatting G, Landmann M, Kull T et al (2005) Internal radionuclide therapy: the ULMDOS software for treatment planning. Med Phys 32:2399–2405
Grimes J, Celler A, Birkenfeld B et al (2011) Patient-Specific Radiation Dosimetry of 99mTc-HYNIC-Tyr3-Octreotide in Neuroendocrine Tumors. J Nucl Med 52:1474–1481
He B, Du Y, Song X, Segars WP, Frey EC (2005) A Monte Carlo and physical phantom evaluation of quantitative In-111 SPECT. Phys Med Biol 50:4169–4185
He B, Wahl RL, Du Y et al (2008) Comparison of residence time estimation methods for radioimmunotherapy dosimetry and treatment planning—Monte Carlo simulation studies. IEEE Trans Med Imaging 27:521–530
He B, Wahl RL, Sgouros G, Du Y, Jacene H, Kasecamp WR (2009) Comparison of organ residence time estimation methods for radioimmunotherapy dosimetry and treatment planning-patient studies. Med Phys 36:1595–1601
Hobbs RF, Baechler S, Senthamizhchelvan S et al (2010) A gamma camera count rate saturation correction method for whole-body planar imaging. Phys Med Biol 55:817–831
Hudson HM, Larkin RS (1994) Accelerated image reconstruction using ordered subsets of projection data. IEEE Trans Med Imaging 13:601–609
Khan S, Krenning EP, van Essen M, Kam BL, Teunissen JJ, Kwekkeboom DJ (2011) Quality of Life in 265 Patients with Gastroenteropancreatic or Bronchial Neuroendocrine Tumors Treated with [177Lu-DOTA0, Tyr3]Octreotate. J Nucl Med 52:1361–1368
Koral KF, Zasadny KR, Kessler ML et al (1994) CT-SPECT Fusion plus conjugate views for determining dosimetry in lodine-131-Monoclonal antibody therapy of lymphoma patients. J Nucl Med 35:1714–1720
Koral KF, Zasadny KR, Ackermann RJ, Ficaro EP (1998) Deadtime correction for two multihead Anger cameras in 131I dual-energy-window-acquisition mode. Med Phys 25:85–91
Koral KF, Dewaraja Y, Li J et al (2000) Initial results for hybrid SPECT-conjugate-view tumor dosimetry in 131I-Anti-B1 antibody therapy of previously untreated patients with Lymphoma. J Nucl Med 41:1579–1586
Kwekkeboom DJ, de Herder WW, Kam BL et al (2008) Treatment with the radiolabeled somatostatin analog [177 Lu-DOTA 0, Tyr3]octreotate: toxicity, efficacy, and survival. J Clin Oncol 26:2124–2130
Ljungberg M, Sjogreen-Gleisner K (2011) The accuracy of absorbed dose estimates in tumours determined by quantitative SPECT: a Monte Carlo study. Acta Oncol 50:981–989
Loudos G, Tsougos I, Boukis S et al (2009) A radionuclide dosimetry toolkit based on material-specific Monte Carlo dose kernels. Nucl Med Commun 30:504–512
Matthay KK, Panina C, Huberty J et al (2001) Correlation of tumor and whole-body dosimetry with tumor response and toxicity in refractory neuroblastoma treated with 131I-MIBG. J Nucl Med 42:1713–1721
Minarik D, Sjogreen-Gleisner K, Linden O et al (2010) 90Y Bremsstrahlung imaging for absorbed-dose assessment in high-dose radioimmunotherapy. J Nucl Med 51:1974–1978
Mut F, Glickman S, Marciano D, Hawkins RA (1988) Optimum processing protocols for volume determination of the liver and spleen from SPECT imaging with technetium-99m sulfur colloid. J Nucl Med 29:1768–1775

Nicolas G, Giovacchini G, Muller-Brand J, Forrer F (2011) Targeted radiotherapy with radiolabeled somatostatin analogs. Endocrinol Metab Clin North Am 40:187–204, ix–x

O'Donoghue JA (1999) Implications of nonuniform tumor doses for radioimmunotherapy. J Nucl Med 40:1337–1341

Pauwels S, Barone R, Walrand S et al (2005) Practical dosimetry of peptide receptor radionuclide therapy with (90)Y-labeled somatostatin analogs. J Nucl Med 46(Suppl 1):92S–98S

Rajendran JG, Fisher DR, Gopal AK, Durack LD, Press OW, Eary JF (2004) High-dose 131I-Tositumomab (Anti-CD20) radioimmunotherapy for Non-Hodgkin's lymphoma: adjusting radiation absorbed dose to actual organ volumes. J Nucl Med 45:1059–1064

Rufini V, Calcagni ML, Baum RP (2006) Imaging of neuroendocrine tumors. Semin Nucl Med 36:228–247

Shcherbinin S, Celler A, Belhocine T, Vanderwerf R, Driedger A (2008) Accuracy of quantitative reconstructions in SPECT/CT imaging. Phys Med Biol 53:4595

Shcherbinin S, Celler A (2011) Assessment of the severity of partial volume effects and the performance of two template-based correction methods in a SPECT/CT phantom experiment. Phys Med Biol 56(16):5355–5371

Shcherbinin S, Piwowarska-Bilska H, Grimes J et al (2011) Quantitative SPECT reconstructions for combined Lu-177/Y-90 radionuclide therapy: phantom experiments [abstract]. J Nucl Med 52(Suppl 1):1745

Shen S, DeNardo GL, Yuan A, DeNardo DA, DeNardo SJ (1994) Planar gamma camera imaging and quantitation of yttrium-90 bremsstrahlung. J Nucl Med 35:1381–1389

Siegel JA, Thomas SR, Stubbs JB et al (1999) MIRD pamphlet no. 16: techniques for quantitative radiopharmaceutical biodistribution data acquisition and analysis for use in human radiation dose estimates. J Nucl Med 40:37S–61S

Siegel JA (2005) Establishing a clinically meaningful predictive model of hematologic toxicity in nonmyeloablative targeted radiotherapy: practical aspects and limitations of red marrow dosimetry. Cancer Biother Radiopharm 20:126–140

Stabin MG (2003) Developments in the internal dosimetry of radiopharmaceuticals. Radiat Prot Dosimetry 105:575–580

Stabin MG, Sparks RB, Crowe E (2005) OLINDA/EXM: the second-generation personal computer software for internal dose assessment in nuclear medicine. J Nucl Med 46:1023–1027

Stabin MG, Sharkey RM, Siegel JA (2011) RADAR commentary: evolution and current status of dosimetry in nuclear medicine. J Nucl Med 52:1156–1161

Strigari L, Menghi E, D'Andrea M, Benassi M (2006) Monte Carlo dose voxel kernel calculations of beta-emitting and Auger-emitting radionuclides for internal dosimetry: a comparison between EGSnrcMP and EGS4. Med Phys 33:3383–3389

van Essen M, Krenning EP, Kam BL, de Jong M, Valkema R, Kwekkeboom DJ (2009) Peptide-receptor radionuclide therapy for endocrine tumors. Nat Rev Endocrinol 5:382–393

Vandervoort E, Celler A, Wells G, Blinder S, Dixon K, Pang Y (2005) Implementation of an analytically based scatter correction in SPECT reconstructions. IEEE Trans Nucl Sci 52: 645–653

Visser E, Postema E, Boerman O, Visschers J, Oyen W, Corstens F (2007) Software package for integrated data processing for internal dose assessment in nuclear medicine (SPRIND). Eur J Nucl Med Mol Imaging 34:413–421

Wehrmann C, Senftleben S, Zachert C, Muller D, Baum RP (2007) Results of individual patient dosimetry in peptide receptor radionuclide therapy with 177Lu DOTA-TATE and 177Lu DOTA-NOC. Cancer Biother Radiopharm 22:406–416

Williams LE, DeNardo GL, Meredith RF (2008) Targeted radionuclide therapy. Med Phys 35:3062–3068

Wiseman GA, Kornmehl E, Leigh B et al (2003) Radiation dosimetry results and safety correlations from 90Y-Ibritumomab Tiuxetan Radioimmunotherapy for relapsed or refractory Non-Hodgkin's Lymphoma: combined data from 4 clinical trials. J Nucl Med 44:465–474

The Bad Berka Dose Protocol: Comparative Results of Dosimetry in Peptide Receptor Radionuclide Therapy Using ^{177}Lu-DOTATATE, ^{177}Lu-DOTANOC, and ^{177}Lu-DOTATOC

Christiane Schuchardt, Harshad R. Kulkarni, Vikas Prasad, Carolin Zachert, Dirk Müller and Richard P. Baum

Abstract

Purpose: The objective of this study is to analyze the in vivo behavior of the ^{177}Lu-labeled peptides DOTATATE, DOTANOC, and DOTATOC used for peptide receptor radionuclide therapy (PRRNT) of neuroendocrine tumors (NETs), by measuring organ and tumor kinetics and by performing dosimetric calculations. *Methods*: Two hundred fifty-three patients (group 1) with metastasized NET who underwent PRRNT were examined. Out of these, 185 patients received ^{177}Lu-DOTATATE, 9 were treated with ^{177}Lu-DOTANOC, and 59 with ^{177}Lu-DOTATOC. Additionally, 25 patients receiving, in consecutive PRRNT cycles, DOTATATE followed by DOTATOC (group 2) and 3 patients receiving DOTATATE and DOTANOC (group 3) were analyzed. Dosimetric calculations (according to MIRD scheme) were performed using OLINDA software. *Results*: In group 1, DOTATOC exhibited the lowest and DOTANOC the highest uptake and therefore mean absorbed dose in normal organs (whole body, kidney, and spleen). In group 2, there was a significant difference between DOTATATE and DOTATOC concerning kinetics and normal organ doses. ^{177}Lu-DOTATOC had the lowest uptake/dose delivered to normal organs and highest tumor-to-kidney ratio. There were no significant differences between the three peptides concerning tumor kinetics and mean absorbed tumor dose. *Conclusions*: The study demonstrates a

C. Schuchardt · H. R. Kulkarni · V. Prasad · C. Zachert · D. Müller · R. P. Baum (✉)
Department of Nuclear Medicine and Centre for PET/CT, ENETS Center of Excellence, Zentralklinik Bad Berka, 99437 Bad Berka, Germany
e-mail: richard.baum@zentralklinik.de
URL: www.zentralklinik-bad-berka.de

R. P. Baum and F. Rösch (eds.), *Theranostics, Gallium-68, and Other Radionuclides*, Recent Results in Cancer Research 194, DOI: 10.1007/978-3-642-27994-2_30,

correlation between high affinity of DOTANOC in vitro and high uptake in normal organs/whole body in vivo, resulting in a higher whole-body dose. DOTATOC exhibited the lowest uptake and dose delivered to normal tissues and the best tumor-to-kidney ratio. Due to large interpatient variability, individual dosimetry should be performed for each therapy cycle.

Keywords
PRRNT · DOTATATE · DOTATOC · DOTANOC · Affinity · Dosimetry

Contents

1 Introduction

There are few treatment options for inoperable or metastasized gastroenteropancreatic (GEP) neuroendocrine tumors (NETs). The majority of well-differentiated NETs express somatostatin receptors (SSTR) and can therefore be visualized and treated with radiolabeled somatostatin analogs (SSTA) (Rufini et al. 2006; Prasad et al. 2010). Due to encouraging clinical results, peptide receptor radionuclide therapy (PRRNT) with radiolabeled SSTA is now established as a treatment modality in advanced NETs (De Jong et al. 2002; Kwekkeboom et al. 2005a; Cremonesi et al. 2006; Otte et al. 1998).

Most NETs predominantly overexpress SSTR subtype 2. Hence, it is important to use a somatostatin analog with high affinity to SSTR2. The different subtype receptor affinity profiles of the various somatostatin analogs result in different uptake and kinetics in normal tissues and tumors. This has important therapeutic implications, since the goal of any internal radiation therapy is to deliver the maximal dose to the tumor while sparing normal organs from damage. In addition, the large variability in biodistribution and tumor uptake among individual patients must be taken into account. For this reason, accurate and individualized dosimetry is essential to ensure maximal tumor doses while preserving normal organ function. This is especially true for the kidneys and bone marrow, which are the dose-limiting organs when performing PRRNT.

Most frequently, the radionuclides ^{90}Y and ^{177}Lu are used for PRRNT (Kwekkeboom et al. 2005a). In contrast to ^{90}Y, which is a pure β-emitter, ^{177}Lu is also a γ-emitter of low emission abundance. These characteristics enable imaging and therapy with the same compound and also allow dosimetry during treatment. The most commonly used peptides for PRRNT are DOTATOC and DOTATATE. In vitro, DOTATATE has the highest affinity to SSTR2 (Reubi et al. 2000). Labeled with ^{177}Lu, DOTATATE was shown to be successful in terms of tumor regression and survival in an animal model. Partial (and some complete) remissions were described in patients undergoing PRRNT (Kwekkeboom et al. 2005b; Erion et al. 1999). The peptide DOTANOC has the highest affinity to SSTR3 and 5, and also high affinity to SSTR2 (Wild et al. 2003). In previous studies we have shown that ^{90}Y-DOTANOC is more toxic than ^{90}Y-DOTATATE, probably because of the higher uptake in normal tissues. When comparing ^{177}Lu-DOTANOC with ^{177}Lu-DOTATATE, we again observed higher uptake of ^{177}Lu-DOTANOC in whole body and normal tissues, but no significantly higher tumor uptake and resulting tumor dose was found (Prasad et al. 2007; Wehrmann et al. 2007). Therefore, DOTANOC is no longer used for PRRNT at our center. However, for comparison with DOTATATE and DOTATOC, results obtained when using DOTANOC were also taken into consideration for the purpose of this study.

Calculating the absorbed dose is important for determination of risk and therapeutic benefit of internal radiation therapy. Because direct measurements are difficult to perform in clinical routine, the absorbed dose is calculated by measuring uptake and retention of the administered radiopharmaceutical. The MIRD scheme provides, together with measurements of the biologic distribution, a method for calculating absorbed doses of radionuclides (Siegel et al. 1999; Bolch et al. 2009). Optimal dose estimation requires time-consuming and sophisticated methods which are difficult due to practical (e.g., patient status) and physical reasons. Nevertheless, to make dosimetry available for most of the patients, we have developed a specific dosimetry procedure used in daily clinical routine (Wehrmann et al. 2007).

The aim of this study is to compare the pharmacokinetics and dosimetry of ^{177}Lu-DOTATATE, ^{177}Lu-DOTATOC, and ^{177}Lu-DOTANOC considering inter- and intrapatient variability in a large cohort of patients undergoing PRRNT.

2 Patients and Methods

2.1 Patients

All patients enrolled in this study were suffering from metastatic NETs with liver, lymph node, bone, or other organ involvement. Intense SSTR expression of (inoperable) primary tumors and metastases had been verified before therapy

Table 1 Patients treated with different peptides (group 1)

	DOTATATE	DOTANOC	DOTATOC
Therapy cycles	185	9	59
	83 male, 102 female	3 male, 6 female	35 male, 24 female
	59.7 ± 10.6 years	64.4 ± 9.9 years	62.3 ± 10.0 years
	27.5–79.7 years	47.9–77.5 years	41.2–81.7 years
Activity per cycle in GBq	5.7 ± 1.1	5.6 ± 1.5	7.3 ± 0.8
	2.5–8.5	3.6–7.4	5.5–8.6

Table 2 Patients treated with DOTATATE and DOTATOC (group 2)

	DOTATATE	DOTATOC
25 patients; 13 male, 12 female	60.2 ± 9.1 years	61.7 ± 9.1 years
	45.3–75.2 years	45.6–75.5
Activity per cycle (GBq)	6.5 ± 1.1	7.3 ± 0.7
	5.0–9.5	5.5–8.5

by using ^{68}Ga-DOTANOC, ^{68}Ga-DOTATOC, or ^{68}Ga-DOTATATE PET/CT. Before PRRNT, each patient was extensively informed about the therapeutic procedure and possible adverse effects. All patients provided written informed consent to undergo treatment and follow-up. The study was approved by the local Ethics Committee and performed in accordance with German regulations concerning radiation safety. Three groups of patients receiving PRRNT were included in this study. The first group consisted of 253 patients (group 1, Table 1), treated with 1–6 cycles of ^{177}Lu-labeled DOTATATE, DOTANOC, or DOTATOC. Differences with respect to kinetics, biodistribution, and mean absorbed doses between the three different peptides were analyzed on the basis of dosimetric data obtained in this group (interindividual comparison). Group 2 consisted of 25 patients (Table 2) who received PRRNT first using ^{177}Lu-DOTATATE and in a following cycle using ^{177}Lu-DOTATOC, to compare kinetics and mean absorbed dose in the same patient (intraindividual variability). The mean time between these therapy courses was 18 months. In case of more than one cycle with each peptide, two consecutive cycles were chosen for dosimetric analyses. Additionally, kinetics and biodistribution were analyzed in three patients (group 3) treated using both ^{177}Lu-DOTANOC and ^{177}Lu-DOTATATE, to assess the intrapatient variability when using these two peptides. The administered activity was 4.5, 4, and 4.2 GBq ^{177}Lu-DOTANOC and 6.5, 4.3, and 4.8 GBq of ^{177}Lu-DOTATATE, respectively.

2.2 Radiopharmaceuticals

The radiopharmaceuticals were prepared in our GMP-certified radiopharmacy. ^{177}Lu-labeling of DOTA peptides was performed according to the following procedure: A solution of 500 μg 2,5-dihydroxybenzoic acid and 20 μg of the corresponding DOTA peptide in 50 μL 0.4 M sodium acetate buffer (pH 5.5) was added to a solution of 1 GBq ^{177}Lu in 30 μL 0.05 M HCl. The mixture was heated to 90°C for 30 min and then diluted with 0.9% saline solution followed by sterile filtration. Quality control was performed by RP-18 HPLC [solvent A: water; solvent B: acetonitrile (both with 0.1% TFA); gradient: 0–2 min 95% A, 20 min 95% B; flow rate: 1.2 mL/min; column: LiChrospher 100 RP 18 EC-5 μm 250 × 4 mm]. The radiochemical purity was always greater than 99%. Samples were taken for sterility and pyrogenicity testing.

2.3 Infusion and Renal Protection

For kidney protection, every patient was infused with 1500 mL of a renoprotective amino acid mixture of 5% lysine HCl and 10% L-arginine HCl. Infusion was started 30 min prior to administration of the therapeutic dose and continued for 4 h thereafter. This co-infusion of amino acids reduces renal exposure significantly (Jamar et al. 2003). The radiopharmaceutical was co-administered over 10–15 min by using a second infusion pump system. The activity to administer was individually chosen based on the uptake in the tumor lesions as shown by Ga-68 SSTR PET/CT (performed before each treatment cycle), kidney function (tubular extraction rate determined by Tc-99m MAG3 scintigraphy and glomerular filtration by Tc-99m DTPA clearance, and serum creatinine), hematological reserve, previous treatments, general status of the patient (Karnofsky Performance Scale), and experience reported by other groups (Kwekkeboom et al. 2005a).

2.4 Dosimetry

In this study, the dosimetric approach is based on the MIRD scheme, where the absorbed dose depends on two main parameters:

1. Time-independent physical factors: so-called *S*-values, which were tabulated by the MIRD committee and include type, size of emitted energies, and geometric aspects (size, type, and structure of source and target regions);
2. Time-dependent biokinetic factors: these describe the cumulated activity, uptake, and retention in the regions of interest, and include the physical half-life of the radionuclide and the biologic half-life of the radiopharmaceutical (expressed as residence time, which also depends on the half-life of the radionuclide and its distribution) (Siegel et al. 1999).

The dose estimation requires an accurate determination of the time-dependent activity of the source regions. Thus, the main objective of the dosimetry is correct evaluation of the distribution and kinetics of the administered radiopharmaceutical

(Sgouros 2005; Stabin and Siegel 2003). For the dose estimations, we developed a convenient procedure which is based on the MIRD scheme and practicable in daily clinical routine (Wehrmann et al. 2007). In short, the kinetics of the radiopharmaceutical is determined on the basis of five planar whole-body scintigraphies in defined time order after administration of the radiopeptide (p.i.). After the first scan acquired immediately after infusion, further scans are obtained at 3, 20, 44, and 68 h p.i. The camera parameters were the following: MEDISO spirit DH-V dual-headed gamma camera, MeGP collimator, 15% energy window, peak at 208 keV, speed 15 cm/min. Scintigraphies were analyzed by the use of regions of interest (ROI). After geometric mean and background correction, time-dependent time–activity curves were obtained and fitted to mono- or biexponential functions (software ORIGIN PRO 8.1G). The residence time and cumulated activity as well as the uptake and effective half-life were then calculated, and the mean absorbed doses were estimated by using the OLINDA/EXM software (Stabin et al. 2005).

Finally, uptake values were calculated as fraction of administered activity (%IA), and effective half-lives, residence times, and mean absorbed organ and tumor doses were obtained for whole body, normal tissues, kidneys, spleen, and tumor lesions of all patients in the different groups. The ROIs for normal tissue and background were placed over those regions showing no tumor involvement. For interpatient comparison, they were scaled to 10% of the whole-body ROI. Estimation of mean absorbed tumor dose requires the lesions' volume. These were obtained from the CT data of the pretherapy ^{68}Ga-DOTA-SSTR PET/CT. Volumes of normal organs were assumed to have standard size as given by OLINDA/EXM.

Organs showing tumor involvement or overlaying with other source regions were not included for dosimetric analysis. For this reason, normal liver was excluded from the analysis in this study because nearly all patients had extensive liver metastases. Some patients had liver lesions superimposing on the right kidney, allowing only analysis of the left kidney. In these cases, it was assumed that the mean absorbed dose would be identical for both kidneys (which was also checked and confirmed by prior Tc-99m MAG3 scintigraphy proving that there was no significant difference in the differential renal function). Also, kinetics and mean absorbed dose of the spleen could not be estimated for all patients as several patients had undergone splenectomy.

2.5 Comparison and Statistics

Dosimetric parameters were determined for whole body, kidneys, spleen, and normal tissues/organs as well as for tumor lesions. Results are expressed as median values. To describe differences between the various radiolabeled peptides, the following parameters were chosen: uptake at 20 h p.i. (max. uptake for tumor lesions), half-life, residence time, and mean absorbed dose. Interpatient variability was estimated by comparing the three peptides in all patients. To describe significant differences among the peptides, nonparametric tests for independent samples were used. In group 2, statistically significant differences were evaluated by nonparametric signed-rank tests for paired samples. All statistical tests were performed using ORIGINPRO 8.1 G; p-values ≤ 0.05 were considered to be significant.

3 Results

3.1 Normal Organs

Dosimetry results are given in Table 3; corresponding uptake and time–activity curves are shown in Fig. 1.

3.1.1 Whole Body

Because the total whole-body counts from the first scan represent the total administered activity, whole-body kinetics start with an initial uptake of 100% for all three peptides. Initially, the curves show a rapid decline followed by a second, slower decline. Therefore, time–activity curves for whole body were fitted by a biexponential function. The highest initial whole-body (WB) uptake was observed for DOTANOC and the lowest for DOTATOC. At 20 h p.i., WB uptake was again highest for DOTANOC, followed by DOTATATE and DOTATOC, correlating with the first half-life, which was shorter for DOTATATE and DOTATOC as compared with DOTANOC. Similar results were calculated regarding the second half-life: DOTANOC exhibited the longest WB residence time, while DOTATOC had the fastest washout. The estimated whole-body dose was therefore highest with DOTANOC, followed by DOTATATE and DOTATOC. There were significant differences in all parameters, when comparing DOTATATE with DOTATOC (Table 4). Except for the second half-life, parameters were also significantly different between DOTATATE and DOTANOC. When comparing DOTANOC with DOTATOC, there were significant differences with respect to uptake, residence time, and mean absorbed dose. The following results were obtained in the 25 patients receiving DOTATATE and DOTATOC: 24 out of the 25 patients (96%) exhibited higher WB uptake for DOTATATE as compared with DOTATOC at 20 h p.i. First half-life was longer for DOTATOC in 22 patients (88%) whereas for DOTATATE second half-life was longer in 17 (68%), and residence time in 23 patients (92%). In 22 patients (88%) whole-body dose was slightly, but statistically significantly, higher when using DOTATATE as compared with DOTATOC. In group 3, i.e., patients treated with DOTATATE and DOTANOC, the following results were obtained: in two out of three patients, DOTANOC had higher uptake at 20 h p.i., and longer first half-life and residence time. One patient also showed longer second half-life and higher mean absorbed WB dose when using DOTANOC.

3.1.2 Normal Tissues

Comparable results were obtained for whole-body kinetics and normal tissues. DOTATOC showed the lowest uptake and DOTANOC the highest uptake, with the exception of the values directly after injection and 3 h p.i. First half-life of the

Table 3 Dosimetric results of 253 patients in group 1 (median and range of variation); for kidneys, spleen, and tumor lesions only the second half-life was calculated because of the fit to a monoexponential function

	DOTA-	Whole body	Normal tissue	Kidneys	Spleen	Tumor lesions
Uptake 20 h p.i.	TATE	27.7 (14.1–58.7)	1.8 (0.9–5.1)	2.4 (0.9–6.7)	1.7 (0.4–14.3)	0.05 (0.001–0.8)
	NOC	38.5 (22.6–70.1)	2.7 (1.9–5.3)	3.2 (2.2–3.6)	1.6 (1.0–4.8)	0.02 (0.004–0.3)
	TOC	19.5 (10.2–52.2)	1.4 (0.7–3.6)	1.6 (0.7–3.3)	1.0 (0.3–4.6)	0.04 (0.001–0.4)
First half-life (h)	TATE	2.2 (0.9–6.8)	2.2 (1.0–8.4)	–	–	–
	NOC	3.0 (0.8–4.2)	2.6 (1.6–3.9)	–	–	–
	TOC	2.7 (1.4–5.9)	2.8 (1.7–8.6)	–	–	–
Second half-life (h)	TATE	55.3 (33.1–94.5)	46.6 (32.4–160.3)	62.7 (36.0–160.3)	67.5 (42.9–160.3)	73.2 (31.1–160.3)
	NOC	57.3 (40.2–69.1)	43.4 (36.4–47.7)	70.3 (49.7–94.1)	79.3 (69.4–101.6)	61.2 (40.5–139.8)
	TOC	51.1 (30.3–82.4)	43.1 (20.1–160.3)	63.4 (37.7–142.0)	72.5 (45.8–160.3)	79.0 (31.1–160.3)
Residence time (h)	TATE	32.2 (17.7–78.6)	2.2 (1.1–7.8)	2.7 (1.0–8.3)	2.1 (0.5–16.1)	0.7 (0.02–54.7)
	NOC	50.0 (22.8–73.0)	2.9 (2.0–5.5)	3.8 (2.0–4.6)	2.3 (1.1–7.1)	0.8 (0.01–34.0)
	TOC	23.3 (14.6–66.2)	1.8 (1.2–4.4)	1.9 (0.9–5.0)	1.3 (0.3–5.9)	0.4 (0.03–36.8)
Absorbed dose (mGy/MBq)	TATE	0.05 (0.02–0.1)	–	0.8 (0.3–2.6)	1.1 (0.2–9.3)	5.2 (0.1–89.6)
	NOC	0.07 (0.04–0.1)	–	1.1 (0.6–1.5)	1.3 (0.7–3.4)	2.0 (0.5–31.7)
	TOC	0.03 (0.02–0.08)	–	0.6 (0.3–1.6)	0.7 (0.2–2.8)	4.9 (0.3–39.7)

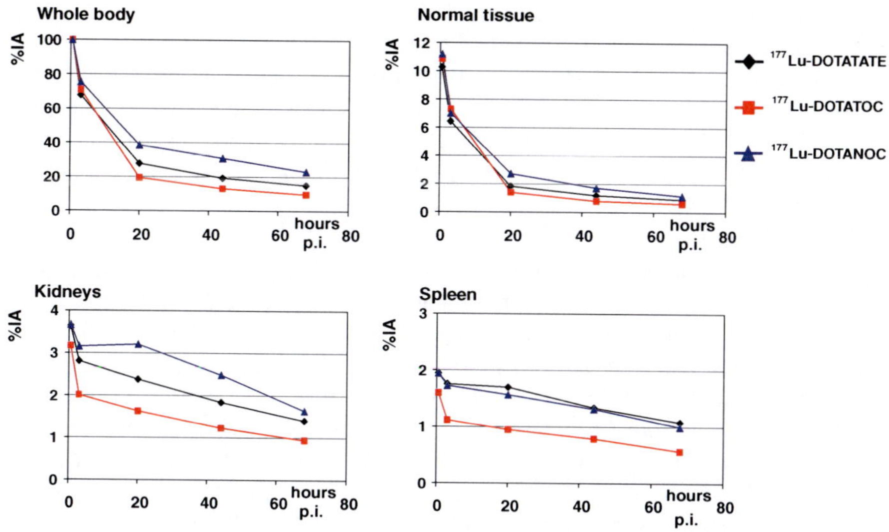

Fig. 1 Kinetics of normal organs and whole body in patients treated with different peptides (group 1)

Table 4 Significant differences between patients (group 1) treated with different peptides (indicated for respective pairs of peptides by •)

	Whole body					Normal tissue				Kidneys				Spleen			
	Up	HL1	HL2	RT	Dose	Up	HL1	HL2	RT	Up	HL	RT	Dose	Up	HL	RT	Dose
TATE–TOC	•	•	•	•	•	•	•	•	•	•		•	•	•	•	•	•
TATE–NOC	•	•		•	•	•		•	•						•		
NOC–TOC	•			•	•	•			•	•		•	•	•		•	•

Up uptake, *HL1* first half-life, *HL2* second half-life

biexponential curve was longest for DOTATOC, followed by DOTANOC and DOTATATE. Otherwise, the second half-life was almost similar for DOTATOC and DOTANOC in contrast to the longer second half-life of DOTATATE. The shortest residence time was calculated for DOTATOC followed by DOTATATE and DOTANOC, which exhibited the longest residence time. As shown in Table 4 and similar to the results for whole body, all parameters were significantly different when comparing DOTATATE and DOTATOC. Except for the first half-life, the results were significantly different for DOTATATE versus DOTANOC; however, for DOTANOC versus DOTATOC only uptake at 20 h p.i. and residence time were found to be significantly different. Results in group 2 were comparable: 24 out of 25 patients had higher WB uptake at 20 h p.i. when injected with

DOTATATE; second half-life and residence time were longer in 16 (64%) and 22 (88%) patients, respectively. However, first half-life was longer for DOTATOC in 21 patients. For normal tissues, all differences between DOTATATE and DOTATOC in the same patient were statistically significant. Higher values were found for uptake, first half-life, and residence for DOTANOC in two out of three patients when comparing DOTANOC and DOTATATE in the same patient.

3.1.3 Kidneys

The kidneys are the dose-limiting organs for PRRNT. Kidneys were analyzed in 171 patients having undergone treatment with DOTATATE, in 7 treated with DOTANOC, and in 58 patients receiving PRRNT with DOTATOC. Renal uptake was highest for DOTANOC and lowest for DOTATOC. For all three peptides, renal uptake showed a rapid decline between the first scan and 3 h p.i. From 20 h p.i. the curves were fitted to a monoexponential function, with the longest half-life for DOTANOC and the shortest for DOTATATE. Similarly, residence time was longest for DOTANOC and shortest for DOTATOC. Therefore, the highest renal dose was calculated when using DOTANOC for PRRNT, followed by DOTATATE and DOTATOC. Direct comparison between DOTATATE and DOTANOC revealed no significant differences. For DOTATOC versus DOTATATE and DOTANOC, significant differences were found for uptake, residence time, and mean absorbed renal dose. In group 2 (analysis in 22/25 patients), higher values were observed for DOTATATE in 19 of 22 patients (86%) for uptake, residence time, and mean absorbed renal dose. These results were also statistically significant. Half-life was found to be similar for both peptides (Table 2). In group 3, only two out of three patients could be evaluated because of superimposition of the liver lesions on the kidney: One patient had higher values for DOTANOC concerning uptake, half-life, residence time, and renal dose. The second patient was found to have higher uptake for DOTANOC, whereas half-life, residence time, and renal dose were higher for DOTATATE.

3.1.4 Spleen

Dosimetric parameters for the spleen were calculated in 132 patients who underwent therapy with DOTATATE, in 7 patients using DOTANOC, and in 49 patients treated with DOTATOC. In contrast to other normal organs, spleen uptake was almost similar for DOTATATE and DOTANOC. The lowest uptake was found for DOTATOC. After an initial decrease between the first two scans, the uptake of all three peptides showed a slight decrease and followed a monoexponential function 20 h p.i. The corresponding half-life was the longest for DOTANOC, followed by DOTATOC and DOTATATE. The resulting residence time was longest for DOTANOC and shortest for DOTATOC. Consequently, the highest dose to the spleen was calculated for DOTANOC and the lowest for DOTATOC. Half-life of DOTATATE and DOTANOC were significantly different. Comparing DOTANOC and DOTATOC, significant differences were found for uptake, residence time, and dose. For DOTATOC versus DOTATATE, the results were similar for whole body and normal tissue (Table 4). In group 2, the spleen dose was calculated in 17/25

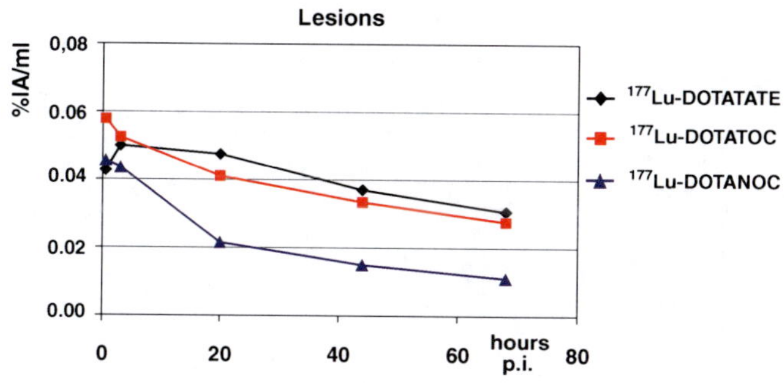

Fig. 2 Kinetics of tumor lesions in patients treated with different peptides (group 1)

patients. In 14 (82%), significantly higher uptake, longer residence time, and higher dose were observed for DOTATATE. In 13 (76%) patients, half-life was significantly longer for DOTATOC. In group 3, the comparison between DOTANOC and DOTATATE showed higher values for uptake, half-life, residence time, and mean absorbed dose for DOTANOC in one of the three patients, whereas the other two patients showed higher values for DOTATATE.

3.2 Tumor Lesions

For better comparison, uptake in tumor lesions is presented as percent of injected activity per unit volume (%IA/mL). This relation allows for comparison of tumor lesions among different peptides, because the volume dependency is eliminated. Additionally, all values are expressed as median values.

Tumor kinetics is shown in Fig. 2. In contrast to the kinetics in normal organs, DOTATATE revealed the highest uptake at 20 h p.i. DOTATOC had the highest initial uptake followed by a fast decline. Initial uptake of DOTATATE and DOTANOC were almost similar, but the retention thereafter was different. While the uptake of DOTATATE increased between the first two scans, a fast decline was found for DOTANOC. All time–activity curves were fitted by monoexponential functions from 20 h p.i. resulting in the longest half-life for DOTATOC and the shortest for DOTANOC. The longest median residence time was determined for DOTANOC and the shortest for DOTATOC. Thus, the resulting absorbed lesion doses were the highest for DOTATATE, followed by DOTATOC and DOTANOC. The differences in uptake and mean absorbed dose were not statistically significant. Only half-life and residence times of DOTATATE as compared with DOTATOC were significantly different as well as the half-life of DOTANOC versus DOTATOC. In patients from group 2, 46 tumor lesions were analyzed: 39 (85%) showed higher uptake at 20 h p.i. and 40 (87%) patients showed longer residence time for DOTATATE, while the tumor lesions of 23 (50%) patients showed longer half-life for DOTATATE. The mean absorbed dose to lesions was higher for DOTATATE in 30 patients (65%). These results are

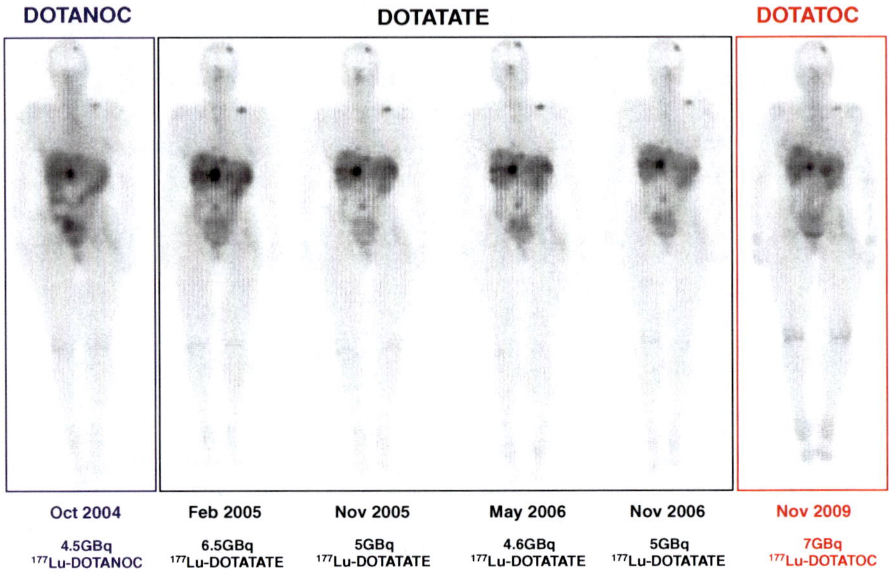

Fig. 3 Anterior whole-body scans at 20 h p.i. during six cycles of PRRNT in one patient (scaled to the maximum pixel of all scans)

statistically significant for uptake, residence time, and mean absorbed dose, but not concerning half-life.

3.3 Tumor-to-Kidney Ratio

The ratio for the three different peptides in patients from group 1 revealed the following results: DOTATOC showed the highest ratio (12), followed by DOTATATE (10) and DOTANOC (6). In patients who underwent therapy using DOTATATE and later DOTATOC (group 2), the ratio was higher for DOTATOC in 23 of 43 (53%) lesions, which was not statistically significant. Therefore, the tumor-to-kidney ratio in patients from group 2 was comparable for both peptides. Concerning group 3, the tumor-to-kidney ratio was calculated in two out of three patients: both exhibited a higher ratio for DOTANOC as compared with DOTATATE.

3.4 Variability

The data shown in Table 3 and the dosimetric results of patients in group 2 reveal high variability among patients. Moreover, high intrapatient variability was observed for patients receiving more than one cycle of therapy (data not shown). Figures 3 and 4 demonstrate the whole-body scans and the kinetics in a patient who received six cycles of therapy using all three peptides. The highest whole-body

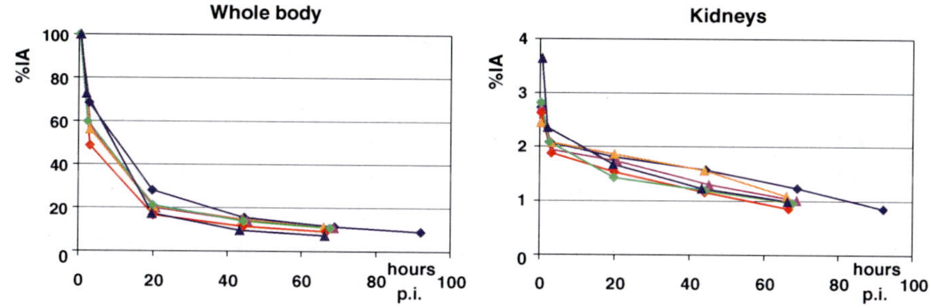

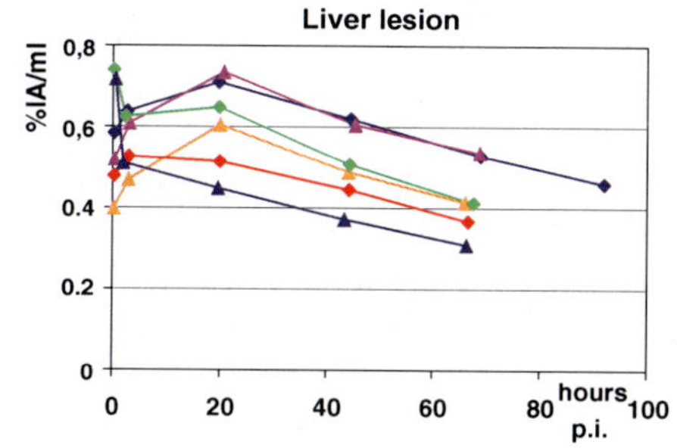

Mean absorbed dose in mGy/MBq

Dosimetry	1	2	3	4	5	6
Whole body	0.04	0.04	0.04	0.03	0.04	0.03
Kidneys	0.9	0.8	0.8	0.6	0.7	0.6
Spleen	1.2	1.5	1	0.6	1.1	0.4
Liver lesion	11	7	4	3	7	3

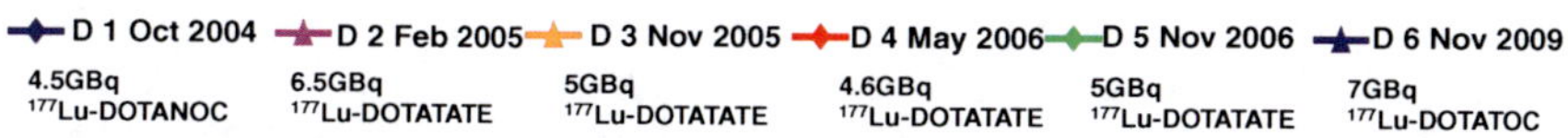

Fig. 4 Dosimetric results of six cycles of PRRNT in one patient using three different peptides

uptake was observed during the first therapy cycle when using DOTANOC, while the highest renal uptake was found during the third cycle. For the liver lesions, maximum uptake was observed during the first two therapies. DOTATOC revealed the lowest whole-body uptake. Also noticeable were the differences in the initial renal uptake; similar trend is seen for the liver lesions and the spleen (data not shown). There was no systematic pattern of uptake or mean absorbed dose in consecutive therapies.

4 Discussion

This study reports results of dosimetric analyses obtained after PRRNT of NETs. All three peptides, ^{177}Lu-DOTATATE, ^{177}Lu-DOTATOC, and ^{177}Lu-DOTANOC, showed high specific uptake in somatostatin receptor-positive tumors. Significant differences were found for all calculated parameters (uptake, half-life, residence time, and mean absorbed dose) concerning whole body, normal tissue, kidneys, and spleen for DOTATATE and DOTATOC in 25 patients receiving both peptides (group 2); similar results were obtained for all parameters in normal organs on comparison of DOTATATE and DOTATOC in different patients (group 1): uptake and mean absorbed doses were lowest for DOTATOC. The dose to whole body, spleen, and kidneys was highest for DOTANOC.

In patients who underwent treatment using DOTATATE and DOTANOC (group 3), uptake, half-life, and residence time for whole body and normal tissue, as well as the whole-body dose, were higher with DOTANOC. The preclinical studies by Wild et al. comparing ^{111}In-DOTANOC and ^{111}In-DOTATOC showed that DOTANOC had higher affinity to SSTR2, 3, and 5 (Wild et al. 2003). DOTANOC has in fact the highest affinity to SSTR3 and 5, which would imply higher uptake in normal organs or whole body in vivo and therefore higher whole-body dose, as was also demonstrated in a previous study comparing DOTATATE and DOTANOC (Wehrmann et al. 2007).

In patients treated with all three peptides, the second half-life of each peptide was longer for the spleen in contrast to the kidneys. Together with the higher renal uptake and despite the shorter half-life, a longer residence time for the kidneys was calculated. However, the highest mean absorbed doses were obtained for the spleen (1.4–39.9 Gy) as compared with whole body and kidneys. The range of the estimated mean dose to the kidney in this study was 1.5–18.2 Gy, as compared with the study by Valkema et al., who reported a renal dose of 1.8–7.8 Gy (Valkema et al. 2005). The large variability in our study could be due to a different patient population (including patients with impaired renal function). However, in comparison with ^{90}Y-labeled peptides (DOTATATE/-TOC), the renal dose with ^{177}Lu was significantly lower, which translates into lower renal toxicity (Forrer et al. 2004; Bodei et al. 2003; Helisch et al. 2004).

The mean absorbed kidney dose was significantly higher for DOTATATE as compared with DOTATOC in patient groups 1 and 2. Additionally, when comparing DOTANOC and DOTATOC among different patients, DOTATOC had a significantly lower renal dose. Since the kidney is the dose-limiting organ in PRRNT, the safe therapeutic window would be best determined by the tumor-to-kidney ratio for the absorbed doses. In this study, this ratio was comparable for DOTATATE and DOTATOC when individual lesions were considered (group 2). Forrer et al. (2004) also found a significant difference between the mean values for the two peptides.

There was no statistically significant difference concerning uptake and mean absorbed dose of tumor lesions when comparing the three peptides in group 1, i.e., in different patients. Even though a significant difference could not be demonstrated, the mean absorbed tumor dose was the highest for DOTATATE and lowest for DOTANOC. This finding is consistent with a previous study comparing ^{177}Lu-DOTATATE and ^{177}Lu-DOTANOC, in which the difference could not be statistically proven (Wehrmann et al. 2007). In patients receiving DOTATATE and DOTATOC (group 2), there was a significant difference in mean absorbed tumor dose between ^{177}Lu-DOTATATE and ^{177}Lu-DOTATOC. This is consistent with the results of Esser et al. (2006) in a study performed in seven patients.

In a preclinical study comparing the effects of ^{177}Lu-DOTATATE and ^{177}Lu-DOTATOC in nude mice xenografted with human midgut carcinoid tumor cell line (GOT1), Swärd et al. (2008) had also demonstrated a significantly higher mean absorbed dose to the tumor by using DOTATATE. Forrer et al. (2004), however, in a comparison between ^{111}In-DOTATOC and ^{111}In-DOTATATE in five patients

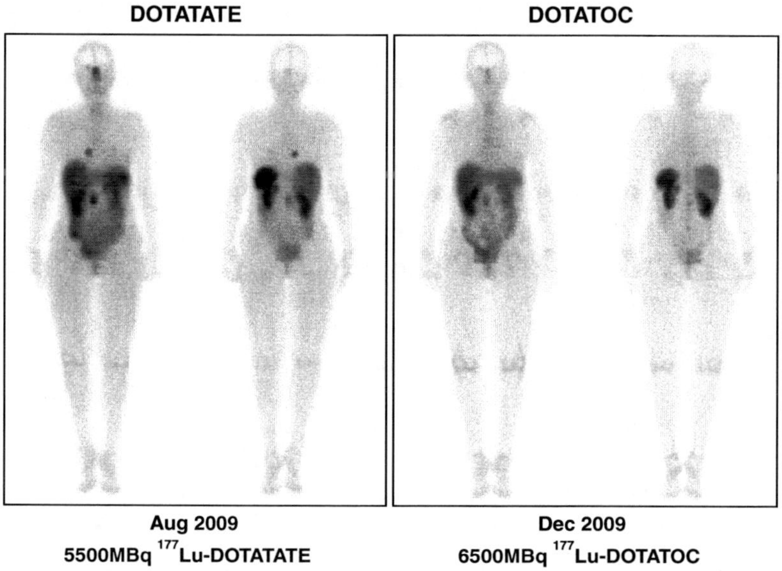

Fig. 5 Whole-body scans at 20 h p.i. in a patient treated with ^{177}Lu-DOTATATE and ^{177}Lu-DOTATOC (scaled to the maximum pixel of both scans)

with metastasized NETs, did not find a significant difference in the doses delivered. Interestingly, they found a higher mean tumor dose with ^{111}In-DOTATOC as compared with ^{111}In-DOTATATE, which is surprising since DOTATATE among all the peptides has the highest affinity to SSTR2. Kwekkeboom et al. found 3–4-fold higher uptake with ^{177}Lu-DOTATATE in comparison with ^{111}In-DTPA^{0}–octreotide. This is in agreement with the higher uptake of DOTATATE found in our study and could explain the higher mean absorbed dose delivered by DOTATATE to the tumor lesions (Kwekkeboom et al. 2001); for example, Fig. 5 shows whole-body scans from a patient (group 2) who was treated using ^{177}Lu-DOTATATE and DOTATOC. The whole-body and organ uptake, as well as the uptake in the tumor lesions, is obviously lower for DOTATOC.

Furthermore, there were significant differences concerning half-life and residence time when comparing DOTATATE and DOTATOC, and for half-life when comparing DOTANOC and DOTATOC (group 1). In patients treated with DOTATATE and DOTATOC (group 2), significantly longer tumor residence time was noted for DOTATATE, which explains the higher mean absorbed tumor dose delivered. Esser et al. also found significantly longer tumor residence time for DOTATATE as compared with DOTATOC and consequently concluded that it should be the preferred peptide for PRRNT. Their results in seven patients were comparable to our findings in a larger group of patients, confirming also the accuracy of our methodology as compared with the results published in the literature (Esser et al. 2006).

High interpatient variability was found for the mean absorbed doses. This is not unexpected, since this was a heterogeneous group of patients having varying receptor densities and tumor burden. In addition, the results showed high intra-patient variability in the same patients undergoing therapy with different peptides. As this is true even for a larger group of 253 patients studied, it leads to the conclusion that the median value of a dosimetric parameter is not representative for different patients or different therapy cycles in the same patient. This variability could be well appreciated in one patient who underwent PRRNT with all three peptides (Fig. 4). Although the variability may be attributed to the difference in the biological behavior of the peptides, the fact that there might also have been an influence of previous radiopeptide therapies or other treatment modalities must be taken into account. The possible effects of previous treatments on the outcome of the current PRRNT (e.g., effect on tumor radiosensitivity) are well known from the literature (Koral and Kaminski 2003; Sgouros et al. 2003).

Moreover, the results obtained for one patient treated with six cycles of PRRNT using different peptides showed variable kinetics and mean absorbed doses, for which no ascending or descending order for consecutive therapies was found. This effect was also seen in patients who received more than one cycle of therapy using ^{177}Lu-DOTATATE (data not shown). Consequently, dosimetry for one cycle of PRRNT should not be used alone to predict the outcome of future following cycles, even if the same peptide is used.

5 Conclusions

Comparing the somatostatin analogs DOTATATE, DOTANOC, and DOTATOC radiolabeled with ^{177}Lu, the following conclusions can be drawn from this study:

- The in vitro higher affinity of DOTANOC correlates with the in vivo higher uptake for whole body and normal tissue, which results in a higher whole-body dose. Therefore, this peptide is not ideal for PRRNT.
- Concerning kidney uptake and mean absorbed dose to normal organs and whole body, DOTATOC revealed the highest tumor-to-kidney ratio and is very appropriate for PRRNT.
- DOTATATE was shown to deliver the highest tumor dose (due to the longer residence time in the malignant lesions) and is also very suitable.

Additionally, the finding of large variability should be addressed in further studies. It is recommended that median values of absorbed doses among patients should not be the only criterion used to plan PRRNT. Beside the described methods for individual dosimetry, interindividual differences should be taken into account, particularly organ functionality, metabolism, or receptor density in organs and tumor lesions.

The results of this study demonstrate further that calculation of mean absorbed doses to critical organs and tumor lesions should be considered for estimation of possible toxicity from PRRNT. In conclusion, individual dosimetry is essential for optimal PRRNT.

References

Bodei L, Cremonesi M, Zoboli S (2003) Receptor-mediated radionuclide therapy with ^{90}Y-DOTATOC in association with amino acid infusion: a phase I study. Eur J Nucl Med 30:207–216

Bolch W, Eckermann KF, Sgouros G, Thomas SR (2009) MIRD pamphlet no. 21: a generalized schema for radiopharmaceutical dosimetry-standardization of nomenclature. J Nucl Med 50:477–484

Cremonesi M, Ferrari M, Bodei L, Giampiero T, Paganelli G (2006) Dosimetry in peptide receptor therapy: a review. J Nucl Med 47:1467–1475

De Jong M, Valkema R, Jamar F (2002) Somatostatin receptor-targeted radionuclide therapy of tumours: Preclinical and clinical findings. Semin Nucl Med 32:133

Erion JL, Bugaj JE, Schmidt MA et al (1999) High radiotherapeutic efficacy of 177Lu-DOTA-Y3- octreotate in a rat tumour model. [Abstract]. J Nucl Med 40:223

Esser JP, Krenning EP, Teunissen JJM (2006) Comparison of [^{177}Lu-DOTA0, Tyr^{3}] octreotate and [^{177}Lu-DOTA0, Tyr^{3}] octreotide: which peptide is preferable for PRRT? Eur J Nucl Med 33:1346–1351

Forrer F, Uusijärvi H, Waldherr C (2004) A comparison of ^{111}In-DOTATOC and ^{111}In-DOTATATE: biodistribution and dosimetry in the same patients with metastatic neuroendocrine tumours. Eur J Nucl Med 31:1257–1262

Helisch A, Förster GJ, Reber H (2004) Pre-therapeutic dosimetry and biodistribution of ^{86}Y-DOTA-Phe^{1}- Tyr^{3}-octreotide versus ^{111}In-pentetreotide in patients with advanced neuroendocrine tumours. Eur J Nucl Med 31:1386–1392

Jamar F, Barone R, Matthieu I et al (2003) 86Y-DOTA0-D-Phe1-Tyr3-octreotide (SMT487) -a phase 1 clinical study: Pharmacokinetics, biodistribution, renal protective effect of different regiments of amino acid coinfusion. Eur J Nucl Med Mol Imaging 30:510

Koral KF, Kaminski MS (2003) Correlation of tumour radiation-absorbed dose with response is easier to find in previously untreated patients. Letter to the editor. J Nucl Med 44:1541–1543

Kwekkeboom DJ, Bakker WH, Kooij PM (2001) [^{177}Lu-DOTA^{0}, Tyr3] octreotate: comparison with [^{111}In- DTPA^{0}] octreotide in patients. Eur J Nucl Med 28:1319–1325

Kwekkeboom DJ, Mueller-Brand J, Paganelli G (2005a) Overview of results of peptide receptor radionuclide therapy with 3 radiolabeled somatostatin analogues. J Nucl Med 46(Suppl 1):62S–66S

Kwekkeboom DJ, Teunissen JJ, Bakker WH et al (2005b) Radiolabeled somatostatin analog [^{177}Lu-DOTA^{0}, Tyr^{3}]-Octreotate in patients with endocrine gastroenteropancreatic tumours. J Clin Oncol 23:2754

Otte A, Mueller-Brand J, Dellas S (1998) Yttrium-90 labelled somatostatin analogue for cancer treatment. Lancet 351:417

Prasad V, Fetscher S, Baum RP (2007) Changing role of somatostatin receptor targeted drugs in NET: nuclear medicine's view. J Pharm Pharm Sci 10(2):321–337

Prasad V, Ambrosini V, Hommann M, Hörsch D, Fanti S, Baum RP (2010) Detection of unknown primary neuroendocrine tumours (CUP-NET) using ^{68}Ga-DOTA-NOC receptor PET/CT. Eur J Nucl Med Mol Imaging 37:67–77

Reubi JC, Schär J, Waser B, Wenger S, Heppeler A, Schmitt J, Mäcke HR (2000) Affinity profiles for human somatostatin receptor subtypes SST1–SST5 of somatostatin radiotracers selected for scintigraphic and radiotherapeutic use. Eur J Nucl Med 27:273–282

Rufini V, Calcagni ML, Baum RP (2006) Imaging of neuroendocrine tumours. Semin Nucl Med 36:228

Sgouros G, Squeri S, Ballangrud AM (2003) Patient-specific 3-dimensional dosimetry in non-Hodgkin's lymphoma patients treated with ^{131}I-anti-B1 antibody: assessment of tumour dose response. J Nucl Med 44:260–268

Sgouros G (2005) Dosimetry of internal emitters. J Nucl Med 46:18S–27S

Siegel JA, Thomas SR, Stubbs JB (1999) MIRD Pamphlet 16: techniques for quantitative radiopharmaceutical biodistribution data acquisition and analysis for use in human radiation dose estimates. J Nucl Med 40:37S–61S

Stabin MG, Siegel JA (2003) Physical models and dose factors for use in internal dose assessment. Health Phys 85(3):294–310

Stabin MG, Sparks RP, Crowe E (2005) OLINDA/EXM: The second-generation personal computer software for internal dose assessment in nuclear medicine. J Nucl Med 46: 1023–1027

Swärd C, Bernhardt P, Johanson V, Schmitt A, Ahlman H, Stridsberg M, Forssell-Aronsson E, Nilsson O, Kölby L (2008) Comparison of [177Lu-DOTA0, Tyr3]-octreotate and [177Lu-DOTA0, Tyr3]- octreotide for receptor-mediated radiation therapy of the xenografted human midgut carcinoid tumour GOT1. Cancer Biother Radiopharm 23(1):114–120

Valkema R, Pauwels SA, Kvols LK (2005) Long-term follow-up of renal function after peptide receptor radiation therapy with ^{90}Y-DOTA0, Tyr3-Octreotide and ^{177}Lu-DOTA0, Tyr3-Octreotate. J Nucl Med 46:83S–91S

Wehrmann C, Senftleben S, Zachert C, Mueller D, Baum RP (2007) Results of individual patient dosimetry in peptide receptor radionuclide therapy with ^{177}Lu DOTA-TATE and ^{177}Lu DOTANOC. Cancer Biother Radiopharm 22(3):406–416

Wild D, Schmitt JS, Ginj M (2003) DOTA-NOC, a high-affinity ligand of somatostatin receptor subtypes 2, 3 and 5 for labeling with various radiometals. Eur J Nucl Med 30:1338–1347

4D SPECT/CT Acquisition for 3D Dose Calculation and Dose Planning in ^{177}Lu-Peptide Receptor Radionuclide Therapy: Applications for Clinical Routine

Kalevi Kairemo and Aki Kangasmäki

Abstract

Molecular radiotherapy combines the potential of a specific tracer (vector) targeting tumor cells with local radiotoxicity. Designing a specific tumor-targeting/killing combination is a tailoring process. Radionuclides with imaging capacity serve best in the selection of the targeting molecule. The potential of targeted therapy with radiolabeled peptides has been reported in many conditions; peptide receptor radionuclide therapy (PRRT) is already part of Scandinavian guidelines for treating neuroendocrine tumors. Lu-177- and Y-90-labeled somatostatin analogs, including DOTATOC, DOTANOC, and DOTATATE, are most the commonly used and have turned out to be effective. For routine use, an efficient, rapid, and reliable dose calculation tool is needed. In this chapter we describe how serial pre- and posttherapeutic scans can be used for dose calculation and for predicting therapy doses. Our software for radionuclide dose calculation is a three-dimensional, voxel-based system. The 3D dose calculation requires coregistered SPECT image sets from several time points after infusion to reconstruct time-activity curves for each voxel. Image registration is done directly by SPECT image registration using the first time point as a target. From the time-activity curves, initial activity and total half-life maps are calculated to produce a cumulated activity map. The cumulated activity map is then convoluted with a voxel-dose kernel to obtain a 3D dose map. We performed dose calculations

K. Kairemo (✉) · A. Kangasmäki
Departments of Nuclear Medicine, Molecular Radiotherapy and Medical Physics, Docrates International Comprehensive Cancer Center, Saukonpaadenranta 2, 00180 Helsinki, Finland
e-mail: kalevi.kairemo@docrates.com
A. Kangasmäki
e-mail: aki.kangasmaki@docrates.com

R. P. Baum and F. Rösch (eds.), *Theranostics, Gallium-68, and Other Radionuclides*, Recent Results in Cancer Research 194, DOI: 10.1007/978-3-642-27994-2_31,

similarly for both therapeutic and preplanning images. Preplanning dose was extrapolated to predict therapy dose using the ratio of administered activities. Our 3D dose calculation results are also compared with those of OLINDA. Our preliminary results indicate that dose planning using pretherapeutic scanning can predict critical organ and tumor doses. In some cases, the dose planning prediction resulted in slight, and slightly dose-dependent, overestimation of final therapy dose. Real tumor dose was similar in both pretherapeutic and posttherapeutic scans using our software. The OLINDA software and our program gave similar normal organ doses, whereas tumor doses could be calculated in a more detailed manner using the 3D program.

Contents

1 Introduction and Background Information

Peptide receptor radionuclide therapies (PRRTs) for somatostatin receptor-positive tumors have become widely used in recent years (Tiensuu Janson et al. 2010; Gabriel et al. 2010; Bodei et al. 2011). Patients receive multiple fractions of ^{177}Lu- or ^{90}Y-labeled somatostatin analogs or their combinations (Konijnenberg et al. 2007; Seregni et al. 2010; Bodei et al. 2008). ^{177}Lu (both a beta and gamma emitter) has the advantage over ^{90}Y (a pure beta emitter) of being directly imageable with a gamma camera, and its beta particles have shorter mean range, potentially increasing the dose to small lesions. Also, the short beta range decreases interorgan (source → target organ) radiation effects (Wessels et al. 2008; Forrer et al. 2009), such as hepatic lesions close to kidneys. ^{90}Y has the advantage when treating larger lesions, because the longer range of ^{90}Y beta radiation reduces the effect of inhomogeneous uptake in the final dose distribution such that the areas of lower uptake receive higher dose. Animal studies have shown the potential of combined ^{177}Lu- and ^{90}Y-labeled treatments, due to the combined advantages of treating small and large lesions with ^{177}Lu and ^{90}Y, respectively (De Jong et al. 2004).

Typically, neuroendocrine tumor (NET) patients undergo only ^{99m}Tc-octreotide, ^{111}In-octreotide, or ^{68}Ga-DOTA imaging prior to ^{177}Lu-DOTA treatment (Konijnenberg et al. 2004; Bakker et al. 2006; Cremonesi et al. 2006). PRRT is already part of Scandinavian guidelines for treating NETs (Tiensuu Janson et al. 2010).

Lu-177- and Y-90-labeled somatostatin analogs, including DOTATOC, DOTA-NOC, and DOTATATE, are most commonly used and have turned out to be effective. This procedure allows visual inspection of lesions and rough identification of tumor-to-background activity ratio. Due to the shorter radionuclide lifetimes and different kinetics of the tracers, it is not possible to obtain reliable dosimetric estimates from diagnostic images. When patient safety and treatment efficacy are of high priority, this is not sufficient.

Usually, the nominal administered activity is 7.4 GBq for all patients and all fractions (Kwekkeboom et al. 2005; Pauwels et al. 2005; Siegel et al. 2010; Cremonesi et al. 2011). The number of fractions is eventually determined by the tumor response and normal organ dose. Because high radiation doses are received by normal tissues, most importantly kidneys but also spleen, justification in the form of good therapeutic ratio is needed to proceed with treatment. For ^{177}Lu-(DOTA^{0}, Tyr^{3})octreotate, i.e., Lu-177-DOTATATE therapy, the maximum dose is determined by bone marrow dose of 2 Gy and kidney dose of 23 Gy, which are based on the Rotterdam experience (Kwekkeboom et al. 2005; Konijnenberg et al. 2007). Therefore, radionuclide treatment planning, similar to that applied in external-beam radiotherapy, is still needed.

Normal practice is, however, not to do preplanning but to proceed directly to treatment based on diagnostic images. Dose evaluation is done with either posttreatment images (Kairemo et al. 2002; Lubberink et al. 2002; Wehrmann et al. 2007) or standard patient kinetic models. During the therapy course, dose monitoring to normal tissues, and treatment efficacy in the form of tumor dose and changes in uptake are needed to justify each new treatment fraction.

Typical imaging for radionuclide therapy dosimetry is done with whole-body images and a transmission scan. Scatter- and attenuation-corrected whole-body (planar) images are summed geometrically to yield images that are used for dose estimation. Whole-body images are repeated at different times to estimate the total half-life of the tracer. Organ/lesion summation is a major problem in this approach. Another approach is to use a single photon emission computed tomography (SPECT) image to obtain better knowledge of the spatial distribution of the tracer, and then use repeated whole-body images to estimate the total half-life of the tracer. Full 3D dose calculation requires repeated SPECT imaging at different time points so that all voxels of the volume of interest are analyzed individually. Dose calculation can be done using Monte Carlo, convolution, or multiplication with a dose conversion constant.

Achieving comprehensive dose data requires a lot of imaging and analysis if treatment planning and patient- and fraction-specific treatment dose monitoring is to be done for each patient. Semiautomated 3D dose calculation is the best method for full characterization of tumor and normal organs.

Although the present work considers ^{177}Lu, the method and programs can be used for all radionuclides that can be imaged with SPECT/CT or PET/CT scanners with known dose-point or voxel-dose kernel (Kangasmäki et al. 2012). Before this automated approach we used planar image-based dosimetry similar to the Bad Berka approach (Wehrmann et al. 2007). In this system, S-factors and mean residence times (MRTs) for each organ have to calculated (Kairemo et al. 2002; Lubberink et al. 2002). Then, absolute uptake and MRTs can be calculated from serial imaging for activity distribution, typically from geometric mean images. This requires precise quantifications for organs and regions of interest. This may cause several uncertainties: (1) Calculations are not necessarily integrated with imagings; (2) Intraorgan distribution is often not taken into account; (3) Individual patient dimensions cannot be considered if the patient differs very much from the standard reference man. This all means that result is an almost real dose distribution. In order to define, e.g., MRT, very precisely, we have worked with a physiology based pharmacokinetic (PBPK) model for radiopharmacokinetics (Heiskanen et al. 2009). In this study, MRTs with three digits for more than 20 organs were calculated, when quantitative whole-body imaging at more than four time points was applied. We obtained more than 200 kinetic constants based on mathematical fitting, but actually this did not contribute much extra for the real dose calculation (Heiskanen et al. 2009).

The patient-specific 3D dose requires the 3D activity distribution at different time points in each patient. In general, exponential clearance in different regions is assumed; then, the imaged activity distribution corresponds to the real activity distribution and a real dose distribution can be calculated with known uncertainty.

This work describes a simple, clinically applicable (time-efficient) method to calculate the 3D dose distribution of ^{177}Lu-DOTA radionuclide therapy. Our method is based on multiple SPECT/CT imaging, voxel-based time-activity curve (TAC) estimation, and a 3D voxel-dose kernel convolution model (Kangasmäki et al. 2012). Additional information, such as biological half-life and initial activity, can be extracted from the same dataset to provide changes in tumor response between treatment fractions. The same approach can be utilized as a method for treatment planning: using a set of small injected activities for pre-planning images it is possible to calculate the 3D dose, which is then scaled to predict the full treatment dose.

2 Methods and Materials

2.1 Dose Calculation

The present 3D dose calculation model was developed for ^{177}Lu-DOTATATE radionuclide therapy. ^{177}Lu emits 113-keV (6%) and 208-keV (11%) gammas, which can be imaged with a gamma camera. The therapeutic dose originates from the emitted beta rays. The mean beta energy is 149 keV, and the maximum beta energy is 497 keV. The mean beta energy corresponds to about 0.25 mm range in water, whereas the maximum beta energy corresponds to about 2 mm range in water. Because of the short-range of ^{177}Lu, a dose per cumulated activity multiplication constant would produce a sufficient 3D dose map, but we constructed a method that can be extended to other radionuclides, such as ^{131}I, which emits high-energy photons. In our case, Lu-177 is produced from Yb-176 using an indirect route via Yb-177, so the byproduct Lu-177m is not formed. With direct irradiation of Lu-176, Lu-177m is formed to some extent in addition to the desired Lu-177. Lu-177m has a long half-life of 160 days.

The method used here is based on a voxel-by-voxel calculation of single exponential time-activity curves. The resulting 3D parameter maps of A_0 and $t_{1/2}$ are used to calculate the cumulated activity in each voxel. The resulting 3D cumulated activity map is then convoluted with a 3D voxel-dose kernel to produce the 3D dose map (Kangasmäki et al. 2012).

Multiple SPECT/CT images are acquired and registered to gain knowledge of voxel time-activity curves. After registering 2–4 SPECT image sets, the registered images are resampled to the target image of the registration (1 h image, or the first image). The registered and resampled images are combined to form a four-dimensional SPECT image that contains spatial and temporal information of the activity distribution.

All SPECT images, to cover at least most of the lesions, kidneys, liver, and spleen, were included. Sometimes, multiple-bed SPECT images were acquired such that also metastatic lesions were included in the images.

To model all voxels in the 4D image set, we used a single-exponential model

$$A(t) = A_0 \times \mathrm{e}^{-\ln 2t/t_{1/2}}$$

to fit A_0 and $t_{1/2}$ for easy calculation of the cumulated activity as

$$A_\mathrm{c} = A_0 \times t_{1/2} \times 1.443.$$

Here, $t_{1/2}$ is the total half-life of the nuclide. A simple time-activity model is needed, because only a small number of activity samples (SPECT/CT images) can be acquired due to time-consuming imaging and inconvenience to patients. A minimum of two time points are needed (because two parameters are fitted: A_0, $t_{1/2}$), and acquiring more than four time points cannot be achieved in our clinical practice. However, the present method does not impose an upper limit on the number of time points, and increasing the number of samples improves the fitted TAC. In our case (a private clinic) we settled for two or three time points depending on the ease of travel for the patients.

The ^{177}Lu voxel-point kernel used here is based on a dose-point kernel described in detail elsewhere (Kangasmäki et al. 2012). After fitting the model, several voxel-dose kernels corresponding to different SPECT image voxel sizes (from 1.2 to 9.59 mm) were created. These different voxel-dose kernels were used in artificial image phantom calculations to check against the results reported by Cremonesi et al. (2006). Only one voxel-dose kernel, with 4.79 mm voxel size, was used in the patient dose calculations, because this is the voxel size of the SPECT/CT images.

The calculation of treatment dose is done by 3D convolution of the voxel-dose kernel and cumulated activity. In the calculation, the patient is assumed to be fully water equivalent; i.e., patient inhomogeneities are not taken into account in the actual dose calculation. This does not impose problems, because we are mostly interested in hepatic lesions, bone marrow and kidney doses, which both are almost water-equivalent tissues.

The 3D cumulated activity distribution is obtained after 2–4 SPECT image sets are registered and the exponential time-activity curve is fitted for all voxels; finally, the cumulated activity is integrated when the initial activity and biologic half-life are known for all voxels (Kangasmäki et al. 2012).

All the calculations were done using MATLAB. All programs were written in house. The whole process of reading multiple SPECT images, calculating 3D initial activity, half-life, and cumulated activity maps, and then calculating the 3D dose distribution takes less than 5 min on a typical personal computer. Image registering and registered image resampling take also less than 5 min for one treatment fraction (three time points).

2.2 Clinical Practice

Patient imaging was done with a Siemens Symbia T2 (Siemens, Erlangen, Germany) dual-head SPECT/CT camera with medium-energy all-purpose collimator (MELP). The imaging protocol consisted of whole-body and SPECT/CT images taken at 1 h and 1, 3, and 7 days after the start of ^{177}Lu-DOTATATE infusion. All imaging utilized two photopeaks at 113 and 208 keV energies (15% energy windows) with scatter correction, the higher energy peak with only lower scatter window and the lower energy peak with both upper and lower scatter windows.

In the whole-body imaging, both AP and PA images were acquired with automatic body contouring enabled. The area of interest for the SPECT/CT imaging was determined from the whole-body images. In SPECT/CT imaging, single or multiple bed positions could be acquired. The bed speed was 7 cm/min. The first whole-body image of the series was acquired immediately after the end of infusion, so that this image contained all of the infused activity (the patient was allowed to empty the bladder only after the whole-body image).

The SPECT images were acquired with 128 × 128 matrix, zoom of 1, 30 s per view, and 64 views. If treatment planning imaging was required, similar image sets were acquired, but with imaging of 60 s per view. The CT images covered the whole SPECT image area; 130 kV, 17 mAs was used with B31 kernel filtering for anatomic information and B08 filtering for attenuation correction. The corresponding slice thicknesses for the two differently filtered CT images were 3 and 5 mm.

SPECT images were reconstructed using a Siemens MMWP multimodality workstation. The reconstruction algorithm was FLASH 3D (3D-OSEM) with 8 subsets and 16 iterations. A 10-mm Gaussian filter was applied. The choice of filtering is a compromise, because the same filtering is used for reconstruction of all SPECT imaging (including imaging with preplanning imaging with nominal injected activity of 200 MBq). CT-based attenuation correction was used in the reconstruction. Also scatter correction was used, and scatter-corrected photopeaks were summed to yield final SPECT images. The FLASH 3D reconstruction contains 3D collimator response modeling.

Whole-body images from the 1 h time point were used to double-check the correctness of the SPECT activity calibration. At 1 h, both whole-body images are acquired before the patient is allowed to empty the bladder, so all the infused activity is contained in the body. In this double-check, the total activity contained in the SPECT-imaged body portion is compared with the activity in the thickness-corrected (attenuation) geometrical mean of whole-body AP and PA images of the same area. A 15% difference in the calculated activities between whole-body and SPECT images is considered acceptable.

The SPECT images from 1, 3, and 7 day imaging times were registered to 1 h images (target in the fusions) and then resampled to 1 h slice locations and saved. Registration and resampling were done to assess the time-activity data for each voxel. These resampled images were then used in the 3D dose calculation. The scanner was calibrated for count to activity conversion using several phantoms, including PTW PET CEC emission phantom L981602 (PTW-Freiburg, Freiburg, Germany) to simulate human body.

Before the radiopeptide infusions, the patients received ondansetron or granisetron orally 30 min before the start of i.v. infusion of amino acids. Amino acids (25 g/l Arg, 25 g/l Lys) were infused with total volume of 1,500 mL, starting for 1 h before ^{177}Lu-DOTATATE was administered and then concomitantly via injection pumps. The mean therapy activity of 7.4 GBq was infused within 15–30 min, and the mean interval between therapies was 8 weeks (range 7–9 weeks), with typically 4–6 cycles of ^{177}Lu-DOTATATE given.

Similar conditions were applied for pretherapeutic scanning after receiving approximately 200 MBq of the same Lu-177-DOTA compound.

3 Results

We used approximately 200 MBq Lu-177-DOTA-FCFWLTCTate, i.e., Lu-177-DOTATATE, for serial imaging at 1, 24, and 72 and/or 168 h using amino acid kidney protection (25 g L/l, 25 g R/l) before the actual PRRT. Similar conditions were applied for posttherapeutic scanning after receiving approximately 7.4 GBq of the Lu-177-labeled compound. We used Organ Level INternal Dose Assessment/EXponential Modeling (OLINDA/EXM) and own software for actual dose calculation. Tumor-to-background ratios based on SPECT/CT in liver varied from 4:1 to 15:1. Tumor doses varied from 2 to 110 Gy, normal organ doses in kidneys from 3 to 12 Gy, normal liver from 2 to 20 Gy, and spleen from 2 to 20 Gy per cycle using posttherapeutic scans. We were also able to calculate the bone marrow dose directly from voxel data.

This type of work requires standardized SPECT/CT imaging; i.e., corrections are needed for attenuation and scatter, in order to create a CT-based attenuation map and iterative reconstructions with scatter corrections, which form the basis of

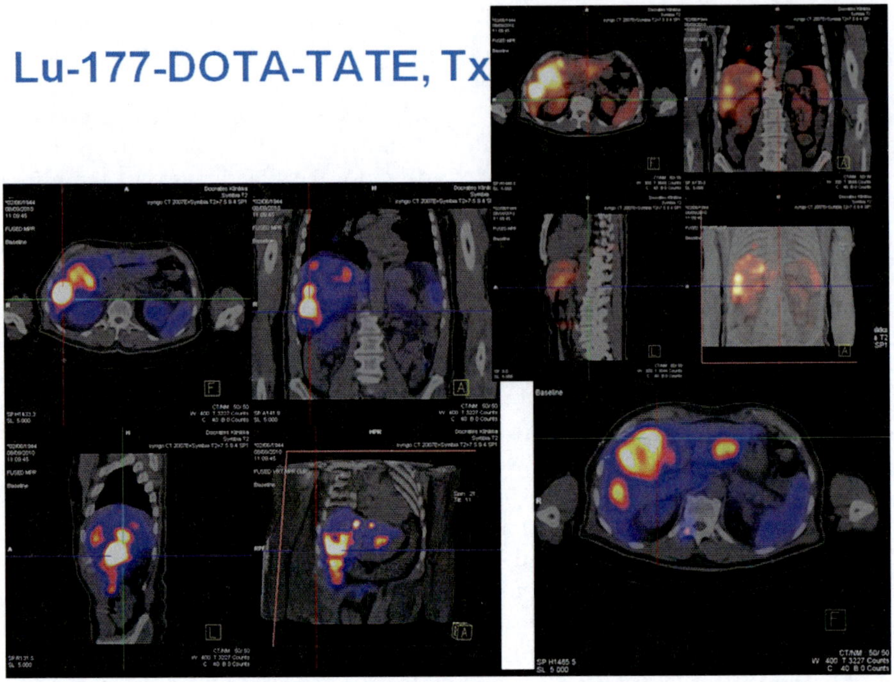

Fig. 1 Typical single photon emission computed tomography (SPECT/CT) findings in a NET patient with multiple liver metastases and single lung and skeletal metastases; this study was performed after a therapeutic Lu-177-DOTA-octreoTATE (DOTATATE) dose

quantitative SPECT imaging. Partial-volume corrections may be taken into account in dose maps. Additionally, the imaging system has to be calibrated using phantom studies. The errors related to uncertainties are described in detail elsewhere, but they are in the range of 10–15% (1 SD) (Kangasmäki et al. 2012).

Figure 1 shows typical SPECT/CT findings in a NET patient with multiple liver metastases and single solitary lung and skeletal metastases; this study was performed after a therapeutic Lu-177-DOTATATE dose. Figure 2 demonstrates serial SPECT registrations. These SPECT/CT registrations are aligned to each other to create a voxel-by-voxel time-activity map, i.e., voxel half-life map. Figure 3 illustrates one of our software tools. The calculated dose distribution can be overlaid, e.g., on CT images, and it is possible to create dose–volume histograms. Figure 4 shows the 3D dose distribution overlaid on the CT part of the SPECT/CT study. Here a relative scale is shown, but it can easily be presented on an absolute scale.

Table 1 demonstrates the pretherapeutic and therapeutic organ doses in various organs. Bone marrow dose was <0.5 Gy in all patients where serial pretherapeutic and posttherapeutic scannings were applied. Kidney doses were very similar.

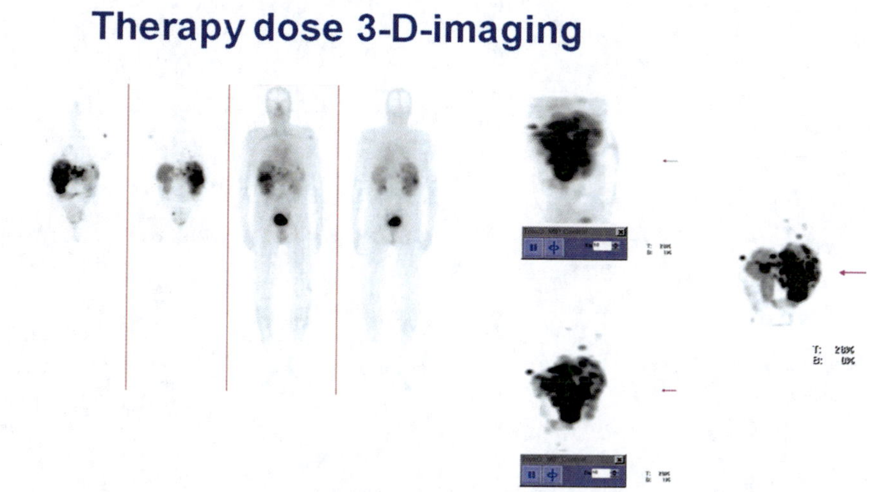

Fig. 2 Serial single photon emission computed tomography (SPECT) registrations, aligned on each other to create a voxel-by-voxel time-activity map, i.e., voxel half-life map

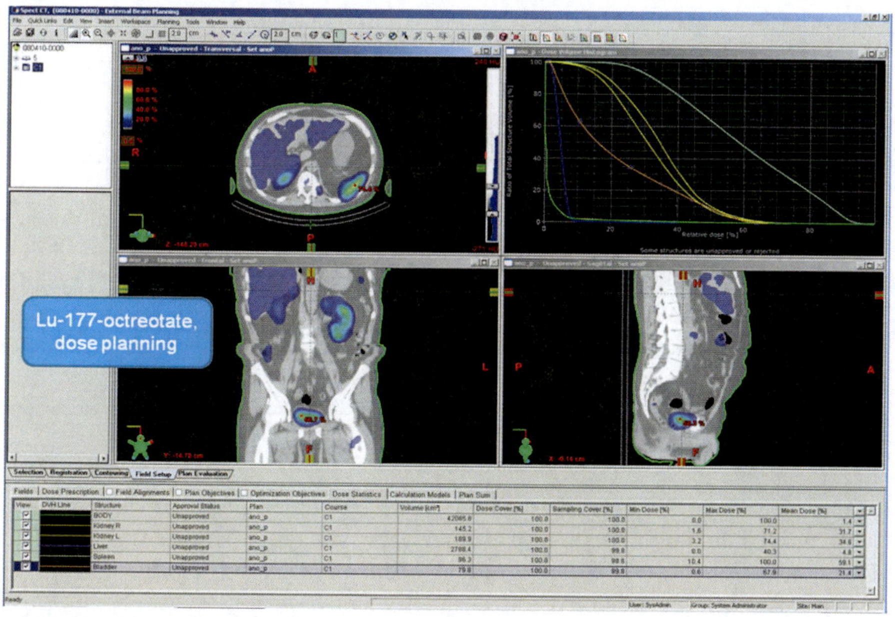

Fig. 3 One of our software tools. The calculated dose distribution can be overlaid, e.g., on CT images, and it is possible to create dose–volume histograms

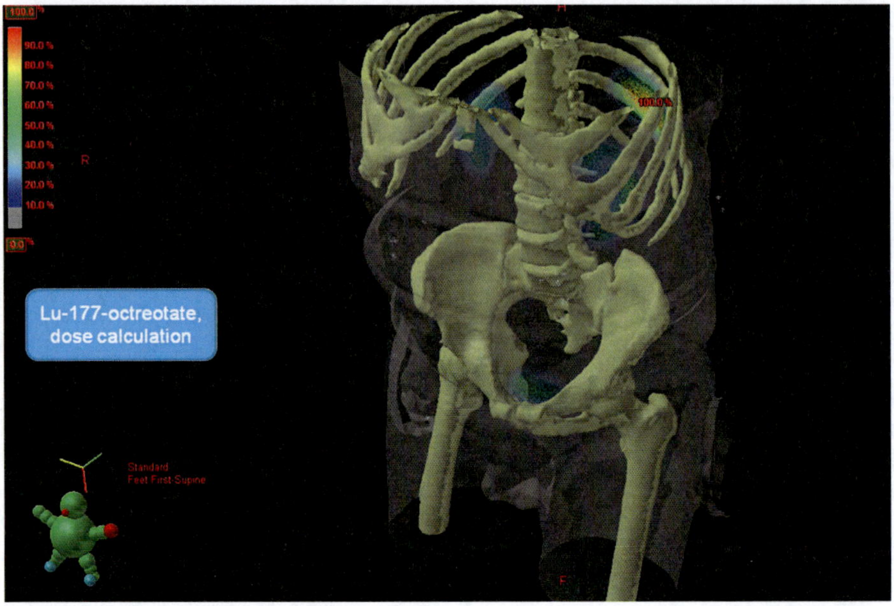

Fig. 4 The 3D dose distribution on the CT part of the single photon emission computed tomography (SPECT/CT). Here a relative scale is shown, to emphasize skeleton on CT, but it can easily be presented on an absolute scale and with other color scales

Table 2 presents the calculated doses in two patients who both received four cycles of Lu-177-DOTATATE treatment, demonstrating how the doses in liver metastases may vary considerably, from 17 to 222 Gy. Cumulative total doses in liver parenchyma in these patients also are very different: 6.7 and 80 Gy, respectively. Anyway, the normal liver doses were quite similar during 1–4 cycles, i.e., 1.1–3.0 Gy and 19.7–20.3 Gy, respectively. It can be further seen that the highest dose was usually obtained during the first cycle of Lu-177-DOTATATE.

4 Discussion

In this chapter we describe a new method for routine clinical PRRT dosimetry. In our hands, the calculations now take on average approximately 15 min per patient. This method offers reliable individualized tumor dosimetry in an arbitrary geometry. This is not yet possible with other existing dosimetry tools, e.g., OLINDA. For this voxel-based calculation, rigid-body registration is usually good enough. If this is not the case, deformable registration or organ of interest-specific registration may be applied. Our method also gives information about intraorgan dose distribution, e.g., about intratumoral or bone marrow dose. With Lu-177-DOTATATE, the bone

Table 1 Calculated pretherapeutic (Dx) and therapeutic (Tx) absorbed radiation doses for Lu-177-DOTATATE in kidneys, spleen, liver, bone marrow, and tumor tissue based on 4D SPECT/CT registration using aligned 3D voxels as basic information (4.8 mm × 4.8 mm × 4.8 mm size, cumulative activity, voxel mean residence times, cumulative dose)

Patient age	Kidney R Dx	Kidney R Tx	Kidney L Dx	Kidney L Tx	Spleen Dx	Spleen Tx	Liver Dx	Liver Tx	Bone marrow Dx	Bone marrow Tx	Tumor Dx	Tumor Tx
1/m 65	10.0	10.0	10.0	10.5	26.0	11.0	8.0	4.0	<0.5	0.5	n.d.	n.d.
2/m 62	8.0	5.0	8.0	5.0	9.0	6.0	5.0	5.0	<0.5	0.5	60–80	60–80
3/m 61	7.0	4.5	6.0	2.5	12.0	5.0	2.0	n.d.	0.5	0.5	25	25
4/f 67	16.0	12.0	16.0	13.5	55.0	20.0	2–8	1–4	<0.5	0.6	n.d.	5
5/m 76	4	4	4	4	9	7	15	15	<0.5	<0.5	30–40	30–50
6/m 36	11	5	8	5	9	2	3	1	n.d	n.d.	15–45	30–50
7/m 66	11	3	9	3	14	10	8	10	n.d	0.5	50	50

Patients were imaged 3–4 times at 1–168 h after both 200 MBq pretherapeutic and 7.4 GBq therapeutic dose of Lu-177-DOTA. Doses are in Gy

Table 2 Calculated therapeutic absorbed radiation doses (in Gy) for Lu-177-DOTATATE in kidneys, spleen, liver, and two liver metastases in two patients based on 4D SPECT/CT registration using aligned 3D voxels as basic information (4.8 mm × 4.8 mm × 4.8 mm size, cumulative activity, voxel mean residence times, cumulative dose)

Organ/patient	Dose planning*	1. Treatment**	2. Treatment	3. Treatment	4. Treatment	Cumulative dose
Patient 1						
Liver parenchyma	+	20.0	20.0	19.7	20.3	80.0
Liver metastasis 1	+	10.0	2.3	2.2	2.5	17.0
Liver metastasis 2	+	100.0	31.2	40.7	50.5	222.2
Kidneys	+	3.4	4.3	4.1	3.7	15.5
Spleen	+	10.0	16.4	29.4	14.0	69.8
Patient 2						
Normal liver	+	3.0	1.1	1.5	1.1	6.7
Liver metastasis 1	+	25.0	16.0	37.0	14.0	92.0
Liver metastasis 2	+	110.0	26.0	38.0	22.0	196.0
Kidneys	+	5.0	5.4	4.0	6.2	20.6

*200 MBq Lu-177-DOTATATE
**1–4 treatment 7.4 GBq Lu-177-DOTATATE
Patients were imaged 3–4 times at 1–168 h after four cycles of 7.4 GBq therapeutic dose of Lu-177-DOTA

marrow dose might be more critical than kidney dose, as our data in Table 1 demonstrate. Usually, kidney dose is critical in PRRT, if protection is not applied or Y-90 is used as a radionuclide (Melis et al. 2005; van Eerd et al. 2006; Vegts et al. 2006).

The results we obtained in dose planning seem to be relevant. Existing data based on OLINDA gave correct tumor and liver doses, but slightly overestimated spleen and kidney doses. Therefore, multicenter trials should be performed. Even though we already have experience of evaluating independent data from other institutions, "better extrapolation factors" for dose planning can only be obtained by analyzing independent, larger datasets.

Based on the data acquired and analyzed here, we can claim that there is a possibility for patient-based PRRT dose planning. This requires test dose-based preplanning and standardized imaging, dose calculation, and an algorithm for projection to full therapy dose. With preplanning it is possible to see: (1) whether the system delivers enough dose to treat tumors, (2) what the critical organ (kidneys, spleen, bone marrow) doses are, and (3) the desired optimal activity.

5 Conclusions and Summary of the Results

Heterogeneous radionuclide distribution of a short-range beta emitter imposes a major problem for planar imaging and the standard-man approach to radionuclide therapy dose calculations. There is a need for practical, fast, and reasonably accurate dose calculation for a variety of radionuclide therapies.

We tested our 3D dose calculation software with simulated image data and patient data. The patient dose calculations were compared with OLINDA/EXM-calculated doses. In both tests the agreement of the mean doses was excellent. In addition to the organ mean dose, our 4D approach yielded a multitude of additional information that can be used for tracer modeling and biological dose modeling.

The present 3D radionuclide dose calculation method is a time-efficient, simple, and clinically applicable and usable method to provide patient- and fraction-specific 3D dose data to plan and document the dose of radionuclide therapies. Furthermore, this method enables dose planning for radionuclide therapies. The 3D dose map allows excellent possibilities in treatment monitoring and radiobiological modeling.

Because peptide receptor radionuclide therapy (PRRT) is already part of Scandinavian guidelines in treating NETs with Lu-177- and Y-90-labeled somatostatin analogs, routine use of an efficient, rapid, and reliable dose calculation tool is needed.

Dose planning in advance requires new tools, this method being one of them. A basic problem is the possible change in the radiopharmacokinetics when the activity is 40-fold higher while the specific activity remains the same. Also, improvement of the preplanning image quality could result in better predictions. In a multicenter study, this extrapolation factor may be calculated in an appropriate manner. Anyway, we encourage investigators to engage in multicenter collaboration in collecting serial Lu-177 SPECT/CT data for 4D measurements and 3D dose calculations.

References

Bakker WH, Breeman WA, Kwekkeboom DJ et al (2006) Practical aspects of peptide receptor radionuclide therapy with [177Lu][DOTA0, Tyr3]octreotate. Q J Nucl Med Mol Imaging 50: 265–271

Bodei L, Cremonesi M, Ferrari M et al (2008) Long-term evaluation of renal toxicity after peptide receptor radionuclide therapy with 90Y-DOTATOC and 177Lu-DOTATATE: the role of associated risk factors. Eur J Nucl Med Mol Imaging 35:1847–1856

Bodei L, Cremonesi M, Grana CM et al (2011) Peptide receptor radionuclide therapy with (177)Lu-DOTATATE: the IEO phase I-II study. Eur J Nucl Med Mol Imaging 38(12): 2125–2135 epub Sept 3

Cremonesi M, Ferrari M, Bodei L et al (2006) Dosimetry in peptide radionuclide receptor therapy: a review. J Nucl Med 47:1467–1475

Cremonesi M, Ferrari M, Di Dia A et al (2011) Recent issues on dosimetry and radiobiology for peptide receptor radionuclide therapy. Q J Nucl Med Mol Imaging 55:155–167

De Jong M, Valkema R, Van Gameren A et al (2004) Inhomogeneous localization of radioactivity in the human kidney after injection of [(111)In-DTPA]octreotide. J Nucl Med 45:1168–1171

Forrer F, Krenning EP, Kooij PP et al (2009) Bone marrow dosimetry in peptide receptor radionuclide therapy with [177Lu-DOTA(0), Tyr(3)]octreotate. Eur J Nucl Med Mol Imaging 36:1138–1146

Gabriel M, Andergassen U, Putzer D et al (2010) Individualized peptide-related-radionuclide-therapy concept using different radiolabelled somatostatin analogs in advanced cancer patients. Q J Nucl Med Mol Imaging 54:92–9

Heiskanen T, Heiskanen T, Kairemo K (2009) Development of a PBPK model for monoclonal antibodies and simulation of human and mice PBPK of a radiolabelled monoclonal antibody. Curr Pharm Des 15:988–1007

Kairemo K, Lubberink M, Garske U et al (2002) Dosimetry of repeated Y-90-octreotide therapy of somatostatin expressing tumours. World J Nucl Med 1:S134–5

Kangasmäki A, Kiljunen T, Pyyry J et al (2012) A simple individualized 3D dose calculation for radionuclide therapy—applied in ^{177}Lu-DOTA receiving patients. (Submitted)

Konijnenberg M, Bijster M, Krenning EP et al (2004) A stylized computational model of the rat for organ dosimetry in support of preclinical evaluations of peptide receptor radionuclide therapy with ^{90}Y, ^{111}In, or ^{177}Lu. J Nucl Med 45:1260–9

Konijnenberg M, Melis M, Valkema R et al (2007) Radiation dose distribution in human kidneys by octreotides in peptide receptor radionuclide therapy. J Nucl Med 48:134–142

Kwekkeboom DJ, Teunissen JJ, Bakker WH et al (2005) Radiolabeled somatostatin analog ^{177}Lu-DOTA^{0}, Tyr^{3}) octreotate in patients with endocrine gastroenteropancreatic tumors. J Clin Oncol 23:2754–2762

Lubberink M, Garske U, Sandström M et al (2002) Dosimetry of repeated Y-90-SMT 487 (Octreother) therapy of somatostatin expressing tumours using Y-90-bremsstrahlung and In-111-octreotide measurements. Eur J Nucl Med 29:S358

Melis M, Krenning EP, Bernard BF et al (2005) Localisation and mechanism of renal retention of radiolabelled somatostatin analogues. Eur J Nucl Med Mol Imaging 32:1136–1143

Pauwels S, Barone R, Walrand S et al (2005) Practical dosimetry of peptide receptor radionuclide therapy with (90)Y-labeled somatostatin analogs. J Nucl Med 46(Suppl 1):92S–8S

Seregni E, Maccauro M, Coliva A et al (2010) Treatment with tandem [(90)Y]DOTA-TATE and [(177)Lu] DOTA-TATE of neuroendocrine tumors refractory to conventional therapy: preliminary results. Q J Nucl Med Mol Imaging 54:84–91

Siegel JA, Stabin MG, Sharkey RM (2010) Renal dosimetry in peptide radionuclide receptor therapy. Cancer Biother Radiopharm 25:581–8

Tiensuu Janson E, Sorbye H, Welin S et al (2010) Nordic guidelines 2010 for diagnosis and treatment of gastroenteropancreatic neuroendocrine tumors. Acta Oncol 49:740–756

van Eerd JE, Vegt E, Wetzels JF et al (2006) Gelatin-based plasma expander effectively reduces renal uptake of 111In-octreotide in mice and rats. J Nucl Med 47:528–533

Vegt E, Wetzels JF, Russel FG et al (2006) Renal uptake of radiolabeled octreotide in human subjects is efficiently inhibited by succinylated gelatin. J Nucl Med 47:432–6

Wehrmann C, Senftleben S, Zachert C et al (2007) Results of individual patient dosimetry in peptide receptor radionuclide therapy with 177Lu DOTA-TATE and 177Lu DOTA-NOC. Cancer Biother Radiopharm 22:406–416

Wessels BW, Konijnenberg MW, Dale RG et al (2008) MIRD pamphlet No. 20: the effect of model assumptions on kidney dosimetry and response–implications for radionuclide therapy. J Nucl Med 49:1884–1899

Peptide Receptor Radionuclide Therapy with ^{177}Lu Labeled Somatostatin Analogs DOTATATE and DOTATOC: Contrasting Renal Dosimetry in the Same Patient

Harshad R. Kulkarni, Christiane Schuchardt and Richard P. Baum

Abstract

Aim: The aim of this study is to correlate the uptake, residence time, and resulting mean absorbed dose in the kidneys with the posttherapy effect on renal function using the two most commonly used somatostatin analogs, ^{177}Lu-DOTATATE and ^{177}Lu-DOTATOC, during consecutive cycles of peptide receptor radionuclide therapy (PRRNT) in the same patient. *Methods*: 22 patients with metastatic neuroendocrine tumors underwent PRRNT with ^{177}Lu-DOTATATE and ^{177}Lu-DOTATOC. Dosimetry (MIRD scheme) was performed using OLINDA software. The patients were followed up for 6–12 months with serum creatinine, BUN, tubular extraction rate (TER) using ^{99m}Tc-MAG3, and glomerular filtration rate (GFR) using ^{99m}Tc-DTPA before and after therapy. Age, hypertension, and diabetes mellitus were the associated risk factors for renal toxicity, which were taken into account. *Results*: Uptake, residence time, and mean absorbed dose to the kidney were slightly, but significantly, higher for DOTATATE (actual absorbed dose 1.9–9.2 Gy) as compared with DOTATOC (dose 2.3–7.8 Gy) in 19 out of the 22 (86%) patients ($p < 0.05$). The tumor-to-kidney ratio was higher for DOTATOC in 23 out of 43 (53%) of the lesions analyzed; however, this difference was not statistically significant. There were no statistically significant changes in serum creatinine, BUN, TER or GFR pre and post-therapy with either DOTATATE or DOTATOC. Five of the 22 patients had mildly elevated serum creatinine after

H. R. Kulkarni · C. Schuchardt · R. P. Baum (✉)
Department of Nuclear Medicine and Center for PET/CT, ENETS Center of Excellence, Zentralklinik Bad Berka, 99437 Bad Berka, Germany
e-mail: richard.baum@zentralklinik.de
URL: www.zentralklinik-bad-berka.de

R. P. Baum and F. Rösch (eds.), *Theranostics, Gallium-68, and Other Radionuclides*, Recent Results in Cancer Research 194, DOI: 10.1007/978-3-642-27994-2_32,

PRRNT, of whom 3 had history of hypertension, 1 had diabetes, and 1 was more than 65 years of age. *Conclusions*: ^{177}Lu-DOTATATE and ^{177}Lu-DOTATOC are safe radiopharmaceuticals concerning renal toxicity. ^{177}Lu-DOTATOC delivers a slightly, but significantly, lower renal dose.

Keywords
Mean absorbed dose · DOTATATE · DOTATOC

Contents

1 Introduction

Treatment with radiolabeled somatostatin analogs is a valid therapeutic option for management of patients with inoperable or metastasized well-differentiated neuroendocrine tumors. Favorable results have been obtained with both ^{90}Y- and ^{177}Lu-labeled peptides in terms of tumor regression (De Jong et al. 2002; Kwekkeboom et al. 2005a, b; Otte et al. 1998).

All the radiopharmaceuticals used for peptide receptor radionuclide therapy (PRRNT) show high uptake in parenchyma of kidneys and hence pose the risk of nephrotoxicity. Renal uptake is not somatostatin receptor mediated, but related primarily to the very rapid clearance of the small radiopeptides that are filtered through the glomeruli and reabsorbed by the tubular cells (Pauwels et al. 2005; De Jong et al. 1998; Behr et al. 1998). Kidneys are therefore the dose-limiting organs for PRRNT, making accurate renal dosimetry absolutely essential to minimize radiation nephropathy (Pauwels et al. 2005; Valkema et al. 2005; Lambert et al. 2004).

The pattern of nephrotoxicity after PRRNT is that of progressive chronic renal disease (Valkema et al. 2005). Age greater than 65 years, hypertension, and diabetes are the risk factors contributing to decline in renal function after PRRNT, in addition to the per-cycle and cumulative renal dose (Valkema et al. 2005; Arora et al. 2012; National Chronic Kidney Disease Fact Sheet 2010; Bodei et al. 2008).

The two radiolabeled peptides commonly used in PRRNT are ^{177}Lu-DOTATATE and ^{177}Lu-DOTATOC. The aim of this study is to compare and correlate the renal uptake, residence time, per-cycle mean absorbed dose, and toxicity to the kidneys in a group of patients having undergone PRRNT with both peptides, taking the additional risk factors into account.

2 Patients and Methods

2.1 Patients

All patients enrolled in this study were suffering from metastasized NETs with liver, lymph node, bone, or other metastases. Intense somatostatin receptor (SSTR) expression of primary tumors and metastases had been verified before therapy by using ^{68}Ga DOTA-somatostatin receptor (SSTR) analog positron emission computed tomography (PET/CT) using DOTANOC/DOTATOC or DOTATATE. Each patient was extensively informed about the therapeutic procedure and possible adverse effects. The study was performed according to guidelines, approved by the local ethics committee, and in accordance with German regulations concerning radiation safety.

Twenty-two patients with neuroendocrine tumors (12 male, 10 female; age 45.3–75.5 years) underwent treatment with ^{177}Lu-DOTATATE (5.0–9.5 GBq) and ^{177}Lu-DOTATOC (5.5–8.5 GBq) in consecutive cycles (Table 1). The time period between cycles was 10–14 months. Data obtained from this group were used to compare kinetics and mean absorbed doses to kidneys with therapy using ^{177}Lu-DOTATATE and ^{177}Lu-DOTATOC in the same patients. The risk factors of chronic renal disease considered in the patient group were age greater than 65 years, hypertension, and diabetes mellitus (Table 2).

2.2 Radiopharmaceuticals

The radiopharmaceuticals were prepared in our own radio pharmacy. ^{177}Lu-labeling of DOTA-peptides was done according to the general procedure: A solution of 500 μg 2,5-dihydroxybenzoic acid and 50 μg of the corresponding DOTA peptide in 50 μL 0.4 M sodium acetate buffer (pH 5.5) was added to a solution of 1 GBq in 30 μL 0.05 M HCl. The mixture was heated to 90°C for 30 min and then diluted with 0.9% saline solution followed by sterile filtration. Quality control settings were the following: RP-18-HPLC, solvent A: water; solvent B: acetonitrile (both with 0.1% TFA); gradient: 0–2 min 100% A, 20 min 100% B; flow rate: 1.2 mL/min; column: LiChrospher 100RP 18EC-5 μm 250 × 4 mm. The radiochemical purity was greater than 99.5%.

Table 1 Characteristics of 22 patients (12 male, 10 female) treated with DOTATATE and DOTATOC included in the study

	DOTATATE	DOTATOC
Age	60.2 ± 9.1 years	
	45.3–75.2 years	
Activity per cycle (GBq)	6.5 ± 1.1	7.3 ± 0.7
	5.0–9.5	5.5–8.5

Table 2 Risk factors present in the patient group

Risk factor	No. of patients
Hypertension	9
Diabetes	2
Age more than 65 years	4

2.3 Infusion and Renal Protection

For kidney protection, every patient was co-infused with 1,500 mL of a renoprotective amino acid mixture of 5% lysine HCL and 10% L-arginine HCL in 250 mL NaCl at pH 7.4 and osmolarity of 400 mosmol/l. This infusion was started 30 min prior to administration of the therapeutic dose and continued for 4 h. The radiopharmaceutical was co-administered over 10–15 min by using a second infusion pump system. This co-infusion of amino acids reduces renal exposure and allows for higher mean absorbed doses to reach tumors (Jamar et al. 2003).

The activity to administer was chosen based on the general status of the patient (e.g., Karnofsky scale), kidney function, hematologic reserve, tumor mass and SSTR expression, previous treatments, and also experience reported by other groups (Kwekkeboom et al. 2005).

2.4 Monitoring of Renal Function

In all patients undergoing PRRNT, follow-up of renal function was carried out after each cycle after a period of 6–12 months with serum creatinine and BUN. GFR was determined using 110–185 MBq ^{99m}Tc-DTPA before and every 3–4 months after therapy, and the tubular extraction rate (TER) determined using ^{99m}Tc-MAG3 was also documented.

2.5 Dosimetry

Dosimetric calculations were performed according to the MIRD scheme from 2D planar whole image sets (Bolch et al. 2009). The time-dependent activity was determined based on conjugated planar whole-body scans acquired 0.5, 3, 20–24, 44–48, and 68–72 h post injection. For estimation of mean absorbed doses,

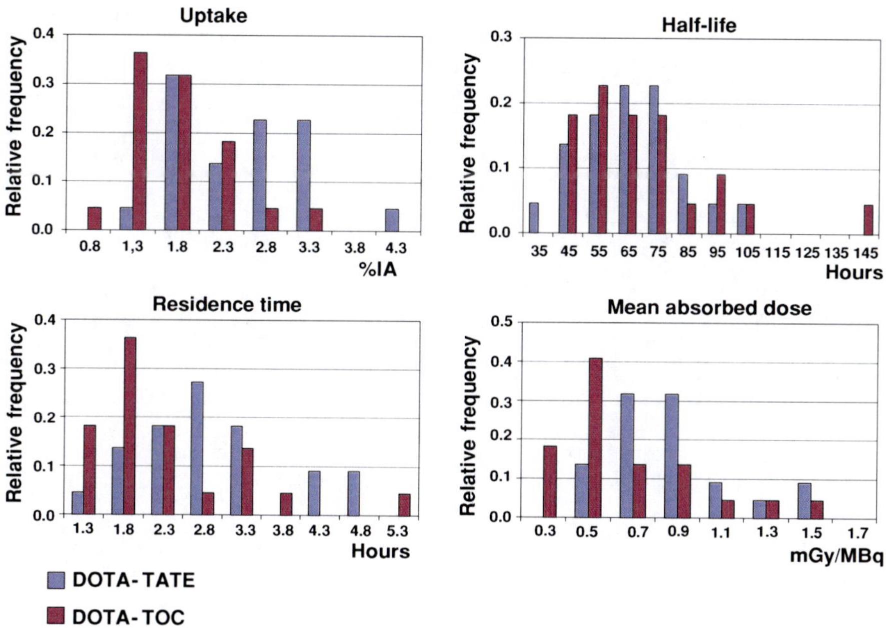

Fig. 1 Comparison of renal dosimetry parameters for DOTATATE and DOTATOC

we used a well-established dosimetry protocol, as was used in a previous study (Wehrmann et al. 2007).

2.6 Comparison and Statistics

The dosimetric parameters determined for kidneys in addition to the mean absorbed dose were uptake, half life, residence time, and tumor-to-kidney ratio. Pre- and post-therapy serum creatinine, GFR, and TER were also compared. The effect of age, diabetes, hypertension, and total administered activity on renal function was determined. For evaluation of statistically significant differences, nonparametric signed-rank tests for paired samples were used. All statistical tests were performed using ORIGINPRO 8.1G; p-values ≤ 0.05 were considered to be significant.

3 Results

The dosimetric parameters for kidneys were determined in 22 patients for both DOTATATE and DOTATOC (Fig. 1). Renal uptake, residence time, and mean absorbed dose per unit administered activity showed higher values for

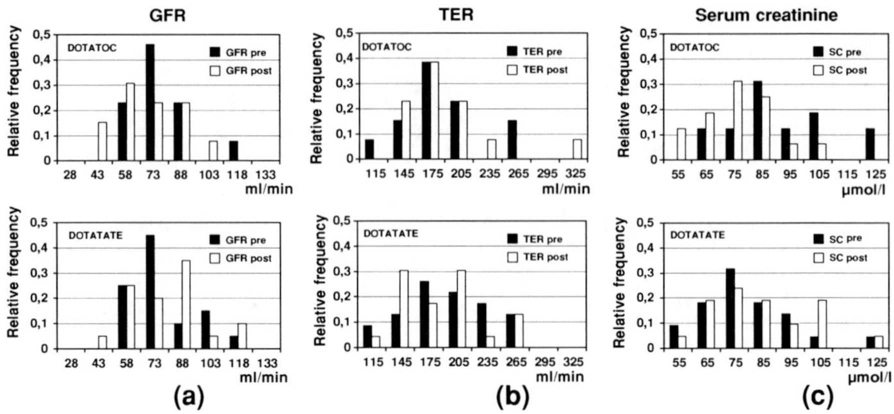

Fig. 2 Comparison of pre- and post-therapy renal parameters in patients treated with DOTATOC and DOTATATE: **a** GFR, **b** TER, and **C** serum creatinine

DOTATATE in 19 of 22 patients (86%, $p < 0.05$). These results were statistically significant. Only half-life was found to be similar for both peptides, where 12 patients (55%) showed longer half-life for DOTATATE ($p > 0.05$).

Tumor-to-kidney ratio was higher for DOTATOC in 23 of 43 (53%) lesions measured; however, this difference was not statistically significant ($p > 0.05$).

There were no statistically significant changes in GFR (Fig. 2a), TER (Fig. 2b), or serum creatinine (Fig. 2c) pre and post-therapy with either DOTATATE or DOTATOC ($p > 0.1$). Five of the 22 patients had mild elevation in serum creatinine, of whom 3 had history of hypertension, 1 had diabetes mellitus, and 1 was aged >65 years. In none of these five patients did any significant fall in serum creatinine occur post-therapy. Thus, no significant changes in renal function were observed in any of the patients irrespective of the amount of administered radioactivity and peptide used for PRRNT.

4 Discussion

Since kidneys are the dose-limiting organs in PRRNT, the safe therapeutic window in our opinion would be best determined by the tumor-to-kidney ratio for absorbed dose. In the present study, this ratio was comparable for DOTATATE and DOTATOC, when individual lesions were considered. However, Forrer et al. (2004), in a study of five patients comparing ^{111}In-DOTATATE and ^{111}In-DOTATOC as surrogates to study the biodistribution of ^{90}Y-labeled peptides, found a significant difference between the mean values for the two peptides and concluded on this basis to continue using DOTATOC for PRRNT.

Esser et al. (2006) compared ^{177}Lu-DOTATATE and ^{177}Lu-DOTATOC in seven patients and found also longer residence time in kidneys with DOTATATE. They concluded, however, that DOTATATE would be the better peptide for PRRNT based on the finding that the ratio of residence times of DOTATATE to DOTATOC in tumor was higher than that for kidneys and hence DOTATATE gives a higher dose to the tumor. On the other hand, Forrer et al. (2004) found no significant difference in mean absorbed dose to kidneys. In our study, the mean absorbed kidney dose was significantly higher for DOTATATE than for DOTATOC due to significantly higher renal uptake and longer residence time in kidneys.

The high interpatient variability in the mean absorbed doses was due to patients' heterogeneity, presenting with varying receptor density and tumor burden. The estimated mean dose to the kidney in this study was 1.9–9.2 Gy, which is comparable to that determined by Valkema et al. (2005), who reported a renal dose of 1.8–7.8 Gy. In addition, the results showed also significant intrapatient variability (i.e., in the same patient undergoing PRRNT with different peptides) with respect to renal pharmacokinetics and renal dose.

However, in comparison with ^{90}Y-labeled peptides (DOTATATE or DOTATOC), the renal dose is significantly lower when using ^{177}Lu, which translates into lower renal toxicity (Forrer et al. 2004; Bodei et al. 2003; Helisch et al. 2004). This corresponds to the clinical experience, where renal impairment occurred more frequently in patients treated with ^{90}Y-peptide as compared with the sporadic incidence observed with ^{177}Lu-DOTATATE PRRNT (despite mean cumulative kidney doses of up to 45 Gy) (Valkema et al. 2005). This can be explained on the basis of the particle range and the site of peptide accumulation. All radiolabeled peptides localize in the proximal tubules, where they are reabsorbed. Since tubular cells are relatively radioresistant and able to repair and regenerate, renal toxicity due to radiation to the renal tubules is quite unlikely, as confirmed by the fact that there was no significant fall in TER in our study (Cremonesi et al. 2006). However, glomerular cells are relatively radiosensitive and not able to regenerate, therefore bearing a high nephrotoxic potential. The long-range β-particles of the ^{90}Y-peptides may increase the toxicity due to cross-fire irradiation of glomerular cells. On the other hand, since the β-particles of ^{177}Lu-peptides are of short range, they irradiate tubular cells more selectively, sparing glomeruli as confirmed by the evidence that there was no significant short-term decline in GFR in our study (Cremonesi et al. 2006).

As previous studies have shown, other contributing risk factors for chronic renal disease must also be considered, the presence of which accelerates the onset of end-stage renal disease (ESRD), especially when using ^{90}Y-labeled peptides (Valkema et al. 2005; Bodei et al. 2008). A dose of 28 Gy has been advocated as the threshold for the biologically effective dose (BED) for patients with risk factors (mainly hypertension and diabetes) to minimize the risk of ESRD following PRRNT (Bodei et al. 2008). In our study we considered age greater than 65 years, diabetes, and hypertension as the most relevant risk factors for chronic renal disease. In fact, all five patients with mild renal dysfunction after PRRNT had one of the risk factors present; however, PRRNT with ^{177}Lu-labeled peptides could be safely administered to these patients without any short-term adverse effects.

5 Conclusions

^{177}Lu-DOTATATE and ^{177}Lu-DOTATOC are safe radiopharmaceuticals concerning renal toxicity. Both are equivalent with respect to tumor-to-kidney ratio. ^{177}Lu-DOTATOC delivers a slightly, but significantly, lower renal mean absorbed dose. The mean absorbed dose to the kidney with ^{177}Lu-labeled peptides is significantly lower than renal mean absorbed doses delivered when using ^{90}Y-labeled DOTATATE or DOTATOC, corresponding to lower renal toxicity. Finally, this study underlines the importance of clinical screening for risk factors of chronic renal disease before PRRNT.

References

Arora P, Verrelli M, Mulloy LL, Talavera F, Aronoff GR, Schmidt RJ, Batuman V. Chronic Renal failure. eMedicine Medscape references Feb 2012. http://emedicine.medscape.com/article/238798-overview

Behr TM, Goldenberg DM, Becker W (1998) Reducing the renal uptake of radiolabeled antibody fragments and peptides for diagnosis and therapy: present status, future prospects and limitations. Eur J Nucl Med 25:201–212

Bodei L, Cremonesi M, Zoboli S (2003) Receptor-mediated radionuclide therapy with ^{90}Y-DOTATOC in association with amino acid infusion: a phase I study. Eur J Nucl Med 30:207–216

Bodei L, Cremonesi M, Ferrari M, Pacifi C, Grana C, Bartolomei M, Baio S, Sansovini M, Paganelli G (2008) Long-term evaluation of renal toxicity after peptide receptor radionuclide therapy with 90Y-DOTATOC and 177Lu-DOTATATE: the role of associated risk factors. Eur J Nucl Med 35(10):1847–1856

Bolch WE, Eckerman KF, Sgouros G, Thomas SR (2009) MIRD pamphlet No. 21: a generalized schema for radiopharmaceutical dosimetry–standardization of nomenclature. J Nucl Med 50:477–484

Cremonesi M, Ferrari M, Bodei L, Tosi G, Paganelli G (2006) Dosimetry in peptide radionuclide receptor therapy: a review. J Nucl Med 47(9):1467–1475

De Jong M, Bakker WH, Breeman WA et al (1998) Pre-clinical comparison of [DTPA0] octreotide, [DTPA0, Tyr3] octreotide and [DOTA0, Tyr3] octreotide as carriers for somatostatin receptor-targeted scintigraphy and radionuclide therapy. Int J Cancer 75:406–411

De Jong M, Valkema R, Jamar F (2002) Somatostatin receptor-targeted radionuclide therapy of tumors: preclinical and clinical findings. Semin Nucl Med 32:133

Esser JP, Krenning EP, Teunissen JJM (2006) Comparison of [^{177}Lu-DOTA^{0}, Tyr3] octreotate and [^{177}Lu-DOTA^{0}, Tyr3] octreotide: which peptide is preferable for PRRT? Eur J Nucl Med 33:1346–1351

Forrer F, Uusijärvi H, Waldherr C (2004) A comparison of ^{111}In-DOTATOC and ^{111}In-DOTATATE: biodistribution and dosimetry in the same patients with metastatic neuroendocrine tumours. Eur J Nucl Med 31:1257–1262

Helisch A, Förster GJ, Reber H (2004) Pre-therapeutic dosimetry and biodistribution of ^{86}Y-DOTA-Phe^{1}-Tyr^{3}-octreotide versus ^{111}In-pentetreotide in patients with advanced neuroendocrine tumours. Eur J Nucl Med 31:1386–1392

Jamar F, Barone R, Matthieu I et al (2003) ^{86}Y-DOTA^{0}-D-Phe^{1}-Tyr^{3}-octreotide (SMT487)—a phase 1 clinical study: pharmacokinetics, biodistribution and renal protective effect of different regiments of amino acid coinfusion. Eur J Nucl Med 30:510

Kwekkeboom DJ, Mueller-Brand J, Paganelli G (2005a) An overview of the results of peptide receptor radionuclide therapy with 3 different radiolabeled somatostatin analogues. J Nucl Med 46:62S

Kwekkeboom DJ, Teunissen JJ, Bakker WH et al (2005b) Radiolabeled somatostatin analog [177Lu-DOTA0, Tyr3]-octreotate in patients with endocrine gastroenteropancreatic tumors. J Clin Oncol 23:2754

Lambert B, Cybulla M, Weiner SM et al (2004) Renal toxicity after radionuclide therapy. Radiat Res 161:607–611

National Chronic Kidney Disease Fact Sheet (2010) CDC website. http://www.cdc.gov/diabetes/pubs/factsheets/kidney.htm

Otte A, Mueller-Brand J, Dellas S (1998) Yttrium-90 labeled somatostatin analogue for cancer treatment. Lancet 351:417

Pauwels S, Barone R, Walrand S et al (2005) Practical dosimetry of peptide receptor radionuclide therapy with ^{90}Y-labeled somatostatin analogs. J Nucl Med 46(suppl 1):92S–98S

Valkema R, Pauwels SA, Kvols LK et al (2005) Long-term follow-up of renal function after peptide receptor radiation therapy with 90Y-DOTA0, Tyr3-octreotide and 177Lu-DOTA0, Tyr3-octreotate. J Nucl Med 46(suppl 1):83S–91S

Wehrmann C, Senftleben S, Zachert C, Mueller D, Baum RP (2007) Results of individual patient dosimetry in peptide receptor radionuclide therapy with 177Lu DOTA-TATE and 177Lu DOTA-NOC. Cancer Biother Radiopharm 22(3):406–416

Is There a Correlation Between Peptide Receptor Radionuclide Therapy-Associated Hematological Toxicity and Spleen Dose?

Harshad R. Kulkarni, Vikas Prasad, Christiane Schuchardt and Richard P. Baum

Abstract

Aim: The spleen receives a high mean absorbed radiation dose during peptide receptor radionuclide therapy (PRRNT). The aim of this study is to correlate the radiation dose to spleen with the effect on blood cell count after PRRNT. *Methods*: Fifty-three neuroendocrine tumor (NET) patients were treated with 3.8–8.5 GBq ^{177}Lu-DOTATATE or ^{177}Lu-DOTATOC. Dosimetry was performed according to MIRD scheme. Eleven NET patients who had undergone splenectomy before PRRNT and who received 4.7–7.6 GBq ^{177}Lu-DOTATATE or ^{177}Lu-DOTATOC were selected as controls. RBC, WBC (total and differential), and platelet counts before and after each cycle of PRRNT were documented. *Results*: The median dose to the spleen in the study group was 6.34 Gy (2.32–20.06 Gy). There was no significant difference in the posttherapy changes in the blood cell counts (RBC, WBC, or platelets) between the study group and the control group. Mild hematological toxicity was found in 7 of the 53 (13.2%) patients in the study group and in 1 out of the 11 patients (9.1%) in the control group. However, there was no correlation between the incidence or grade of hematological toxicity and the dose to the spleen. *Conclusion*: This study demonstrates for the first time that hematological toxicity after PRRNT is not related to the radiation dose to the spleen.

H. R. Kulkarni · V. Prasad · C. Schuchardt · R. P. Baum (✉)
Department of Nuclear Medicine, Center for PET/CT,
ENETS Center of Excellence Zentralklinik Bad Berka, 99437 Bad Berka, Germany
e-mail: richard.baum@zentralklinik.de

R. P. Baum and F. Rösch (eds.), *Theranostics, Gallium-68, and Other Radionuclides*, Recent Results in Cancer Research 194, DOI: 10.1007/978-3-642-27994-2_33,

Contents

1 Background

Peptide receptor radionuclide therapy (PRRNT) is a well-established therapeutic option for metastatic neuroendocrine tumors (NETs) (Krenning et al. 2004; van Essen et al. 2007; Kwekkeboom et al. 2008). The spleen has been found to have very high uptake of somatostatin receptor analogs, thereby receiving a high radiation dose during PRRNT using radiolabeled somatostatin receptor analogs (Wehrmann et al. 2007). It has previously been postulated that this is related to the presence of somatostatin receptors on lymphocytes (Reubi et al. 1990). The exact site and mechanism of the uptake in the spleen have, however, not been clearly elucidated. Even though the spleen is not the site of formation of blood cells, it serves as a reservoir of erythrocytes and platelets, to be made available in the event of an emergency such as hemorrhagic shock, and of leukocytes, particularly undifferentiated monocytes, which are mobilized and deployed at sites of inflammation. Apart from the functions of cellular and humoral immunity, irreversible trapping of particulate matter (e.g., bacteria), and extramedullary hematopoiesis (e.g., in severe anemia in adults), two other important functions of the spleen are removal of damaged and senescent RBCs and sequestration of platelets (a passive process whereby platelets become adhered to the reticular meshwork of splenic cords and can be released by epinephrine). In addition, a recent study showed that spleen acts as a reservoir for undifferentiated monocytes, outnumbering their counterparts in circulation. The reservoir monocytes assemble in clusters in the cords of the subcapsular red pulp and are distinct from macrophages and dendritic cells, into which they differentiate upon tissue entry. In response to ischemic myocardial injury, splenic monocytes increase their motility, exit the spleen en masse, accumulate in injured tissue, and participate in wound healing (Swirski et al. 2009).

Previous studies have demonstrated the effect of external radiation to the spleen on hematological profile (Weinmann et al. 2001). However, there have been no previous studies demonstrating the effect of dose to the spleen during radionuclide (internal radiation) therapy. In spite of the low dose rate, the absolute dose to the spleen is the highest of all the organs during PRRNT (Reubi et al. 1990). Hence, we sought to investigate the effect of this high dose on the blood cells sequestered.

The aim of our study is to correlate the mean absorbed dose to the spleen during peptide receptor radionuclide therapy (PRRNT) with the changes in the blood cell count after therapy.

2 Patients and Methods

2.1 Patients

All patients enrolled in this study were suffering from metastatic NETs with liver, lymph node, bone, or other organ involvement. Intense SSTR expression of (inoperable) primary tumors and metastases had been verified before therapy by using ^{68}Ga-DOTANOC, ^{68}Ga-DOTATOC, or ^{68}Ga-DOTATATE positron emission computed tomography (PET/CT), after which they underwent PRRNT with ^{177}Lu-DOTATATE or ^{177}Lu-DOTATOC. To study the effect of the mean absorbed dose to the spleen on hematological toxicity, the patients were divided into two groups: the study group consisting of patients with intact spleen ($n = 53$), and the control group consisting of patients having undergone splenectomy at time of PRRNT ($n = 11$). One cycle of PRRNT was considered for analysis in each patient. The patients in the control group were patients with neuroendocrine tumor of the tail of the pancreas, having undergone splenectomy in addition to the surgery of the primary tumor, as discussed and decided by our interdisciplinary tumor board. Since chemotherapy also has an adverse effect on the hematological profile, patients with past history of chemotherapy were excluded from the study and the control group.

2.2 Dosimetry

Dosimetric calculations were performed according to the MIRD scheme on the basis of five planar whole-body scans in the following time order: the first scan immediately after administration of the radiopharmaceutical, followed by 3, 24, 48, and 72 h post injection (p.i.). Regions of interest (ROI) were drawn around the spleen and, after consideration of geometric mean and background correction, were analyzed to obtain time-activity curves. From the residence time of the radiopharmaceutical, the mean absorbed dose to the spleen was estimated by OLINDA/EXM software.

2.3 Statistics

To assess significance of differences in incidence and grade of hematological toxicity in the study and control groups, nonparametric tests for independent samples were used; p-values ≤ 0.05 were considered to be significant (ORIGINPRO 8.1 G).

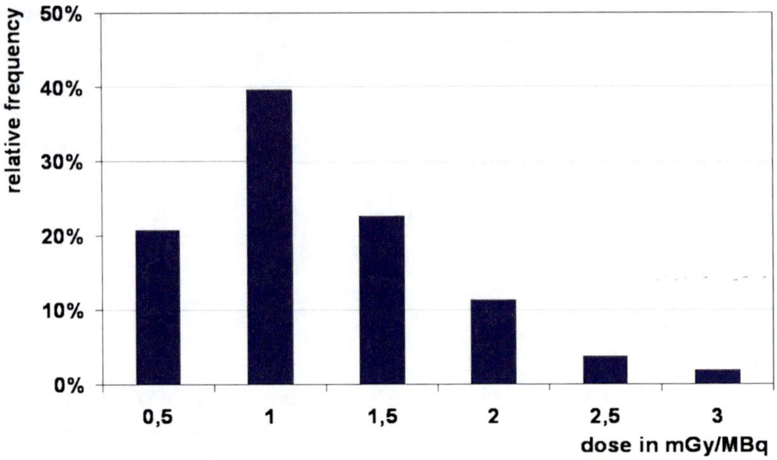

Fig. 1 Frequency distribution of mean absorbed dose to the spleen in the 53 patients in the study group

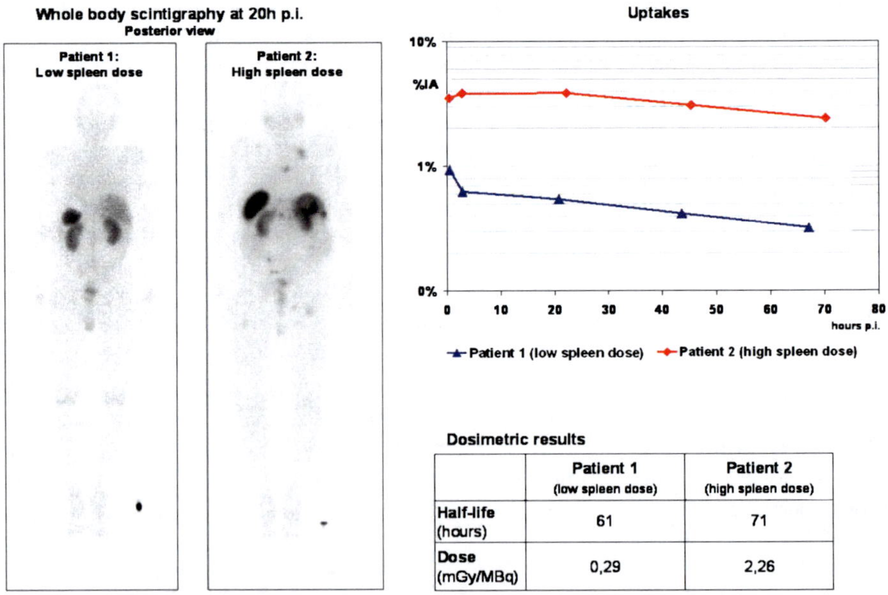

	Patient 1 (low spleen dose)	Patient 2 (high spleen dose)
Half-life (hours)	61	71
Dose (mGy/MBq)	0,29	2,26

Fig. 2 ^{177}Lu posttherapy whole-body scans 20 h p.i. along with corresponding time-activity curves in two patients with high and low mean absorbed dose to the spleen

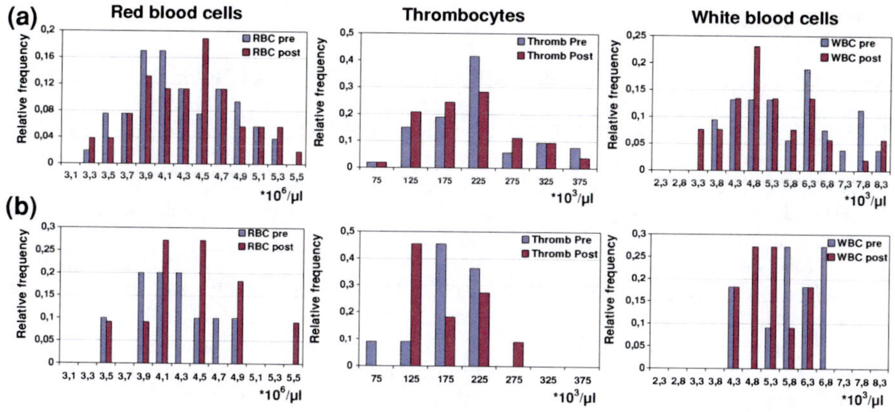

Fig. 3 Comparison between pre- and post-PRRNT blood cell counts in the study group (**a**) and control group (**b**)

3 Results

The median dose to the spleen in the study group was 6.34 Gy (2.32–20.06 Gy). The frequency distribution of the mean absorbed dose to the spleen in the 53 patients in the study group (Fig. 1) demonstrated wide variation. Figure 2 shows ^{177}Lu posttherapy whole-body scans 20 h p.i. along with corresponding time-activity curves in two patients with high and low mean absorbed dose to the spleen.

The analysis of hematological parameters revealed no significant difference ($p > 0.05$) in posttherapeutic changes of blood cell counts (RBC, WBC, or platelets) between the study group (Fig. 3a) and the control group (Fig. 3b). Mild hematological toxicity (erythrocytopenia and thrombocytopenia grade I) was observed in 7/53 (13.2%) of patients with intact spleen. Erythrocytopenia grade I was also observed in 1/11 (9.1%) of patients without spleen after PRRNT. In addition, there was no significant correlation between the incidence of hematological toxicity and the dose to the spleen ($r^2 = 0.029$; $p = 0.5$).

4 Conclusion

PRRNT with ^{177}Lu-labeled peptides is safe and has minor adverse hematological effects, mostly mild erythrocytopenia. However, this is most likely due to the radiation dose delivered to whole body (including bone marrow). This study demonstrates for the first time that hematological toxicity after PRRNT is not related to the radiation dose to spleen.

References

Krenning EP, Kwekkeboom DJ, Valkema R, Pauwels S, Kvols LK, De Jong M (2004) Peptide receptor radionuclide therapy. Ann N Y Acad Sci 1014:234–245

Kwekkeboom DJ, de Herder WW, Kam BL, van Eijck CH, van Essen M, Kooij PP, Feelders RA, van Aken MO, Krenning EP (2008) Treatment with the radiolabeled somatostatin analog [177 Lu-DOTA 0, Tyr3]octreotate: toxicity, efficacy, and survival. J Clin Oncol 26:2124–2130

Reubi JC, Kvols L, Krenning EP, Lamberts SWJ (1990) Distribution of somatostatin receptor in normal and tumour tissue. Metabolism 30(suppl 2):78–81

Swirski FK, Nahrendorf M, Etzrodt M, Wildgruber M, Cortez-Retamozo V, Panizzi P, Figueiredo JL, Kohler RH, Chudnovskiy A, Waterman P, Aikawa E, Mempel TR, Libby P, Weissleder R, Pittet MJ (2009) Identification of splenic reservoir monocytes and their deployment to inflammatory sites. Science 325:612–616

Wehrmann C, Senftleben S, Zachert C, Müller D, Baum RP (2007) Results of individual patient dosimetry in peptide receptor radionuclide therapy with 177Lu DOTA-TATE and 177Lu DOTA-NOC. Cancer Biother Radiopharm 22:406–416

Weinmann M, Becker G, Einsele H, Bamberg M (2001) Clinical indications and biological mechanisms of splenic irradiation in chronic leukaemias and myeloproliferative disorders. Radiother Oncol 58:235–246

van Essen M, Krenning EP, De Jong M, Valkema R, Kwekkeboom DJ (2007) Peptide receptor radionuclide therapy with radiolabelled somatostatin analogues in patients with somatostatin receptor positive tumours. Acta Oncol 46:723–734

Old and New Peptide Receptor Targets in Cancer: Future Directions

Jean Claude Reubi

Abstract

A precise definition of the tumor tissue targets to be selected for in vivo peptide receptor targeting, namely to know which peptide receptor is expressed in which type of cancer, is an important prerequisite for successful clinical application of this technology. In this short review, I give three selected examples of new and promising peptide receptor targets. In the somatostatin receptor field, based on in vitro receptor autoradiography experiments showing that much more sst_2 binding sites are detected in tumors using a ^{177}Lu-labeled sst_2 antagonist than a ^{177}Lu-labeled agonist, it can be proposed that, in addition to neuroendocrine tumors, nonneuroendocrine tumors with lower sst_2 levels such as breast carcinomas, renal cell carcinomas, and non-Hodgkin lymphomas may become potential candidates for sst_2 antagonist targeting. In the gastrin-releasing peptide receptor field, recent in vitro data show that not only tumor cells may overexpress gastrin-releasing peptide receptors but also neoangiogenic tumoral vessels, making tumors expressing high levels of gastrin-releasing peptide receptors in tumor vessels, such as ovarian or urinary tract cancers, attractive new candidates for gastrin-releasing peptide receptor targeting. In the incretin receptor field, it was found in vitro that, apart from glucagon-like peptide 1 receptors overexpressed in benign insulinomas, incretin receptors, especially the glucose-dependent insulinotropic polypeptide receptors, can be overexpressed in medullary thyroid cancers, an unexpected finding making also these tumors potential novel candidates for incretin receptor

J. C. Reubi (✉)
Division of Cell Biology and Experimental Cancer Research,
Institute of Pathology, University of Berne, Murtenstrasse 31,
PO Box 62, 3010 Berne, Switzerland
e-mail: reubi@pathology.unibe.ch

R. P. Baum and F. Rösch (eds.), *Theranostics, Gallium-68, and Other Radionuclides*, Recent Results in Cancer Research 194, DOI: 10.1007/978-3-642-27994-2_34,

targeting. Due to the abundance of peptide receptors in various cancers, it may be possible in the future to define for each tumor type a corresponding overexpressed peptide receptor suitable for targeting.

Abbreviations

GLP-1	Glucagon-like peptide 1
GRP	Gastrin-releasing peptide
VEGF	Vascular endothelial growth factor
GIP	Glucose-dependent insulinotropic polypeptide

Contents

1 Introduction

There are two prerequisites for successful peptide receptor targeting of cancer: (1) a precise definition of the target involved, namely which peptide receptor is overexpressed in which type of cancer (Reubi 2003), and (2) the use of adequate tools; this implies the development of radiolabeled peptide analogs with adequate characteristics in terms of receptor binding and in vivo biodistribution (Reubi and Maecke 2008). In this short review, I primarily focus on some aspects of the target definition and give a number of examples for possible new indications for cancer targeting with peptide radiopharmaceuticals. In the past two decades, numerous peptide receptor targets could be identified, such as somatostatin receptor in neuroendocrine tumors, glucagon-like peptide 1 (GLP-1) receptors in insulinomas, cholecystokinin 2 receptors in medullary thyroid cancers, gastrin-releasing peptide (GRP) receptors in prostate cancers, and neuropeptide Y receptors in breast cancers (Reubi 2003). Those targets can nowadays be considered established targets since, in each case, there is at least an in vivo proof of principle in man that the listed tumors can be targeted with the corresponding radiolabeled peptides (Reubi et al. 2005). For some of these examples, in particular in the somatostatin receptor field, there has been extensive clinical investigation making somatostatin receptor targeting of neuroendocrine tumors a routine application (Oberg et al. 2010).

2 Somatostatin Receptors

Somatostatin receptors have been shown to be expressed in a large variety of human cancers (Reubi 2003). There is, however, wide variability in receptor incidence and their density in various cancers. It is well known to nuclear physicians that neuroendocrine tumors frequently express a high density of somatostatin receptors; this includes pituitary adenomas, gastrointestinal neuroendocrine tumors, pancreatic neuroendocrine tumors such as insulinomas or gastrinomas, bronchial neuroendocrine tumors, and pheochromocytomas. Also brain tumors, such as medulloblastomas, meningiomas, and even neuroblastomas, frequently express somatostatin receptors. In the majority of the cases, the somatostatin receptor subtype sst_{2A} is the most abundant (Reubi 2003).

There is, however, a large variety of nonneuroendocrine cancers which can also overexpress, to various extents, somatostatin receptors (Reubi 2003). In some cases, their incidence is low, making such tumors of little interest to clinicians. In other cases the incidence is rather high, while the density of the receptors is low; this is, among others, the case for lymphomas, breast tumors, renal cell cancers, and gastric carcinomas (Reubi 2003). While neuroendocrine tumors and brain tumors are considered established indications for somatostatin receptor targeting, the nonneuroendocrine and nonbrain tumors mentioned above have barely been considered of significant interest for peptide receptor targeting. This may change, as discussed in the remaining part of this section.

For established indications such as targeting of neuroendocrine tumors, the used somatostatin radioligands are usually potent agonists, which are considered preferable over antagonists because agonists become internalized after binding to the receptor, demonstrating an important mechanism for accumulation and retention in tumor cells (Maecke and Reubi 2011). We have, however, recently shown that sst_2- and sst_3-selective antagonists have higher tumor uptake in mice bearing corresponding tumors and have generally improved pharmacokinetics, including lower kidney retention and faster clearance from the body (Ginj et al. 2006). The higher tumor uptake is explained by the higher number of binding sites recognized by antagonists as compared with agonists, and a longer dissociation time. Recently, it could be shown that imaging of neuroendocrine tumors with sst antagonists is clinically feasible. Indeed, Wild et al. (2011b) showed in five patients with neuroendocrine tumors that the antagonist ^{111}In-DOTA -pNO_2-Phe-c(DCys-Tyr-DTrp-Lys-Thr-Cys)-DTyr-NH_2 (^{111}In-DOTA-BASS) detected a total of 25 of 28 lesions, whereas ^{111}In-DTPA-octreotide detected only 17 of 28 lesions. In the same patient, DOTA-BASS showed higher tumor and lower renal uptake than ^{111}In-DTPA-octreotide. The favorable human biodistribution data suggest that sst antagonists could significantly affect peptide receptor-mediated imaging and therapy in sst_2-expressing neuroendocrine tumors.

We could show in a recent in vitro study that this antagonist strategy may also apply to nonneuroendocrine tumors expressing a lower density of sst_2 than neuroendocrine tumors (Cescato et al. 2011). In this study, we evaluated the

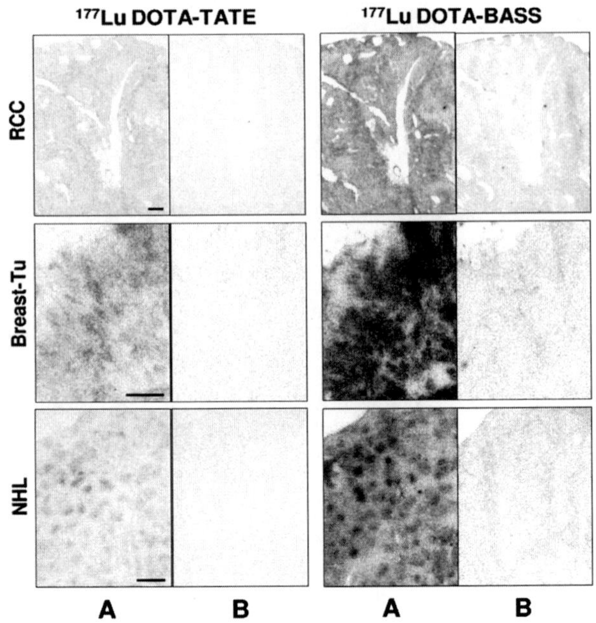

Fig. 1 Receptor autoradiography showing ^{177}Lu-DOTA-BASS antagonist versus ^{177}Lu-DOTATATE agonist binding in renal cancer (*upper row*), breast cancer (*middle row*), and non-Hodgkin lymphoma (*lower row*). **a** Total binding with the respective radioligands; **b** nonspecific binding. Bars = 1 mm

in vitro binding of the ^{177}Lu-DOTA-BASS sst_2 antagonist or the ^{177}Lu-DOTA-TATE agonist to sst_2-expressing human tumor samples. Forty-eight sst_2-positive human tumor tissue samples (9 ileal carcinoids, 10 pheochromocytomas, 7 breast carcinomas, 10 renal cell carcinomas, and 12 non-Hodgkin lymphomas) were analyzed by in vitro receptor autoradiography for expression of sst_2, comparing quantitatively the binding capacity of ^{177}Lu-DOTA-BASS and ^{177}Lu-DOTATATE in successive tissue sections. In all cases, the radiolabeled antagonist bound to more receptor sites than the agonist. The mean ratios of the antagonist ^{177}Lu-DOTA-BASS to the agonist ^{177}Lu-DOTATATE were 4.2 ± 0.5 in the 9 ileal carcinoids, 12 ± 3 in the 10 pheochromocytomas, 11 ± 4 in the 7 breast carcinomas, 5.1 ± 0.6 in the 10 renal cell carcinomas, and 4.8 ± 0.7 in the 12 non-Hodgkin lymphomas (Cescato et al. 2011). A representative example is shown in Fig. 1. These in vitro human data (Cescato et al. 2011), together with previous in vivo animal tumor data (Ginj et al. 2006), are therefore strong arguments indicating that sst_2 antagonists may be worth testing in vivo in patients in a wide range of sst_2-expressing tumors including nonneuroendocrine tumors.

3 Bombesin Receptors

Peptide receptor targeting of tumors is normally based on overexpression of receptors in tumor cells. In the GRP receptor field, this is well documented for prostate and breast cancers (Gugger and Reubi 1999; Markwalder and Reubi 1999). However, we have observed recently that a variety of human tumors can demonstrate massive overexpression of GRP receptors in tumoral and peritumoral vessels, while they rarely express GRP receptors in the tumor cell. This is most impressive in ovarian cancers and urinary tract cancers (Fleischmann et al. 2007, 2009).

We showed for instance that in ovarian carcinomas the GRP receptor protein was expressed in tumoral blood vessels in 84% of cases, but in tumor cells in only 32% of cases (Fleischmann et al. 2007). In contrast, normal ovarian vessels do not express measurable amounts of GRP receptors. GRP-receptor-expressing blood vessels are clearly limited to the tumors and the tumoral interface. These vessels are mainly of small size (30–120 μm) and possess a muscular coat indicating mature vessels; the GRP receptors are usually expressed in high densities, and homogeneously and transmurally distributed in the muscular wall of the vessels (Fleischmann et al. 2007). As muscle cells have the ability to contract, these vascular receptors might play a role in hemodynamics, influencing tumor progression by alteration of the blood flow in the tumoral vasculature. Indeed, bombesin and GRP have been shown to influence the vascular tone under physiological conditions (Bjenning et al. 1991; Clive et al. 2001; Luu et al. 1993); treatment with GRP-receptor antagonists can alter the microvascular perfusion of a tumor in a xenograft model (Heuser et al. 2005). Alternatively, overexpression of GRP receptors in this site might be implicated in blood vessel maturation, defined as the process of recruitment of cells (pericytes, smooth muscle cells) to form the vessel wall, which is an important step in neoangiogenesis. This step involves distinct mechanisms such as cell proliferation, migration, and morphogenesis, all known to be mediated by GRP and the corresponding receptor (Bunnett 1994; Jensen et al. 2001; Kim et al. 1997; Yule and White 1999). The results of recent functional studies propose GRP to be a new angiogenic molecule and link GRP and its receptor to tumor neoangiogenesis; for instance, GRP upregulates the proangiogenic vascular endothelial growth factor (VEGF) A in vitro in prostate and endometrial cancer cell lines (Levine et al. 2003a, b).

GRP-receptor-positive blood vessels are present in all ovarian tumor categories, with a tendency for higher incidence of GRP-receptor-positive vessels in malignant tumors compared with benign or low-grade malignant tumors (Fleischmann et al. 2007). This finding might reflect the different conditions of vascular development in various tumors with variable growth velocities. Most interestingly, these GRP-receptor-positive vessels are detected in particularly high density in tumors of ovarian origin that are usually fatal, namely metastases of primary ovarian carcinomas. This phenomenon points to GRP receptor overexpression in tumor vasculature as a mechanism independent of the primary site of tumor genesis. Interestingly, these vessels are present in very high numbers and with high GRP receptor densities in these metastases, potentially reflecting tumor clones with uppermost angiogenic properties (Fleischmann et al. 2007).

In a follow-up study, selected other human cancers also showed high prevalence of GRP receptors in their tumoral vessels. This is particularly true for invasive urothelial carcinomas, but also for squamous lung carcinomas, colorectal

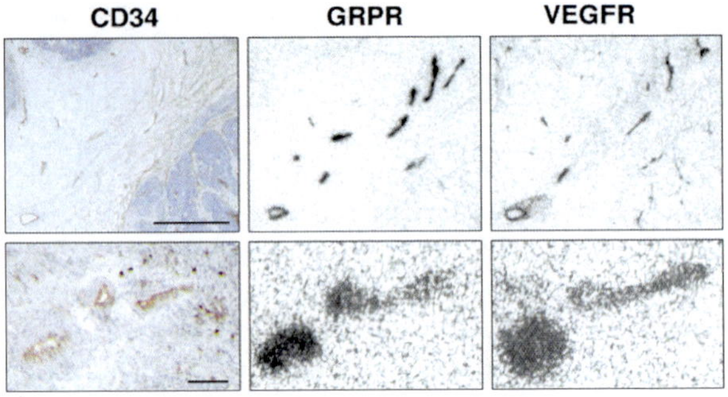

Fig. 2 Tumoral and peritumoral vessels express both GRP receptors and VEGF receptors in autoradiographic experiments. CD34 immunohistochemistry identifies tumoral and peritumoral vessels. Bars = 1 mm (*upper row*) or 0.1 mm (*lower row*)

carcinomas, renal cell carcinomas, or lung adenocarcinomas (Fleischmann et al. 2009).

Recently, we further characterized these GRP receptors by comparing the vascular GRP receptor expression and localization in a selection of human cancers with that of an established biological marker of neoangiogenesis, the VEGF receptor (Reubi et al. 2011). In vitro quantitative receptor autoradiography was performed in parallel for GRP and VEGF receptors in 32 human tumors of various origins, using ^{125}I-Tyr-bombesin and ^{125}I-VEGF$_{165}$ as radioligands, respectively. While all tumors expressed GRP and VEGF receptors in their vascular system, VEGF receptors were expressed in the endothelium in the majority of the vessels and GRP receptors were expressed in a subpopulation of vessels, preferably in their muscular coat (Reubi et al. 2011). The vessels expressing GRP receptors were all VEGF receptor positive, whereas the VEGF-receptor-expressing vessels were not all GRP receptor positive. GRP-receptor-expressing vessels were found immunohistochemically to coexpress VEGF receptor subtype 2. Remarkably, the density of vascular GRP receptors was much higher than that of VEGF receptors. A representative example is shown in Fig. 2. Concomitant expression of GRP and VEGF receptors appears to be a frequent phenomenon in many human cancers. The GRP receptors, localized and expressed in extremely high density in a subgroup of vessels, may function as target for antiangiogenic tumor therapy or angiodestructive targeted radiotherapy with radiolabeled bombesin analogs given alone or preferably together with VEGF-receptor-targeted therapy.

GRP receptor overexpression is the molecular basis for in vivo targeting with radiolabeled bombesin analogs. Clinical proof of principle has been obtained in vivo for targeting GRP-receptor-overexpressing breast and prostate cancers, with a ^{99}Tc-labeled bombesin analog. Further, second-generation bombesin radioligands have been developed, such as ^{177}Lu-DOTA-CH_2CO-G-4-aminobenzoyl-Gln-Trp-Ala-Val-Gly-His-Leu-Met-NH_2 (^{177}Lu-AMBA) or ^{90}Y-DOTA-PEG$_4$-bombesin(7-14) (^{90}Y-DOTA-PESIN), which are bombesin agonists characterized by excellent receptor-mediated internalization into the cell and, therefore, high tumor accumulation (Reubi and Maecke 2008). Recently, however, it was found that radiolabeled GRP receptor antagonists, although they do not internalize easily, are even better tumor markers than agonists (Cescato et al. 2008; Mansi et al. 2009, 2011). Targeted tumor radiotherapy with potent bombesin radiolabeled antagonists may not only include destruction of tumor cells, but also of tumoral and peritumoral vessels, or both, and as such may become a powerful alternative to current oncologic therapy.

Interestingly, despite the strong in vitro evidence for GRP receptor expression in tumoral vessels and the availability of excellent bombesin radioligands, there has been no in vivo study in patients evaluating whether metastatic ovarian cancers or urinary tract cancers can be targeted through their overexpressed vascular GRP receptors. Such a study, even though logistically difficult, is greatly awaited.

4 Incretin Receptors

Incretins such as GLP-1 or glucose-dependent insulinotropic polypeptide (GIP) are important glucose-dependent insulin secretagogues released primarily from the gastrointestinal tract in response to nutrient intake (Holst 2007; Holst et al. 2009; Irwin and Flatt 2009). In addition to their regulation of glucose-dependent insulin secretion, those peptides have other common actions on β-cells, including stimulation of cell proliferation and reduction of β-cell apoptosis (Ehses et al. 2003; Holst et al. 2009; Kim et al. 2008). These effects are mediated by specific GLP-1 and GIP receptors in pancreatic islets. Interestingly, recent data indicate that incretin receptors can also be overexpressed in selected human cancers; for instance, extremely high GLP-1 receptor expression has been reported in insulinomas (Reubi and Waser 2003), leading to the successful development of GLP-1 receptor targeting in these tumors (Christ et al. 2009; Wild et al. 2008, 2011a). Moreover, we recently observed that, unexpectedly, medullary thyroid carcinomas, a tumor originating from an organ unrelated to incretin physiological action, expresses incretin receptors to various extents; GLP-1 receptors are expressed in 27% of medullary thyroid carcinomas, while GIP receptors are expressed in as many as 89% of these carcinomas (Korner et al. 2007; Waser et al. 2011).

The unexpectedly high GIP receptor expression in human medullary thyroid carcinomas might be the molecular basis for GIP receptor targeting in vivo in those patients. At the moment, GIP-derived radioligands are not available for preclinical studies; however, the development of such compounds may be greatly facilitated by our findings of high GIP receptor expression in the TT cell line (Waser et al. 2011).

We may expect that, in the future, incretin receptors, in particular GIP receptor targeting of medullary thyroid carcinomas, may be combined with cholecystokinin 2 receptor targeting that has previously been reported to be successful in imaging medullary thyroid carcinomas in patients, due to the massive overexpression of cholecystokinin 2 receptors in these tumors (Reubi 2007). Figure 3 compares the incidence and density of the three receptors in imaging medullary thyroid carcinomas.

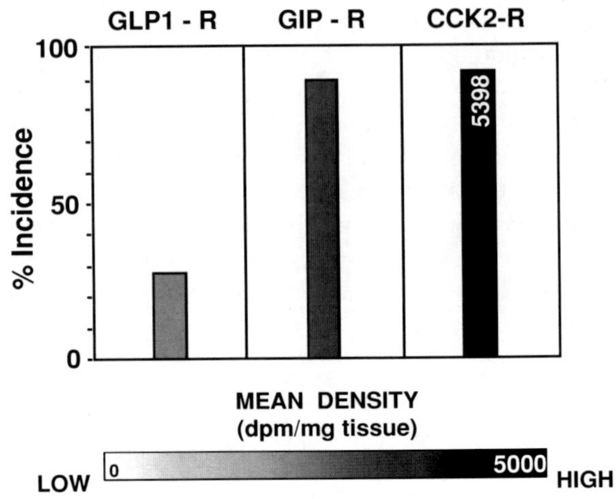

Fig. 3 Incidence and density of GLP-1 receptors, GIP receptors, and cholecystokinin 2 receptors in medullary thyroid carcinomas. Mean density from 0 to 5,000 dpm/mg is represented by the darkness of the bars. Values for mean density exceeding 5,000 dpm/mg tissue are reported in the bars

5 Conclusion

Our recent in vitro data suggest that novel peptide receptor targets may play a role in future developments in nuclear medicine. The three examples selected in this review should give indications for possible and promising new directions which have not yet been investigated in clinical settings.

- Several nonneuroendocrine tumors, known to express often a low density of sst_2, such as lymphomas, renal cell carcinomas, and breast cancers, may turn out to become valid indications for peptide receptor targeting, if radiolabeled sst_2 antagonists are used as radioligands.
- Tumoral and peritumoral vessels expressing high levels of GRP receptors in invasive ovarian and urinary tract cancers are highly attractive targets, as seen in in vitro studies. In vivo GRP receptor targeting should therefore be performed with high priority in these types of tumor patients, in order to establish the proof of principle in vivo that not only tumor cells but, alternatively, tumoral vessels may be adequate targets.
- Medullary thyroid carcinomas appear to overexpress a large variety of peptide receptors, such as CCK_2 receptors or somatostatin receptors, but also the incretin receptors GLP-1 and GIP; those receptors, alone or in combination, may be an attractive molecular basis for novel peptide receptor targeting.

References

Bjenning C, Farrell AP, Holmgren S (1991) Bombesin-like immunoreactivity in skates and the in vitro effect of bombesin on coronary vessels from the longnose skate, Raja rhina. Regul Pept 35:207–219

Bunnett G (1994) Gastrin-releasing peptide. Gut peptides: biochemistry and physiology, New York pp 423–445

Cescato R, Maina T, Nock B et al (2008) Bombesin receptor antagonists may be preferable to agonists for tumor targeting. J Nucl Med 49:318–326

Cescato R, Waser B, Fani M et al (2011) Evaluation of ^{177}Lu-DOTA-SST2-antagonist versus ^{177}Lu-DOTA-SST2-agonist binding in human cancers in vitro. J Nucl Med 52:1886–1890

Christ E, Wild D, Forrer F et al (2009) Glucagon-like peptide-1 receptor imaging for localization of insulinomas. J Clin Endocrinol Metab 94:4398–4405

Clive S, Jodrell D, Webb D (2001) Gastrin-releasing peptide is a potent vasodilator in humans. Clin Pharmacol Ther 69:252–259

Ehses JA, Casilla VR, Doty T et al (2003) Glucose-dependent insulinotropic polypeptide promotes beta-(INS-1) cell survival via cyclic adenosine monophosphate-mediated caspase-3 inhibition and regulation of p38 mitogen-activated protein kinase. Endocrinology 144:4433–4445

Fleischmann A, Waser B, Reubi JC (2007) Overexpression of gastrin-releasing peptide receptors in tumor-associated blood vessels of human ovarian neoplasms. Cell Oncol 29:421–433

Fleischmann A, Waser B, Reubi JC (2009) High expression of gastrin-releasing peptide receptors in the vascular bed of urinary tract cancers: promising candidates for vascular targeting applications. Endocr Relat Cancer 16:623–633

Ginj M, Zhang H, Waser B et al (2006) Radiolabeled somatostatin receptor antagonists are preferable to agonists for in vivo peptide receptor targeting of tumors. Proc Natl Acad Sci USA 103:16436–16441

Gugger M, Reubi JC (1999) GRP receptors in non-neoplastic and neoplastic human breast. Am J Pathol 155:2067–2076

Heuser M, Schlott T, Schally AV et al (2005) Expression of gastrin releasing Peptide receptor in renal cell carcinomas: a potential function for the regulation of neoangiogenesis and microvascular perfusion. J Urol 173:2154–2159

Holst JJ (2007) The physiology of glucagon-like peptide 1. Physiol Rev 87:1409–1439

Holst JJ, Vilsboll T, Deacon CF (2009) The incretin system and its role in type 2 diabetes mellitus. Mol Cell Endocrinol 297:127–136

Irwin N, Flatt PR (2009) Therapeutic potential for GIP receptor agonists and antagonists. Best Pract Res Clin Endocrinol Metab 23:499–512

Jensen JA, Carroll RE, Benya RV (2001) The case for gastrin-releasing peptide acting as a morphogen when it and its receptor are aberrantly expressed in cancer. Peptides 22:689–699

Kim JS, McKinnis VS, White SR (1997) Migration of guinea pig airway epithelial cells in response to bombesin analogues. Am J Respir Cell Mol Biol 16:259–266

Kim SJ, Nian C, Widenmaier S et al (2008) Glucose-dependent insulinotropic polypeptide-mediated up-regulation of beta-cell antiapoptotic Bcl-2 gene expression is coordinated by cyclic AMP (cAMP) response element binding protein (CREB) and cAMP-responsive CREB coactivator 2. Mol Cell Biol 28:1644–1656

Korner M, Stockli M, Waser B et al (2007) GLP-1 receptor expression in human tumors and human normal tissues: potential for in vivo targeting. J Nucl Med 48:736–743

Levine L, Licci JA 3rd, Townsend CM Jr et al (2003a) Expression of gastrin-releasing peptide receptors in endometrial cancer. J Am Coll Surg 196:898–904

Levine L, Lucci JA 3rd, Pazdrak B et al (2003b) Bombesin stimulates nuclear factor kappa B activation and expression of proangiogenic factors in prostate cancer cells. Cancer Res 63:3495–3502

Luu TN, Chester AH, O'Neil GS et al (1993) Different responses of the human gastroepiploic and internal mammary arteries to vasoactive peptides. Am J Physiol 264:H583–H587

Maecke HR, Reubi JC (2011) Somatostatin receptors as targets for nuclear medicine imaging and radionuclide treatment. J Nucl Med 52:841–844

Mansi R, Wang X, Forrer F et al (2009) Evaluation of a 1,4,7,10-tetraazacyclododecane-1,4,7,10-tetraacetic acid-conjugated bombesin-based radioantagonist for the labeling with single-photon emission computed tomography, positron emission tomography, and therapeutic radionuclides. Clin Cancer Res 15:5240–5249

Mansi R, Wang X, Forrer F et al (2011) Development of a potent DOTA-conjugated bombesin antagonist for targeting GRPr-positive tumours. Eur J Nucl Med Mol Imaging 38:97–107

Markwalder R, Reubi JC (1999) Gastrin-releasing peptide receptors in the human prostate: relation to neoplastic transformation. Cancer Res 59:1152–1159

Oberg KE, Reubi JC, Kwekkeboom DJ et al (2010) Role of somatostatins in gastroentero-pancreatic neuroendocrine tumor development and therapy. Gastroenterology 139:742–753 753 e741

Reubi JC (2003) Peptide receptors as molecular targets for cancer diagnosis and therapy. Endocr Rev 24:389–427

Reubi JC (2007) Targeting CCK receptors in human cancers. Curr Top Med Chem 7:1239–1242

Reubi JC, Fleischmann A, Waser B et al (2011) Concomitant vascular GRP-receptor and VEGF-receptor expression in human tumors: molecular basis for dual targeting of tumoral vasculature. Peptides 32:1457–1462

Reubi JC, Macke HR, Krenning EP (2005) Candidates for peptide receptor radiotherapy today and in the future. J Nucl Med 46:67S–75S

Reubi JC, Maecke HR (2008) Peptide-based probes for cancer imaging. J Nucl Med 49: 1735–1738

Reubi JC, Waser B (2003) Concomitant expression of several peptide receptors in neuroendocrine tumors as molecular basis for in vivo multireceptor tumor targeting. Eur J Nucl Med 30:781–793

Waser B, Beetschen K, Pellegata NS et al (2011) Incretin receptors in non-neoplastic and neoplastic thyroid C cells in rodents and humans: relevance for incretin-based diabetes therapy. Neuroendocrinology 94:291–301

Wild D, Caplin M, Christ E et al (2011a) Glucagon-like peptide-1 vs. somatostatin receptor targeting in malignant insulinomas. J Nucl Med 52:1073–1078

Wild D, Fani M, Behe M et al (2011b) First clinical evidence that imaging with somatostatin receptor antagonists is clinically feasible. J Nucl Med 52:1412–1417

Wild D, Mäcke H, Christ E et al (2008) Glucagon-like peptide 1-receptor scans to localize occult insulinomas. N Engl J Med 359:766–768

Yule KA, White SR (1999) Migration of 3T3 and lung fibroblasts in response to calcitonin gene-related peptide and bombesin. Exp Lung Res 25:261–273

MIX
Papier aus verantwortungsvollen Quellen
Paper from responsible sources
FSC® C105338

Printed by Books on Demand, Germany